P9-BJM-580

VETERINARY
Immunology

An Introduction

VETERINARY
Immunology

An Introduction

Ian R. Tizard, PhD, BSc, BVMS

Richard M. Schubot Professor of Exotic Bird Health
and Professor of Immunology
College of Veterinary Medicine
Texas A&M University
College Station, Texas

SEVENTH EDITION

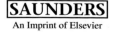

SAUNDERS
An Imprint of Elsevier

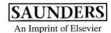

SAUNDERS

An Imprint of Elsevier

The Curtis Center
Independence Square West
Philadelphia, Pennsylvania 19106

VETERINARY IMMUNOLOGY: AN INTRODUCTION,   ISBN 0-7216-0136-7
SEVENTH EDITION
Copyright © 2004, Elsevier (USA). All rights reserved.

No part of this publication may be reproduced or transmitted in any form or by any means, electronic or mechanical, including photocopying, recording, or any information storage and retrieval system, without permission in writing from the publisher. Permissions may be sought directly from Elsevier's Health Sciences Rights Department in Philadelphia, PA, USA: phone: (+1) 215 238 7869, fax: (+1) 215 238 2239, e-mail: healthpermissions@elsevier.com. You may also complete your request on-line via the Elsevier Science homepage (http://www.elsevier.com), by selecting 'Customer Support' and then 'Obtaining Permissions.'

NOTICE

Veterinary Medicine is an ever-changing field. Standard safety precautions must be followed, but as new research and clinical experience broaden our knowledge, changes in treatment and drug therapy become necessary or appropriate. Readers are advised to check the product information currently provided by the manufacturer of each drug to be administered to verify contraindications. It is the responsibility of the treating veterinarian relying on experience and knowledge of the animal to determine dosages and the best treatment for the animal. Neither the publisher nor the editor assumes any responsibility for any injury and/or damage to animals or property.

Previous editions copyrighted 1977, 1982, 1987, 1992, 1996, 2000

International Standard Book Number 0-7216-0136-7

Publishing Director: Linda Duncan
Senior Editor: Teri Merchant
Senior Developmental Editor: Jolynn Gower
Publishing Services Manager: Patricia Tannian
Senior Project Manager: John Casey
Senior Book Designer: Julia Dummitt

Printed in China

Last digit is the print number: 9   8   7   6   5   4   3   2   1

To Claire, Thelma, Robert, Fiona, and Tim

ABBREVIATIONS

ADCC	antibody-dependent cell-mediated cytotoxicity
AIDS	acquired immune deficiency syndrome
AIHA	autoimmune hemolytic anemia
AITP	autoimmune thrombocytopenia
ANA	antinuclear antibodies
APC	antigen-presenting cell
BALT	bronchus-associated lymphoid tissue
BCG	bacillus Calmette–Guerin (*Mycobacterium bovis*)
BCR	B-cell receptor
BLAD	bovine leukocyte adherence deficiency
BLV	bovine leukemia virus
BoLA	bovine leukocyte antigen
C	complement
CAM	cell adhesion molecule
CBH	cutaneous basophil hypersensitivity
CD	cluster of differentiation
CDw	cluster of differentiation (provisional designation)
CDR	complementarity-determining region
CFT	complement fixation test
CID	combined immunodeficiency
CLL	chronic lymphoid leukemia
Con A	concanavalin A
CR	complement receptor
CRP	C-reactive protein
CSF	colony-stimulating factor (or cerebrospinal fluid)
DAF	decay-accelerating factor
DAG	diacylglycerol
DC	dendritic cell
DTH	delayed-type hypersensitivity
EAE	experimental allergic encephalitis
EAN	experimental allergic neuritis
ELISA	enzyme-linked immunosorbent assay
EPO	eosinophil peroxidase
Fab	antigen-binding fragment
Fc	crystallizable fragment (of immunoglobulin)
FCA	Freund's complete adjuvant
FcR	Fc receptor
FeLV	feline leukemia virus
FOCMA	feline oncornavirus cell membrane antigen
FPT	failure of passive transfer
FITC	fluorescein isothiocyanate
FIV	feline immunodeficiency virus

GALT	gut-associated lymphoid tissue
GM-CSF	granulocyte-macrophage colony-stimulating factor
GPI	glycosylphosphatidylinositol
GVH	graft-versus-host (disease)
HAT	hypoxanthine aminopterin thymidine (medium)
HDN	hemolytic disease of the newborn
HEV	high endothelial venule
HI	hemagglutination inhibition
HIV	human immunodeficiency virus
HLA	human leukocyte antigen
HSP	heat-shock protein
Ia	mouse class II MHC molecule
ICAM	intercellular adhesion molecule
IDDM	insulin-dependent diabetes mellitus
IEL	intraepithelial lymphocytes
IFA	indirect fluorescence assay
IFN	interferon
Ig	immunoglobulin
IK	immunoconglutinin
IL	interleukin
ISCOM	immune-stimulating complex
ISG	immune serum globulin
IU	international unit
J	joining
kDa	kilodalton
LAD	leukocyte adherence deficiency
LAK	lymphokine-activated killer (cells)
LBP	lipopolysaccharide-binding protein
LD50	lethal dose 50
LE	lupus erythematosus
LFA	lymphocyte function–associated antigen
LGL	large granular lymphocyte
lpr	lymphoproliferation
LPS	lipopolysaccharide
LT	lymphotoxin (or leukotriene)
β_2M	β_2-microglobulin
MAC	membrane attack complex
MBL	mannose-binding lectin
M-CSF	macrophage colony-stimulating factor
MHC	major histocompatibility complex
MIP	macrophage inflammatory protein
MLC	mixed lymphocyte culture
MLD	minimal lethal dose
MLR	mixed lymphocyte reaction
MLV	modified live virus

MPGN	membranoproliferative glomerulonephritis	SAP	serum amyloid P
NK	natural killer (cell)	SCID	severe combined immunodeficiency
NS	natural suppressor (cell)	SID	single intradermal test
PAF	platelet-activating factor	SLA	swine leukocyte antigen
PAMP	pathogen-associated molecular pattern	SLE	systemic lupus erythematosus
PCA	passive cutaneous anaphylaxis	SMAC	supramolecular activation cluster
PF	protective fraction	TAP	transporter for antigen processing
PFC	plaque-forming cell	TCID$_{50}$	tissue culture infective dose 50
PG	prostaglandin	TCR	T-cell receptor
PHA	phytohemagglutinin	TdT	terminal deoxynucleotidyltransferase
pIgR	receptor for polymeric immunoglobulin	TGF	transforming growth factor
PKC	protein kinase C	Tcs cell	contrasuppressor T cell
PPD	purified protein derivative (of tuberculin)	Th cell	T helper cell
PWM	pokeweed mitogen	TIL	tumor-infiltrating lymphocyte
R	receptor (e.g., IL-2R)	TLR	toll-like receptor
RAST	radioallergosorbent test	TK	thymidine kinase
RF	rheumatoid factor	TNF	tumor necrosis factor
RIA	radioimmunoassay	Ts cell	suppressor T cell
S19	strain 19 *Brucella abortus* vaccine	VLA	very late antigen
SAA	serum amyloid A (protein)	WC	workshop cluster
		ZAP	zeta-associated protein

GREEK LETTERS

Lower case Greek letters are widely used in immunology to denote peptide chains or other molecules. Below is a list of Greek letters with examples of their usage.

EXAMPLES OF GREEK LETTERS IN IMMUNOLOGY

α alpha   α heavy chains (IgA)
β beta β_2-microglobulin
γ gamma   γ globulin, γ interferon
δ delta   δ heavy chains (IgD)

ε epsilon   ε heavy chains (IgE)
ζ zeta   ζ chain of CD3
η eta   η chain of CD3
θ theta   θ antigen (a synonym for CD90)
κ kappa   κ light chains
λ lambda   λ light chains
μ mu   μ heavy chains (IgM)
υ upsilon   υ heavy chain (IgY)
φ phi   φX174, a bacteriophage
ψ psi   a notation for a pseudogene
τ tau   interferon-τ
ω omega   interferon-ω

PREFACE

The first edition of this book was published 27 years ago. In considering the changes in veterinary immunology since that time, certain trends are readily apparent. The most obvious is the volume of available information. Clearly the subject has grown, and the book has grown with it. The second change is in the level of detail available. It is now possible to explain almost all the major immunological processes at the molecular level. Although these processes are complex, they also provide a rational explanation for effects that were previously not understood. At the practical level, this has not resulted in great improvements in the way we treat animals. Certainly, vaccines are more effective, safer, and directed against a broader range of pathogens. Some diagnostic tests have improved significantly. Immunosuppressive and antiinflammatory drugs are more potent, making organ grafting, for example, a relatively safe process. Yet great gaps in our knowledge remain. Tumor immunology has failed to yield significant results. We are still unable to explain the development of allergic diseases. We know of many more autoimmune and immunodeficiency diseases now than we did a generation ago. Yet we cannot explain their appearance, and our treatments, while improved, are not radically better. Thus there is much room for improvement, and veterinary immunology is by no means a mature discipline. On the contrary, many more exciting discoveries remain to be made.

The purpose of this book remains, as always, to provide a first-level textbook for students of veterinary and comparative medicine and to assist veterinarians by informing them about recent developments in immunology, especially as it relates to the major domestic animals.

ORGANIZATION

The overall arrangement of the text is the same as in previous editions. Thus, after the introductory chapter, Chapters 2 through 4 describe the innate defenses. These are the defenses of the body that respond rapidly to invasion and tissue damage and control microbial invaders while the acquired immune system is given time to react and complete the job. Chapters 5 through 18 describe the cellular and molecular basis of the acquired immune system as we currently understand it. Chapters 19 through 25 relate how both the innate and acquired immune systems defend animals against invading microorganisms and how we exploit these mechanisms

by the use of vaccines. Chapters 26 through 36, on the other hand, describe the negative consequences that may occur as a result of the activities of the immune system or a lack thereof. The book concludes with chapters on immunopharmacology and on the evolution of the immune system. The last is a reminder that the species of veterinary interest are but a very small subset of the enormously diverse array of animal life on this planet.

Readers familiar with earlier editions will immediately note that color has been added, greatly increasing the effectiveness of the figures. The number of these illustrations has also been significantly increased, and many older ones have been extensively revised to enhance comprehension of key concepts.

This is not a reference book, and no attempt has been made to provide a comprehensive bibliography. Nevertheless, the chapter references have been expanded, updated, and selected to provide a mixture of key research papers and reviews. They should enable interested students to expand their knowledge of a specific area if desired.

NEW INFORMATION

The most significant recent development in immunology has been the recognition of the importance of the innate immune defenses. Once profoundly unfashionable, innate immunity is now seen as the key to the early defense of the body against microbial invasion. The lag period required for acquired immunity to develop is now recognized as a time when an animal's survival depends on innate immunity. Therefore the thrust of the text as a whole has been modified to emphasize the key role of innate immunity.

The first chapters focus exclusively on mechanisms of innate immunity, whereas related topics are covered in the chapters dealing with specific infectious and parasitic agents. For example, the recognition of mast cells as triggers of inflammation and the identification of toll-like receptors has shown how the animal body recognizes that it is being invaded. Members of the chemokine family are now seen as critical molecules in all aspects of inflammation and immune responses. Chemokine nomenclature, once a disorganized collection of acronyms, has been rationalized with acceptance of a new nomenclature system. Likewise, ongoing studies have revealed the enormous diversity and significance of small antibacterial peptides such as the defensins. There is now much more information on the role of microbial nucleic acids as antigens and as triggers of innate immunity. Some of the areas where the innate and acquired immune systems overlap and interact are also described. These include, for example, the complement system and the functions of natural killer cells. In the case of natural killer cells, we have made progress in understanding how they recognize abnormal cells and how they vary between species.

In the area of acquired immunity, the role and the significance of dendritic cells are increasingly recognized, and there is a growing body of information on the function of these cells in the domestic animal species. This may turn out to be enormously relevant to antigen processing, adjuvant design, and, eventually, vaccine development.

The march of immunological progress can be followed by the expansion of cell surface molecule nomenclature up to CD254. These molecules are expressed very differently in the domestic mammals than in humans or laboratory rodents. As cell populations and their functions are analyzed, there is an increased awareness that many cell types can function as either stimulator or suppressor. This dichotomy is now well recognized in T cells, dendritic cells, and macrophages, and it explains many otherwise complex or anomalous responses.

The naming of new cytokines continues at an accelerating pace; for example, the interleukins have been named up to interleukin-30. Unfortunately the rush to assign new names has outpaced our knowledge of their properties. It is not yet known whether any of these newly identified molecules are biologically or medically significant.

Other basic topics expanded and described in detail include the new nomenclature for immunoglobulin and T-cell antigen receptor genes; the role of γ/δ T cells and their subpopulations in domestic animals; and the processes involved in the development and survival of memory cells, a subject of considerable practical importance with respect to the duration of immunity induced by vaccines.

The widespread use of molecular and genetic techniques has permitted us to define key molecules and genes from domestic animals in great detail. The ongoing development of the bovine, canine, and chicken genome mapping projects will provide us with incredibly potent tools to analyze and compare these immune systems. Comparative genetic studies have already revealed the many different ways by which antibody diversity is generated in the domestic mammals. Patterns are beginning to emerge that may ultimately be of benefit in developing new vaccines. Similarly, new information is available on immunoglobulin genes in domestic animal species. As a result, for example, the equine immunoglobulin genes have been described and renamed in a rational manner. They no longer appear to be as unique as once believed.

Vaccine technology continues to evolve rapidly, and new techniques such as polynucleotide vaccination are being increasingly applied to animal vaccines. Adjuvants are finally being scientifically and rationally tested so that it is now possible to escape the empiricism that has traditionally encompassed their use.

One continuing area of concern is that regarding "overvaccination" and the issue of revaccination frequency. The animal vaccine industry has produced highly effective and incredibly safe vaccines. As a result, infectious diseases have decreased in significance in companion animal species in developed countries. On the other hand, occasional adverse effects have received disproportionate attention, and unrealistic expectations have caused a significant overstatement of the hazards of vaccination. Ever since the days of Edward Jenner, vaccines have been the subject of ill-informed attack. As always, such attacks are best countered with objective, evidence-based data.

Having pointed this out, it is important to note that the animal vaccine industry has matured to the extent that opportunities for new and profitable vaccines are limited. By reducing the impact of the major infectious diseases, the industry has reduced opportunities to expand and has been forced to turn its attention to much less important diseases when generating new products. At the same time, new vaccine technologies are evolving fast. It is difficult to determine how much demand there will be for a new generation of vaccines despite their improved safety and efficacy.

On the other hand, an area that is clearly relevant to veterinarians is the growing awareness of the genetic problems affecting many domestic animal species. Many animal breeds are at great risk of immunological disease as a result of decreased genetic diversity. From an academic viewpoint, these disease models provide fascinating insight into molecular processes. Unfortunately, many could be avoided by prudent breeding practices. It is also unfortunate that in many cases these are blamed on vaccination. As stated above, the appropriate response to this is to generate reliable, objective data.

In the areas of immunopathology and hypersensitivity, new views on the relationship of mast cells to inflammation are examined, as well as the significance of chemokines in determining the composition of cellular infiltrates. Several new immunological diseases have been described, although it has been difficult to avoid simply listing these. Two examples of increased coverage include the cause of severe combined immunodeficiency in Jack Russell terriers and the molecular basis of the *CLAD* mutation.

Comparative immunological studies have proven very useful in explaining why different mammals employ very different "antigen" receptors on their natural killer cells. Likewise, our views of the broader phylogenetic picture have been clarified with the concept of the "immunological big bang" described in the last chapter of the book.

ACKNOWLEDGMENTS

As always it is a pleasure to publicly acknowledge my enormous debt to those colleagues who assisted materially in the preparation of this book. Among the individuals who reviewed the manuscript and provided critical and insightful recommendations are Dr. Robert Kennis and his colleagues who analyzed the text in great detail. Likewise I am greatly obliged to Dr. Lauren Skow and his students who played a key role in sorting out my confusion regarding things genetic. To this I must add my thanks to my colleagues, Dr. Yawei Ni, Ms. Debra Turner, and Ms. Marilyn Rubach, for their tolerance and patience while I concentrated on the book.

Most important, and as always, I must express my ongoing appreciation for the wonderful support of my wife, Claire.

Ian Tizard
Department of Veterinary Pathobiology
Texas A&M University
College Station, Texas 77843
email: itizard@cvm.tamu.edu
February 2004

CONTENTS

VETERINARY
Immunology
An Introduction

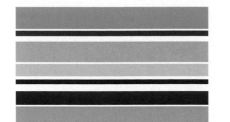

The Defense of the Body

CHAPTER 1

The living animal body contains all the components necessary to sustain life. It is warm, moist, and rich in many different nutrients. As a result, animal tissues are extremely attractive to microorganisms that seek to invade the body and exploit these resources for themselves. The magnitude of this microbial attack can be readily seen when an animal dies. Within a few hours, especially when warm, a body decomposes rapidly as microbes invade its tissues. On the other hand, the tissues of living, healthy animals are highly resistant to microbial invasion. This resistance is due to multiple interlinked defense mechanisms. Indeed, the survival of an animal depends on its successful defense against microbial invaders. This defense is encompassed by the discipline of immunology and is the subject of this book.

Because effective resistance to infection is critical, the body dare not rely on a single defense mechanism. To be effective and reliable, multiple defense systems must be available. Some may be effective against many different invaders. Others may only destroy specific organisms. Some act at the body surface to exclude invaders. Others act deep within the body to destroy organisms that have breached the outer defenses. Some defend against bacterial invaders, some against viruses that live inside cells, and even some against large invaders such as fungi or parasitic worms and insects. The protection of the body comes from a complex system of overlapping and interlinked defense mechanisms that together can destroy or control almost all invaders. A failure in these defenses, either because the immune system is destroyed (as occurs in acquired immune deficiency syndrome, AIDS) or because the invading organisms can overcome or evade the defenses, will result in disease and possibly death. An effective immune system is not simply a useful system to have around. It is essential to life itself.

A BRIEF HISTORY OF VETERINARY IMMUNOLOGY

Our awareness of the importance of the defense of the body against microbial invasion could only develop after the medical community accepted the concept of infectious disease. When infections such as smallpox or plague spread through early human societies, although many people died, some individuals recovered. It was rarely noticed that these recovered individuals remained healthy during subsequent outbreaks—a sign that they had developed effective immunity. Nevertheless, by the 12th century the Chinese had observed that those individuals who recovered from smallpox were resistant to further attacks of this disease. Being practical people, they therefore deliberately infected infants with smallpox by rubbing the scabs from infected individuals into small cuts in their skin. Those infants who survived the resulting disease were protected from smallpox in later life. The risks inherent in this procedure were acceptable in an era of high infant mortality. On gaining experience with the technique it was found that using scabs from the mildest smallpox cases minimized the hazards. As a result, mortality due to smallpox inoculation (or variolation) dropped to about 1% as compared to a mortality of about 20% in clinical smallpox cases. Knowledge of

1

variolation spread westward to Europe by the early 18th century, and was soon widely employed.

Outbreaks of rinderpest (then called cattle plague) had been a common occurrence throughout western Europe since the ninth century and inevitably killed huge numbers of cattle. Since none of the traditional remedies appeared to work and the skin lesions in affected animals vaguely resembled those seen in smallpox, it was suggested in 1754 that inoculation might help. This process involved soaking a piece of string in the nasal discharge from an animal with rinderpest and then inserting the string into an incision in the dewlap of the animal to be protected. The resulting disease was usually milder than natural infection, and the inoculated animal became resistant to the disease. The process proved very popular, and skilled inoculators traveled throughout Europe inoculating cattle and branding them to show that they were protected against rinderpest.

In 1798, Edward Jenner, an English physician, demonstrated that material from cowpox lesions could be substituted for smallpox in variolation. Since cowpox does not cause severe disease in humans, its use reduced the risks incurred by variolation to insignificant levels. The effectiveness of this procedure, called vaccination (*vacca* is Latin for "cow") was such that it was eventually used in the 1970s to eradicate smallpox from the world.

Once the general principles of inoculation were accepted (even although nobody had the faintest idea how it worked), attempts were made to use similar procedures to prevent other animal diseases. Some of these techniques were effective. Thus, material derived from sheep pox was used successfully to protect sheep in a process called ovination and was widely employed in Europe. Likewise, inoculation for bovine pleuropneumonia consisted of inserting a small piece of tissue from an infected lung into a cut in the tail. The tail fell off within a few weeks, but the animal became immune! Although the process was effective, infected material from the tail also spread the disease and so delayed its eradication. On the other hand, administration of cowpox material to the nose of puppies to prevent canine distemper, though widely employed, was a complete failure.

The general implications of Jenner's observations on cowpox and the importance of reducing the ability of an immunizing organism to cause disease were not realized until 1879. In that year, Louis Pasteur in France investigated fowl cholera, a disease caused by the bacterium now called *Pasteurella multocida* (Figure 1-1). Pasteur had a culture of this organism that was accidentally allowed to age on a laboratory bench while his assistant was on vacation. When the assistant returned and tried to infect chickens with this aged culture, the birds remained healthy (Figure 1-2). Being frugal, Pasteur retained these chickens and subsequently used them for a second experiment in which they were challenged again, this time with a fresh culture of *P. multocida* known to be capable of killing chickens. To Pasteur's surprise the birds were

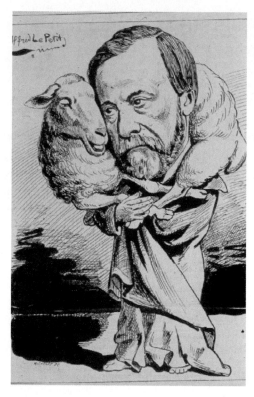

Figure 1-1. Louis Pasteur made the key discoveries that led to the development of vaccines against infectious agents. This drawing shows him as the good shepherd "Le bon Pasteur," reflecting his discovery of a vaccine against anthrax, 1882. (Copyright Institut Pasteur. With permission.)

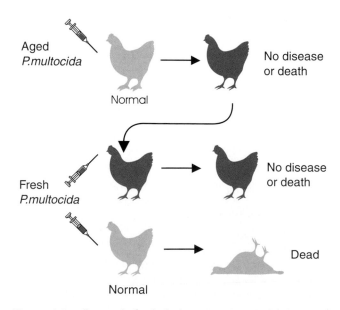

Figure 1-2. Pasteur's fowl cholera experiment. Birds inoculated with an aged culture of *P. multocida* did not die. However, when subsequently inoculated with a fresh culture of virulent *P. multocida* the birds were found to be protected.

resistant to the infection and did not die. In a remarkable intellectual jump, Pasteur immediately recognized that this phenomenon was similar in principle to Jenner's use of cowpox for vaccination. In vaccination, exposure of an animal to a strain of an organism that will not cause disease (an avirulent strain) can provoke an immune response. This immune response will protect the animal against a subsequent infection by a disease-producing (or virulent) strain of the same, or closely related, organism. Having established the general principle of vaccination, Pasteur first applied it to anthrax. He made anthrax bacteria (*Bacillus anthracis*) avirulent by growing them at an unusually high temperature. These attenuated organisms were then used as a vaccine to protect sheep against challenge with virulent anthrax bacteria. Pasteur subsequently developed a successful rabies vaccine by drying spinal cords taken from rabies-infected rabbits and using the dried cords as his vaccine material. The drying process effectively rendered the rabies virus avirulent (and probably killed much of it).

Although Louis Pasteur used only living organisms in his vaccines, it was not long before Daniel Salmon and Theobald Smith, working in the United States, demonstrated that dead organisms could also be used as vaccines. They showed that a heat-killed culture of a bacterium called *Salmonella enterica choleraesuis* (then called *Bacillus suipestifer* and believed to be the cause of hog cholera) could protect pigeons against the disease caused by that organism. A little later, Von Behring and Kitasato in Germany showed that filtrates taken from cultures of the tetanus bacillus (*Clostridium tetani*) could protect animals against tetanus even although they contained no bacteria. Thus bacterial products, in this case tetanus toxin, were also protective.

By 1900 the existence of immunity to infectious diseases of animals was well recognized. Over the past century immunologists have succeeded in identifying the molecular and cellular basis of this antimicrobial immunity. With this understanding has come the ability to use immune mechanisms to enhance resistance to infectious diseases. The role of the immune system in many different disease processes has been clarified. While much has been learned, much remains to be investigated. It is the current state of immunology as it relates to those species of interest to veterinarians that is the subject of this book.

MICROBIAL INVASION

The world is full of a diverse array of microorganisms. These include bacteria, viruses, fungi, protozoa, and helminths (worms). As they struggle to survive, many of these microorganisms see the animal body as a rich source of nutrients and a place to shelter. They will thus seek to invade animal tissues. This is normally prevented by our immune defenses. Sometimes, however, these organisms may overcome the immune defenses and cause

disease. Organisms that cannot evade or overcome the immune defenses are unable to invade the body, cannot cause tissue damage, and cannot therefore cause disease. An organism that can cause disease is said to be a pathogen. It is important to point out, however, that only a small proportion of the world's microorganisms are associated with animals and that only a very small proportion of these have the ability to overcome the immune defenses and become pathogens.

These pathogens vary greatly in their ability to cause disease (or to evade the body's defenses). This ability is termed *virulence*. Thus a highly virulent organism has a greater ability to defeat the immune system and cause disease than an organism with low virulence. If a bacterium can cause disease almost every time it invades a healthy individual, even in low numbers, then it is considered a primary pathogen. Examples of primary pathogens include distemper virus; the human immunodeficiency virus (HIV), which causes AIDS; and *Brucella abortus*, the cause of contagious abortion in cattle. Other pathogens may be of such low virulence that they will only cause disease if administered in very high doses or if the immune defenses of the body are impaired first. These are opportunistic pathogens. Examples of opportunistic pathogens are those that invade animals whose immune systems have been destroyed or suppressed. They include bacteria such as *Mannheimia hemolytica* and fungi such as *Pneumocystis carinii*. These organisms rarely, if ever, cause disease in healthy animals.

THE BODY'S DEFENSES

Physical Barriers

Because the successful exclusion of microbial invaders is essential for survival, it is not surprising that animals use many different defense strategies. Indeed, the body employs multiple layers of defense (Figure 1-3). As a result,

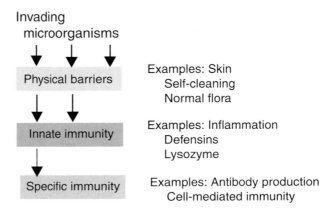

Figure 1-3. The three general ways by which the animal body defends itself against microbial invasion.

an organism that has succeeded in breaking through the first defensive layer is then confronted with the need to overcome a second, higher barrier, and so forth. The first and most obvious of these layers are the physical barriers to invasion. Thus intact skin provides an effective barrier to microbial invasion. If it is damaged, infections may occur; however, wound healing ensures that it is repaired very rapidly. On other body surfaces, such as in the respiratory and gastrointestinal tracts, simple physical defenses include the "self-cleaning" processes: coughing, sneezing, and mucus flow in the respiratory tract; vomiting and diarrhea in the gastrointestinal tract; and urine flow in the urinary system. The presence of an established normal flora on the skin and in the intestine also excludes many potential invaders. Well-adapted organisms adapted to living on body surfaces can easily outcompete poorly adapted pathogenic organisms.

Innate Immunity

Physical barriers, though very helpful in excluding invaders, cannot be entirely effective in themselves. Given time and persistence an invading microorganism will eventually overcome mere physical obstacles. However, given that most animals are not perpetually sick, it is likely that most of these infections are terminated quickly before the onset of disease. This is the task of the innate immune system. This second layer of defenses therefore consists of preexisting or rapidly responding chemical and cellular defense mechanisms (Table 1-1). Innate immunity relies on the fact that invading microorganisms are chemically very different from normal body components. Thus animals have enzymes that can digest bacterial cell walls and carbohydrate-binding proteins that will coat bacteria and hasten their destruction. Animals also have cells that can recognize the molecules associated with invading microorganisms and kill them. One key aspect of innate immunity is the body's ability to focus these innate defense mechanisms on sites of microbial invasion. This focused defensive

response is called inflammation. During inflammation, changes in tissues brought about by microbial invasion or tissue damage result in increased blood flow and the local accumulation of cells that can attack and destroy the invaders. These cells, called neutrophils and macrophages, can destroy most invading organisms and prevent their spread to uninfected areas of the body. The body also uses enzymes that are triggered by the presence of invaders to cause microbial destruction. These enzymes form what is known as the complement system. Some of the cells involved in inflammation may also repair damaged tissues once the invaders have been destroyed.

Animals also possess natural antimicrobial molecules such as the carbohydrate-digesting enzyme lysozyme and many carbohydrate-binding proteins. Some of these molecules circulate all the time; others are induced by the presence of bacteria or damaged tissues. These proteins can bind to invading organisms and accelerate their destruction.

The innate immune system lacks any form of memory. As a result the intensity and duration of processes such as inflammation remain unchanged no matter how often a specific invader is encountered. On the other hand, it is always ready to respond immediately once an invading pathogen is encountered.

Acquired Immunity

Inflammation and the other components of the innate immune system contribute significantly to the defense of the body. Animals that cannot mount an effective innate response will die from overwhelming infections. Nevertheless, these innate mechanisms cannot offer the ultimate solution to the defense of the body. What is really needed is a defense system that can recognize invaders, destroy them, and then learn from the process. The animal body requires a "smart" system that can recognize and remember invaders so that when it encounters them on subsequent occasions it can respond more rapidly and effectively. Therefore, the more often an individual encounters an invader, the more effective will be its defenses against that organism. This type of adaptive response is the function of the acquired immune system. The acquired immune system takes at least several days to become effective (Figure 1-4). Although it develops rather slowly, this is an incredibly effective defense system. As a result, when an animal eventually develops acquired immunity to an invader, the chance of successful invasion by that organism will be reduced to a very low level. The acquired immune system is a complex and sophisticated system that provides the ultimate defense of the body. Its importance is readily seen when it is destroyed. Thus in human AIDS patients, loss of acquired immunity leads inevitably to death as a result of uncontrolled infections. The main distinction between the innate and acquired immune systems lies in their use of receptors to recognize foreign invaders. The innate

TABLE 1-1		
A Comparison of Innate and Acquired Immunity		
	Innate Immunity	**Acquired Immunity**
Cells engaged	Macrophages, dendritic cells neutrophils, NK cells	T and B cells
Evolutionary history	Ancient	Recent
Onset	Rapid (min-hr)	Slow (days-weeks)
Specificity	Common microbial structures	Unique antigens

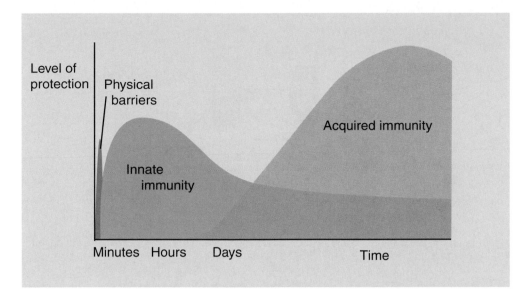

Figure 1-4. The time course of innate and acquired immunity. Surface barriers provide immediate protection. Innate mechanisms provide rapid protection that keeps microbial invaders at bay until acquired immunity can develop. It may take several days or weeks for acquired immunity to become effective.

system uses preexisting receptors that can bind to molecules and molecular patterns commonly found on many different microbial pathogens. In contrast, the cells of the acquired immune system randomly generate enormous numbers of structurally unique receptors. These receptors can bind to an enormous array of foreign molecules. Because the binding repertoire of these receptors is generated randomly, they are not predestined to recognize any specific foreign molecule but collectively can recognize almost any invading microorganism.

The acquired immune system can recognize foreign invaders, destroy them, and retain the memory of the encounter. If the animal encounters the same organism a second time the immune system responds more rapidly and more effectively. Such a sophisticated system must of necessity be complex. One reason for this complexity is the enormous diversity of potential invaders. Microbial invaders fall into two broad categories. One category consists of the organisms that originate outside the body. This includes most bacteria and fungi, as well as many protozoa and invading helminths. The second category consists of the organisms that originate or live inside the body's own cells. These include viruses and intracellular bacteria or protozoa. The acquired immune system therefore consists of two major branches that defend against each of these two categories of invaders. Thus one branch of the immune system is directed against the extracellular or exogenous invaders. Proteins called antibodies destroy these invaders. This type of immune response is sometimes called the "humoral immune response" since antibodies are found in body fluids (or "humors"). The other major branch of the immune system is directed against the intracellular or endogenous invaders that invade cells. Specialized cells destroy these infected or abnormal cells. This type of response is therefore called the "cell-mediated immune response."

ANTIBODY-MEDIATED IMMUNE RESPONSES

Soon after Louis Pasteur discovered that it was possible to produce immunity to infectious agents by vaccination, it was recognized that the substances that provided this immunity could be found in the blood serum (Figure 1-5). For example, if serum is taken from a horse that has been vaccinated against tetanus (or has recovered from tetanus) and injected into a normal horse, the recipient animal will become resistant to tetanus for several weeks (Figure 1-6).

The protective molecules found in the serum of an immunized animal are proteins called antibodies. Antibodies against tetanus toxin are not found in the serum of normal horses but are produced following exposure to tetanus toxin as a result of infection or vaccination. Tetanus toxin is an example of a foreign substance that stimulates an immune response. The general term for such a substance is antigen. If an antigen is injected into an animal, then antibodies will be produced which can bind to that antigen and ensure its destruction. Antibodies are specific and only bind to the antigen that stimulates their production. For example, the antibodies produced in response to tetanus toxin bind only tetanus toxin. If serum containing these antibodies is mixed with a solution of tetanus toxin, the antibodies bind and "neutralize" the toxin so that it is no longer toxic for animals. In this way antibodies protect animals against the lethal effects of the toxin.

The time course of the antibody response to tetanus toxin can be followed by taking blood samples from a horse at intervals after injection of the toxin (or injection of chemically detoxified toxin called tetanus toxoid, a much safer procedure). The blood is allowed to clot and the clear serum removed. The amount of antibody in the serum may be estimated by measuring the ability of the

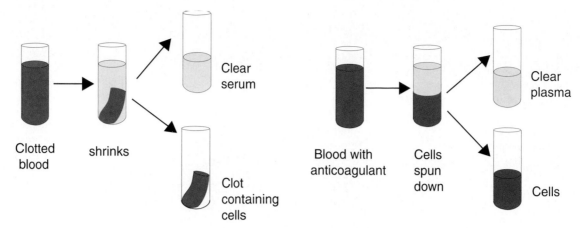

Figure 1-5.   The difference between serum and plasma. Plasma contains blood-clotting components that are absent from serum.

serum to neutralize a standard amount of toxin. Following a single injection of toxin into a horse that has never been previously exposed to it, no antibody is detectable for several days (Figure 1-7). This lag period lasts for about one week. When antibodies eventually appear in serum their level climbs to reach a peak by 10 to 20 days before declining and disappearing within a few weeks. The amount of antibody formed, and therefore the amount of protection conferred, during this first or primary response is relatively small.

If sometime later a second dose of toxin or toxoid is injected into the same horse and the antibody response followed, then the lag period lasts for no more than 2 or 3 days. The amount of antibody in serum then rises rapidly to a high level before declining slowly. Antibodies may be detected for many months or years after this injection. A third dose of the antigen given to the same

animal results in an immune response characterized by an even shorter lag period and a still higher and more prolonged antibody response. As will be described later in this book, the antibodies produced after repeated injections are better able to bind and neutralize the toxin than those produced early in the immune response. The stimulation of the immune responses to infectious agents by repeated injections of antigen forms the basis of vaccination.

The response of an animal to a second dose of antigen is very different from the first in that it occurs much more quickly, antibodies reach much higher levels, and it lasts for much longer. This secondary response is specific in that it can be provoked only by a second dose of an antigen. A secondary response may be provoked many months or years after the first injection of antigen, although its size tends to decline as time passes.

Figure 1-6.   Transfer of immunity to tetanus by means of serum derived from an immunized horse. This clearly demonstrates that antibodies in serum are sufficient to confer immunity to tetanus.

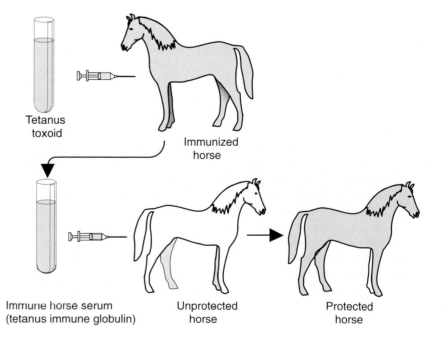

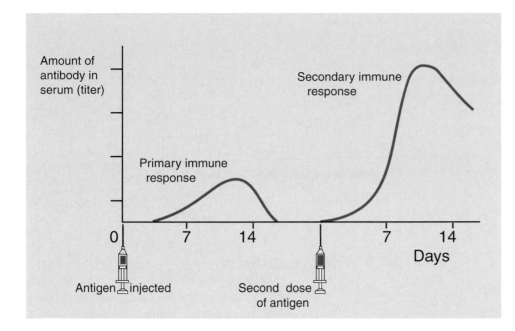

Figure 1-7. The characteristic time course of the immune response to an antigen as measured by serum antibody levels. Note the key differences between a primary and a secondary immune response.

A secondary response can also be induced even though the response of the animal to the first injection of antigen was so weak as to be undetectable. These features of the secondary response indicate that the antibody-forming system possesses the ability to "remember" previous exposure to an antigen. For this reason, the secondary immune response is sometimes called an anamnestic response (*anamnesko* is Greek for "memory"). It should be noted, however, that repeated injections of antigen do not lead indefinitely to greater and greater immune responses. The level of antibodies in serum is regulated, so that they eventually stop rising, even after multiple doses of antigen or exposure to many different antigens.

CELL-MEDIATED IMMUNE RESPONSES

If a piece of living tissue such as a kidney or a piece of skin is surgically removed from one animal and grafted onto another of the same species, it usually survives for a few days before being rejected by the recipient. This process of graft rejection is significant because it demonstrates the existence of a mechanism whereby foreign cells, differing only slightly from an animal's own normal cells, are rapidly recognized and destroyed. Even cells with minor structural abnormalities may be recognized as foreign by the immune system and destroyed though they are otherwise apparently healthy. These abnormal cells include aged cells, virus-infected cells, and some cancer cells. The immune response to foreign cells as shown by graft rejection demonstrates that the immune system can identify and destroy abnormal cells.

If a piece of skin is transplanted from one dog to a second, unrelated dog, it will survive for about 10 days. The grafted skin will initially appear to be healthy, and blood vessels will develop between the graft and its host.

By one week, however, these new blood vessels will begin to degenerate, the blood supply to the graft will be cut off, and the graft will eventually die and be shed (Figure 1-8). If a second graft is taken from the original donor and placed on the same recipient, then that second graft will survive for no more than a day or two before being rejected. Thus the rejection of a first graft is relatively weak and slow and analogous to the primary antibody response, whereas a second graft stimulates very rapid and powerful rejection similar in many ways to the secondary antibody response. Graft rejection, like antibody formation, is a specific immune response in that a rapid secondary reaction occurs only if the second graft is from the same donor as the first. Like antibody formation, the graft rejection process also involves memory, since a second graft may be rapidly rejected many months or years after loss of the first.

However, graft rejection is not entirely identical to the process involved in protection against tetanus toxin because it cannot be transferred from a sensitized to a normal animal by means of serum antibodies. The ability to mount a secondary reaction to a graft can only be transferred between animals by living cells. The cells that do this are called lymphocytes and are found in the spleen, lymph nodes, and blood. The process of graft rejection is mediated primarily by lymphocytes and not by serum antibodies. It is a good example of a cell-mediated immune response.

MECHANISMS OF ACQUIRED IMMUNITY

In some ways the acquired immune system may be compared to a totalitarian state in which foreigners are expelled, citizens who behave themselves are tolerated, but those who "deviate" are eliminated. While this analogy must

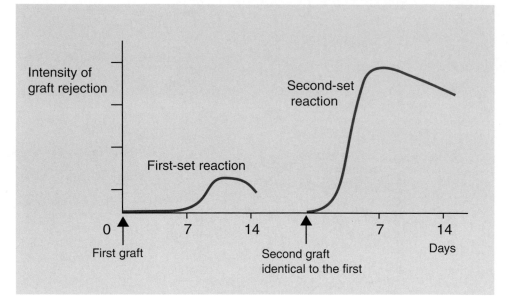

Figure 1-8. The characteristic time course of the rejection of a foreign skin graft. Notice how similar this diagram is to Figure 1-7.

not be carried too far, clearly such regimes possess a number of characteristic features. These include border defenses and a police force that keeps the population under surveillance and promptly eliminates dissidents. In the case of the acquired immune system, the antibody-mediated responses would be responsible for keeping the foreigners out whereas the cell-mediated responses would be responsible for stopping internal dissent. Organizations of this type also tend to develop a pass system, so that foreigners or dissidents not possessing certain identifying features are rapidly detected and dealt with.

Similarly, when a foreign antigen enters the body it first must be trapped and processed so that it can be recognized as being foreign. If so recognized, then this information must be conveyed either to the antibody-forming system or to the cell-mediated immune system. These systems must then respond by the production of specific antibodies and/or cells that are capable of eliminating the antigen. The acquired immune system must also remember this event so that the next time an animal is exposed to the same antigen, its response will be faster and more efficient. The immune system also learns how to make antibodies or cells that can bind more strongly to the invader. In our totalitarian state analogy, the police force would be trained to recognize selected foreigners or dissidents and respond more promptly when they are encountered.

We can therefore consider that the acquired immune system includes four major components (Figure 1-9).
1. Cells that can trap and process antigen and then present it for recognition to the cells of the immune system.
2. Cells that have receptors for the processed antigen. These cells can thus bind and respond to the antigen (antigen-sensitive cells.)

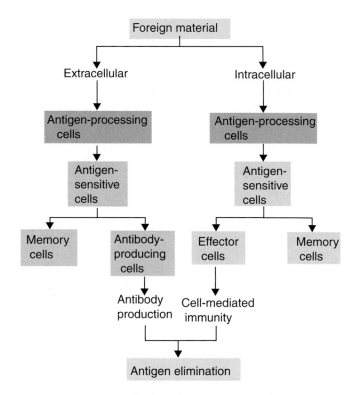

Figure 1-9. A simple flow diagram showing the essential features of the acquired immune responses.

3. Cells that, once activated by antigen, will produce specific antibodies or will participate in the cell-mediated immune responses against the antigen (effector cells).
4. Cells that will retain the memory of the event and react rapidly to that specific antigen if it is encountered at a later time.

A fifth type of cell is also required if the acquired immune system is to function correctly. These cells regulate the immune system so that the response is at an appropriate level.

All of these cell populations can be recognized within the body. Antigen is trapped, processed, and presented by several cell types, including dendritic cells and macrophages. Lymphocytes called B and T cells have specific receptors for foreign antigen and are thus able to bind the processed antigen and respond appropriately. Lymphocytes also function as memory cells and therefore initiate a secondary immune response. The lymphocytes that mediate the cell-mediated responses are T cells. The lymphocytes that mediate the antibody-mediated responses are B cells. The immune response is mainly regulated by populations of T cells. Those that promote immune responses are called helper T cells. Those that inhibit immune responses are called regulatory T cells.

In subsequent chapters we will first review the mechanisms involved in innate immunity. Following that, we will review acquired immunity in detail and examine each of its basic components in turn. We will then examine the role of the immune system in protecting animals against microbial invasion. We will also see what happens when the immune system functions abnormally, either excessively or inadequately.

WHERE TO GO FOR ADDITIONAL INFORMATION

Many veterinary journals carry articles of interest to immunologists. Some of the most important are as follows: *Acta Veterinaria Scandinavica, American Journal of Veterinary Research, Australian Veterinary Journal, The Veterinary Journal, Canadian Journal of Comparative Medicine, Journal of the American Veterinary Medical Association, Journal of Comparative Pathology, Research in Veterinary Science, Veterinary Immunology and Immunopathology, Veterinary Pathology,* and *The Veterinary Record.*

For information on new developments on basic immunology (with occasional papers on subjects of veterinary interest), the reader should review journals such as *Nature, Science, Journal of Immunology, Trends in Immunology, Proceedings of the National Academy of Sciences of the United States of America, New England Journal of Medicine, Infection and Immunity, Immunity, Immunogenetics,* and *Immunology.*

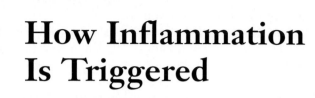

How Inflammation Is Triggered

Infectious agents such as bacteria or viruses can grow very rapidly. A single bacterium with a doubling time of 50 minutes can produce about 500 million offspring within 24 hours. Thus if a microorganism invades the body it must be rapidly recognized and destroyed before it overwhelms the defenses. Time is of the essence and delay can be fatal. The animal body must therefore rely on preexisting innate immune mechanisms as its first line of defense against microbial invasion. The most important of these innate mechanisms is acute inflammation.

Inflammation is the response of tissues to invading microorganisms or tissue damage. It is also a vital protective process because it is the means by which defensive cells and molecules are concentrated rapidly at sites of microbial invasion. Inflammation involves the activation and directed migration of many different cells, especially neutrophils and macrophages, from the bloodstream to sites of invasion. Cells such as neutrophils are normally restricted to the bloodstream. They must migrate into tissues in order to destroy invaders. Likewise, many protective molecules, such as antibodies and complement components, are normally found only in blood. These large molecules can only escape into the tissues at sites of inflammation. Inflammation thus provides a mechanism by which key protective processes are focused on a localized region of tissue (Figure 2-1). The first priority is for these processes to attack and eliminate invaders. Later, when the danger is past, they initiate the repair of tissue damage.

HOW INVADERS ARE RECOGNIZED

The first step in innate immunity is for the body to sense that it is being invaded. This involves recognizing the presence of microorganisms, as well as molecules released by damaged cells.

The presence of invading microbes and the resulting tissue damage is detected by "sentinel cells." The three major types of sentinel cells are macrophages, dendritic cells, and mast cells. These cells have surface receptors that can recognize molecules that are normally expressed by microbes and never found in higher animals. For example, most bacteria are covered in a cell wall largely composed of complex carbohydrates. Thus the cell walls of gram-positive organisms are largely composed of peptidoglycans (chains of alternating *N*-acetylglucosamine and *N*-acetylmuramic acid cross-linked by short peptide side chains) (Figure 2-2). Gram-positive bacterial cell walls also contain lipoteichoic acids. The cell walls of gram-negative organisms consist of peptidoglycans covered by a layer of lipopolysaccharide (LPS). Acid-fast bacteria are covered in glycolipids. Yeasts are also covered by a carbohydrate wall. Other important molecules unique to microorganisms include their DNA and some proteins.

Microbes not only grow fast, but also are highly diverse and can mutate and change their molecular structures much faster than an infected animal can respond. Thus the sentinel cell receptors are not designed to recognize all possible microbial molecules. Rather, the cells use

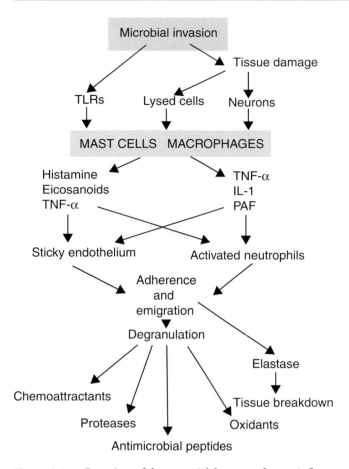

Figure 2-1. Overview of the essential features of acute inflammation. An innate mechanism for focusing cells and other defensive mechanisms at sites of microbial invasion and tissue damage.

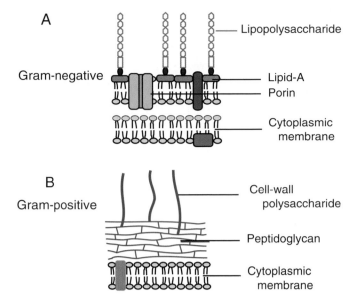

Figure 2-2. The major structural features of the cell walls of Gram-negative and Gram-positive bacteria.

receptors that recognize highly conserved molecules or molecular patterns that are widespread in many different microorganisms. Collectively, these are called pathogen-associated molecular patterns (PAMPs). PAMPs include the LPS of gram-negative bacteria, the lipoteichoic acids of gram-positive bacteria, the mannans of yeasts and the glycolipids of mycobacteria, as well as bacterial DNA. All of these molecules are restricted to microorganisms and are not found in animal tissues. They tend to be essential for microbial survival and are commonly shared by entire classes of pathogens. The most important of the sentinel cell receptors are called toll-like receptors.

Toll-like Receptors

Toll-like receptors (TLRs) play a central role in recognizing invading microbes and in triggering inflammation. These receptors are expressed on macrophages and mast cells, as well as on dendritic cells, eosinophils, and epithelial cells in the respiratory tract and intestine (Figure 2-3). They owe their curious name to a closely related receptor called "Toll," which was first identified in the fruit fly, *Drosophila*. In mammals, binding of microbial molecules

to TLRs induces the cells to produce molecules that trigger innate immunity, especially inflammation. A cell such as a macrophage thus uses its TLRs to identify the presence of an invader and respond appropriately.

There are at least 10 different TLRs, and each serves as a receptor for one or more specific microbial molecules (Table 2-1). For example, TLR4 can bind lipopolysaccharides from the surface of gram-negative bacteria. TLR2, on the other hand, recognizes many different bacterial components, including peptidoglycans, lipoproteins, and a glycolipid called lipoarabinomannan from *Mycobacterium tuberculosis*. Another TLR, termed TLR5, binds to flagellin, the protein from bacterial flagella. TLR9, on the other hand, is a cytoplasmic receptor for bacterial DNA. Bacteria must therefore be disrupted if the bacterial DNA is to be recognized. Both TLR3 and TLR7 bind double-stranded ribonucleic acid (RNA) from viruses. A deficiency of TLR4 increases the susceptibility of mice to some viral infections, implying that TLR4 may also play a role in antiviral immunity. In addition, TLR2 can associate with TLR6, and the dual receptor complex can then recognize another ligand, bacterial lipopeptide. Likewise, TLR1 associates with TLR2 to recognize mycobacterial lipoprotein. It is believed that the presently known TLRs can collectively recognize almost all infectious agents.

Once a TLR binds a molecule from an invading microorganism, a signal passes into its cell and activates the genes for proteins called cytokines. Different TLRs trigger the production of different combinations of cytokines, and different microbial products trigger distinctly different responses even within one cell type. For example, TLRs that recognize bacterial molecules will trigger the production of cytokines optimized to combat bacteria,

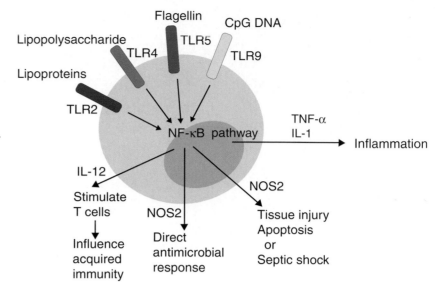

Figure 2-3. Toll-like receptors and the consequences of ligand binding.

those that recognize viral will produce antiviral cytokines, and so forth.

TLRs not only trigger innate immune defenses such as inflammation but also begin the process of "turning on" the acquired immune system. For example, stimulation of TLR4 makes macrophages and its close relative, the dendritic cell, produce cytokine molecules that are potent stimulators of immune cells (Chapter 6).

In addition to recognizing molecules from invading microorganisms, TLRs also recognize molecules produced by damaged tissues. Thus broken cells generate fragments of heparan sulfate. This molecule is normally restricted to cell membranes and the extracellular matrix but is shed into tissue fluids following injury. Heparan sulfate binds to TLR4 and so activates sentinel cells.

Fibrinogen, a clotting protein, also stimulates macrophages through TLR4. Other molecules released from damaged cells, such as heat-shock proteins, can trigger macrophage activation through TLR2 and TLR4.

Other PAMP Receptors

While the TLRs are the most prominent of these receptors, it is clear that macrophages, mast cells, and dendritic cells have many other surface receptors that recognize microbial molecules. These include CD14, which binds bacterial LPS; the mannan and glucan receptors, which bind microbial carbohydrates; scavenger receptors such as CD36, which can bind bacterial lipoproteins, and CD1, which binds microbial glycolipids.

Bacterial DNA

Bacterial deoxyribonucleic acid (DNA) is a significant stimulator of innate immunity. It differs from eukaryotic DNA in that it contains a large proportion of the dinucleotide cytosine-guanosine (CpG). In addition, while the cytosine in eukaryotic DNA is normally methylated, this is not the case in bacterial DNA (Figure 2-4). Thus unmethylated CpG dinucleotides can trigger innate immune responses. The biological activity of these CpG dinucleotides is influenced by the flanking nucleotides found on each side of the CpG motif. CpG dinucleotides can bind and activate many different cell types, including macrophages, dendritic cells, and mast cells, through their receptor TLR9. (Different sequences activate different cell types.) Bacterial DNA also contains deoxyguanosine (dG) residues. These dG residues form unconventional base pairs and, as a result, form structures other than the usual double helix. One structure that they form is called quadriplex DNA. This binds to TLR9 and stimulates production of the cytokine interleukin-12 (IL-12). Bacterial DNA also triggers increased

---

TABLE   2-1
Products Recognized by the Mammalian Toll-like Receptors

TLR	NATURAL LIGANDS
TLR1	Diacylated lipoproteins
TLR2	Peptidoglycan, bacterial lipoproteins, zymosan Some LPS, spirochetes, mycobacteria, lipoteichoic acid, heat-shock protein, necrotic cells
TLR3	Viral double-stranded RNA
TLR4	LPS, lipoteichoic acid, viral protein, heat-shock protein, fibrinogen, saturated fatty acids, β-defensins, heparan sulfate
TLR5	Flagellin and flagellated bacteria
TLR6	Necrotic cells, diacylated lipoprotein, peptidoglycan (with TLR2)
TLR7	Small antiviral molecules
TLR8	Small antiviral molecules
TLR9	Unmethylated CpG bacterial DNA
TLR10	A pseudogene

TLR, Toll-like receptor; *LPS,* lipopolysaccharide; *CpG,* cytosine-guanosine.

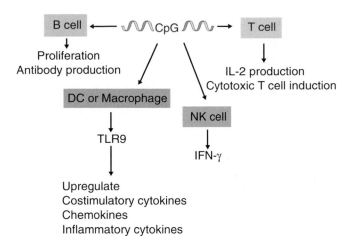

Figure 2-4. The immunostimulating functions of bacterial CpG DNA. *DC*, Dendritic cell; *NK*, natural killer cells.

production of the cytokines tumor necrosis factor-α (TNF-α) and interleukin-6 (IL-6) by macrophages.

Bacterial Lipopolysaccharides

Bacterial lipopolysaccharides are very potent inducers of innate immunity. They are released by invading gram-negative bacteria. They do not act directly on cells by themselves but first bind to LPS-binding protein (LBP) in serum (Figure 2-5). LBP immediately transfers LPS molecules to a protein called CD14 located on the surface of macrophages (Box 2-1). CD14 cannot penetrate cell membranes and so is unable to signal to cells directly. CD14 therefore binds to TLR4 on the cell surface. Binding of LPS to the CD14/TLR4 complex activates macrophages and triggers cytokine production. The LPS subsequently dissociates from CD14 and binds to lipoproteins where its toxic activities are lost. CD14 not only binds LPS but also binds to many other microbial molecules including lipoarabinomannans from mycobacteria, manuronic acid polymers from *Pseudomonas*, and peptidoglycans from *Staphylococcus aureus*.

The Complement System

Another innate protective system that can recognize microbes is the complement system. This system consists of a set of enzymes and other proteins found in the blood. When activated by exposure to invading bacteria, the complement system kills invading microorganisms. The complement system is activated by the presence of bacterial cell walls through a pathway called the alternative complement pathway. Once activated, complement components can either kill microbes directly or prepare them for capture by phagocytic (eating) cells. A second complement pathway is activated when a protein called mannose-binding lectin binds to microbial surfaces.

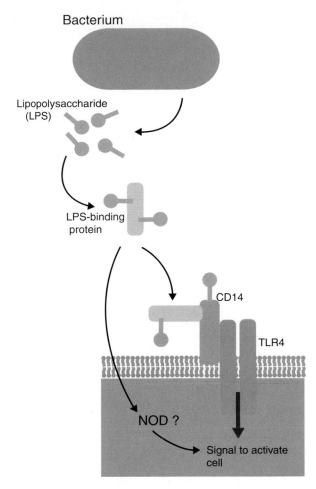

Figure 2-5. The processing and fate of bacterial lipopolysaccharide.

It too results in microbial killing. The complement system is described in detail in Chapter 15.

SENTINEL CELLS

The major sentinel cells, macrophages, dendritic cells, and mast cells, are scattered throughout the body. They are found in highest numbers just below body surfaces at

---

BOX 2–1

The CD System

When advances in immunology made it possible to make highly specific antibodies against individual cell surface proteins (Chapter 11), it was soon shown that cells possessed hundreds of different surface proteins. To classify these proteins, a system was established that gave each molecule a specific number. Thus each protein was assigned to a numbered cluster of differentiation (CD). In many cases, a defined CD denotes a protein of specific function. For example, the protein CD14 binds bacterial lipopolysaccharide. More than 240 of these CD molecules have now been identified, and the number will assuredly grow.

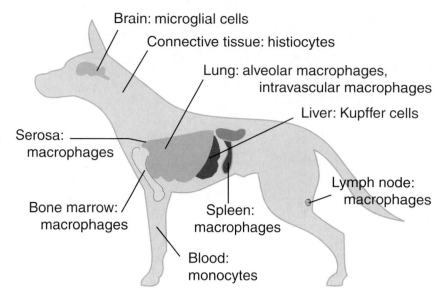

Figure 2-6. The location of the cells of the mononuclear phagocyte system.

locations where invading microorganisms are likely to be encountered.

Macrophages

Macrophages participate in many aspects of the defense of the body. Thus not only can they act as sentinel cells and sense the presence of invading microorganisms, but they can also kill invading organisms and play an essential role in triggering acquired immunity. When stimulated, they secrete cytokines that promote both innate and acquired immune responses; they control inflammation; they contribute directly to the repair of damaged tissues by removing dead, dying, and damaged cells and so assist the healing process. Their name is derived from the fact that they are "large-eating" cells (Greek *macro, phage*).

Immature macrophages are found in the blood where they are called monocytes. As monocytes mature they migrate into tissues and become macrophages. Mature macrophages are found in connective tissue, where they are called histiocytes; those found lining the sinusoids of the liver are called Kupffer cells; those in the brain are microglia. The macrophages found in the alveoli of the lungs are called alveolar macrophages, whereas those in the capillaries of the lung are called pulmonary intravascular macrophages. Large numbers are found in the sinusoids of the spleen, bone marrow, and lymph nodes. Irrespective of their name or location, they are all macrophages and all are part of the mononuclear phagocyte system (Figure 2-6).

Structure

Macrophages change their shapes in response to their environment. In suspension, however, they are round cells of about 15 mm diameter. They possess abundant cytoplasm, at the center of which is a single nucleus that may be round, bean shaped, or indented (Figure 2-7). Their central cytoplasm contains mitochondria, large numbers of lysosomes, some rough endoplasmic reticulum, and a Golgi apparatus, indicating that they can synthesize and secrete proteins (Figures 2-8 and 2-9). In living cells, the peripheral cytoplasm is in continuous movement, forming and reforming veil-like ruffles. Some macrophages show variations from this basic structure. Peripheral blood monocytes have round nuclei, which elongate as the cells mature. Alveolar macrophages rarely possess rough endoplasmic reticulum, but their cytoplasm is full of granules. The microglia of the central nervous system have rod-shaped nuclei and very long cytoplasmic

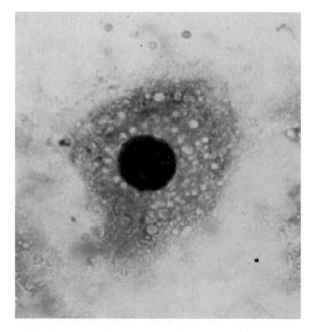

Figure 2-7. A typical macrophage, original magnification ×500.

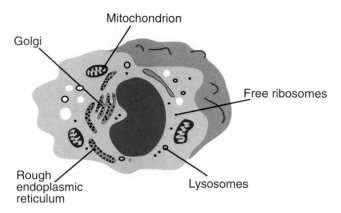

Figure 2-8. The major structural features of a macrophage.

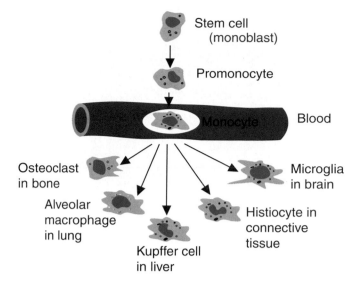

Figure 2-10. Origin and development of macrophages. Monocytes in blood can differentiate into many different types of macrophage.

processes that are lost when the cell is stimulated by tissue damage.

Life History

All the cells of the mononuclear phagocyte system arise from stem cells in the bone marrow called monoblasts (Figure 2-10). Monoblasts develop into promonocytes, and promonocytes develop into monocytes—all under the influence of cytokines called colony-stimulating factors. Monocytes then enter the blood and circulate for about 3 days before entering tissues and developing into macrophages. They form about 5% of the total leukocyte population in blood. Tissue macrophages either originate from monocytes or divide within tissues. They are

relatively long-lived cells, replacing themselves at a rate of about 1% per day unless activated by inflammation or tissue damage. (Some monocytes may develop into a different cell type, called dendritic cells, discussed in Chapter 6.) Macrophages may live for a long time after ingesting chemically inert particles, such as the carbon injected in tattoo marks, although they may fuse together to form multinucleated giant cells in an attempt to eliminate the foreign material.

Mast Cells

Structure

Mast cells are very large, round cells (15 to 20 μm in diameter) scattered throughout the body in connective tissue, under mucosal surfaces, in the skin, and around nerves (Figure 2-11). They are found in highest numbers

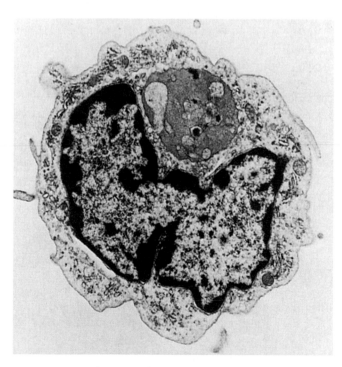

Figure 2-9. Transmission electron micrograph of a normal rabbit macrophage. The nature of the large inclusion is unknown. (Courtesy Dr. S. Linthicum.)

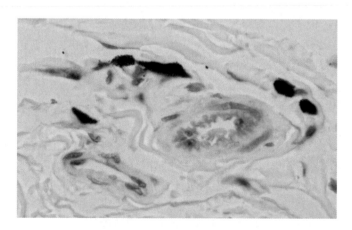

Figure 2-11. A section of canine skin stained to show mast cells. The mast cells stain intensely because of the heparin in their cytoplasmic granules.

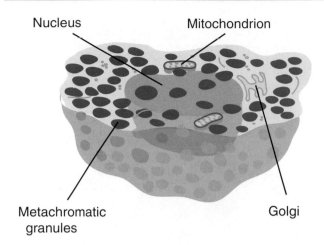

Figure 2-12. A diagram of the structural features of a connective tissue mast cell. The term "metachromatic" simply means that the granules stain intensely.

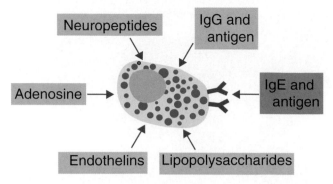

Figure 2-13. Some of the stimuli that make mast cells degranulate. Antigen bound through IgE causes rapid complete degranulation. The other stimuli shown cause a more gradual, piecemeal degranulation. Thus in normal inflammatory responses the degree of mast cell degranulation is tailored to local defensive needs.

under body surfaces. They are easily recognizable because their cytoplasm is densely packed with large granules that stain very strongly with dyes such as toluidine blue. These granules often mask the large, bean-shaped nucleus (Figure 2-12). (Mast cells are so called because, being full of granules, they were considered to be "well-fed cells" [German *Mastzellen*]). Mast cells from connective tissue and skin and from the intestinal walls differ both chemically and structurally (Table 2-2). For example, connective tissue and skin mast cells are rich in the molecules histamine and heparin, whereas intestinal mast cells contain chondroitin sulfate and have little histamine in their granules.

Life History
Mast cells originate from stem cells in the bone marrow. The mast cell precursors emigrate to tissues where they mature and survive for several weeks or months. Although connective tissue mast cells remain at relatively constant levels, intestinal mast cells can proliferate. It has been suggested that the intestinal mast cells respond specifically to invasion by parasitic worms.

Mast cells have a key role in innate immunity because when appropriately stimulated they release a complex

mixture of molecules that trigger acute inflammation. These inflammatory molecules are normally confined to the mast cell granules. Several different mechanisms stimulate mast cell degranulation. The best recognized of these is through the antibody called IgE (Chapter 26). IgE and antigen can trigger an explosive release of mast cell granule contents, which is responsible for the severe inflammation that occurs in allergic diseases. However, allergies are a special case. In normal inflammation, mast cells release their granule contents relatively slowly in a process called piecemeal degranulation. They may also release some mediators without any degranulation.

Mast cells undergo piecemeal degranulation in response to many different stimuli (Figure 2-13). For example, bacteria and bacterial products will trigger degranulation. Many small peptides, such as the defensins, neuropeptides, and endothelins (small peptides from endothelial cells), also trigger mast cell degranulation. Dead and dying cells release the nucleotide adenosine that activates and degranulates mast cells.

Stimulation of different TLRs causes mast cells to release different mixtures of mediators. Thus bacterial peptidoglycans acting through TLR2 stimulate histamine release, whereas lipopolysaccharides acting through TLR4 do not. Mast cells at inflammatory sites probably adjust their release of mediators to specific needs.

PRODUCTS OF SENTINEL CELLS

Macrophages and mast cells are activated when microbial products or products from broken cells bind to their TLRs. They respond by secreting a mixture of cytokines and releasing a complex mixture of small molecules that affect the functions of blood vessels. Dendritic cells respond somewhat differently. This is described in Chapter 6.

TABLE 2-2
Comparison of Two Major Types of Mast Cell

	Connective Tissue Mast Cells	Mucosal Mast Cells
Structure	Few, variable-sized granules	Many uniform granules
Size	9 to 10 μm diameter	19 to 20 μm diameter
Proteoglycan	Chondroitin sulfate	Heparin
Histamine	1.3 pg/cell	15 pg/cell
Life span	<40 d	>6 mo
Location	Peritoneal cavity, skin	Intestinal wall, lung

Cytokines

When exposed to infectious agents or their PAMPs, the sentinel cells secrete many different molecules. These molecules include the major cytokines interleukin-1 (IL-1) and tumor necrosis factor-α (TNF-α) as well as others, such as IL-6, IL-12, and IL-18. They also secrete oxidants, such as O_2^-, H_2O_2, $^\bullet OH$, and $NO^\bullet$, and lipids, such as the leukotrienes and prostaglandins. When released in sufficient quantities these molecules can also cause a fever, sickness behavior, and promote an acute-phase response (Chapter 4).

Tumor Necrosis Factor-α

TNF-α is a protein produced mainly by activated macrophages and mast cells. The precursor TNF-α molecule is cleaved from the macrophage surface by a protease called TNF-α convertase. Its production is stimulated not only through TLRs but also by molecules secreted by nerves such as the neurotransmitter substance P. TNF-α is produced very early in inflammation, and this is followed by IL-1 and then by IL-6.

TNF-α is an essential mediator of inflammation because in combination with IL-1 it triggers critical changes in the cells that line small blood vessels (vascular endothelial cells). A local increase in TNF-α causes the "cardinal signs" of inflammation, including heat, swelling, pain, and redness. Systemic increases in TNF-α depress cardiac output, induce microvascular thrombosis, and cause capillary leakage. TNF-α acts on neutrophils (key defensive cells in inflammation; see Chapter 3) to enhance their ability to kill microbes. It is a potent attractant for neutrophils, drawing them to sites of tissue damage and increasing their adherence to vascular endothelium (Figure 2-14). TNF-α acts on macrophages to stimulate their production of IL-1 and the inflammatory

lipid, prostaglandin E_2 (PGE_2). It also stimulates macrophage phagocytosis and oxidant production. It amplifies and prolongs inflammation by activating other cells to release IL-1, inflammatory lipids, nitric oxide, and oxidants. TNF-α also activates mast cells.

Interleukin-1

When activated through CD14 and TLR4, macrophages produce two glycoproteins called IL-1α and IL-1β. Ten- to 50-fold more IL-1β is produced than IL-1α, and while IL-1β is secreted, IL-1α remains attached to the cell. Therefore IL-1α can only act on target cells that come into direct contact with the macrophage (Figure 2-15). Transcription of IL-1 mRNA occurs within 15 minutes of exposure to a stimulus. It reaches a peak 3 to 4 hours later and levels off for several hours before declining. Like TNF-α, IL-1 acts on vascular endothelial cells to make them adhesive for neutrophils.

During severe infections, some IL-1 escapes into the bloodstream (Figure 2-16) where, in association with TNF-α, it is responsible for sickness behavior. Thus it acts on the brain to cause fever, lethargy, malaise, and lack of appetite. It acts on muscle cells to mobilize amino acids causing pain and fatigue. It acts on liver cells to induce the production of new proteins, called acute-phase proteins, that assist in the innate defense of the body (Chapter 4.)

As will be described in detail in Chapter 10, IL-1 can activate lymphocytes (the cells that mediate the acquired immune response) and is necessary for the successful initiation of some forms of acquired immunity.

Interleukin-6

IL-6 is also produced by macrophages and mast cells. Its production is stimulated by bacterial endotoxins,

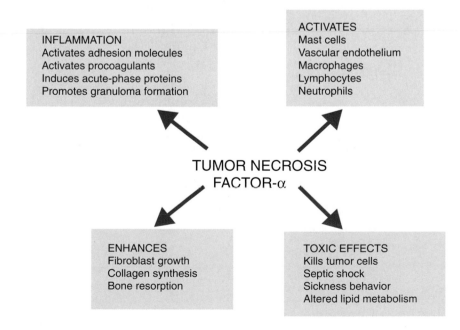

Figure 2-14. Some of the properties of tumor necrosis factor-α.

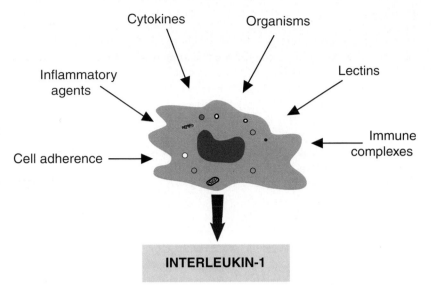

Figure 2-15. The wide variety of stimuli that promote the release of interleukin-1 from macrophages.

IL-1, and TNF-α. IL-6 affects many different functions, including both inflammation and acquired immunity. It is a major mediator of the acute-phase reaction and of septic shock (Chapter 4). It has been suggested that IL-6 regulates the transition from a neutrophil-dominated process early in inflammation to a macrophage-dominated process later on.

Chemokines

Chemokines are a family of chemotactic cytokines that serve as attractants for specific cell populations and so dictate the natural course of an inflammatory response (Table 2-3). They are small proteins (8 to 10 kDa) produced by diverse cell types including macrophages and

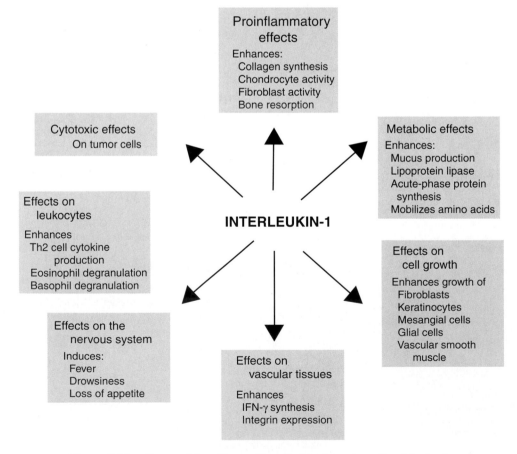

Figure 2-16. Some of the effects of interleukin-1 on the cells of the body.

TABLE 2-3
The Nomenclature of Some Selected Chemokines and Their Receptors

New Name	Old Name	Receptor
α FAMILY		
CCL2	MCP-1	CCR2
CCL3	MIP-1α	CCR1, CCR5
CCL4	MIP-1β	CCR5
CCL5	RANTES	CCR1, CCR3, CCR5
CCL7	MCP-3	CCR3
CCL8	MCP-2	CCR3
CCL11	Eotaxin	CCR3
CCL13	MCP-4	CCR3
CCL20	MIP-3α	CCR6
CCL22	MDC	CCR4
CCL26	Eotaxin 3	CCR3
CCL28	MEC	CCR3
β FAMILY		
CXCL1	GRO-1	CXCR2
CXCL7	MDGF	CXCR2
CXCL8	IL-8	CXCR1, CXCR2
CXCL12	SDF	CXCR4
CXCL13	BCA-1	CXCR5
γ FAMILY		
XCL1	Lymphotactin	XCR1
δ FAMILY		
CX3CL1	Fractalkine	CX3CR1

mast cells. At least 50 chemokines have been identified. They are classified into four families according to the spacing of their cysteine residues (Figure 2-17). For example, the CC, or α, chemokines have two contiguous cysteine residues, whereas the CXC, or β, chemokines have two cysteine residues separated by another amino acid. [Chemokine nomenclature is based on this classification, each molecule or receptor receiving a numerical

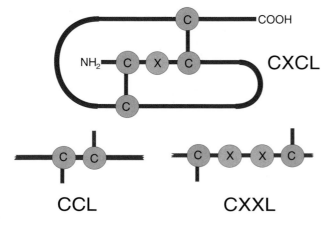

Figure 2-17. The classification of chemokines is based on the location and spacing of their cysteine residues.

designation. Ligands have the suffix "L" (e.g., CXCL8), whereas receptors have the suffix "R" (e.g., CXCR1).]

CXCL8 (or IL-8) is a typical example of a CXC chemokine produced by stimulation of macrophages. CXCL8 will attract and activate neutrophils, releasing their granule contents, and stimulating the respiratory burst and leukotriene release (see Chapter 3). Another important CXC chemokine is CXCL2 (macrophage inflammatory protein-2, MIP-2), which is secreted by macrophages and also attracts neutrophils.

CC chemokines act predominantly on macrophages and dendritic cells. Thus CCL3 and CCL4 (MIP-1α and -1β) are produced by macrophages and mast cells. CCL4 attracts CD4+ T cells, whereas CCL3 attracts B cells, eosinophils, and cytotoxic T cells. CCL2 (monocyte chemotactic protein-1, MCP-1) is produced by macrophages, T cells, fibroblasts, keratinocytes, and endothelial cells. It attracts and activates monocytes, stimulating their respiratory burst and lysosomal enzyme release. CCL5 (RANTES) is produced by T cells and macrophages. It is chemotactic for monocytes, eosinophils, and some T cells. It activates eosinophils and stimulates histamine release from basophils. Regakine-1 is a CC chemokine found in bovine serum that acts together with CXCL8 and C5a to attract neutrophils and enhance inflammation.

Two chemokines fall outside the CC and CXC families. A C (only one cysteine residue) or γ chemokine, called XCL1 (or lymphotactin), is chemotactic for lymphocytes. Its receptor is XCR1. The CXXXC (two cysteines separated by three amino acids) or δ chemokine called CX3CL1 (or fractalkine) triggers adhesion by T cells and monocytes. Its receptor is CX3CR1.

Most chemokines are produced in inflamed or damaged tissues and attract other cells to sites of inflammation or microbial invasion. It is probable that several different chemokines serve to attract different cell types to inflammatory sites. Indeed it is likely that the chemokine mixture produced in damaged tissues regulates the precise composition of the inflammatory cell populations. In this way the body can adjust the inflammatory response to provide the most effective way of destroying different microbial invaders. Many chemokines, such as CXCL4, CCL20, and CCL5, are structurally similar to defensins and, like them, have significant antibacterial activity. Chemokines have a major role in infections and inflammation in domestic animal species. They have been detected in many inflammatory diseases, including pneumonia (bovine pasteurellosis), bacterial mastitis, arthritis, and endotoxemia.

INCREASED VASCULAR PERMEABILITY

Acute inflammation can develop within minutes after a tissue is damaged. The damaged tissue triggers three types of signal. First, pain causes nerves to release bioactive

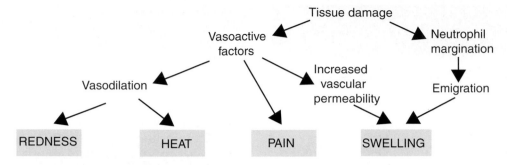

Figure 2-18.   The cardinal signs of acute inflammation and how they are generated.

peptides. Second, broken cells release intracellular proteins that trigger the release of cytokines from sentinel cells. Third, microbes release products that trigger sentinel cell responses, including the production of cytokines and other inflammatory mediators.

In its classical form, acute inflammation has five cardinal signs: heat, redness, swelling, pain, and loss of function . All these signs result from changes in small blood vessels (Figure 2-18). Immediately after injury the blood flow through small capillaries at the injection site is decreased to give leukocytes an opportunity to bind to the blood vessel walls. Shortly thereafter, the small blood vessels in the damaged area dilate and blood flow to the injured tissue increases. While the blood vessels are dilated, they begin to leak so that fluid moves from the blood into the tissues, where it causes edema and swelling.

At the same time as these changes in blood flow are occurring, cellular responses are taking place. The changes in cells lining blood vessel walls permit neutrophils and monocytes to adhere to the vascular endothelial cells. If the blood vessels are damaged, then blood platelets

may also bind to the injured sites and release vasoactive and clotting molecules.

Inflamed tissues swell as a result of leakage of fluid from blood vessels. This leakage occurs in two stages. First there is an immediate increase in leakage mediated by vasoactive molecules released by mast cells, by damaged tissues, and by nerves (Table 2-4). The second phase of increased leakage occurs several hours after the onset of inflammation, at a time when the leukocytes are beginning to emigrate. The endothelial and perivascular cells contract so that they are pulled apart and fluid escapes through the intercellular spaces.

VASOACTIVE MOLECULES

Mast cells respond to signals from damaged tissues by releasing a mixture of molecules that affect blood vessel walls (vasoactive molecules). These include histamine, inflammatory lipids, enzymes (tryptase and chymase), cytokines, and chemokines. Histamine, the lipids, and

TABLE   2-4
Some Vasoactive Molecules Produced During Acute Inflammation

Mediator	Major Source	Function
Histamine	Mast cells and basophils, platelets	Increased vascular permeability, pain
Serotonin	Platelets, mast cells, basophils	Increased vascular permeability
Kinins	Plasma kininogens and tissues	Vasodilation
		Increased vascular permeability, pain
Prostaglandins	Arachidonic acid	Vasodilation, increased vascular permeability
Thromboxanes	Arachidonic acid	Increased platelet aggregation
Leukotriene B$_4$	Arachidonic acid	Neutrophil chemotaxis
		Increased vascular permeability
Leukotrienes C, D, E	Arachidonic acid	Smooth muscle contraction
		Increased vascular permeability
Platelet-activating factor	Phagocytic cells	Platelet secretion
		Neutrophil secretion
		Increased vascular permeability
Fibrinogen breakdown products	Blood clot contraction	Smooth muscle
		Neutrophil chemotaxis
		Increased vascular permeability
C3a and C5a	Serum complement	Mast cell degranulation
		Smooth muscle contraction
		Neutrophil chemotaxis (C5a)

tryptases cause vasodilation and blood vessel leakage of fluid. The tryptases activate receptors on mast cells, sensory nerve endings, vascular endothelial cells, and neutrophils. As a result, the blood vessel walls become sticky for neutrophils. Once activated neutrophils release a lipid called platelet-activating factor (PAF). The PAF makes endothelial cells even more sticky and so enhances neutrophil adhesion and emigration.

The most important of the vasoactive molecules released by mast cells is histamine (Figure 2-19). The effects of histamine are mediated through several different receptors. H1 and H2 receptors are expressed on nerve cells, smooth muscle cells, endothelial cells, neutrophils, eosinophils, monocytes, dendritic cells, and T and B cells. Histamine binding to H1 receptors stimulates endothelial cells to convert L-arginine to nitric oxide, a very potent vasodilator. At the same time, histamine causes vascular leakage, leading to fluid accumulation and local edema.

Serotonin (5-hydroxytryptamine, 5-HT), a derivative of the amino acid tryptophan, is released from the mast cells of some rodents and the large domestic herbivores. Serotonin normally causes a vasoconstriction that results in a rise in blood pressure (except in cattle where it is a vasodilator). It has little effect on vascular permeability, except in rodents where it induces acute inflammation.

Although these two amines are very important mediators of inflammation, they are only a fraction of the complex mixture of molecules released when mast cells degranulate. More than half the protein in mast cell granules consists of proteases called tryptases and chymases. These enzymes sensitize smooth muscle to histamine; they stimulate proliferation of fibroblasts, smooth muscle, and epithelial cells; generate kinins; up-regulate expression of adherence proteins; and stimulate the

release of the chemokine CXCL8. Mast cell tryptases can activate some receptors on sensory nerves, neutrophils, mast cells, and endothelial cells.

Vasoactive Lipids

When tissues are damaged or stimulated, phospholipases act on cell wall phospholipids to release arachidonic acid. Under the influence of the enzyme 5-lipoxygenase, the arachidonic acid is converted to biologically active lipids called leukotrienes (Figure 2-20). Under the influence of the enzyme cyclooxygenase, arachidonic acid is converted to a second group of active lipids called prostaglandins. The collective term for all these complex lipids is eicosanoids.

Four leukotrienes play a central role in inflammation. Leukotriene B_4 stimulates neutrophil and eosinophil chemotaxis and random motility, whereas leukotrienes C_4, D_4, and E4 increase vascular permeability.

There are four groups of proinflammatory prostaglandins: PGE_2, PGF_2, the thromboxanes (TxA_2, PGA_2), and the prostacyclins (PGI_2). The enzymes that generate the prostacyclins are found in vascular endothelial cells; the thromboxanes are found in platelets; and the other prostaglandins can be generated by most nucleated cells. The biological activities of the prostaglandins vary widely, and since many different prostaglandins are released in inflamed tissues, their net effect may be very complex.

As neutrophils enter inflammatory sites, they use the enzyme 5-lipoxygenase to produce lipoxins from arachidonic acid. These oxidized eicosanoids bind cellular receptors and block neutrophil migration. Thus there is a gradual switch in production from proinflammatory leukotrienes to anti-inflammatory lipoxins. The rise in PGE_2 in tissues also gradually inhibits 5-lipoxygenase activity and so eventually suppresses inflammation.

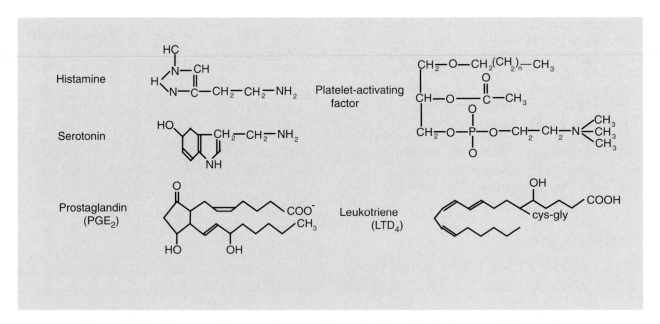

Figure 2-19. Structure of some major vasoactive molecules active during acute inflammation.

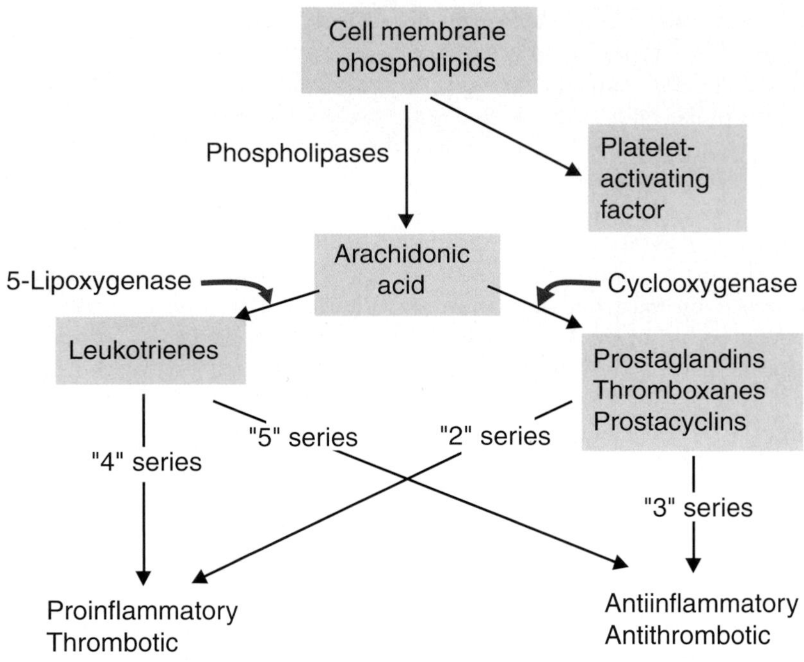

Figure 2-20. Production of leukotrienes and prostaglandins by the actions of lipoxygenase and cyclooxygenase on arachidonic acid. Both prostaglandins and leukotrienes may have proinflammatory or antiinflammatory activity depending on their chemical structure.

PAF is a phospholipid closely related to lecithin. It is synthesized by mast cells, platelets, neutrophils and eosinophils. PAF aggregates platelets and makes them release their vasoactive molecules and synthesize thromboxanes. It acts on neutrophils in a similar fashion. Thus it promotes neutrophil aggregation, degranulation, chemotaxis, and release of oxidants.

Vasoactive Polypeptides

Mast cell proteases can act on the complement components C3 and C5 to generate small, biologically active peptides called anaphylatoxins (C3a and C5a). They both promote histamine release from mast cells. In addition, C5a is a very potent attractant for neutrophils and monocytes. Mast cell granules also contain proteases called kallikreins. These act on proteins called kininogens to generate small peptides called kinins. Both the kinins and the anaphylatoxins cause blood vessel dilation and leakage. The most important of the kinins is bradykinin. Kinins not only increase vascular permeability, but also stimulate neutrophils and trigger pain receptors.

Proteoglycans such as heparin from connective tissue mast cells and chondroitin sulfate from intestinal mast cells are also released on mast cell degranulation. These proteoglycans regulate the storage and release of many vasoactive mediators.

The Coagulation System

When fluid leaks from the bloodstream into the tissues, the coagulation system is activated. Platelet aggregation and activation accelerate this process. Activation of the coagulation system leads to a series of enzyme reactions as a result of which large quantities of thrombin, the main clotting enzyme, are formed. Thrombin acts on fibrinogen in tissue fluid and plasma to produce insoluble strands of fibrin. Fibrin is therefore deposited in inflamed tissues and capillaries, forming an effective barrier to the spread of infection. Activation of the coagulation cascade also initiates the fibrinolytic system. This leads to activation of plasminogen activator, which in turn generates plasmin, a potent fibrinolytic enzyme. In destroying fibrin, plasmin releases peptide fragments that are chemotactic for neutrophils.

SOURCES OF ADDITIONAL INFORMATION

Ahmad-Nejad P, Häcker H, Rutz M, et al: Bacterial CpG-DNA and lipopolysaccharides activate toll-like receptors at distinct cellular compartments, *Eur J Immunol* 32:1958-1968, 2002.

Akira S: Mammalian toll-like receptors, *Curr Opin Immunol* 15:5-11, 2003.

Andersson U, Erlandsson-Harris H, Yang H, Tracey KJ: HMGB1 as a DNA-binding cytokine, *J Leukoc Biol* 72: 1084-1091, 2002.

Baggiolini M: Chemokines and leukocyte traffic, *Nature* 392: 565-568, 1998.

Baggiolini M: Chemokines in pathology and medicine, *J Intern Med* 250:91-104, 2001.

Beg AA: Endogenous ligands of toll-like receptors: implications for regulating inflammatory and immune responses, *Trends Immunol* 23:509-511, 2002.

Dabbagh K, Dahl ME, Stepick-Biek P, Lewis DB: Toll-like receptor 4 is required for optimal development of Th2 immune responses: role of dendritic cells, *J Immunol* 168:4524-4530, 2002.

Gangur V, Birmingham NP, Thanesvorakul S: Chemokines in health and disease, *Vet Immunol Immunopathol* 86:127-136, 2002.

Gordon S: Pattern recognition receptors: doubling up on the innate immune response, *Cell* 111:927-930, 2002.

Heeg K, Zimmerman S: CpG DNA as a Th1 trigger, *Int Arch Allergy Immunol* 121:87-97, 2000.

Johnson GB, Brunn GJ, Kodaira Y, Platt JL: Receptor-mediated monitoring of tissue well-being via detection of soluble heparan sulfate by toll-like receptor 4, *J Immunol* 168:5233-5239, 2002.

Kaplanski G, Marin V, Montero-Julian F, et al: IL-6: a regulator of the transition from neutrophil to monocyte recruitment during inflammation, *Trends Immunol* 24:25-30, 2003.

Krieg AM: Now I know my CpGs, *Trends Microbiol* 9:249-251, 2001.

Malaviya R, Abraham SN: Mast cell modulation of immune responses to bacteria, *Immunol Rev* 179:16-24, 2001.

Medzhitov R, Janeway C Jr: Innate immunity, *N Engl J Med* 343:338-343, 2000.

O'Neill LA: Toll-like receptor signal transduction and the tailoring of innate immunity: a role for Mal? *Trends Immunol* 23:296-300, 2002.

Rehli M: Of mice and men: species variations of toll-like receptor expression, *Trends Immunol* 23:375-378, 2002.

Stassen M, Hultner L, Schmitt E: Classical and alternative pathways of mast cell activation, *Crit Rev Immunol* 22:115-140,2002.

Strom H, Thomsen HK: Effects of proinflammatory mediators on canine neutrophil chemotaxis and aggregation, *Vet Immunol Immunopathol* 25: 209-218, 1990.

Takeuchi O, Sato S, Horiuchi T, et al: Role of toll-like receptor 1 in mediating immune response to microbial lipoproteins, *J Immunol* 169:10-14, 2002.

Zhu FG, Marshall JS: CpG-containing oligodeoxynucleotides induce TNF-alpha and IL-6 production but not degranulation from murine, bone-marrow derived mast cells, *J Leukoc Biol* 69:253-262, 2001.

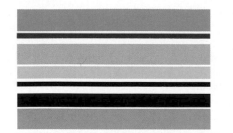

Neutrophils and Their Products

CHAPTER 3

Although physical barriers such as the skin can exclude many organisms, such barriers are not impenetrable, and microbial invaders often gain access to body tissues. These invaders must be promptly attacked and destroyed. Some are killed by antimicrobial peptides or complement, but many are eaten and killed by cells. This uptake of microbes by cells is called phagocytosis (Greek for "eating by cells"). Phagocytosis is central to the whole inflammatory process.

The defensive cells of the body are found in blood, where they are called leukocytes (white cells). The blood cells of mammals derive from stem cells known as myeloid stem cells located in the bone marrow (*myelos* is Greek for "bone marrow") (Figure 3-1). All the different types of leukocytes originate from myeloid stem cells, including granulocytes, monocytes, and dendritic cells, and all have key roles in the defense of the body. Two types of leukocytes are specialized for killing and eating invading microorganisms. These cells, called neutrophils and macrophages, originate from a common stem cell but look very different and have different, but complementary, roles. Thus neutrophils respond and eat invading organisms very rapidly but are incapable of sustained phagocytic effort. The macrophages, in contrast, have multiple roles. They act as sentinel cells but are also capable of repeated phagocytosis. In this chapter we will review the properties of neutrophils and their role in inflammation and innate immunity.

LEUKOCYTE CLASSIFICATION

Some leukocytes have a cytoplasm filled with granules; these are called granulocytes (Figure 3-2). Likewise, many of these cells have characteristic lobulated, irregular nuclei, so that they are described as "polymorphonuclear" (as opposed to the single rounded nuclei of "mononuclear" cells). Granulocytes are classified into three populations based on the staining properties of their granules. Cells whose granules take up basic dyes such as hematoxylin are called basophils; those whose granules take up acidic dyes such as eosin are called eosinophils; and those that take up neither basic nor acidic dyes are called neutrophils. All have important roles in the defense of the body.

NEUTROPHILS

The major cell blood leukocyte is the polymorphonuclear neutrophil granulocyte, otherwise called the neutrophil (Figure 3-3). Neutrophils are formed in the bone marrow (at a rate of about 8 million per minute in humans), migrate to the bloodstream, and about 12 hours later move into the tissues. They die after a few days. Neutrophils constitute about 60% to 75% of the blood leukocytes in most carnivores but only about 50% in the horse and 20% to 30% in cattle, sheep, and laboratory

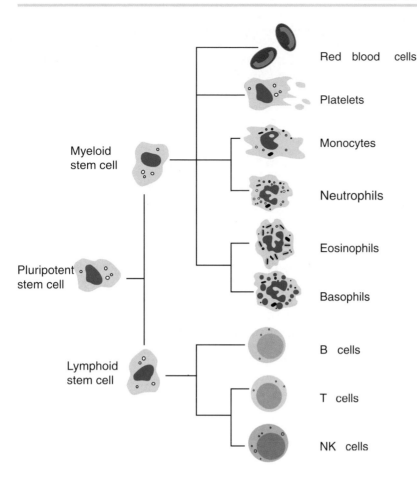

Figure 3-1. The origin of cells from the bone marrow. Note that lymphoid cells originate from different stem cells than the cells of the myeloid system. Note too that cells such as eosinophils and basophils are probably closely related despite significant morphological differences.

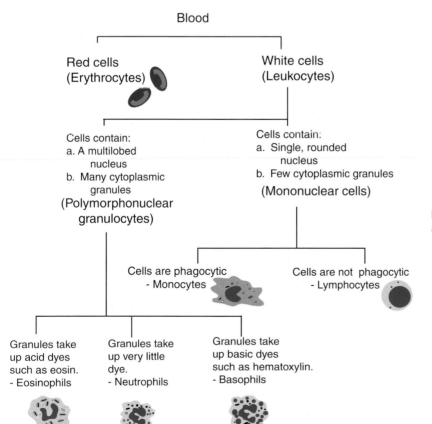

Figure 3-2. Differentiation and nomenclature of the cells found in blood.

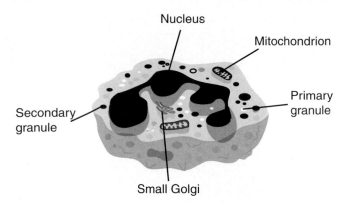

Figure 3-3.   Major structural features of a neutrophil.

rodents. There are two pools of neutrophils in blood: a circulating pool and a pool of cells sequestered in capillaries. During bacterial infections the numbers of circulating neutrophils may increase 10-fold as they are released from the bone marrow and the sequestered pool.

Structure

Neutrophils suspended in blood are round cells about 10 to 20 µm in diameter. They have a finely granular cytoplasm at the center of which is an irregular sausage-like or segmented nucleus (Figure 3-4). The chromatin in the nucleus is compacted and assumes a segmented shape because the cell cannot divide. Electron microscopy shows two types of enzyme-rich granules in their cytoplasm (Figure 3-5). Primary granules contain enzymes such as myeloperoxidase, lysozyme, elastase, β-glucuronidase, and cathepsin B. Secondary granules contain lysozyme and collagenase and the iron-binding protein lactoferrin. Mature neutrophils have a small Golgi apparatus, some mitochondria, and a few ribosomes or rough endoplasmic reticulum.

CHANGES IN VASCULAR ADHERENCE

As pointed out earlier, neutrophils are normally confined to the bloodstream. Thus if they are to defend tissues against a microbial invasion, they must first leave the

bloodstream. In normal tissues, neutrophils are carried by the flow, like other blood cells. In inflamed tissues they must be able to bind to blood vessel walls and then leave blood vessels by penetrating these walls. This process of emigration is mediated by changes both in the endothelial cells that line blood vessel walls and in the neutrophils.

Changes in Endothelial Cells

Bacterial products such as lipopolysaccharide (LPS), or molecules produced by damaged tissues such as thrombin or histamine, cause capillary endothelial cells to express a glycoprotein called P-selectin (CD62P). P-selectin is normally stored in granules but it moves to the cell surface within minutes after the cells are stimulated. Once on the endothelial cell surface, P-selectin binds to carbohydrate side chains on a protein called L-selectin (CD62L) expressed on passing neutrophils. This binding is transient because the neutrophils readily shed their L-selectin. As a result, the neutrophils gradually slow down, rolling along the endothelial cell surface as they lose speed and eventually come to a complete stop (Figure 3-6).

Changes in Neutrophils

As the neutrophils roll along the endothelial surface, the second stage of adhesion occurs. A lipid called platelet-activating factor (PAF), secreted by the endothelial cells, activates the rolling neutrophils. As a result, the neutrophils express a protein called CD11a/CD18 or LFA-1. CD11a/CD18 is an adhesive protein or integrin, and it binds strongly to a glycoprotein called intercellular adhesion molecule-1 (ICAM-1; CD54) expressed on inflamed endothelial cells (Figure 3-7). This strong binding makes the neutrophil come to a complete stop and attaches it firmly to the vessel wall despite the shearing force of the blood flow. Neutrophils are also activated by tumor necrosis factor-α (TNF-α) and leukotrienes secreted by activated mast cells. Adherent neutrophils secrete small amounts of elastase. The elastase cleaves CD43 (leukosialin), an antiadhesive protein, from the neutrophil surface, which allows the integrins to bind to the endothelial cells even more strongly.

Figure 3-4.   Neutrophils in peripheral blood smears. **A**, Horse. **B**, Cat. **C**, Dog. These cells are about 10 µm in diameter. Giemsa stain. (Courtesy Dr. MC Johnson.)

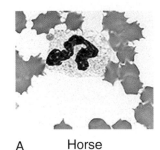

A   Horse

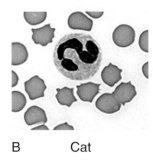

B   Cat

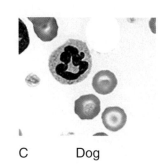

C   Dog

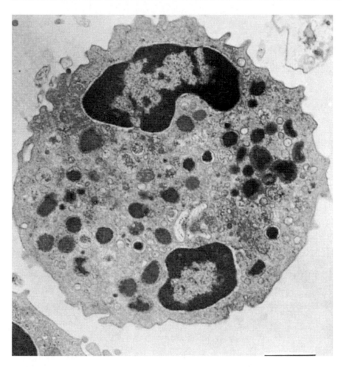

Figure 3-5. Transmission electron micrograph of a rabbit neutrophil. (Courtesy Dr. S Linthicum.)

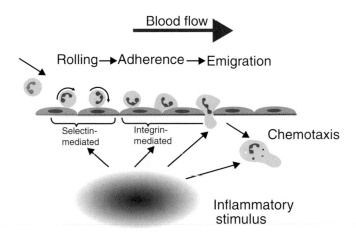

Figure 3-6. Stages of neutrophil adhesion and emigration from blood vessels. Selectins on endothelial cells tether neutrophils and stimulate them to roll. When they come to a halt, integrins bind them firmly to vascular endothelial cells and signal them to emigrate into tissues.

A third stage of increased leukocyte–endothelial cell adhesion takes several hours to develop and is mediated by cytokines and chemokines. Thus endothelial cells activated by interleukin-1 (IL-1) or TNF-α express E-selectin (CD62E), which enhances neutrophil adhesiveness even further. IL-1 also induces the production of the chemokine CXCL8 from endothelial cells, and this in turn attracts more neutrophils. TNF-α stimulates endothelial cells to secrete IL-1. It also promotes vasodilation, procoagulant activity, and thrombosis, and increases both expression of cell adherence proteins and production of chemotactic molecules.

Integrins

Many cell surface proteins make cells stick together, but the most important of these are the integrins. There are several families of integrins. Each consists of paired protein chains (heterodimers) using a unique α chain linked to a common β chain. For example, three β_2-integrins are found on neutrophils. The α chain, called CD11a, b, or c, is linked to a common β_2 chain (CD18). So these three integrins are called CD11a/CD18, CD11b/CD18, and CD11c/CD18. As described above, CD11a/CD18 expressed by activated neutrophils binds to CD54 (ICAM-1) expressed on capillary endothelial cells. CD11b/CD18 also binds leukocytes to endothelial cells and is a receptor for some components of the complement system (complement receptor 3, CR3), (Chapter 15).

Emigration

After adhering to blood vessel walls, neutrophils emigrate into the surrounding tissues (Figure 3-8). The neutrophils squeeze between the endothelial cells and the basement membrane. Since neutrophils are the most mobile of all the blood leukocytes, they are the first cells to arrive at the damaged tissues.

PHAGOCYTOSIS

Once they reach sites of microbial invasion and inflammation, neutrophils capture and destroy foreign particles such as invading bacteria through phagocytosis.

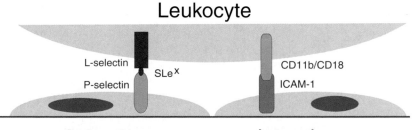

Figure 3-7. Simplified view of the proteins and their ligands engaged in neutrophil-vascular endothelial cell binding. Selectins are carbohydrate-binding proteins that bind other glycoproteins through a carbohydrate called sialyl Lewis^X (SLe^X). This selectin-mediated binding is weak and temporary. Subsequently integrins on leukocytes, especially CD11a/18, bind strongly to their ligand ICAM-1 on vascular endothelial cells.

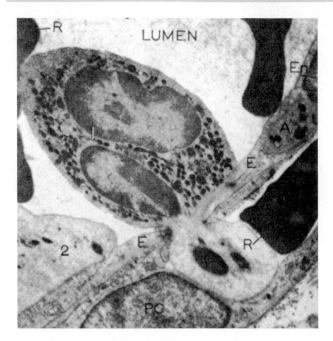

Figure 3-8. Inflamed venule of a rat. Cell 1 is a neutrophil pushing its way through a capillary wall to reach the surrounding tissues. *R,* Red blood cells; *E,* endothelium; *PC,* periendothelial cell; cells 2 and 3 are also neutrophils. (From Marchesi VT, Florey HW: *Q J Exp Physiol* 45:343, 1960.)

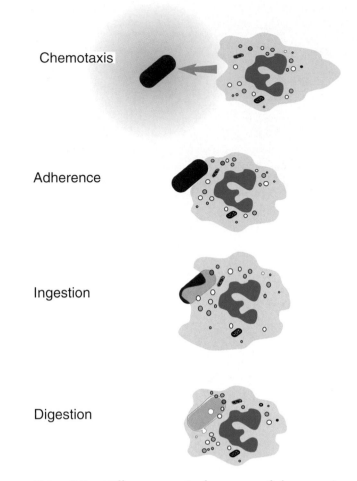

Figure 3-9. Different stages in the process of phagocytosis.

Although a continuous process, phagocytosis can be divided into discrete stages: activation, chemotaxis, adherence, ingestion, and digestion (Figure 3-9).

Activation

Although neutrophils are always ready to attack and destroy invading organisms, they can, under some circumstances, become "activated." Thus, when neutrophils receive the dual signal of integrin binding together with stimulation by TNF-α, CXCL8, or C5a, they are triggered to degranulate, mount a respiratory burst, and release elastase, defensins, and oxidants. The elastase released promotes their adhesiveness. The oxidants activate tissue metalloproteases, which in turn cleave more TNF-α from macrophages. The TNF-α, in turn, attracts more neutrophils.

Chemotaxis

The directed migration of neutrophils is called chemotaxis. Bacterial invasion and the resulting tissue damage generate many different attractants. These include a peptide called C5a, generated by activation of complement (Chapter 15); a peptide called fibrinopeptide B, derived from fibrinogen; and a peptide called azurocidin related to the defensins. Also produced are many different chemokines (Chapter 2) and lipids such as leukotriene B_4.

In addition, invading bacteria release peptides with formylated methionine groups that are very attractive to the neutrophils of some mammals.

As chemotactic molecules diffuse from sites of a microbial invasion they form a concentration gradient. When neutrophils detect these molecules, they crawl toward the area of highest concentration—the source of the material. The cells generate projections (lamellipodia) at their leading edge. Chemoattractant receptors are distributed over the neutrophil surface, but the formation of lamellipodia is driven by the selective concentration of attractants at the cell's leading edge.

Adherence and Opsonization

Once a neutrophil encounters a bacterium, it must "catch" it. This does not happen spontaneously because both cells and bacteria suspended in body fluids usually have a negative charge (zeta potential) and so repel each other. The charge on bacteria must be neutralized by coating them with positively charged molecules. Molecules that coat bacteria in this way and so promote phagocytosis are called opsonins. This word is derived from the Greek word for "sauce," implying perhaps that they make the bacterium "tastier" for the neutrophil. Examples of such charged molecules include innate molecules such as mannose-binding lectin and complement components. They also include antibody molecules (Chapter 13).

Antibody receptor–mediated phagocytosis (or type I phagocytosis) involves the use of specific antibody receptors on neutrophils (Figure 3-10). Thus CD32 is a neutrophil receptor that can bind to antibody-coated bacteria. This binding triggers polymerization of F-actin so that F-actin-rich processes (lamellipodia) will extend to engulf the particle. CD32 is found on many cell types in addition to neutrophils. As an antibody receptor it binds the Fc region of antibody molecules (Chapter 13). CD32 is therefore called an Fc receptor (FcR). (Since there are several different Fc receptors, it is classified as FcγRII.)

In complement-mediated phagocytosis (type II phagocytosis) particles sink into the neutrophil without lamellipodia formation, suggesting that the ingestion process is fundamentally different from the antibody-mediated process. CD35 (or CR1) is a receptor for the complement component C3b. It is found not only on neutrophils but also on other granulocytes, monocytes, red cells, and B cells. Binding of C3b-coated particles to CD35 on neutrophils leads to their attachment but may not necessarily trigger ingestion.

Antibodies, the major proteins of the acquired immune system, are by far the most effective opsonins. They coat bacteria, link them to receptors on phagocytic cells, and provoke their ingestion. However, as pointed out previously, they are not produced until several days after the onset of an infection, and the body must therefore rely on innate opsonins for immediate protection.

Another important mechanism that promotes contact between bacteria and neutrophils is trapping. Normally bacteria are free to float away when they encounter a neutrophil suspended in blood plasma. If, however, a bacterium is lodged in tissues, or trapped between a neutrophil and another cell surface and thus prevented from floating away, it can be readily ingested. This process is called surface phagocytosis.

Ingestion

As neutrophils crawl toward a chemotactic source, a pseudopod advances first, followed by the main portion of the cell. The cytoplasm of the neutrophil pseudopod contains a filamentous network of proteins called actin and myosin whose state determines the fluidity of the cytoplasm. When a neutrophil meets a bacterium, its pseudopod flows over and around it, and binding occurs between opsonins on the organism and receptors on the neutrophil (Figure 3-11). Binding of these receptors enables a cup-like pseudopod to cover the particle. The bacterium is eventually drawn into the cell and, as the cytoplasm engulfs it, becomes enclosed in a vacuole called a phagosome. The ease of this engulfment depends, in part, on the properties of the bacterial surface. Neutrophil cytoplasm readily flows over

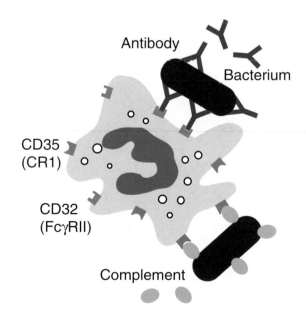

Figure 3-10. Opsonization of a bacterium by antibodies and complement. The combination of these ligands with their appropriate receptors triggers ingestion and the respiratory burst. The antibody receptor is called CD32 and the complement receptor is called CD35. Type 1 phagocytosis is mediated by antibodies through CD32. Type 2 phagocytosis is mediated by complement through CD35.

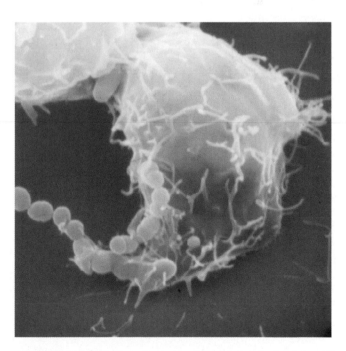

Figure 3-11. Scanning electron micrograph of a bovine milk neutrophil ingesting *Streptococcus agalactiae*. Note how a film of neutrophil cytoplasm appears to flow over the surface of the bacterium. Original magnification ×5000.

hydrophobic lipid surfaces so that hydrophobic bacteria, such as *Mycobacterium tuberculosis*, are readily ingested. In contrast, *Streptococcus pneumoniae*, a cause of pneumonia in humans, has a hydrophilic carbohydrate capsule. It is poorly phagocytosed unless made hydrophobic by a coating of antibodies or C3b. The progressive covering of a particle by the linkage of cell receptors with particle ligands has been likened to a zipper. An alternative process is called coiling phagocytosis. In this case a single pseudopod may wrap itself several times around the organism. This is associated with bacteria such as *Legionella pneumophila* and *Borrelia burgdorferi*.

Ingestion may or may not be dependent on opsonization. Thus neutrophils may possess cell surface receptors such as mannose receptors or integrins that can bind directly to bacteria. Alternatively, neutrophils may require opsonins such as antibodies or complement that must first coat a particle. The coated particles can then bind to antibody or complement receptors.

Destruction

Destruction of the ingested bacterium occurs through two distinct processes. One involves the generation of potent oxidants—the respiratory burst. The other involves release of lytic enzymes and antimicrobial peptides from intracellular granules.

The Respiratory Burst

Within seconds of binding to a bacterium, neutrophils increase their oxygen consumption nearly 100-fold. This increase is a result of activation of a cell surface enzyme complex called NADPH oxidase (NOX). The components of the NOX complex remain separated in resting cells. When the neutrophil is triggered by adherence of an opsonized bacterium to an Fc receptor, these components are assembled together (Figure 3-12). Once assembled, the activated NOX converts NADPH (the reduced form of NADP, nicotinamide adenine dinucleotide phosphate) to NADP$^+$ with the release of electrons. One molecule of oxygen accepts a single donated electron, resulting in the generation of one molecule of a superoxide anion (the dot in $^{\bullet}O_2^-$ denotes the presence of an unpaired electron).

$$NADPH + 2O_2 \xrightarrow{\text{NOX}} NADP^+ + H^+ + 2^{\bullet}O_2^-$$

The NADP$^+$ accelerates the hexose monophosphate shunt, a metabolic pathway that converts sucrose to a pentose and CO_2, and releases energy for use by the cell. The two molecules of $^{\bullet}O_2^-$ interact spontaneously (dismutate) to generate one molecule of H_2O_2 under the influence of the enzyme superoxide dismutase.

$$2^{\bullet}O_2^- + 2H^+ \rightarrow H_2O_2 + O_2$$

Because this reaction occurs so rapidly, superoxide anion does not accumulate but H_2O_2 does. The hydrogen peroxide is converted to bactericidal compounds through the action of myeloperoxidase, the most significant respiratory burst enzyme in neutrophils. Myeloperoxidase is found in large amounts in the primary granules. It catalyzes the reaction between hydrogen peroxide and intracellular halide ions (Cl^-, Br^-, I^-, or SCN^-) to produce hypohalides:

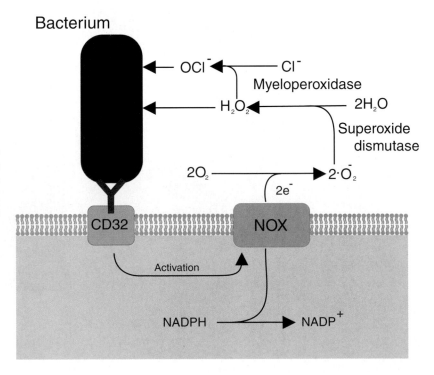

Figure 3-12. The major features of the respiratory burst pathway in neutrophils. The process is triggered by antibody binding to its receptor CD32. It results in the generation of bactericidal products such as hydrogen peroxide (H_2O_2) and hypochloride ions (OCl^-).

$$H_2O_2 + Cl^- \xrightarrow{\text{myeloperoxidase}} H_2O + OCl^-$$

Cl⁻ is probably used at most inflammatory sites except in milk and saliva where SCN⁻ is also employed. OCl⁻ is the major product of neutrophil oxidative metabolism. Because of its intense reactivity, OCl⁻ does not accumulate in biological systems but instantly disappears in multiple reactions. As long as H_2O_2 is supplied, and neutrophils can generate H_2O_2 for up to 3 hours after triggering, myeloperoxidase will use plasma Cl⁻ to generate OCl⁻. OCl⁻ kills bacteria by oxidizing their proteins and enhances the bactericidal activities of the lysosomal enzymes. (Remember that HOCl is the active ingredient of household bleach and is commonly used to prevent bacterial growth in swimming pools.) There are minor quantitative differences in neutrophil activity between the domestic species, especially in the intensity of the respiratory burst. For example, sheep neutrophils appear to produce less superoxide than human or bovine neutrophils. Neutrophils also have defense mechanisms to detoxify oxidants. Thus they contain large amounts of glutathione, which reduces them. Redox-active metals such as iron can be bound to lactoferrin to minimize OH formation, and antioxidants such as ascorbate or vitamin E interrupt these reactions.

ANTIMICROBIAL MOLECULES

Lytic Enzymes

While many bacteria are killed by oxidation, the phagosomes undergo maturation. They progressively acidify their contents, raising their pH to an optimal level for granule proteases as well as providing ideal ionic conditions for their activity.

Once a bacterium is attached to the neutrophil membrane, the primary granules (or lysosomes) migrate through the cytoplasm, fuse with the maturing phagosome, and release their enzymes. (The complete vacuole is then called a phagolysosome.) The rise in ionic strength within phagosomes releases lysosomal enzymes such as elastase and cathepsin G from their sulfated proteoglycan matrix (Figure 3-13). Other lysosomal enzymes include lysozyme, proteases, acid hydrolases, and myeloperoxidase. The enzymes that accumulate in phagosomes can digest bacterial walls and kill most microorganisms, but, as might be expected, variations in susceptibility are observed. Gram-positive bacteria susceptible to lysozyme are rapidly destroyed. Gram-negative bacteria such as *Escherichia coli* survive somewhat longer, since their outer wall is relatively resistant to digestion. Lactoferrin, by binding iron, may also prevent bacterial growth. Some organisms such as *Brucella abortus* and *Listeria monocytogenes* can interfere with phagosomal maturation in such a way that they do not come into contact with the lysosomal enzymes and can therefore grow inside phagocytic cells. The second major granule type (secondary granules) contains collagenase, lysozyme, and lactoferrin.

Neutrophil enzymes released into tissues promote tissue breakdown. They cleave membrane-bound TNF-α from macrophages. The TNF-α attracts and activates yet more neutrophils.

Peptides

Antimicrobial peptides are widely distributed throughout the plant and animal kingdoms, and more than 800 have been identified to date. Although structurally diverse, these peptides have a net cationic charge due to the presence of multiple arginine and lysine residues and the ability to form amphipathic structures; that is, they

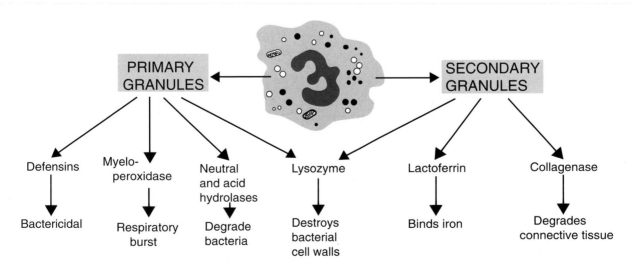

Figure 3-13. Contents of the cytoplasmic granules and their functions in neutrophils.

have both hydrophobic and hydrophilic regions. The hydrophobic regions can insert themselves into the lipid-rich membranes of bacteria whereas the other regions can form channel-like pores or simply cover the membrane. This results in membrane disruption and microbial death.

The cationic antimicrobial peptides have a broad spectrum of antimicrobial activity and can kill most species of bacteria as well as some fungi, protozoa, enveloped viruses, and tumor cells. The fact that they kill microorganisms rather than host cells is thought to be due to their interactions with microbial phospholipids, LPSs, or teichoic acids.

Antimicrobial peptides are concentrated in sites where microbes are most likely to be encountered. These include intracellular locations such as within neutrophils and macrophages (Chapter 4); and within lymphocytes (Chapter 9) such as natural killer cells and cytotoxic T cells. Epithelial cells of the skin and respiratory, alimentary, and genitourinary tracts also synthesize antimicrobial peptides.

The defensins are typical antimicrobial peptides that have been characterized in many different vertebrates, insects, and plants. More than 50 mammalian defensins have been identified. In cattle at least 13 different β-defensins are produced by neutrophils alone. Defensins contain 28 to 42 amino acids including six to eight conserved cysteine residues. These cysteines form three or four pairs of intramolecular disulfide bonds. The vertebrate defensins are classified as α, β, or θ defensins based on their origin and on the number and position of these disulfide bonds. The α defensins are found in large amounts in neutrophils and in the Paneth cells of the small intestine; β defensins are found in many different tissues including the epithelial cells that line the airways, skin, salivary gland, and urinary system. The θ defensins have only been described in primate phagocytes. Defensins can be produced at a constant rate (constitutively) or in response to microbial infection. They are major constituents of the granules in neutrophils where they account for about 15% of the total protein. Some defensins are chemoattractants for monocytes, immature dendritic cells, and T cells. All defensins identified so far can kill or inactivate some bacteria, fungi, or enveloped viruses.

Although present in normal tissues, defensins can increase in response to infections. For example, calves infected with *Cryptosporidium parvum* show a fivefold increase in cryptdin production. Likewise cows infected with *Mycobacterium paratuberculosis* have increased levels of cryptdins. *Mannheimia hemolytica* infection in bovine lungs induces an increase in defensin expression in airway epithelium. Other classes of antibacterial peptides found in neutrophil granules are variously called serprocidins, cathelicidins, and protegrins. Granulysins are toxic peptides produced by cytotoxic T cells and NK cells (Chapters 17 and 31).

Two other important antibacterial proteins include bactericidal permeability–increasing protein (BPI) and calprotectin. BPI is a major constituent of the primary granules of human and rabbit neutrophils. It kills gram-negative bacteria by binding to LPSs and damaging their inner membrane. Calprotectin is found in neutrophils, monocytes, macrophages, and epidermal cells. It forms about 60% of neutrophil cytoplasmic protein and is released in large amounts into blood and tissue fluid in inflammatory lesions.

Lysozyme

The enzyme lysozyme destroys bacterial peptidoglycans. Lysozyme is found in all body fluids except cerebrospinal fluid, sweat, and urine. It is absent from bovine neutrophils and tears. It is found in high concentrations in tears of other mammals and in egg white. Although many of the bacteria killed by lysozyme are nonpathogenic, it might reasonably be pointed out that this susceptibility could account for their lack of pathogenicity. Lysozyme is found in high concentrations in neutrophil granules and so accumulates in areas of acute inflammation, including sites of bacterial invasion. Lysozyme is also a potent innate opsonin, binding to bacterial surfaces and so facilitating phagocytosis in the absence of specific antibodies and under conditions where its enzyme activity is ineffective.

Lectins

Lectins are proteins that bind carbohydrates. Given that carbohydrates are major components of bacterial cell walls, lectins often bind to bacteria. Mammalian lectins are classified by the structure of their carbohydrate recognition site.

The C-type lectins include the collectins found in plasma and the selectins found on the surface of endothelial cells and leukocytes. They require calcium to bind to carbohydrates. The collectins range in size from 600 to 1000 kDa. Each end of a collectin molecule has a distinct function; the C-terminal domain binds to bacterial carbohydrates whereas the N-terminal domain interacts with cells and complement components, thereby exerting the biological effect. It is their ability to recognize foreign carbohydrates that makes collectins a part of the innate host defense systems.

The most important lectin in the innate immune system is mannose-binding lectin (MBL), a collectin found in serum. MBL has multiple carbohydrate-binding sites that bind many oligosaccharides, including N-acetylglucosamine, mannose, glucose, galactose, and N-acetylgalactosamine. The binding is relatively weak, but multiple binding sites give a high functional activity. Most of the ligands of MBL are present at high levels on microbial surfaces. As a result, MBL binds very strongly to bacteria such as *Salmonella enterica, Listeria monocytogenes,*

Haemophilus influenzae, and *Neisseria meningitidis*. It binds to *Streptococcus* and *Escherichia coli* with moderate affinity, but it does not bind to encapsulated *N. meningitidis*, *H. influenzae*, or *Streptococcus agalactiae*. MBL binds strongly to yeasts such as *Candida albicans* and *Cryptococcus neoformans*. It can bind viruses such as human immunodeficiency virus and influenza A as well as the protozoa *Leishmania*. MBL plays an important role in activating the complement system (Chapter 15).

Collectins such as MBL can bind to leukocytes, platelets, endothelial cells, and fibroblasts. Bacteria coated by MBL are readily ingested by phagocytic cells through interaction with surface receptors. Thus the collectins act as innate opsonins. Collectins are especially important in young animals whose acquired immune system is not fully capable of mounting an efficient response. For example, a congenital deficiency of MBL makes children highly susceptible to infections.

Five different collectins [conglutinin, MBL, pulmonary surfactant proteins (SP-A, SP-D), and collectin-43 (CL-43)] have been identified in mammals. However, conglutinin and CL-43 have only been identified in bovids. Bovine conglutinin is produced in the liver. It binds to receptors on macrophages, dendritic cells, and glial cells. The level of conglutinin in plasma decreases in infections such as mastitis.

The pentraxins are also lectins. They include two important molecules: C-reactive protein (CRP) and serum amyloid P (SAP). These are called acute-phase proteins because their blood levels climb greatly during infections or following trauma. Pentraxins have multiple biological functions, including activation of the complement system and stimulation of leukocytes. Each pentraxin molecule consists of five protein subunits arranged in a ring. Pentraxins bind to carbohydrates such as LPSs in a calcium-dependent manner. Both CRP and SAP can activate the classical complement pathway by interacting with C1q (Chapter 15). They also interact with neutrophils, monocytes/macrophages, and natural killer cells and augment their activities. For example, CRP not only binds to phosphatidylcholine, a molecule found in all cell membranes, but its major receptor on leukocytes is FcγRII (CD32). It can bind to invading organisms and promote their phagocytosis. SAP binds to galactose polymers and glycosaminoglycans.

Iron-Binding Proteins

One of the most important innate factors that determines the success or failure of bacterial invasion is the level of iron in body fluids. Many bacteria, such as *Staphylococcus aureus*, *E. coli*, *Pasteurella multocida*, and *Mycobacterium tuberculosis*, require considerable amounts of iron for growth. If iron concentrations are low the bacteria cannot grow. Thus, one effective defensive strategy is to remove iron from sites of bacterial invasion. Within the body, iron is associated with several iron-binding proteins including transferrin, lactoferrin, haptoglobin, and ferritin. When bacteria invade the body, intestinal iron absorption ceases. Liver cells are stimulated to secrete transferrin and haptoglobin, and there is increased incorporation of iron into the liver. This effectively reduces the availability of iron. A similar situation occurs in the mammary gland when, in response to bacterial invasion, milk neutrophils release their stores of lactoferrin. The lactoferrin binds any free iron and makes it unavailable to the bacteria. In spite of the reduced availability of iron, some bacteria, such as *M. tuberculosis* and *E. coli*, can successfully invade the body. This is because they in turn produce potent iron-binding proteins that withdraw iron from serum proteins and make it available to the bacteria. When serum iron levels are elevated, as occurs following red cell destruction, animals may become more susceptible to bacterial infections.

SURFACE RECEPTORS

Cells must interact with many molecules in their environment. To this end they have many different cell surface receptors. As mentioned in Chapter 2, cell surface glycoproteins are classified by the cluster of differentiation (CD) system. Neutrophils carry many different CD molecules on their surface (Figure 3-14). The most relevant of these proteins are the receptors for opsonins and those that mediate neutrophil attachment to blood vessel walls. Other neutrophil surface molecules include receptors for inflammatory mediators such as leukotrienes, complement components such as C5a, chemokines, and cytokines.

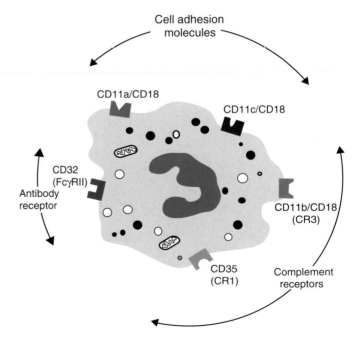

Figure 3-14. Some of the major surface receptors on neutrophils and their functions.

FATE

Neutrophils have a limited reserve of energy that cannot be replenished. They are therefore active immediately after being released from the bone marrow, but are rapidly exhausted and can undertake only a limited number of phagocytic events. Neutrophils survive for only a few days. Thus they may be considered a first line of defense, moving rapidly toward invading organisms and destroying them promptly but being incapable of sustained effort. The second line of defense is the mononuclear phagocyte system.

SOURCES OF ADDITIONAL INFORMATION

Baggiolini M, Dewald B: The neutrophil, *Int Arch Allergy Appl Immunol* 76 (suppl 1):13-20, 1985.

Bertram TA: Neutrophil leukocyte structure and function in domestic animals, *Adv Vet Sci Comp Med* 30:91-129, 1985.

Boxer GJ, Curnutte JT, Boxer LA: Polymorphonuclear leukocyte function, *Hosp Pract* 20:69-90, 1985.

Brown EJ: Phagocytosis, *Bioessays* 17:109-117, 1995.

Buchta R: Functional and biochemical properties of ovine neutrophils, *Vet Immunol Immunopathol* 24:97-112, 1990.

Condliffe AM, Hawkins PT: Moving in mysterious ways, *Nature* 404:135-137, 2000.

Durr M, Peschel A: Chemokines meet defensins: the merging concepts of chemoattractants and antimicrobial peptides in host defense, *Infect Immun* 70:6515-6517, 2002.

Eagleson JS, Moriarty KM: Neutrophils, oxidative killing mechanisms and chemiluminescence, *N Z Vet J* 32:41-43, 1984.

Foster AP, Lees P, Cunningham FM: Platelet activating factor is a mediator of equine neutrophil and eosinophil migration in vitro, *Res Vet Sci* 53:223-229, 1992.

Ganz T: Versatile defensins, *Science* 298:977-979, 2002.

Hancock REW, Diamond G: The role of cationic antimicrobial peptides in innate host defences, *Trends Microbiol* 8: 402-409, 2000.

Lewis RA, Austen KF, Soberman RJ: Leukotrienes and other products of the 5-lipoxygenase pathway. Biochemistry and relation to pathobiology in human diseases, *N Engl J Med* 323:645-655, 1990.

Luscinskas FW, Lawler J: Integrins as dynamic regulators of vascular function, *FASEB J* 8:929-938, 1994.

Osborn L: Leukocyte adhesion to endothelium in inflammation, *Cell* 62:3-6, 1990.

Salmon JE, Cronstein BN: Fcγ receptor-mediated functions in neutrophils are modulated by adenosine receptor occupancy, *J Immunol* 145:2235-2240, 1990.

Reeves EP, Lu H, Jacobs HL, et al: Killing activity of neutrophils is mediated through activation of proteases by K^+ flux, *Nature* 416:291-297, 2002.

Rittig MG, Burmester G-R, Krause A: Coiling phagocytosis: when the zipper jams, the cup is deformed, *Trends Microbiol* 6:384-388, 1998.

Roos D, Winterbourn CC: Lethal weapons, *Science* 296: 669-670, 2002.

Rosen GM, Pou S, Ramos CI, et al: Free radicals and phagocytic cells, *FASEB J* 9:200-209, 1995.

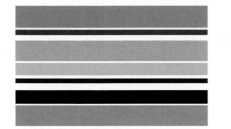

Macrophages and the Later Stages of Inflammation

Although neutrophils act as a first line of defense, mobilizing rapidly and eating and killing invading microorganisms with enthusiasm, they cannot, by themselves, ensure that all invaders are killed. The body therefore employs a "backup" system. This backup system consists of a second population of cells called macrophages. Macrophages differ from neutrophils in their speed of response, which is slower; in their antimicrobial abilities, which are greater; and in their ability to trigger acquired immune responses. Unlike neutrophils, which are specialized for a single task—the killing of invading organisms—monocytes and macrophages have a much greater diversity of roles. These include not only triggering inflammation by acting as sentinel cells, but also cleaning up the mess afterward.

MACROPHAGE FUNCTIONS

Sensors of Invasion

As described in Chapter 2, macrophages possess toll-like receptors and so can detect invading bacteria and viruses. They respond by producing cytokines, the most important of which are interleukin-1 and tumor necrosis factor-alpha (TNF-α).

Phagocytosis

Similar processes to those that affect neutrophils mediate monocyte adhesion to vascular endothelial cells. Thus cell rolling is mediated by selectin binding, and the cells are eventually brought to a halt by monocyte integrins binding to their ligands on blood vessel walls. The monocytes bind strongly to the endothelial cells, using $\beta2$ integrins binding to ICAM-1, and emigrate through the vessel walls. Within the tissues these cells are now called macrophages. Several hours after neutrophils have arrived at an inflammatory site, the macrophages begin to arrive.

Macrophages are attracted not only to bacterial products and the products of complement activation such as C5a, but also to molecules released from damaged cells and tissues. Dying neutrophils release elastase and collagenase and so generate chemotactic factors. Defensins and other peptides released by neutrophils attract monocytes and macrophages. Activated neutrophils and endothelial cells produce the selective attractant chemokine called monocyte chemoattractant protein-1 (CCL2) under the influence of IL-6. Neutrophils are thus the martyrs of the immune system: they reach and attack foreign material first, and in dying they attract macrophages to the site of invasion. Phagocytosis by macrophages is similar to the process in neutrophils. Macrophages destroy bacteria by both oxidative and nonoxidative mechanisms. In contrast to neutrophils, however, macrophages can undertake sustained, repeated phagocytic activity. An important additional function of macrophages is the removal of dead and dying cells.

Generation of Nitric Oxide

In some mammals, especially rodents, cattle, sheep, and horses (but not in humans, pigs, goats, or rabbits), microbial products trigger macrophages to synthesize inducible nitric oxide synthase (NOS2). This enzyme uses NADPH and oxygen to act on L-arginine to produce large amounts of nitric oxide (NO) and citrulline (Figure 4-1). Although nitric oxide itself is not highly toxic, it can react with superoxide anion to produce highly reactive and toxic oxidants such as peroxynitrite and nitrogen dioxide radical.

$$NO + O_2^- \rightarrow OONO^- \rightarrow HOONO \rightarrow OH + NO_2^-$$

| Nitric oxide | Peroxynitrite anion | Nitrogen dioxide radical |

The sustained production of NO permits macrophages to kill bacteria, fungi, protozoa, some helminths, and tumor cells very efficiently. Nitric oxide binds to metal-containing enzymes such as ribonucleotide reductase and impedes DNA synthesis. It also blocks mitochondrial heme-containing respiratory enzymes.

It must be noted that not all macrophages can generate nitric oxide as described above (these are classified as M1 cells). Other populations of macrophages, called M2 cells, convert arginine to ornithine using the enzyme arginase, and NO is not generated. It is believed that these two macrophage populations play distinctly different roles in defending the body. If M1 cells are activated, they defend against microbial invaders and produce proinflammatory cytokines. M2 cells have opposite effects: they reduce inflammation and produce cytokines that tend to suppress immune responses. These M2 cells

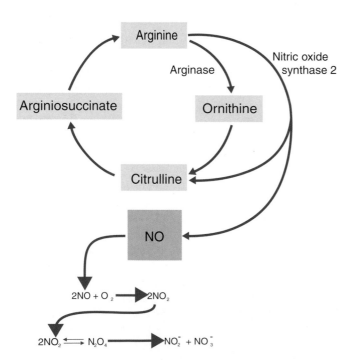

Figure 4-1. The two pathways of arginine metabolism in macrophages. The production of nitric oxide through the use of nitric oxide synthase is a major antimicrobial pathway and the key feature of M1 macrophages. The use of arginase to produce ornithine, however, reduces the antimicrobial activities of M2 cells.

may play a key role in wound healing by promoting blood vessel formation, tissue remodeling, and tissue repair. It is likely that M1 cells are produced early in the inflammatory process when inflammation is required. M2 cells, on the other hand, appear late in the process when healing is required.

Activation

Although monocytes and resting macrophages are fairly effective phagocytes, their activities can be greatly enhanced by innate mechanisms. Triggers include the ligands for toll-like receptors such as lipopolysaccharides, CpG DNA, microbial carbohydrates, and heat shock proteins as well as inflammatory products. Different levels of activation are recognized, depending on the triggering agent, and some bacteria, such as *M. tuberculosis*, are better able to activate macrophages than others. Thus when monocytes first move into inflamed tissues, they produce increased amounts of lysosomal enzymes, increase phagocytic activity, increase the expression of antibody and complement receptors, and secrete more proteases (Figure 4-2). The cytokines produced by these inflammatory macrophages, especially TNF-α and interleukin-12, activate a population of lymphocytes called natural killer (NK) cells. The NK cells in turn secrete the cytokine interferon-γ, which then activates macrophages still further. Interferon-γ upregulates many different genes, especially the gene for inducible nitric oxide synthase (NOS2). Thus the NOS2 gene can be upregulated 400-fold by a combination of IFN-γ and mycobacteria. As a result of increased NO production, activated macrophages become very potent killers of bacteria.

Receptors

Macrophages have many different receptor proteins on their surface (Figure 4-3). We have already described the toll-like receptors that recognize microbial components. Macrophages also possess receptors for antibodies. For example, CD64 (FcγRI) is a high-affinity antibody receptor expressed on monocytes and macrophages and to a lesser extent on neutrophils. Like other antibody receptors, CD64 binds to the Fc region of antibody molecules and so is called an Fc receptor (FcR). Its expression is enhanced by interferon-γ–induced activation. Human macrophages also carry two low-affinity antibody receptors, CD32 (FcγRII) and CD16 (FcγRIII). Cattle macrophages have a unique Fc receptor called Fcγ2R, which can bind particles coated with a specific type of antibody called IgG2.

Macrophages also have receptors for complement components. They include CD35 (CR1), the major receptor for C3b, and the integrin CD11b/CD18, which is also a receptor for fragments of C3b. These receptors permit organisms coated with C3b to bind to macrophages (Box 4–1).

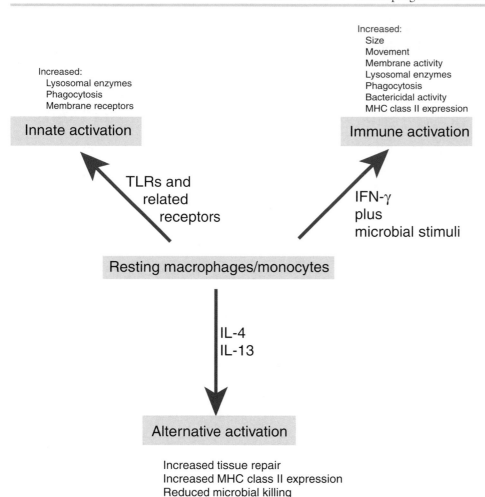

Increased:
    Size
    Movement
    Membrane activity
    Lysosomal enzymes
    Phagocytosis
    Bactericidal activity
    MHC class II expression

Increased:
    Lysosomal enzymes
    Phagocytosis
    Membrane receptors

Innate activation

Immune activation

TLRs and related receptors

IFN-γ plus microbial stimuli

Resting macrophages/monocytes

IL-4 IL-13

Alternative activation

Increased tissue repair
Increased MHC class II expression
Reduced microbial killing

Figure 4-2. The progressive activation of macrophages can involve three different pathways. Thus macrophages can be activated by pathways involving toll-like receptors. They can be activated by acquired pathways involving IFN-γ, or they may undergo "alternative activation" and so become suppressive.

The integrins described in the previous chapter are responsible for binding macrophages to other cells, to connective tissue molecules such as collagen and fibronectin, and to some complement components. A novel integrin called $\alpha_d\beta_2$ has been identified on dog macrophages. Its ligand and function are unknown. Macrophages also have mannose-binding receptors

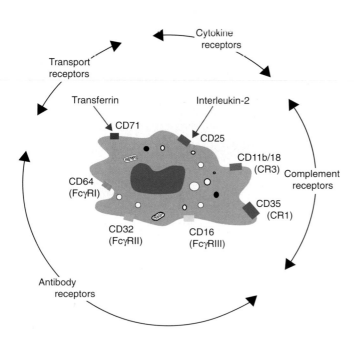

Transport receptors

Cytokine receptors

Transferrin

Interleukin-2

CD71

CD25

CD11b/18 (CR3)

Complement receptors

CD64 (FcγRI)

CD35 (CR1)

CD32 (FcγRII)

CD16 (FcγRIII)

Antibody receptors

Figure 4-3. Some of the major surface receptors expressed on macrophages and their functions.

BOX 4–1

Genes That Control Innate Immunity

Innate resistance to mycobacteria, *Brucella, Leishmania,* and *Salmonella enterica typhimurium* is controlled by a gene called N*ramp,* which has been identified in humans, dogs, mice, sheep, bison, red deer, cattle, and chickens. N*ramp* codes for an ion transporter protein in macrophages called natural resistance–associated transporter protein (Nramp1). After phagocytosis, Nramp1 is acquired by the phagosomal membrane. It then acts to pump divalent metals out of the phagosome and so inhibits the growth of intracellular parasites by depriving them of metal ions. Cattle with the resistant allele effectively activate their macrophages and so control the in vitro growth of *Brucella abortus*. The difference between the resistant and susceptible alleles appears to be associated with a single nucleotide substitution in the Nramp gene.

(CD206). These are proteins that can bind to mannose or fucose in the capsule or lipopolysaccharide of invading bacteria and so permit macrophages to bind and ingest nonopsonized bacteria.

Another important macrophage receptor is CD40. This glycoprotein is used to communicate between macrophages and lymphocytes. Its ligand is called CD40 ligand (CD154, or CD40L) and is present on T cells. Macrophages can also receive activation signals via CD40. When activated in this way, they increase their cytokine synthesis and the production of nitric oxide. They also live longer.

THE FATE OF FOREIGN MATERIAL

Macrophages are found scattered throughout the body and hence can capture invaders entering by many different routes. For example, if bacteria are injected intravenously, they are rapidly removed from the blood. Their precise fate depends on the species of animal involved. In dogs, laboratory rodents, and humans, bacteria and other particles are predominantly (80%-90%) trapped and removed in the liver. The mechanisms of this liver clearance have recently been analyzed. It was believed for many years that circulating bacteria were removed from the bloodstream through phagocytosis by the macrophages (Kupffer cells) that line the sinusoids of the liver. However, the process is much more complex than this. Circulating bacteria are indeed trapped by Kupffer cells, but they bind to the outside of the cells! Bacterial products then interact with their TLRs and stimulate the Kupffer cells to secrete TNF-α and IL-1. These cytokines attract circulating neutrophils that bind to the Kupffer cells through cell-surface integrins. The bound neutrophils then ingest and kill the bacteria. After phagocytosis the neutrophils begin to degenerate and undergo apoptosis. The intact apoptotic neutrophils

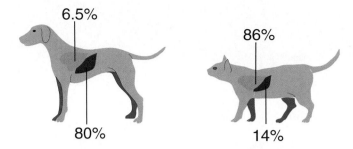

Figure 4-4. The different routes by which bacteria are cleared from the bloodstream in the dog and cat. Dogs mainly use Kupffer cells in the liver. Cats mainly employ pulmonary intravascular macrophages.

are then ingested and destroyed by the Kupffer cells so that toxic metabolic products and proteases cannot escape. These processes within the liver thus resemble those in acute inflammation where neutrophils are primarily responsible for destruction of invaders while the macrophages are responsible for preventing damage caused by the escape of neutrophil breakdown products. In contrast, in calves, sheep, goats, deer, llamas, pigs, horses, and cats, particles are mainly removed by the macrophages that line small blood vessels in the lungs (pulmonary intravascular macrophages) (Table 4-1 and Figure 4-4). These pulmonary intravascular macrophages are attached to the endothelium of lung capillaries (Figure 4-5).

In species where hepatic clearance is important, large viruses or bacteria may be cleared completely by a single

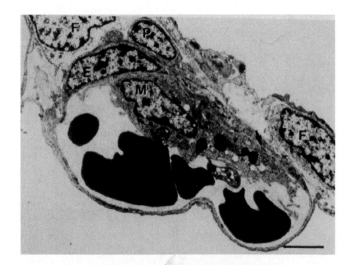

Figure 4-5. An intravascular macrophage *(M)* from the lung of a 7-day-old pig. The cell has numerous pseudopods, electron-dense siderosomes, phagosomes and lipid droplets. It is closely attached to the thick portion of the air-blood tissue barrier that contains fibroblasts *(F)* and a pericyte *(P)* between basal laminae of the capillary endothelium *(E)* and the alveolar epithelium. At sites of close adherence, intercellular junctions with subplasmalemmal densities are seen *(arrow)*. Bar = 2 μm (×8000). (From Winkler GC, Cheville NF: *Microvasc Res* 33:224-232, 1987.)

TABLE   4-1
Sites of Clearance of Particles From the Blood in Domestic Mammals

Species	Localization (%)	
	Lung	Liver/Spleen
Rabbit	0.6	83
Dog	6.5	80
Guinea pig	1.5	82
Rat	0.5	97
Mouse	1.0	94
Cat	86	14
Calf	93	6
Sheep	94	6

Selected data from Winkler GC: *Am J Anat* 181:223, 1988; and from Chitko-McKown CG, Blecha F: *Ann Rech Vet* 23:201-214, 1992.

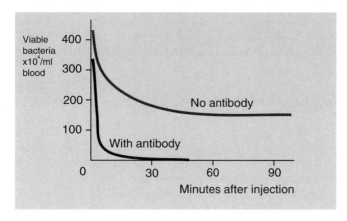

Figure 4-6. The clearance of bacteria from the blood (in this case *E. coli* from piglets). In the absence of antibodies, bacteria are slowly and incompletely removed.

passage through the liver (Figure 4-6). The spleen is a more effective filter than the liver, but since it is a much smaller organ, it traps much less material. There is also a difference in the types of particle removed by the liver and spleen. Splenic macrophages have antibody receptors (CD64); thus particles coated with antibody tend to be preferentially removed in the spleen. In contrast, phagocytic cells in the liver express complement receptors (CD35) so that particles coated with complement are preferentially removed in the liver. The rate of clearance of particles from the blood is regulated by opsonins such as fibronectin, or mannose-binding lectin. If an animal is injected intravenously with a very large dose of colloidal carbon, its opsonins will be temporarily depleted and other particles (such as bacteria) will not be removed from the bloodstream. In this situation the mononuclear-phagocytic system is said to be "blockaded."

Removal of organisms from the blood is greatly enhanced if specific antibodies are also present, since opsonization increases the trapping efficiency of neutrophils and macrophages. If antibodies are absent or the bacteria possess an antiphagocytic polysaccharide capsule, the rate of clearance is decreased. Some compounds, such as bacterial endotoxins, estrogens, and simple lipids, stimulate macrophage activity and therefore also increase the rate of bacterial clearance. Steroids and other drugs that depress macrophage activity also depress the clearance rate.

Soluble Proteins Given Intravenously

Unless carefully treated, protein molecules in solution tend to aggregate spontaneously. If a protein solution is injected intravenously, neutrophils and macrophages rapidly remove these protein aggregates. The unaggregated proteins remain in solution and are distributed evenly through the animal's blood. Small proteins (less than 60 kDa) are also distributed throughout the extravascular tissue fluids. Once distributed, the protein is treated like other body proteins and catabolized, resulting in a slow but progressive decline in its concentration. Within a few days, however, the animal makes an immune response to the protein. Antibodies combine with the foreign antigen to form antigen-antibody complexes. Phagocytic cells remove these antigen-antibody complexes from the blood, and all the foreign protein is eliminated (Figure 4-7).

This triphasic clearance pattern of distribution, catabolism, and immune elimination may be modified under certain circumstances. For example, if the animal has not been previously exposed to the antigen, it takes between 5 and 10 days before antibodies are produced and immune elimination occurs. If, on the other hand, the animal has been primed by previous exposure to the antigen, a secondary immune response will occur in 2 to 3 days, and the stage of progressive catabolism will therefore be relatively short. If antibodies are already circulating at the time of antigen administration, immune elimination will occur immediately, and no phase of catabolism is seen. If the injected material is not antigenic, or if the immune response does not occur, catabolism will continue until all the material is eliminated.

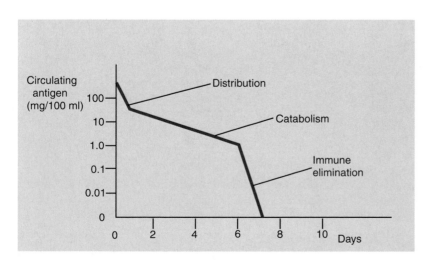

Figure 4-7. The clearance of a soluble antigen from the bloodstream. Note the three phases of this clearance.

Fate of Material Administered by Other Routes

When foreign material is injected into a tissue, some damage and inflammation are bound to occur. As a result, neutrophils and macrophages migrate toward the injection site under the influence of chemotactic factors released from the damaged tissue. These cells phagocytose the injected material. The material taken up by macrophages and dendritic cells is processed and may eventually stimulate an immune response. Antibodies and complement (Chapter 15) interact with the antigenic material, generating more chemotactic factors that attract still more phagocytic cells, thus hastening its final elimination. In a sensitized animal, a web of antigen-trapping dendritic cells called Langerhans cells, located within the skin, may trap foreign molecules and present the antigen directly to lymphocytes. For this reason intradermal injection of antigen may be most effective in stimulating an immune response.

Soluble material injected into a tissue is redistributed by the flow of tissue fluid through the lymphatic system. It eventually reaches the bloodstream, so its final fate is similar to intravenously injected material. Any aggregated material present is phagocytosed by blood neutrophils or tissue macrophages or by the macrophages and dendritic cells of lymph nodes through which the tissue fluid flows.

Digestive Tract

Normally, digestive enzymes break down molecules passing through the intestine into small fragments. However, some foreign molecules may remain intact and pass through the intestinal epithelium. Bacterial polysaccharides and those molecules that associate with lipids are especially effective in this respect, since they are absorbed in chylomicrons. Particles that enter the blood from the intestine are promptly removed by macrophages in the liver, whereas those particles entering the intestinal lymphatics are trapped in the mesenteric lymph nodes.

Respiratory Tract

The fate of inhaled particles depends on their size. Large particles (greater than 5 µm in diameter) are deposited on the mucous layer over the respiratory epithelium from the trachea to the terminal bronchioles (see Figure 20-3). These particles are then removed by the flow of mucus toward the pharynx or by coughing. Most particles that reach the lung alveoli are ingested by alveolar macrophages, which carry them back to the bronchoalveolar junction; from there they are also removed from the lung by the flow of mucus. Nevertheless, some particles may be absorbed from the alveoli. Small particles absorbed in this way are cleared to the draining lymph nodes, whereas soluble molecules enter the bloodstream and are distributed throughout the body. When large quantities of particles are inhaled, as occurs in workers exposed to industrial dusts or in cigarette smokers, the alveolar macrophage system may be temporarily blockaded and the lungs made more susceptible to microbial invasion.

CHRONIC INFLAMMATION

If foreign material is not destroyed but persists for long periods within the body, the inflammatory process may also persist and become chronic. Examples of such persistence include infections with bacteria such as *Mycobacterium tuberculosis*, fungi such as *Cryptococcus*, parasites such as liver fluke, or the presence of inorganic material such as asbestos crystals. Macrophages, fibroblasts, and lymphocytes may accumulate in large numbers around the persistent material. Because they resemble epithelium in histological sections, these accumulated macrophages are called epithelioid cells. Epithelioid cells may fuse and form multinucleated giant cells if they attempt to enclose particles too large to be ingested by a single macrophage. Epithelioid cells and giant cells are a prominent feature of tubercles, the persistent inflammatory lesions that develop in individuals suffering from tuberculosis (Chapter 29).

In all these cases, the persistence of foreign material results in the continual arrival of new macrophages and fibroblasts and excessive deposition of collagen in affected tissues. The lesion that surrounds the foreign material is called a granuloma (Figure 4-8). Granulomas consist of granulation tissue—an accumulation of macrophages, lymphocytes, fibroblasts, loose connective

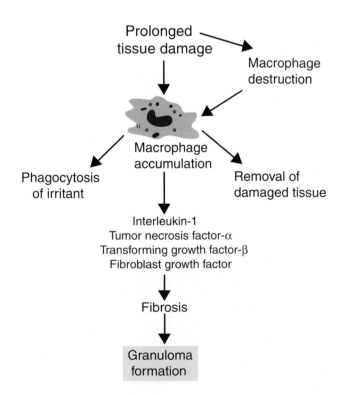

Figure 4-8.   The pathogenesis of chronic inflammation.

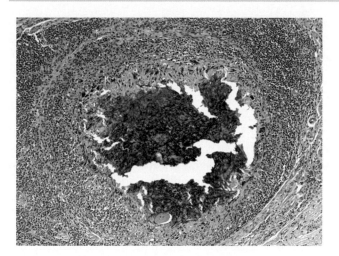

Figure 4-9. A granulomatous inflammatory reaction around a degeneration tapeworm cyst in a bovine heart. The mass of cells around the central organism is a mixture of macrophages and fibroblasts serving to wall it off from the rest of the body (×250). (Courtesy Dr. John Edwards.)

tissue, and new blood vessels. The term *granulation tissue* is derived from the granular appearance of this tissue when cut. The "granules" are in fact new blood vessels.

If the persistent irritant is a nonantigenic "foreign body" (for example, silica, talc, or mineral oil), few neutrophils or lymphocytes will be attracted to the lesion. Epithelioid and giant cells, however, are formed in an attempt to destroy the offending material. If the material is toxic for macrophages (as is asbestos), macrophage enzymes may be released, leading to excessive tissue damage and eventually to local fibrosis and severe scarring.

If the irritant is antigenic, as a result of the release of cytokines and of persistent immune stimulation, the granuloma will contain many lymphocytes as well as macrophages, fibroblasts, and probably some neutrophils, eosinophils, and basophils (Figure 4-9). The chronically activated macrophages within these granulomas will also secrete IL-1, which can stimulate collagen deposition by fibroblasts and eventually "wall-off" the lesion from the rest of the body. Antigens that provoke this form of reaction include bacteria such as the mycobacteria and *Brucella abortus* and parasites such as liver fluke and schistosomes. Chronic granulomatous reactions, whether due to immunological or foreign body reactions, are important since they may enlarge and destroy normal tissues. In liver fluke infestations, for example, death may result from the gradual replacement of normal liver cells by fibrous tissue as a result of chronic irritation.

RECOVERY FROM INFLAMMATION

Since acute inflammation may cause severe tissue damage, it must be carefully controlled. Likewise, once the invading organisms have been destroyed, the tissue

response must switch from a killing process to a repair process. The timing of this switch is very important—to stop killing invaders before all have been destroyed would cause problems.

As inflammation progresses, the cells involved, especially macrophages, change their properties. They gradually begin to secrete SLP1, a serine protease inhibitor. This molecule inhibits the release of elastase and oxidants by TNF-stimulated neutrophils, and inhibits the activity of elastase. SLP1 also protects the anti-inflammatory cytokine TGF-β from breakdown. Neutrophils also change. They secrete TNF receptor fragments that bind and neutralize the TNF-α. TNF-α induces macrophages to secrete IL-12, which induces lymphocytes to secrete IFN-γ. The IFN-γ acts as a macrophage activator early in the inflammatory process but later becomes suppressive. Neutrophil-derived lipoxins suppress leukotriene synthesis. The neutrophil and macrophage-derived oxidants destroy chemotactic factors. Antiinflammatory cytokines such as TGF-β and IL-10 inhibit the release of TNF-α. Steroids, adrenalin, and other "stress" hormones produced as a response to neuronal stimulation suppress cytokine synthesis and signal transduction.

Neutrophils are short-lived cells that usually die during an inflammatory response. If, however, the dead cells were to rupture and release their lysosomal enzymes, they could cause severe tissue damage. This does not normally occur because as neutrophils undergo programmed cell death (apoptosis), they are phagocytosed by macrophages (Figure 4-10).

Even in normal healthy animals, many cells die every day and must be promptly removed. Much of this task is

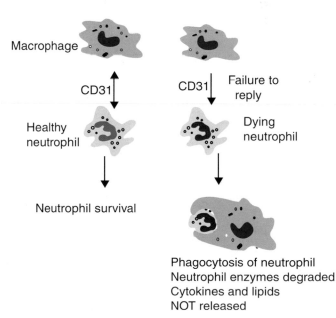

Figure 4-10. The removal of apoptotic neutrophils. The reaction is initiated by interactions between CD31 on neutrophils and macrophages. If the neutrophil fails to reply when interrogated by a macrophage, it will be ingested and destroyed.

the function of macrophages. A good example of this is the daily removal of enormous numbers of aged neutrophils. It appears that macrophages methodically palpate any neutrophils that they encounter. If the neutrophil is healthy, it quickly detaches from the macrophage. If, however, the cell is dead or dying, as reflected in the expression of phosphatidyl serine on the plasma membrane, the macrophage remains in contact and eats the neutrophil.

The molecular basis of this interaction operates through the adhesion protein CD31 (see Figure 4-10). Thus CD31 on a neutrophil binds to CD31 on a macrophage. If the neutrophil is healthy, a signal sent to the macrophage causes it to disengage. On the other hand, dead and dying neutrophils fail to signal to macrophages and get eaten. It is interesting to note that failure in CD31 signaling occurs well before a neutrophil becomes so degraded that its enzyme contents can leak and cause damage. The macrophages that consume these neutrophils do not release cytokines or vasoactive lipids. Ingestion of apoptotic neutrophils does cause the macrophages to secrete more TGF-β, which in turn promotes tissue repair. Clearly, phagocytosis of apoptotic cells is an efficient way of removing unwanted cells without causing additional tissue damage or triggering unwanted inflammation.

Plasma contains several molecules that either inactivate inflammatory mediators or inhibit the enzymes that generate these mediators. Thus α_1-antitrypsin and α_2-macroglobulin block the enzymes released from neutrophil granules. C-reactive protein blocks platelet aggregation. Highly reactive oxidants (superoxide and hydrogen peroxide) released during the neutrophil respiratory burst are inhibited by free radical scavengers. Catalases and peroxidases scavenge peroxides while superoxide dismutase, ceruloplasmin, and free copper ions scavenge superoxide.

Once they reach inflammatory sites, macrophages also phagocytose and destroy damaged cells and tissues. Macrophages secrete collagenases and elastases that directly destroy connective tissue (Figure 4-11). They also release plasminogen activator that generates plasmin, another potent protease. Thus macrophages can "soften-up" the local connective tissue matrix. By releasing IL-1, macrophages attract and activate fibroblasts. The fibroblasts migrate into the damaged area and secrete collagen. Initially they secrete collagen III, but this is later replaced by collagen I. This production of collagen is stimulated by multiple cytokines and by mast cell tryptase. Once sufficient collagen has been deposited, its synthesis stops. This collagen is then gradually remodeled over several weeks or months as the area returns to normal. In addition, the reduced oxygen tension in the middle of dead tissues stimulates macrophages to secrete molecules that promote the growth of new blood vessels. Once the oxygen tension is restored to normal, new blood vessel formation ceases.

The final result of this healing process depends to a large extent on the effectiveness of the inflammation. If the cause is rapidly and completely removed, healing will follow uneventfully.

SICKNESS BEHAVIOR

When the animal body is invaded by microorganisms, there is not only a local inflammatory response, but also a generalized response to the infection that we call sickness. The subjective feelings of sickness—malaise, lassitude, fatigue, loss of appetite, and muscle and joint pains—along with a fever, are part of a highly organized strategy to fight infection. They reflect a change in the body's priorities as it seeks to fight off invaders. Microbial molecules acting on the toll-like receptors of phagocytic cells stimulate the production of a mixture of cytokines (IL-1, IL-6, and TNF-α) that affect many different organ systems, including the brain(Figure 4-12). These cytokines provide signals that reach the brain by two routes. One route is a direct pathway from neurons that serve damaged tissue. Interleukin-1 receptors are found on sensory neurons on the vagus nerve, and vagal sensory stimulation can thus trigger sickness responses in the brain. (IL-1 can make the vagus nerve excessively sensitive and so trigger nausea.)

The second route is a humoral pathway involving circulating cytokines. These blood cytokines either diffuse

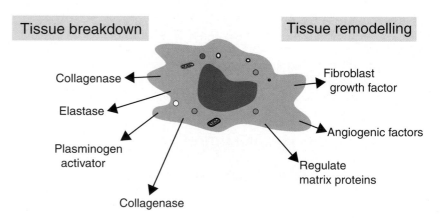

Figure 4-11. Diagram showing the role of macrophages in wound healing.

Tissue breakdown

Tissue remodelling

Collagenase

Elastase

Plasminogen activator

Collagenase

Fibroblast growth factor

Angiogenic factors

Regulate matrix proteins

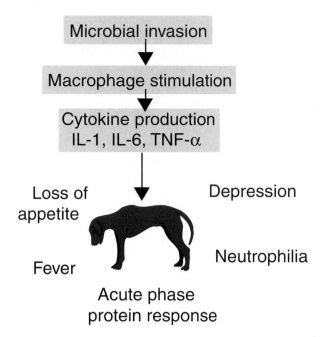

Microbial invasion

↓

Macrophage stimulation

↓

Cytokine production
IL-1, IL-6, TNF-α

↓

Loss of appetite   Depression

Fever   Neutrophilia

Acute phase
protein response

Figure 4-12. Sickness behavior is part of the response of the body to inflammatory stimuli. Multiple systemic effects are due to the three major cytokines secreted by macrophages IL-1, IL-6, and TNF-α.

to brain target areas, or brain macrophages are triggered to produce cytokines. These signals act on the brain to modify an animal's behavior (Box 4–2).

One of the most significant features of the brain's response to infection is the development of a fever. IL-1, IL-6 and TNF-α all diffuse into the brain's temperature-regulating center, where they raise body temperature, induce sleep, and suppress appetite. These cytokines induce prostaglandin production, which causes the body's thermostatic set-point to rise. In response, animals increase heat conservation by vasoconstriction and heat

production by shivering, thus causing the body temperature to rise until it reaches the new set-point. This fever promotes some key components of the immune responses. For example, elevated body temperatures cause dendritic cells to mature; enhance the circulation of lymphocytes; and promote the secretion of the key cytokine interleukin-2. The cytokines released during inflammation, especially IL-1, are also responsible for the reduction in social behavior seen in sickness; they promote the release of sleep-inducing molecules in the brain. Increased lethargy is commonly associated with a fever and may, by reducing the energy demands of an animal, enhance the efficiency of defense and repair mechanisms. IL-1 also suppresses the hunger centers of the brain and so induces the loss of appetite associated with infections. The benefits of this are unclear but it may permit the animal to be more selective about its food. If the anorexia persists, it can have an adverse effect on growth.

Metabolic Changes

In addition to their effects on the nervous and immune systems, IL-1, IL-6 and TNF-α act on skeletal muscle to enhance protein catabolism and thus mobilize a pool of available amino acids. Although this eventually results in muscle wastage, the newly available amino acids are available for increased antibody synthesis. Other systemic responses include the development of a neutrophilia (elevated blood neutrophils), weight loss due to muscle wasting and loss of adipose tissue, and the production of many new proteins (acute-phase proteins) that help fight infection.

Acute-Phase Proteins

Under the influence of IL-1, TNF-α, and especially IL-6, liver cells increase protein synthesis and secretion. Their response begins within a few hours of injury and usually subsides within 24 to 48 hours. The levels of these new proteins may climb enormously under appropriate stimulation (Figure 4-13). Because this synthesis is associated with acute infections and inflammation, these proteins are called acute-phase proteins. Many of the acute-phase proteins are important components of the innate immune system. They include complement components, clotting molecules, protease inhibitors, and metal-binding proteins. Different mammal species produce different acute-phase proteins (Table 4-2). Thus C-reactive protein (CRP) is the major acute-phase protein in primates, pigs, rabbits, hamsters, and dogs (Figure 4-14). CRP belongs to the pentraxin family of lectins. It was first identified and named for its ability to bind and precipitate the C-polysaccharide of *Streptococcus pneumoniae*. CRP binds to phosphatidylcholine, a molecule found in all cell membranes. As a result, it can bind to activated lymphocytes, to invading organisms, and to damaged tissues, where it activates complement. CRP is an opsonin.

BOX 4–2

HMG-1 and Sickness

High-mobility group protein 1 (HMG-1) was long known as a small chromosomal protein that served to bend DNA molecules. Unexpectedly, this molecule has now been recognized as a potent sickness-inducing cytokine. As described in the text, IL-1, IL-6 and TNF-α have long been known to be mediators of septic shock and sickness behavior. It is now clear that these three molecules, in association with interferon-γ, induce HMG-1 release from macrophages several hours after initiation of sickness. It enters secretory lysosomes and is released slowly from the cells. HMG-1 has been implicated in food aversion and weight loss by its actions on the hypothalamic-pituitary axis. It also mediates endotoxin lethality, arthritis, and macrophage activation. It is likely that the inflammation induced by necrotic cells is caused by the release of HMG-1 from disrupted nuclei.

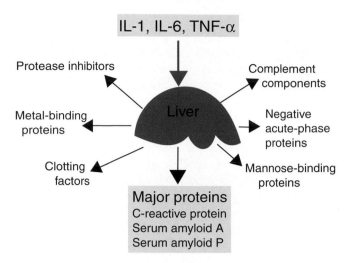

Figure 4-13. The acute-phase proteins. Under the influence of IL-1, IL-6, and TNF-α, hepatocytes secrete a large number of proteins. Almost all of these help the body control infection.

It binds to neutrophils through their Fc receptors and promotes the phagocytosis and removal of damaged, dying, or dead cells and organisms. It also has an antiinflammatory role since it inhibits neutrophil superoxide production and degranulation. CRP may therefore promote tissue healing by reducing damage and enhancing the repair of damaged tissue. (In cattle, CRP is a lactation-associated protein whose level rises two- to five-fold in lactating cows.)

Serum amyloid A (SAA) is the major acute-phase protein in cattle, cats, and horses and is also important in humans and dogs. Thus equine SAA concentrations rise several hundred-fold during noninfectious arthritis, while canine SAA concentrations increase up to 20-fold after bacterial inoculation. Since SAA protein is immunosuppressive, it has been suggested that SAA regulates immune responses. SAA is a chemoattractant for neutrophils, monocytes, and T cells.

In cattle lipopolysaccharide-binding protein is an acute-phase protein that rises very rapidly after infection.

TABLE   4-2
The Major Acute-Phase Proteins in Domestic Animals

Species	Major Proteins
Human	CRP, SAA
Bovine	SAA, haptoglobin, lipopolysaccharide binding protein
Sheep	Haptoglobin
Pig	MAP, CRP, haptoglobin
Horse	SAA
Dog	CRP, α_1-acid glycoprotein, haptoglobin
Cat	SAA, α_1-acid glycoprotein, haptoglobin
Chicken	SAA, transferrin, fibrinogen

Serum amyloid P (SAP) is the major acute-phase protein in rodents. It is a pentraxin structurally and functionally related to CRP. Like CRP it can bind nuclear constituents such as DNA, chromatin, and histones. It can also bind and activate C1q, the first component of the complement system.

The major acute-phase protein in pigs is called MAP (major acute-phase protein!). MAP is a substrate for the proteolytic enzyme kallikrein and so can release potent inflammatory peptides called kinins. Other major acute-phase proteins in pigs include C-reactive protein, haptoglobin, and ceruloplasmin.

Haptoglobin is a major acute-phase protein in ruminants, horses, and cats. It can rise from virtually undetectable levels in normal calves to as high as 1 mg/ml in calves with acute respiratory disease. Haptoglobin binds iron molecules and makes them unavailable to invading bacteria, thus inhibiting bacterial proliferation and invasion. Haptoglobin also reduces iron availability for red blood cell production so that anemia is commonly associated with severe or chronic infections. It is possible to identify animals with severe infections or inflammatory conditions by measuring serum haptoglobin levels. This may be of benefit in antemortem meat inspections to identify those animals that are not fit to eat. Other iron-binding acute-phase proteins include transferrin (important in birds) and hemopexin.

Some serum protease inhibitors such as α_1-antitrypsin, α_1-antichymotrypsin, and α_2-macroglobulin are acute-phase proteins in many mammalian species. All of these may inhibit the tissue damage caused by neutrophil proteases in sites of acute inflammation.

Some protein levels fall during acute inflammation. These are called "negative" acute-phase proteins. In the pig, for example, these include albumin, α-lipoprotein, fetuin, and transferrin.

SYSTEMIC INFLAMMATORY RESPONSE SYNDROME

Under some conditions, especially in response to severe infections or massive tissue damage, very large amounts of cytokines and oxidants escape into the bloodstream and may cause a lethal form of shock known as systemic inflammatory response syndrome (SIRS).

Bacterial Septic Shock

Septic shock is the name given to the systemic inflammatory response syndrome caused by bacterial endotoxins. Thus animals infected with gram-negative bacteria such as *Escherichia coli* or *Salmonella enterica* develop fevers, rigors, myalgia, headache, and nausea. More severe infections cause acidosis, fever, lactate release in tissues, an uncontrollable drop in blood pressure, elevation of plasma catecholamines, and renal, hepatic, and lung

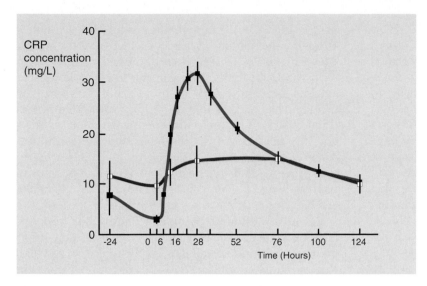

Figure 4-14. The rise in C-reactive protein levels in six dogs following anesthesia and surgery *(red line)* and in six dogs undergoing anesthesia alone *(blue line)*. (From Burton SA, Honor DJ, Mackenzie AL, et al: *Am J Vet Res* 55:615, 1994.)

injury. Endothelial procoagulant activity is enhanced, leading to intravascular coagulation and capillary thrombosis (Figure 4-15). All these effects arc mediated by a massive release of inflammatory cytokines, a "cytokine storm," from endotoxin-stimulated macrophages and neutrophils. The most important cytokines involved are TNF-α and IL-1β. Other cytokines involved include IFN-γ, IL-6, and CXCL8. This cytokine storm is accompanied by an increase in serum nitric oxide and myeloperoxidase. The cytokines act directly on vascular endothelial cells, activating them so that their expression of integrins and procoagulant activity is enhanced.

Multiple organ dysfunction syndrome (MODS) is the end stage of severe septic shock. It is characterized by hypotension, insufficient tissue perfusion, uncontrollable bleeding and organ failure caused by hypoxia, tissue acidosis, tissue necrosis, and severe local metabolic disturbances. The severe bleeding is due to disseminated intravascular coagulation and involves blood vessels and platelets as well as excessive fibrinolysis.

The sensitivity of mammals to septic shock varies greatly. Thus in species with pulmonary intravascular macrophages (cat, horse, sheep, and pig), low doses of gram-negative bacteria or endotoxins can cause extensive lung injury. In contrast, dogs and rodents lack pulmonary intravascular macrophages and are relatively insusceptible to lung injury in septic shock.

Toxic effects are also induced when animals are exposed to chronic, sublethal doses of TNF-α. They lose weight and become anemic and protein-depleted. The weight loss occurs because TNF-α inhibits the synthesis of enzymes necessary for the uptake of lipids by preadipocytes and causes mature adipocytes to lose stored lipids. TNF-α also stimulates the catabolism of muscle cells and hepatocytes. It is thus responsible for the severe weight loss seen in animals with cancer or chronic parasitic and bacterial diseases.

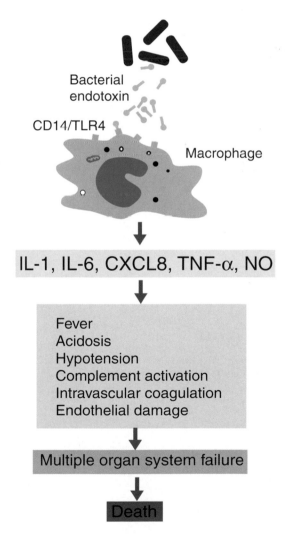

Figure 4-15. The pathogenesis of the systemic inflammatory response syndrome.

Bacterial Toxic Shock

Although endotoxin from gram-negative bacteria plays a major role in inducing SIRS, some gram-positive bacteria can do the same. Thus some strains of *Staphylococcus aureus* produce enterotoxins that bind specifically to certain T cell receptors (Figure 4-16). These toxins may bind and stimulate up to 20% of an animal's T cells. As a result of this stimulation, the T cells secrete very large quantities of the cytokines IL-2 and IFN-γ. These in turn stimulate production of TNF-α and IL-1. This leads to the development of a fever, hypotension, collapse, skin lesions, and damage to the liver, kidney and intestines with multiple organ dysfunction syndrome. This disease is called toxic shock syndrome. A similar syndrome has also been observed in some streptococcal infections.

Graft-Versus-Host Disease

Another condition characterized by excessive production of cytokines, especially TNF-α, is graft-versus-host disease. In this disease, described in more detail in Chapter 30, grafted lymphocytes attack the tissues of the graft recipient. TNF-α secreted by these cells causes mucosal destruction, leading to mucosal ulceration, diarrhea, and liver destruction.

PROTEIN MISFOLDING DISEASES

Amyloidosis is the name given to the abnormal deposition of insoluble proteins in tissues. These appear as amorphous, eosinophilic, hyaline proteins in cells and tissues (Figure 4-17). Amyloid is produced as a result of errors in the folding of newly formed protein chains. These incorrectly folded chains eventually aggregate to form insoluble fibrils. Electron microscopy shows that amyloid proteins consist of protein fibrils, formed by peptide chains cross-linked to form β-pleated sheets (Figure 4-18). This molecular conformation makes amyloid proteins extremely insoluble and almost totally resistant to proteases. Consequently, once deposited in cells or tissues, amyloid deposits are almost impossible to remove. Excessive amyloid infiltration leads to gradual cell loss, tissue destruction, and death.

At least 20 different amyloid precursor proteins have been identified. One of the most common forms occurring in domestic animals is called reactive amyloid. Reactive amyloid usually consists of deposits of a protein called amyloid A (AA) derived from the acute-phase protein SAA. During chronic inflammation certain isoforms of SAA are partially cleaved into fragments that misfold and tend to be deposited in tissues as amyloid. Reactive amyloidosis is therefore associated with chronic inflammation in diseases such as mastitis, osteomyelitis, abscesses, traumatic pericarditis, and tuberculosis (Figure 4-19). Reactive amyloidosis is a major cause of death in animals repeatedly immunized for commercial antiserum production. Familial amyloidosis of Shar-Pei dogs is also due to amyloid A deposition following chronic immune-mediated arthritis.

A second common form of amyloidosis, called immunogenic amyloid, consists of misfolded antibody light chains (AL) (Chapter 13). In animals with plasma cell tumors (myelomas), excessive amounts of these light

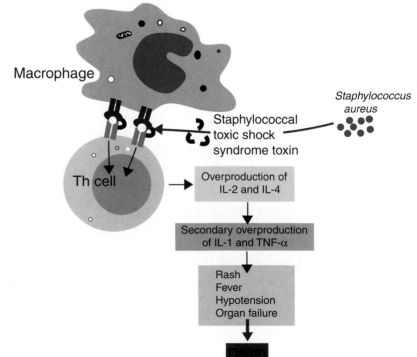

Figure 4-16.   The pathogenesis of staphylococcal toxic shock syndrome.

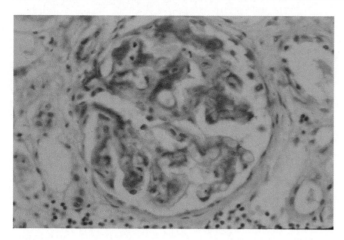

Figure 4-17. Secondary amyloid deposited in a glomerulus. The red dye (Congo red) specifically binds to amyloid fibrils (×400).

chains are produced, and misfolding results in amyloid deposition. Several other well-defined forms of amyloidosis are recognized in domestic animals; for example, old dogs may suffer from vascular amyloidosis, in which amyloid is deposited in the media of leptomeningeal and cortical arteries. An inherited form of amyloid has been described in Abyssinian cats. Tumor-like amyloid nodules and subcutaneous amyloid have been reported in horses, but in general, amyloid deposits are found in the liver, spleen, and kidneys, particularly within glomeruli. In humans, amyloid fibrils are deposited in the neurons of patients with Alzheimer's disease, whereas misfolded prion proteins appear to be the cause of spongiform encephalopathies. Indeed, it is of interest to note that even reactive amyloidosis is somewhat "transmissible," since inoculation of AA proteins into an animal will hasten

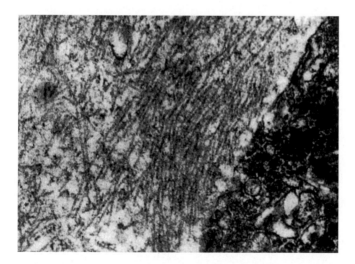

Figure 4-18. Amyloid fibrils. An electron micrograph showing bundles of paired amyloid fibrils deposited parallel to a cell membrane. (Courtesy Dr. EC Franklin. From Franklin EC: *Adv Immunol* 15:25, 1972.)

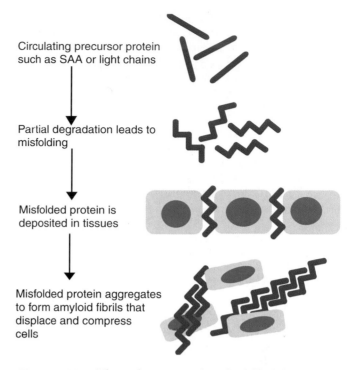

Figure 4-19. The pathogenesis of amyloid fibril deposition.

the development of amyloidosis. They seem to act by providing a substrate upon which other misfolded proteins can be deposited. Thus silk, a protein high in β-sheets, will also cause amyloidosis when injected into mice!

SOURCES OF ADDITIONAL INFORMATION

Alava MA, Gonzales-Ramon N, Heegaard P, et al: Pig MAP, porcine acute phase proteins and standardisation of assays in Europe, *Comp Haematol Int* 7:208-213, 1997.

Altet L, Francino O, Solano-Gallego L, et al: Mapping and sequencing of the canine *NRAMP1* gene and identification of mutations in leishmaniasis-susceptible dogs, *Inf Immun* 70:2763-2771, 2002.

Campbell GA, Adams LG, Sowa BA: Mechanisms of binding of *Brucella abortus* to mononuclear phagocytes from cows naturally resistant or susceptible to brucellosis, *Vet Immunol Immunopathol* 41:295-306, 1994.

Chitko-McKown CG, Blecha F: Pulmonary intravascular macrophages: a review of immune properties and functions, *Ann Rech Vet* 23:201-214, 1992.

Danilenko DM, Rossito PV, Van der Vieren M, et al: A novel canine leukointegrin, a_db_2, is expressed by specific macrophage subpopulations in tissue and a minor CD8+ lymphocyte subpopulation in peripheral blood, *J Immunol* 155:35-44, 1995.

Eckersall PD, Saini PK, McComb C: The acute phase response of α_1-acid glycoprotein, ceruloplasmin, haptoglobin and C-reactive protein, in the pig, *Vet Immunol Immunopathol* 51:377-385, 1996.

Gabay C, Kushner I: Acute-phase proteins and other systemic responses to inflammation, *N Engl J Med* 340:448-453, 1999.

González-Ramón N, Alava MA, Sarsa JA, et al: The major acute phase serum protein in pigs is homologous to human plasma kallikrein sensitive PK-120, *FEBS Letters* 371:227-230, 1995.

Gregory SH, Wing EJ: Neutrophil-Kupffer cell interaction: a critical component of host defenses to systemic bacterial infections, *J Leukocyte Biol* 72:239-248, 2002.

Gruys E, Obwolo MJ, Toussaint MJM: Diagnostic significance of the major acute phase proteins in veterinary clinical chemistry: a review, *Vet Bull* 64:1009-1018, 1994.

Hulten C, Gronlund U, Hirvonen J, et al: Dynamics in serum of the inflammatory markers serum amyloid A (SAA), hapto-globin, fibrinogen and α2-globulins during induced nonin-fectious arthritis in the horse, *Equine Vet J* 34:699-704, 2002.

Kent J: Acute phase proteins: their use in veterinary diagnosis, *Br Vet J* 148:279-282, 1992.

Konsman JP, Parnet P, Dantzer R: Cytokine-induced sickness behaviour: mechanisms and implications, *Trends Neurosciences* 25:154-159, 2002.

Kovacs EJ: Fibrogenic cytokines: the role of immune mediators in the development of scar tissue, *Immunol Today* 12:17-23, 1991.

Kushner I: C-reactive protein and the acute-phase response, *Hosp Pract* 25:13-28, 1990.

Longworth KE, Jarvis KA, Tyler WS, et al: Pulmonary intravascular macrophages in horses and ponies, *Am J Vet Res* 55:382-385, 1994.

Schroedl W, Fuerll B, Reinhold P, et al: A novel acute-phase marker in cattle: lipopolysaccharide binding protein, *J Endotoxin Res* 7:49-52, 2001.

Sigurdsson EM, Wisniewski T, Frangione B: Infectivity of amyloid diseases, *Trends Mol Med* 8:411-413, 2002.

Stone MJ: Amyloidosis: a final common pathway for protein deposition in tissues, *Blood* 75:531-545, 1990.

Winkler GC: Pulmonary intravascular macrophages in domestic animal species: review of structural and functional properties, *Am J Anat* 181:217-234, 1988.

Yamashita K, Fujinaga T, Miyamoto T, et al: Canine acute phase response: relationship between serum cytokine activity and acute phase protein in dogs, *J Vet Med Sci* 56:487-492, 1994.

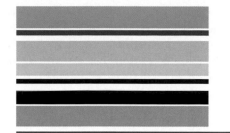

Antigens: Triggers of Acquired Immunity

Up to now we have considered only the body's innate reactions to a microbial invasion. Innate immunity is initiated by recognition of conserved microbial molecules such as CpG DNA and lipopolysaccharide. The triggering of inflammation and the mobilization of phagocytic cells such as neutrophils and macrophages induced by these molecules contribute to the rapid destruction of microbial invaders. Although this is usually a very effective response and is often sufficient to protect the body, it cannot always provide the level of immunity required to ensure resistance to infection. Thus a more potent immune response should recognize all the foreign molecules on an invading microbe. In addition, an ideal defensive response would be able to learn from this experience and, given time, develop more efficient procedures to combat subsequent invasions. This adaptive response is the function of the acquired immune system.

During an acquired immune response, molecules from invading organisms are captured, processed, and presented to the cells of the immune system. When appropriately presented, this antigen will trigger a powerful protective immune response that ensures an animal's survival. In addition, the immune system "remembers" these antigens and responds even more effectively if it encounters them subsequently.

ANTIGENS

Since the function of the acquired immune system is to defend the body against invading microorganisms, it is essential that these organisms be recognized as soon as they invade the body. The body must be able to recognize that these are foreign (and dangerous) if they are to stimulate an immune response. The innate immune system recognizes certain key molecules (the PAMPs) that are characteristic of major groups of pathogens. The acquired immune system, however, can recognize and respond to a vast array of foreign molecular structures. These molecular structures are called antigens.

MICROBIAL ANTIGENS

Bacterial Antigens

Bacteria are ovoid or spherical organisms consisting of a cytoplasm containing the essential elements of cell structure surrounded by a lipid-rich cytoplasmic membrane (Figure 5-1). Outside the cytoplasmic membrane is a thick, carbohydrate-rich cell wall. The major components of the bacterial surface thus include the cell wall, and its associated protein structures, the capsule, the pili, and the flagella. The cell wall of gram-positive organisms is largely composed of peptidoglycan (chains of alternating N-acetyl glucosamine and N-acetyl muramic acid cross-linked by short peptide side chains) (see Figure 2-2). Gram-positive cell walls also contain lipoteichoic acids that are involved in transport of ions across the cell wall. The cell wall in gram-negative organisms consists of a thin layer of peptidoglycan covered by an outer membrane consisting of a lipopolysaccharide. Most of the antigenicity of gram-negative bacteria is associated with

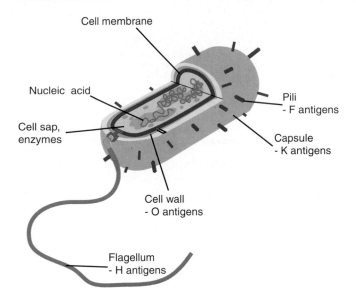

Figure 5-1. The structure of a typical bacterium and the location of its most important antigens.

this component. It consists of an oligosaccharide attached to a lipid (lipid A) and to a series of repeating trisaccharides. The structure of these trisaccharides determines the antigenicity of the organism. Many bacteria are classified according to this antigenic structure. For example, the genus *Salmonella* contains a major species, *S. enteritica*, that is then divided into more than 2300 serovars based on antigenicity. Their polysaccharide antigens are called O antigens. The outer cell wall lipopolysaccharides of gram-negative bacteria bind to toll-like and other receptors and so induce the release of a mixture of cytokines when an animal is infected. These cytokines induce toxic effects. As a result, bacterial lipopolysaccharides are also called endotoxins.

Bacterial capsules consist of polysaccharides (except in *Bacillus anthracis*, where the capsule consists of proteins). These polysaccharides are usually good antigens. Capsules protect bacteria against phagocytosis (Chapter 3), and anticapsular antibodies can protect an infected animal. Capsular antigens are collectively called K antigens.

Pili and fimbriae are short projections that cover the surfaces of some gram-negative bacteria; they are classified as F or K antigens. Pili attach the bacteria to other bacteria and play a role in bacterial conjugation. Fimbriae attach bacteria to surfaces. Antibodies to fimbriae may have an important protective function since they can prevent bacterial adherence to body surfaces. Bacterial flagella consist of a single protein called flagellin. Flagellar antigens are collectively called H antigens.

Other significant bacterial antigens include the porins, the heat-shock proteins, and the exotoxins. The porins are proteins that form the pores on the surface of gram-negative organisms. Heat-shock proteins are generated in large numbers in stressed bacteria. The exotoxins are toxic proteins secreted by bacteria or released into the surrounding environment when they die. Exotoxins are highly immunogenic proteins and stimulate the production of antibodies called antitoxins. Many exotoxins, when treated with a mild protein-denaturing agent such as formaldehyde, lose their toxicity but retain their antigenicity. Toxins modified in this way are called toxoids. Toxoids may be used to prevent disease caused by toxigenic bacteria such as *Clostridium tetani*. Bacterial nucleic acids rich in unmethylated CpG sequences serve both as effective antigens for the acquired immune system and as potent stimulators of innate immunity.

Viral Antigens

Viruses are very small organisms that can grow only inside living cells. They are thus "obligate," intracellular parasites. Viruses have a relatively simple structure consisting of a nucleic acid core surrounded by a protein layer (Figure 5-2). This protein layer is termed the capsid, and it consists of multiple subunits called capsomeres. The capsid proteins are good antigens, highly capable of provoking antibody formation. Some viruses may also be surrounded by an envelope containing lipoproteins and glycoproteins. A complete viral particle is called a virion. When a virus infects an animal, the proteins in the virions act as antigens and trigger an acquired immune response. Viruses, however, are not always found free in the circulation but live within cells, where they are protected from

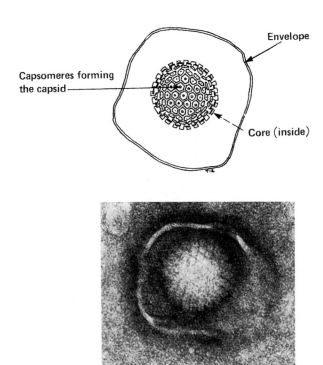

Figure 5-2. The structure of a virus. This is an electron micrograph of equine herpesvirus type 4 magnified 184,000 times. The virus is negatively stained—that is, the electron-dense "dye" has filled the low areas on the virion, leaving the higher areas unstained. (Courtesy Dr. J. Thorsen.)

the unwelcome attentions of antibodies. Indeed, viral nucleic acid can be integrated into a cell's genome. In this situation, the viral genes code for new proteins, some of which are carried to the surface of infected cells. These proteins, although they are synthesized within an animal's cells, are still considered foreign and can provoke strong immune responses. These newly synthesized foreign proteins are called endogenous antigens to distinguish them from the foreign antigens that enter from the outside and are called exogenous antigens.

Other Microbial Antigens

In addition to bacteria and viruses, animals may be invaded by fungi, protozoan parasites, and even by parasitic worms (helminths). Each of these organisms consists of many different structures composed of proteins, carbohydrates, lipids, and nucleic acids. Some of these can serve as antigens and trigger acquired immunity. However, their antigenicity does vary, and the immune responses triggered by these organisms are not always successful in protecting an animal or eliminating the invader.

NONMICROBIAL ANTIGENS

Invading microorganisms are not the only source of foreign material entering the body. Food may contain foreign molecules, which under some circumstances may trigger an immune response and cause an allergic reaction. Likewise, inhaled dusts can contain foreign particles such as fungal spores or pollen grains, and antigens from these may enter the body through the respiratory system. Foreign molecules may be injected directly into the body through a snake bite (or mosquito bite), or they may be injected deliberately by a veterinarian administering a vaccine or a blood transfusion. Furthermore, foreign proteins may be injected into animals for experimental purposes. Organ grafts are an effective way of administering a large amount of foreign material to an animal.

Cell-Surface Antigens

The cytoplasmic membrane of every mammalian cell consists of a mosaic of protein molecules immersed in a fluid lipid bilayer. Most of these proteins can act as antigens if they are injected into an animal of another species or even into a different animal of the same species. For example, glycoproteins known as blood-group antigens are found on the surface of red blood cells. Early attempts to transfuse blood between unrelated individuals usually met with disaster, because the transfused cells were rapidly destroyed even though the recipient had never before received a transfusion. Investigation revealed that the problem was due to the presence of naturally occurring antibodies against these red cell glycoproteins (Chapter 27).

Nucleated cells, such as leukocytes, possess hundreds of different protein molecules on their cytoplasmic membrane. These proteins are good antigens and readily provoke an immune response when injected experimentally into an animal of a different species. These surface molecules are classified by the CD system (Chapter 2). Other cell surface proteins may provoke an immune response (such as graft rejection) if transferred into a genetically different individual of the same species. The most important cell-surface proteins that trigger graft rejection are called MHC molecules. These molecules are of such importance in immunology that they warrant a complete chapter of their own (Chapter 7).

Autoantigens

In some situations (and not always abnormal ones), an immune response may be directed against normal body components. This is called an autoimmune response. Antigens that induce this autoimmunity are called autoantigens. They can include hormones such as thyroglobulin; structural components such as basement membranes; complex lipids such as myelin; intracellular components, such as the mitochondrial proteins, nucleic acids, or nucleoproteins; and cell surface proteins, such as hormone receptors. The production of these autoantibodies and the consequences of this production are discussed in detail in Chapter 32.

WHAT MAKES A GOOD ANTIGEN?

Molecules vary in their ability to act as antigens (their antigenicity) and stimulate an immune response (Figure 5-3). In general, foreign proteins make the best antigens, especially if they are big (a molecular weight greater than

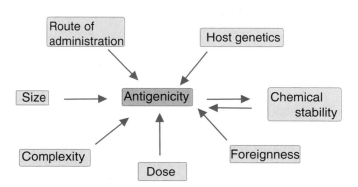

Figure 5-3. The factors that significantly influence the antigenicity of a molecule. Of these, either excessive or insufficient stability will reduce antigenicity. The best antigens are large, complex, and foreign. However, their ability to stimulate an immune response is also determined by their route of administration, by the amount of antigen administered, and by the genetic makeup of the immunized animal.

1000 daltons (Da) is best.) Many of the major antigens of microorganisms such as the clostridial toxins, bacterial flagella, virus capsids, and protozoan cell membranes are proteins. Other important antigenic proteins include components of snake venoms, serum proteins, cell surface proteins, milk and food proteins, hormones, and even antibody molecules themselves.

Simple polysaccharides, such as starch or glycogen, are not good antigens simply because they are degraded before the immune system has had time to respond to them. More complex carbohydrates, however, may be of immunological importance, especially if bound to proteins. These include the major cell-wall antigens of gram-negative bacteria and the blood-group antigens of red blood cells. Many of the so-called natural antibodies found in the serum of unimmunized animals are directed against polysaccharides and probably arise as a result of exposure to glycoproteins or carbohydrates from the normal intestinal flora or from food. To this extent they can also be considered to be part of the innate immune system.

Lipids tend to be poor antigens because of their wide distribution, relative simplicity, structural instability, and rapid metabolism. Nevertheless, when linked to proteins or polysaccharides, lipids may be able to trigger immune responses.

Mammalian nucleic acids are very poor antigens because of their relative simplicity and flexibility and because they are very rapidly degraded. Microbial nucleic acids, on the other hand, have a structure very different from that found in eukaryotes with many unmethylated CpG sequences. As a result, they can stimulate a potent immune response. It is perhaps for this reason that autoantibodies to nucleic acids are a characteristic feature of several important autoimmune diseases (Chapter 34).

Proteins are the most effective antigens because they have properties that best trigger an immune response. (More correctly, the acquired immune system is optimized to trap, process, and then recognize foreign proteins.) Thus large molecules are better antigens than small molecules, and proteins can be very large indeed (Figure 5-4). For example, hemocyanin, a very large protein from invertebrate blood (670 kDa), is a potent antigen. Serum albumin from other mammals (69 kDa) is a fairly good antigen but may also provoke tolerance. The peptide hormone angiotensin (1031 Da) is a poor antigen.

Similarly, the more complex an antigen is, the better. For example, starch and other simple repeating polymers are poor antigens, but complex bacterial lipopolysaccharides are good. Complex proteins containing many different amino acids, especially aromatic ones, are better antigens than large, repeating polymers, such as the lipids, carbohydrates, and nucleic acids.

Structural stability is an important feature of good antigens, especially those that trigger antibody responses. To bind to a foreign molecule, the cell surface receptors of the immune system must recognize its shape.

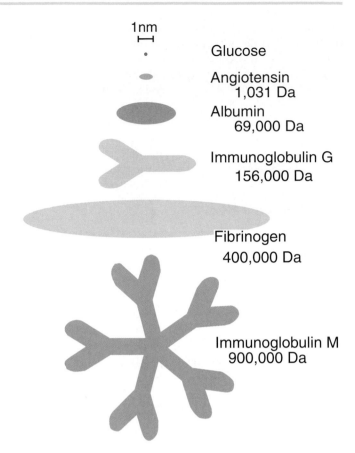

Figure 5-4. The relative sizes of several significant antigens. Size does matter! Big molecules are generally much more antigenic than small molecules. Molecules as small as angiotensin are poor antigens.

Consequently, highly flexible molecules that have no fixed shape are poor antigens. For example, gelatin, a protein well known for its structural instability (which is why it can wobble), is a poor antigen unless it is stabilized by the incorporation of tyrosine or tryptophan molecules, which cross-link the peptide chains. Similarly, flagellin, the major protein of bacterial flagella, is a structurally unstable, weak antigen. Its stability, and thus its antigenicity, is greatly enhanced by polymerization.

Remember too that the route of antigen administration, its dose, and the genetics of the recipient animal also influence antigenicity.

Clearly not all foreign molecules can stimulate an immune response. Stainless steel bone pins and plastic heart valves, for example, are commonly implanted in humans without triggering an immune response. The lack of antigenicity in the large organic polymers, such as the plastics, is due not only to their molecular uniformity but also to their inertness. These polymers cannot be degraded and processed by cells to a form suitable for triggering an immune response. Conversely, since immune responses are antigen-driven, foreign molecules that are unstable and destroyed very rapidly may not persist for a sufficient time to stimulate an immune response.

Foreignness

The cells that respond to antigens (antigen-sensitive cells) are selected so that their antigen receptors do not normally bind to molecules originating within an animal (self-antigens). They will bind and respond, however, to foreign molecules that differ even in minor respects from those normally found within the body. This lack of reactivity of the specific immune system to normal body components occurs because those cells whose receptors bind self-antigens are selectively killed. During their development, the cells are exposed to self-antigens, and those cells that respond are killed in a process called "negative selection."

The immunogenicity of a molecule also depends on its degree of foreignness. The greater the difference in structure between a foreign antigen and an animal's own antigens, the greater will be the intensity of the immune response. For example, a kidney graft from an identical twin will be readily accepted because its proteins are identical to those on the recipient's own kidney. A kidney graft from an unrelated animal of the same species will be rejected in about 10 days unless drugs are used to control the rejection. A kidney graft between different species such as one from a pig to a dog will be rejected within a few hours despite the use of immunosuppressive drugs.

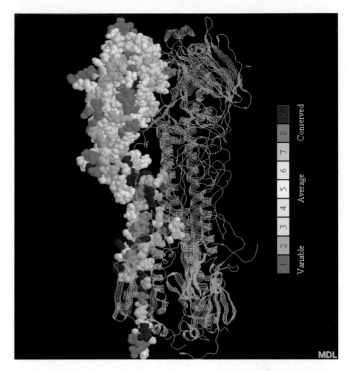

Figure 5-5. A molecular model of an antigen. This is an important influenza virus antigen called the hemagglutinin. It consists of two chains, one of which is lightly drawn so that the details of the other can be seen. The irregular surface forms characteristic shapes that can be recognized by the cells of the immune system. Influenza virus constantly changes the shape of this molecule, and this is denoted by the color coding. (Courtesy Dr. Fabian Glaser.)

EPITOPES

Foreign particles, such as bacteria, nucleated cells, and red blood cells, are a complex mixture of proteins, glycoproteins, polysaccharides, lipopolysaccharides, lipids, and nucleoproteins. The acquired immune response against such a foreign particle is, therefore, a mixture of many simultaneous immune responses against each of the foreign molecules in the mixture.

A single large molecule such as a protein can also be shown to stimulate multiple immune responses. Large molecules have specific regions, against which immune responses are directed. These regions, usually on the surface of the molecule, are called epitopes, or antigenic determinants (Figure 5-5). In a large, complex protein molecule, many different epitopes may be recognized by the immune system, but some are much more immunogenic than others. Thus animals may respond to a few favored epitopes, and the remainder of the molecule is virtually nonimmunogenic. Such epitopes are said to be immunodominant. In general, the number of epitopes on a molecule is directly related to its size and there is usually about one epitope for each five kDa of a protein. When we describe a molecule as "foreign," therefore, we are implying that it contains epitopes that are not found

on self-antigens. The cells of the immune system recognize and respond to foreign epitopes.

Haptens

A small molecule such as a drug or a hormone with a molecular weight of less than 1000 Da is far too small to be appropriately processed and presented to the immune system. As a result, it is not immunogenic. If, however, the small molecule is chemically linked to a large protein molecule, completely new epitopes will be formed on the surface of the larger molecule (Figure 5-6). If this complex is injected into an animal, immune responses will be triggered against all its epitopes. Some of the antibodies made in response to the complex will be directed against new epitopes formed by the small molecule. Small molecules or chemical groups that can function as epitopes when bound to other larger molecules are called haptens (in Greek *haptein* means "to grasp or fasten"). The antigenic molecule to which the haptens are attached is called the carrier. Many drug allergies occur because the drug molecules, although small, can bind covalently to normal body proteins and so act as haptens.

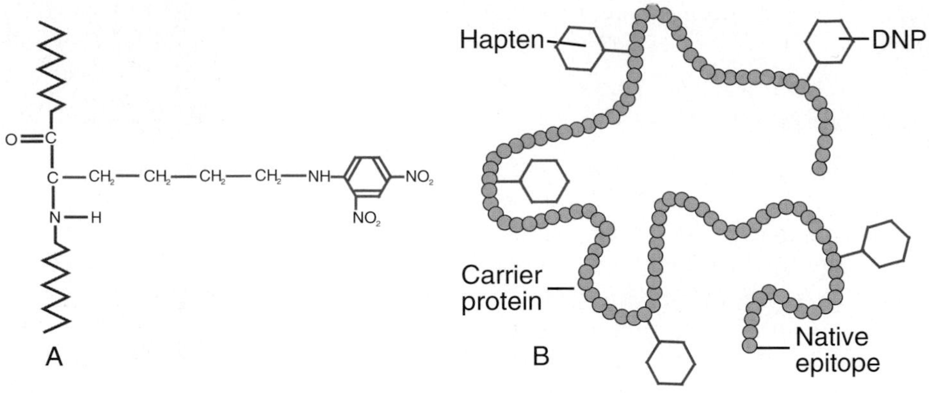

Figure 5-6. **A,** A typical hapten, in this case, dinitrophenol attached to a lysine side-chain. **B,** When several haptens are attached to a peptide chain, they serve as new epitopes and will stimulate immune responses.

By using haptens of known chemical structure, it is possible to study the interaction between antibodies and epitopes in great detail. For example, antibodies raised against one hapten can be tested for their ability to bind to other, structurally related molecules. Simple tests have shown that any alteration in the shape, size, or charge of a hapten alters its ability to bind to antibodies. Even very minor modifications to the shape of a hapten, such as the difference between stereoisomers, may influence its ability to be bound by an antibody. Since there exists an enormous variety of potential haptens, and since each hapten can provoke its own specific antibodies, it follows that animals must be able to generate an extremely large variety of specific antibody molecules.

Some Examples of Haptens

Although the concept of haptens and carrier molecules provides the basis for much of our knowledge concerning the specificity of the antibody response, haptens may also be of clinical importance. For example, the antibiotic penicillin is a small nonimmunogenic molecule. Once degraded within the body, however, it forms a very reactive "penicilloyl" group, which can bind to serum proteins such as albumin, to form penicilloyl-albumin complexes (Figure 5-7). The penicilloyl hapten can be recognized as a foreign epitope in some individuals and so provokes an immune response. Antibodies generated against it may cause an allergic response to penicillin (Chapter 26).

A second example of a naturally occurring reactive chemical that binds spontaneously to normal proteins and so acts as a hapten is the toxic component of the poison ivy plant (*Rhus radicans*). The resin of this plant, called urushiol, will bind to any protein with which it comes into contact—including the skin proteins of a person who rubs against the plant. The modified skin proteins are then regarded as foreign and attacked by lymphocytes in a manner similar to the rejection of a skin graft. The result is the uncomfortable skin rash called allergic contact dermatitis (Chapter 29).

CROSS-REACTIONS

Identical or similar epitopes may sometimes be found on apparently unrelated molecules. As a result, antibodies directed against one antigen may react unexpectedly with an unrelated antigen. In another situation, the epitopes on a protein may differ in only minor respects from those on the same protein obtained from an animal of a related species. Consequently, antibodies directed against a protein in one species may also react in a detectable manner with the homologous or similar protein in another species. Both phenomena are called cross-reactions.

An example of a cross-reaction of the first type is seen when blood-typing. Many bacteria possess cell-wall glycoproteins with carbohydrate side-chains that are identical to those found on mammalian red blood cell glycoproteins. For example, some intestinal bacteria possess glycoproteins with A or B side-chains on their cell walls (Chapter 27). These glycoproteins are absorbed

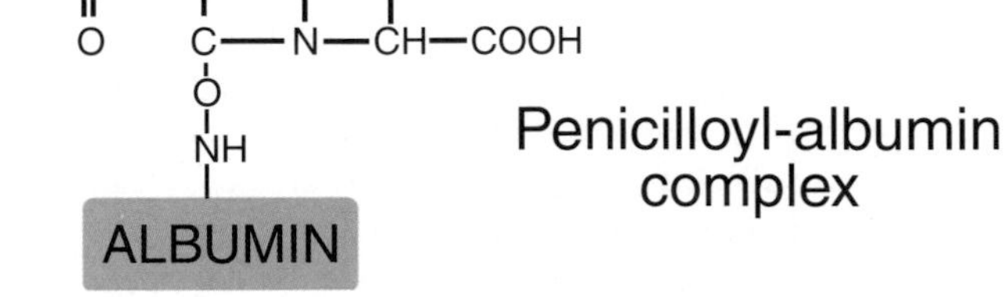

Figure 5-7. Penicillin as a hapten. Penicillin can break down in vivo by several different pathways. The most important derivative is a penicillenic acid that combines with amino groups in a protein such as serum albumin to form a penicilloyl-protein complex. This complex may provoke an immune response and result in a penicillin allergy.

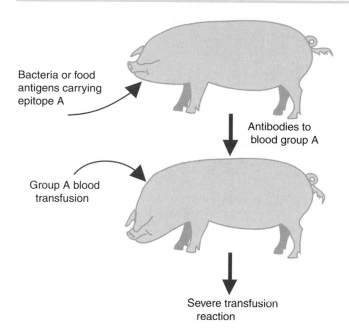

Figure 5-8. Food or bacterial antigens encountered in the diet carry epitopes that cross-react with blood group glycoprotein A. As a result, pigs of blood group O make antibodies to the A epitope despite never having received group A red cells. Should these animals be inadvertently transfused with A blood, they will suffer an immediate and severe transfusion reaction.

through the intestinal wall into the bloodstream and trigger an antibody response. For example, blood-group glycoprotein side-chain A is foreign to a pig of blood group O (Figure 5-8). Pigs of blood group O therefore develop antibodies that react with red cells from pigs of blood group A. These antibodies arise not as a response to previous immunization with group A red cells, but following exposure to the glycoproteins that originate in the intestinal bacteria. Cross-reacting antibodies of this type are called heterophile antibodies.

Another example of cross-reactivity occurs between *Brucella abortus* and some strains of *Yersinia enterocolitica*. *Y. enterocolitica*, a relatively unimportant organism, may provoke cattle to make antibodies that cross-react with *B. abortus*. Since *Brucella*-infected animals are detected by testing for the presence of serum antibodies, a *Yersinia*-infected animal may be wrongly thought to carry *B. abortus* and so be killed. In another example, cross-reactivity occurs between the virus of feline infectious peritonitis (FIP) and the virus of pig transmissible gastroenteritis (TGE). It is very difficult to grow the FIP virus in the laboratory. TGE virus, on the other hand, is readily propagated. By detecting antibodies to TGE in cats, it is possible to diagnose FIP without having to culture the FIP virus.

The second type of cross-reactivity, which occurs between related proteins, may be demonstrated in many different biological systems. One example is the method used to detect relationships between mammalian species. Thus antisera to bovine serum cross-react well

TABLE 5-1

The Degree of Cross-Reaction Between a Specific Antibody (Antibovine Light Chain Antibodies) and Related Proteins (Light Chains) From Other Mammals

Cow	*Bos taurus*	100
Bison	*Bos bison*	100
Sheep	*Ovis aires*	100
Yak	*Pocphagus grunniens*	68
Goat	*Capra hircus*	68
Elk	*Cervus canadensis*	64
Buffalo	*Bubalus bubalus*	54
Reindeer	*Rangifer tarandus*	37
Human	*Homo sapiens*	17
Horse	*Equus caballus*	10
Rat	*Rattus rattus*	10
Mouse	*Mus musculus*	10
Pig	*Sus scrofa*	8
Camel	*Camelus dromedarius*	7

Data from Henning D, Nielsen K: *Vet Immunol Immunopathol* 34: 235-243, 1992.

with sheep and bison serum proteins but react much more weakly with serum proteins from other mammals (Table 5-1). Presumably, this reflects the degree of structural similarity between the epitopes on serum proteins and is thus a useful tool in determining evolutionary relationships.

SOURCES OF ADDITIONAL INFORMATION

Atassi MZ: Precise determination of the entire antigenic structure of lysozyme, *Immunochemistry* 15:909-936, 1978.
Borek F: *Immunogenicity, Frontiers of Biology Series*, Amsterdam, 1972, Elsevier North-Holland.
Green N, Alexander H, Olsen A, et al: Immunogenic structure of the influenza virus hemagglutinin, *Cell* 28:477-487, 1982.
Katz ME, Maizels RM, Wicker L, et al: Immunological focusing by the mouse major histocompatibility complex: mouse strains confronted with distantly related lysozymes confine their attention to very few epitopes, *Eur J Immunol* 12: 535-540, 1982.
Landsteiner K: *The specificity of serological reactions*, Cambridge, 1945, Harvard University Press.
Marx JL: Do antibodies prefer moving targets? *Science* 226: 819- 821, 1984.
Mason D, Andre P, Bensussan A, et al: CD antigens, 2001, *Immunology* 103:401-406, 2001.
Sela M: Antigenicity: some molecular aspects, *Science* 166: 1365-1374, 1969.
Sercarz E, ed: *Antigenic determinants and immune regulation, Chemical immunology*, vol 46, Basel, Switzerland, 1989, Karger.
Tizard I: Antigen structure and immunogenicity, *JAVMA* 181:978-982, 1982.
Wilson IA, Niman HL, Houghten RA, et al: The structure of an antigenic determinant in a protein, *Cell* 37:767-778, 1984.

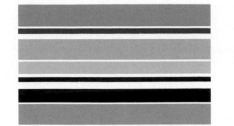

Dendritic Cells and Antigen Processing

CHAPTER 6

The innate immune defenses are designed to destroy microbial invaders as they enter the body. They perform this role well, and most invaders, especially if they are of low virulence, are rapidly eliminated. However, in addition to being uncomfortable and damaging to normal tissues, inflammation is not a foolproof process. If the body is to be defended effectively, an animal must have a defense system that automatically detects and eliminates invaders without the damage and discomfort associated with inflammation. It should also ensure the destruction of all microbial invaders. This is the task of the acquired immune system.

In order to trigger an acquired immune response, a sample of foreign material must first be captured, processed, and presented in the correct fashion to the cells that can recognize it. The first steps in this process are the responsibility of antigen-processing cells.

Antigen-processing cells are attracted to inflammatory sites and activated by the same stimuli that trigger inflammation. Indeed, dendritic cells and macrophages are both sentinel cells for innate immunity and effective antigen-processing cells. This means that antigen-processing can proceed at the same time as the invader is being eliminated by the innate defenses. When an invader has been eliminated, the body can proceed to strengthen its defenses against a second attack by the same organism.

Antigen processing involves the fragmentation of antigen molecules into small peptides. These peptides are then attached to specialized, antigen-presenting molecules called MHC molecules. The complex of antigen plus MHC is then carried to the cell surface, where it is recognized by the cells called lymphocytes. There are two different classes of MHC molecules—MHC I and MHC II—and each binds a different type of antigen. Acquired immune responses are triggered when antigen fragments bind to specific receptors on lymphocytes. Some of these lymphocytes (called T cells) can respond only to antigen fragments that have been correctly processed. This is because the T cells must also be stimulated by signals originating in the antigen-processing cells.

The organisms that trigger acquired immunity are of two distinct types. First, there are foreign microorganisms such as bacteria that invade the body from outside and grow in the tissues and extracellular fluid. Their antigens are called exogenous antigens, and these are processed by specialized antigen-processing cells. A second type of invading organism is actually made within the body. For example, when viruses invade a cell, they force the cell to make new viral proteins. These new proteins are called endogenous antigens. Endogenous antigens are processed and presented to antigen-sensitive cells by the cells in which they are formed.

Three types of cells are employed to sample and process exogenous antigens. These cells are dendritic cells, macrophages, and B cells. The most effective, by far, are the dendritic cells (Figure 6-1).

DENDRITIC CELLS

Dendritic cells are a family of cells that have no known function other than to present antigens to T cells. Indeed they appear to be at least 100 times more potent in this role than the other two major antigen-processing cell populations, macrophages and B cells. Dendritic cells can take up many different antigens, including dead microorganisms, soluble antigens in tissue fluids, and antigens released by dying cells, and present them to the cells of the immune system. Dendritic cells are the only antigen-processing cells that can activate those T cells that have never previously encountered an antigen (naive cells) and thus are essential for initiating primary immune responses.

Origin

Dendritic cells (DCs) are produced from bone marrow stem cells (Figure 6-2). These immature dendritic cells then migrate around the body, where they form lattice-like networks in virtually every tissue. DCs are found in

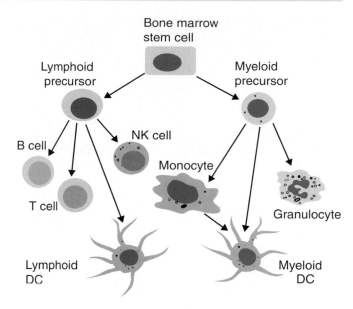

Figure 6-2. The origin of dendritic cells. Although all DCs originate from bone marrow stem cells, they can originate from either myeloid or lymphoid precursors. These two major dendritic cell subpopulations may have very different properties and roles.

all organs except the brain, parts of the eye, and the testes. They are especially prominent in lymph nodes, skin, and mucosal surfaces where invading microbes might be encountered. They die within 2 to 4 days if they fail to encounter antigens.

Structure

Dendritic cells are characterized by having a relatively small cell body and many long cytoplasmic processes. These processes, often many times the length of the cell body, are known as dendrites (Figure 6-3). It is believed that the dendrites increase the efficiency of antigen trapping and maximize contact between dendritic cells and other cells.

Subpopulations

DC subpopulations differ in their origin, location, and function. Thus in humans there are two major subpopulations—myeloid and lymphoid DCs (Figures 6-2 and 6-4). The myeloid DCs include Langerhans cells (epidermal DCs) and other tissue dendritic cells. They are derived from blood monocytes. Lymphoid DCs, in contrast, are found in blood and lymphoid organs.

In mice there are at least three major DC subpopulations. They are known as myeloid DCs, lymphoid DCs, and Langerhans cells. Myeloid DCs arise from the same precursors as neutrophils and monocytes, whereas lymphoid DCs arise from lymphoid stem cells. Both are heterogeneous cell populations with subsets that differ in

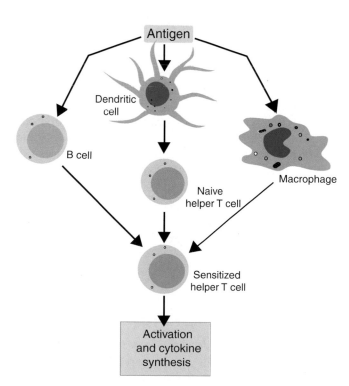

Figure 6-1. The three major populations of antigen-presenting cells: B cells, dendritic cells, and macrophages. Of these, only dendritic cells can activate naive T cells and trigger a primary immune response.

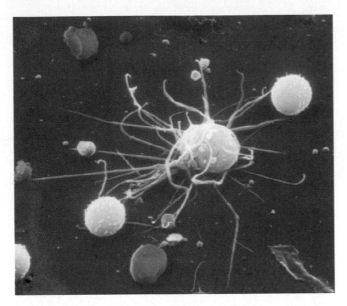

Figure 6-3. A scanning electron micrograph of a dendritic cell from a guinea pig lymph node. Note the relatively small cell body and the numerous long dendrites (×4000).

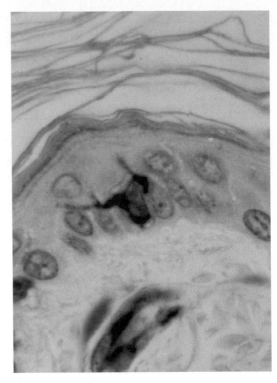

Figure 6-5. This red in the midepidermis of a dog is a Langerhans cell stained for the protein vimentin. Note its dendrites extending between the epidermal cells. (Courtesy Dr. KM Credille.)

their surface markers, in the cytokines that they secrete, and in their functions.

Langerhans cells are specialized dendritic cells found in the epidermis, where they trap and process antigens that penetrate the skin (Figure 6-5). These include topically applied antigens, such as the resins of poison ivy, or intradermally injected antigens, such as mosquito saliva. Langerhans cells influence the development of skin immune responses, such as delayed hypersensitivity and allergic contact dermatitis (Chapter 29). Langerhans cells contain characteristic granules called Birbeck granules.

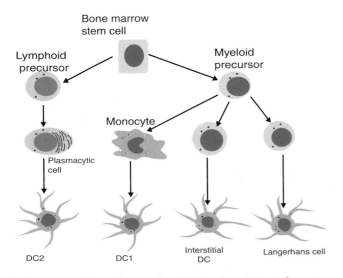

Figure 6-4. Not only can dendritic cells originate from two distinct precursors, but their properties are also determined by their location. The major functional subpopulations are DC1 and DC2 cells.

Blood monocytes are the immediate precursors of both tissue macrophages and myeloid DCs. Which cell type is produced depends on interactions between cytokines and cells encountered by the monocyte as it matures. Each cell type can convert to the other until late in the differentiation process. In domestic animals myeloid (monocyte)-derived dendritic cells have been characterized in pigs, cattle, horses, chickens and dogs. Langerhans cells have been described in pigs, cattle, horses, dogs, and cats. Lymphoid dendritic cells have only been described in mice.

Although there are different subpopulations of dendritic cells, the most important division is based on their state of maturity (Figure 6-6). Thus immature dendritic cells are highly specialized and efficient antigen-trapping cells. When they mature, dendritic cells change their role and become specialized and efficient antigen-processing cells.

Immature Dendritic Cells

Most newly generated dendritic cells move from the bone marrow through the blood to the lymph and eventually to lymph nodes or tissues. Here they serve as "sentinels" whose role is to capture invading microbes. With their short life-span, they can be regarded as disposable antigen-trapping cells. If they do not encounter antigens, they die in a few days. If, however, they encounter

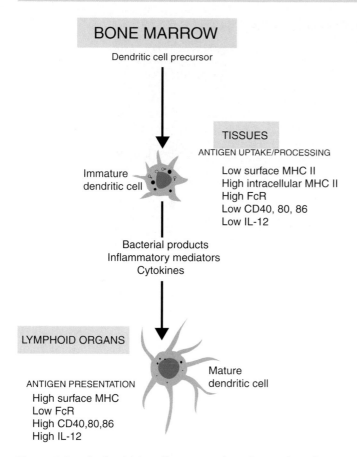

BONE MARROW

Dendritic cell precursor

TISSUES

ANTIGEN UPTAKE/PROCESSING

Immature dendritic cell

Low surface MHC II
High intracellular MHC II
High FcR
Low CD40, 80, 86
Low IL-12

Bacterial products
Inflammatory mediators
Cytokines

LYMPHOID ORGANS

ANTIGEN PRESENTATION
High surface MHC
Low FcR
High CD40,80,86
High IL-12

Mature dendritic cell

Figure 6-6. As dendritic cells mature, they change their function. Immature dendritic cells are specialized antigen-trapping cells. Mature dendritic cells, on the other hand, are specialized antigen-processing cells.

antigens together with tissue damage or inflammation, they become activated and mature rapidly.

Dendritic cell activation occurs in response to molecules produced by tissue damage or invading microorganisms. Thus injured and inflamed tissues release large amounts of soluble heparan sulfate that binds to TLR4 and activates dendritic cells. Breakdown of nucleic acids generates uric acid, a potent dendritic cell activator. Dendritic cell activation is also triggered by an elevated body temperature, such as occurs with fever. Immature dendritic cells have receptors for inflammatory chemokines and so are attracted to areas of inflammation. Neutrophil-derived defensins have the same effect. Mast cell–derived vesicles (exosomes) are potent stimulators of dendritic cell activation. Other molecules that activate dendritic cells include inflammatory cytokines such as TNF-α and IL-1, microbial products such as lipopolysaccharide, bacterial DNA, and double-stranded RNA from viruses.

Immature dendritic cells specialize in capturing antigens in peripheral tissues. They capture antigens by phagocytosis, by pinocytosis (the uptake of fluid droplets—cell drinking), and by interaction with various cell surface receptors. They also capture apoptotic cell bodies. If they ingest bacteria, they can usually kill them.

Dendritic cells have many different surface receptors that help them carry out their functions. These include cytokine receptors such as IL-1R and TNFR; chemokine receptors; C-type lectins, Fc receptors (FcγR and FcεR), mannose receptors (CD206), heat shock protein receptors, and the toll-like receptors, TLR2 and TLR4.

Mature Dendritic Cells

Once they come into contact with an antigen, dendritic cells mature rapidly and this maturation radically boosts their antigen-presenting abilities. Thus MHC molecules are redistributed from intracellular locations to the cell surface. There is an increased expression of costimulatory molecules, cytoskeletal reorganization, shape changes, and the secretion of cytokines, chemokines, and proteases. Fc and mannose receptors are down-regulated, and endocytosis is reduced.

After they have captured and processed antigens, mature dendritic cells have to carry the antigen to sites where it can be recognized by the antigen-sensitive cells called T cells. Thus the dendritic cells migrate via the blood or lymph to organs such as lymph nodes or spleen. Activated DCs are attracted to lymphoid organs by the chemokine, CCL20, which is released by mature DCs within the node. Infection or damage to tissues also promotes the migration of antigen-bearing dendritic cells from tissues to lymph nodes or the spleen. Stimulated dendritic cells found within lymphatics are called veiled cells. When they enter a draining lymph node, they become mature dendritic cells.

Once within the lymphoid organs, the mature DCs are examined by T cells. These T cells will bind to antigens on the dendritic cell surface only if their receptors match. This dendritic cell–T cell interaction forms visible clusters (Figure 6-7). A cluster of T cells forms around each dendritic cell, and synthesis of cytokines occurs, leading to an immune response.

Mature dendritic cells attract T and B cells by secreting chemokines. For example, Langerhans cells that migrate from sensitized skin secrete CCL22. This attracts T cells, which consequently accumulate in clusters around the antigen-presenting dendritic cell. As dendritic cells mature, MHC molecules are redistributed from intracellular compartments to the cell surface. Cell surface expression of costimulatory molecules is also enhanced. MHC molecules and MHC-peptide complexes are found at levels 100 times higher on dendritic cells than on other antigen-processing cells such as B cells or macrophages, and their expression of costimulatory molecules such as CD86 (Chapter 10) may also rise 100-fold.

Mature dendritic cells are the only cells that can trigger a primary T cell response. One reason for this efficiency is that these cells may preassemble a complete T cell activation complex (antigen-loaded MHC plus activation molecules such as CD80) within the cell before

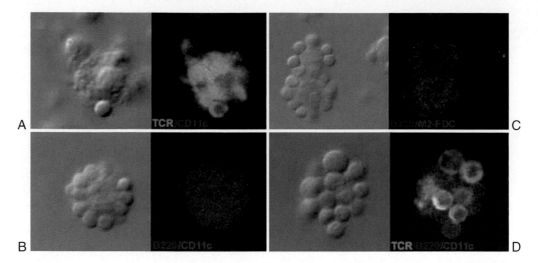

Figure 6-7. When dendritic cells and T cells interact, they form visible clusters as the cells converse among themselves. Thus in these figures, dendritic cells are stained with a blue fluorescent dye (anti-CD11c), T cells are stained with a green dye (anti-CD3), and B cells are stained with a red dye (anti-B220). **A,** T cells are interacting with a dendritic cell. **B,** B cells are binding to a dendritic cell. **C,** B cells are binding to a follicular dendritic cell. **D,** There is a mixed B and T cell cluster. Note that some B cells appear to be attached to T cells. (From Hommel M, Kyewski B: *J Exp Med* 197:269-280, 2003.)

it arrives at the cell surface. Because of their potency only a few dendritic cells are required to trigger a strong response. Indeed, one dendritic cell may activate as many as 3000 T cells.

Mature dendritic cells bind strongly to T cells through ligands such as DC-SIGN, a C-type lectin, which binds to ICAM-3 expressed on naive T cells. DC-SIGN is unique in that it not only captures antigen but also mediates transient binding between dendritic cells and T cells. It permits a dendritic cell to screen thousands of T cells in order to find the few that are expressing a compatible antigen receptor.

Tolerance Induction

Under steady state conditions a few immature dendritic cells spontaneously mature and migrate to lymphoid tissues, carrying tissue antigens with them. If this "normal" antigen is recognized by a T cell, the T cell is triggered to undergo apoptosis and die! Thus the processing of normal body components leads to T cell deletion and immunological tolerance. The spontaneously mature dendritic cells may present T cells with some sort of unique signal, or perhaps the signal they deliver is insufficient to trigger a full T cell response.

DC1 and DC2 Cells

When a microorganism invades the body, a decision must be made as to the best way to respond to the organism. This decision is made by dendritic cells based on the nature of the invader. As pointed out earlier, the acquired

immune system has two major branches, the antibody-mediated and cell-mediated immune responses. The type of immune response mounted by an animal is determined by the type of helper T cell triggered to respond to an antigen. Thus helper T (Th) cells fall into two subpopulations (Figure 6-8). One subpopulation called Th1 cells stimulates cell-mediated immune responses designed to protect animals against intracellular organisms. The other subpopulation, Th2 cells, stimulates antibody-mediated immune responses designed to protect animals against extracellular invaders. This raises a question—how does the body select which T cell population to employ? It appears that this selection results from the use of distinct dendritic cell subpopulations.

Thus when dendritic cells stimulate T cells, they provide three signals. The first is mediated by contact with an antigen associated with an MHC molecule. The second signal provides costimulation through molecules such as CD40 and CD80/86. The third signal determines the polarization of naive Th cells. This third signal can be mediated by various soluble or membrane-bound molecules, including the cytokines IL-12, IL-18, and interferon-α (IFN-α), as well as a surface receptor called OX40-ligand. The expression of these third signals is governed by the conditions under which the dendritic cells are activated.

Some microbial molecules promote the generation of dendritic cells that secrete IL-12 on activation. These IL-12–producing dendritic cells are called DC1 cells. Their IL-12 favors activation of Th1 cells. In contrast, other microbial molecules induce dendritic cells to produce the cytokines IL-1, IL-6, and IL-4. These

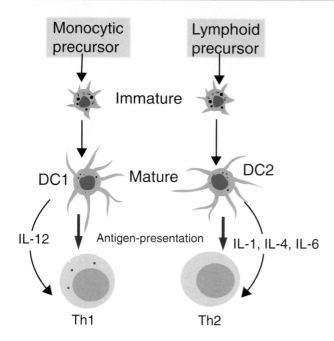

Figure 6-8. Two subpopulations of dendritic cells appear to favor different T cell subpopulations. Th1 cells promote cell-mediated immunity, whereas Th2 cells promote antibody formation. The helper cell population employed depends on the use of dendritic cell subpopulations. These cells have different origins and secrete different costimulatory cytokines.

cytokines preferentially stimulate Th2 cells. These IL-4–producing dendritic cells are called DC2 cells.

Molecules derived from invading organisms such as CpG DNA, lipopolysaccharide, double-stranded viral RNA, and *B pertussis* toxin promote the development of DC1 cells. On the other hand, inflammatory mediators, such as IL-10, TGF-β, PGE2, histamine, extracts of the parasitic worm *Schistosoma mansoni*, or the toxin of *V. cholerae*, all promote a DC2 response. It thus appears that different antigens (or pathogens) determine the development of specific types of dendritic cells by provoking tissues to release the molecules that determine polarization.

A similar division of macrophages has also been identified. Thus one macrophage population (M1 cells) appears to have a distinctly different metabolic program than another population (M2 cells). M1 cells, for example, are easily activated to produce nitric oxide (NO), whereas M2 cells are not—although they do produce ornithine using the enzyme arginase (see Figure 4-1). Because NO inhibits cell replication and ornithine has an opposite effect, it is postulated that they also have differential effects on T helper cells.

One possible clue to the activity of dendritic cell subsets may lie in the fact that they possess different toll-like receptors (TLRs) (Chapter 2). Thus TLR4 is expressed on myeloid dendritic cells, and TLR9 is expressed on lymphoid dendritic cells. As a result the TLR4+ population responds to lipopolysaccharides, whereas the

TLR9+ population responds to CpG DNA. Stimulation of TLR4 or TLR9 induces IL-12 production and expression of costimulatory molecules such as CD40. Likewise, different TLRs employ different signal-transducing pathways. TLR3, for example, uses a different signaling pathway than TLR4. It is possible that the differences lie in the signal transduction pathways used.

It may be that the same DC can promote either a Th1 or Th2 response, depending on the dose and type of antigen. The response may also depend on the environment of the DCs when they encounter the antigen. For example, DCs from the intestine or airways seem to preferentially secrete IL-4 and thus promote Th2 responses. In those cases, perhaps the intestinal microenvironment provides the Th2-polarizing signals.

Other Dendritic Cell Populations

Thymic Dendritic Cells

A specialized population of dendritic cells found in the thymus may recognize and kill self-reactive T cells and induce unresponsiveness in immature T cells (Chapter 18). Some of these cells may express CD95L (CD178) and so stimulate apoptosis in T cells. These dendritic cells may arise from a lymphoid precursor since their production is driven by IL-3 and they lack myeloid cell markers. These thymic dendritic cells have a very short life span.

Follicular Dendritic Cells

These cells are found in lymphoid follicles in the B cell areas of lymphoid tissues. They are a specialized population of dendritic cells used to trigger B cells.

Follicular dendritic cells present antigens in two different ways. In an unprimed animal (that is, an animal that has not previously been exposed to the antigen) antigen presentation is a passive process. The dendritic cells simply provide a surface on which antigen can be presented. In animals that have previously been exposed to an antigen and so possess antibodies, the antigen and antibody combine to form antibody-antigen complexes (also called immune-complexes). Follicular dendritic cells take up these immune complexes on their surface and then shed them in round beaded structures from their processes. These cell fragments called exosomes are taken up by B cells. The B cells ingest the antigen and, after processing, they present it to antigen-sensitive T cells. Follicular dendritic cells can retain antigens on their surface for more than 3 months.

Interferon-Producing Dendritic Cells

The type I interferons (IFN-α and IFN–β) have long been known to be produced by white blood cells. However, only recently has the source of these cytokines been shown to be dendritic cells. Although relatively rare in the blood, these cells seem to be able to produce massive amounts of these important cytokines. Their numbers increase during infection. It is possible that these cells serve as a form of early warning system for viral infections since they are rapidly turned on by microbial DNA.

DENDRITIC CELLS IN DOMESTIC ANIMALS

Pigs

Dendritic cells derived from pig bone marrow can be generated by culture using GM-CSF plus TNF-α. Monocyte-derived dendritic cells can also be generated by growing these cells in the presence of GM-CSF and interleukin 4. Both types of dendritic cells are SWC3+, CD1+, CD80/86+, CD14+, and CD16+.

Dogs

Dendritic cells derived from canine bone marrow can be generated by exposure to GM-CSF and TNF-α. There are two main populations of DC in the dog. One is MHC class II+, CD34+, CD14–; the other is MHC class II+, CD34+, CD14+.

Cats

Feline Langerhans cells are CD18+, MHC class II+, CD1a+, and CD4+. They also contain the Birbeck granules characteristic of these cells. Dendritic cells obtained from feline blood mononuclear cells are CD1+, CD14+, and MHC classes I and II+.

Cattle

Bovine dendritic cells express not only the normal costimulatory molecules CD80, CD86, and CD40 (Figure 6-9) but also other molecules restricted to the bovine. These include the ligand to CD47, called MyD-1 (CD172a), a molecule that mediates binding to T cells and augments intracellular signaling by dendritic cells. CD26 found on a subset of bovine dendritic cells is also costimulatory for lymphocytes. Analysis of the dendritic cells in bovine afferent lymph shows the presence of two major subpopulations that differ in their ability to stimulate CD4 and CD8 T cells. One population synthesized more IL-12, whereas the other population produced more IL-1 and IL-10; these are likely to represent DC1 and DC2 subpopulations, respectively.

Sheep

Ovine dendritic cells have been derived from peripheral blood monocytes; they are MHC class II+, CD11c+, CD14–. Sheep DCs show high levels of endocytosis and are able to present antigens to CD4+ T cells.

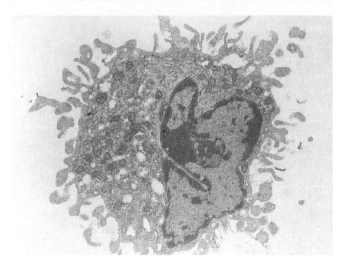

Figure 6-9. A transmission electron micrograph of a dendritic cell from bovine afferent lymph. It has been stained with a monoclonal antibody specific for bovine CD1b. (The antibody is linked to colloidal gold particles, which are visible as small, electron dense dots around the outside of the cell.) (Courtesy Dr. CJ Howard and Dr. P Bland, Institute for Animal Health, Compton, UK.)

Horses

Dendritic cells have been isolated from horse blood; these are MHC class II+, CD11+, EqWC1+, and EqWC2+. They do not express any T or B cell markers but do express antigens also found in macrophages. Langerhans cells have been described in horses.

OTHER ANTIGEN-PROCESSING CELLS

Naive T cells can bind to dendritic cells and divide in response to antigens. Once activated, these T cells gain the ability to respond to antigens presented by macrophages or B cells. Thus naive T cells first respond only to dendritic cells. Once activated, they become responsive to macrophages and B cells. The type of antigen-processing cell employed thus depends on whether the body has been exposed to an antigen previously.

Macrophages

Antigen processing by macrophages is inefficient, since much of the ingested antigen is destroyed by lysosomal proteases and oxidants. Indeed, macrophages and B cells can be considered to be cells with other priorities (some call them "semi-professional" antigen-processing cells). Macrophages are the most accessible and best understood of the antigen-processing cells. Their properties have been described in Chapter 4. Once antigens are taken up by macrophages, a portion is processed and presented to sensitized T cells.

B Cells

B cells are also antigen-processing cells and have receptors that can bind whole antigen molecules. They then ingest and process antigens before presenting them, in association with MHC class II molecules, to sensitized T cells. B cells probably play a very minor role in antigen processing for the primary immune response but a much more significant one for the secondary response when their numbers have increased.

Other Cells

It has been generally believed that only the "professional" antigen-processing cells are capable of stimulating T cell responses, since only these professional cells can load antigen fragments on their surfaces and provide the correct costimulatory signals. However, T cells may be activated by a variety of other "nonprofessional" cell types. These include neutrophils, eosinophils, T cells, endothelial cells, fibroblasts, natural killer cells, smooth muscle cells, astrocytes, microglial cells, and some epithelial cells such as thymic epithelial cells and corneal cells. Their effectiveness may depend on the local environment. Thus fibroblasts can be very effective antigen-processing cells when located within lymphoid organs. Presumably costimulation can come from other nearby cells in this cytokine-rich environment. Vascular endothelial cells can also take up antigens, synthesize IL-1, and under the influence of interferon-γ, express MHC class II molecules on their surface. Even skin keratinocytes can secrete cytokines similar to IL-1, express MHC class II molecules, and present antigen to T cells. In pigs, a subpopulation of circulating γδ T cells can act as professional antigen-processing cells. These cells can recognize antigens directly and present them to helper T cells via MHC class II.

PROCESSING OF EXOGENOUS ANTIGEN

The presentation of exogenous antigen is mediated through MHC class II molecules. Although many cells can phagocytose foreign particles, only those that express MHC class II molecules can process this material in such a way that it can stimulate an immune response. The most efficient antigen-processing cells are thus mature MHC II+ dendritic cells. Unlike those in macrophages, dendritic cell lysosomes have limited proteolytic activity and do not degrade internalized antigens rapidly. As a result, antigens may persist for extended periods within dendritic cells. The MHC class II molecules can bind fragments of these ingested molecules and present them to helper T cells (Figure 6-10). Helper T cells can recognize a foreign antigen and respond to it only if it is bound to an MHC class II molecule. If an antigen is

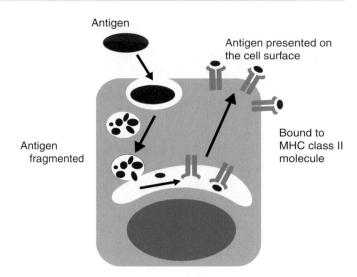

Figure 6-10. The processing of exogenous antigen by macrophages. This involves proteolytic digestion and linkage to a MHC class II antigen for presentation to a helper T cell.

presented to T cells without being linked to an MHC class II molecule, the T cells may be turned off or die, and tolerance may result (Chapter 18).

Multiple steps occur in exogenous antigen processing. First, the antigen must be phagocytosed and taken into the phagosome. The phagosome then fuses with granules (lysosomes) containing proteases. Ingested peptides are broken down by these proteases into fragments of varying length. The endosomes containing these peptide fragments then fuse with other endosomes carrying newly synthesized MHC class II molecules.

MHC class II chains are translocated to the endoplasmic reticulum, where they are assembled into a large complex together with a peptide called the invariant chain (Ii) or γ chain. This complex travels to an endocytic compartment, where the invariant chain molecules are proteolytically digested, leaving a small peptide called class II–associated Ii Peptide (CLIP), which remains associated with the MHC molecule. The CLIP chains occupy the antigen-binding site of the MHC molecule. The antigen peptides are then exchanged for CLIP. The presence of the CLIP chains prevents the MHC class II molecule from being transported to the cell surface as soon as it is made. Thus, unlike most transmembrane proteins that are expressed minutes after assembly, MHC class II molecules are retained inside the cell for several hours. The CLIP chain redirects the MHC molecule to endosomes, where it can associate with antigen fragments.

Once the antigen fragment and MHC molecule have combined, they move toward the cell surface in a vesicle. The MHC antigen-binding sites can hold a peptide of 12 to 24 amino acids as a straight, extended chain that projects out of both ends of the binding site. Side chains from the peptide bind in pockets on the walls of the binding site. Once they reach the cell surface, the vesicle fuses with the cell membrane and the MHC-peptide complex is presented on the cell surface.

It has been calculated that an antigen-processing cell carries about 2×10^5 MHC class II molecules that are capable of presenting antigen fragments to T cells. If costimulation is provided, a T cell can be activated by exposure to 200 to 300 peptide-MHC complexes; therefore it is possible for one antigen-processing cell to present many different antigens simultaneously.

Since the helper T cells must be stimulated in order for most immune responses to occur, the MHC class II molecules effectively determine whether or not an immune response will occur in response to any antigen. Class II molecules specifically bind some, but not all, peptides created during antigen processing, thereby selecting the epitopes that are to be presented to T cells. (Further coverage of MHC molecules is provided in Chapter 7.)

PROCESSING OF ENDOGENOUS ANTIGEN

As previously pointed out, some of the antigens that trigger an immune response originate within the body's own cells. These are called endogenous antigens; examples include the new proteins made by virus-infected cells. These proteins are handled in a different manner than exogenous antigens: after being chopped up by proteases, their fragments are bound to MHC class Ia molecules and carried to the cell surface. Peptides bound to MHC class Ia molecules can then be recognized by lymphocytes called cytotoxic T cells, not by helper T cells. These cytotoxic T cells respond to antigens by destroying

virus-infected cells. The key difference lies in the nature of the MHC molecules used to present the antigen to the T cells.

One function of the T cell–mediated immune response is the identification and destruction of cells producing abnormal or foreign proteins. The best examples of such cells are those infected by viruses. Viruses take over the protein-synthesizing machinery of the cell and use it to make new viral proteins (Figure 6-11). To control infection, cytotoxic T cells must respond to the viral proteins expressed on the surface of infected cells. They will respond to these proteins only if they are processed and their fragments bound to a binding site on an MHC class Ia molecule. Cytotoxic T cells recognize protein-MHC class Ia complexes. This can be demonstrated experimentally by showing that cytotoxic T cells will destroy virus-infected target cells only if the T cells can recognize the MHC class Ia molecules on the target cell (Chapter 10). These cells are thus said to be MHC-restricted.

The MHC class Ia α chain is folded in such a way that a large antigen-binding site is formed on its outermost surface (see Figures 7-5 and 7-6). This binding site, however, differs from that on class II molecules in that it is closed at each end with deep pockets. As a result, bound peptides cannot project out of the ends of the site. Because the binding site is closed at each end, MHC class Ia molecules can only bind peptides containing nine amino acids. Indeed, in order to do this, these peptides must bulge out in the middle. Overall, however, the antigen-binding sites on class II and class Ia molecules function in a very similar manner.

The processing of endogenous peptides is very different from that associated with class II molecules. Living cells

Figure 6-11. The processing of endogenous antigen. Newly synthesized proteins are sampled by attachment to MHC class I molecules and carried to the cell surface where they encounter cytotoxic T cells.

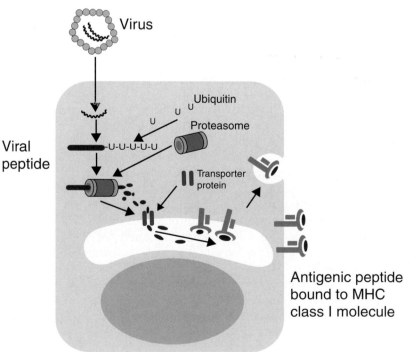

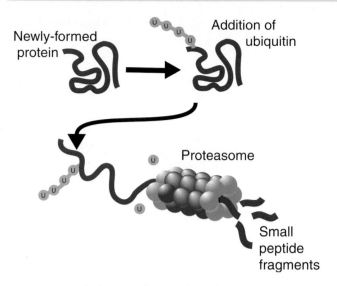

Newly-formed protein

Addition of ubiquitin

Proteasome

Small peptide fragments

Figure 6-12. A diagram showing how the proteasome acts as a powerful protease. Ubiquinated proteins are fed into its central channel, where they are cut into small peptides.

continually break down and recycle proteins. As a result, abnormal proteins are removed, regulatory peptides are not allowed to accumulate, and amino acids are made available for other purposes. As a first step, the protein molecules to be recycled are linked to ubiquitin, a small stable protein found in all eukaryote cells (Figure 6-12). Usually a chain of at least four ubiquitin molecules is added to the target protein-like beads on a string. Ubiquinated proteins are marked for destruction. The ubiquitin chains are then recognized by a large enzyme complex called a proteasome. Proteasomes are tubular structures consisting of an inner cylinder and two outer rings. Ubiquinated proteins bind to an outer ring. This unfolds the protein, releases the ubiquitin for reuse, and passes the peptide chain into the cylinder, where it is broken into fragments between 8 and 15 amino acids long (like a meat grinder). The activity of proteasomes is regulated by cytokines such as IFN-γ.

Most of these fragmented peptides are recycled into new proteins. For about one in a million molecules, however, the peptides are rescued from further breakdown by attachment to transporter proteins. Two transporter proteins have been identified—TAP-1 and TAP-2 (*TAP* standing for "*t*ransporter for *a*ntigen *p*rocessing"). TAP-1 and TAP-2 select the peptides and carry them from the cytoplasm, across the endoplasmic reticulum, into its lumen. Here the peptides are attacked by an aminopeptidase, which shortens them, one amino acid at a time, until they are completely degraded—unless an intermediate, 9-amino-acid-peptide precisely fits the binding site on an empty MHC class I molecule. In this case, degradation stops and the MHC-peptide complexes are carried to the cell surface, where they are displayed for many hours.

A cell can express about 10^6 MHC-peptide complexes, and about 200 MHC class I molecules loaded with the same viral peptide are required to activate a cytotoxic T cell. Thus the MHC-peptide complexes provide fairly complete information on virtually all the proteins being made by a cell. Cytotoxic T cells can screen these peptides to determine whether any are "foreign" and bind to their TCRs.

Cross-Priming

Although it is usual for the two antigen-processing pathways to remain completely separate, under some circumstances exogenous antigens may enter the cytoplasm, join the endogenous antigen pathway, and be presented on MHC class Ia molecules. Thus in antigen-presenting cells such as macrophages and dendritic cells, endocytosed viral antigen can be transported from the phagosomes into the cytoplasm where it is degraded by proteasomes and processed as an endogenous antigen. This antigen thus becomes associated with MHC class Ia molecules and is recognized by cytotoxic T cells. This may be important in immunity to viruses, since it implies that the antigens from dead virions may still be able to trigger a response by cytotoxic T cells (Chapter 17). In general, however, cells that ingest an antigen through phagocytosis present it through MHC I–associated pathways.

HISTIOCYTOSIS AND HISTIOCYTOMAS

Domestic animals suffer from several diseases in which macrophage or dendritic cells proliferate excessively. These are called histiocytomas or histiocytosis. Histiocytomas are common in the dog but rare in goats and cattle. Their occurrence in cats is debated. Langerhans cell histiocytosis is a reactive lesion whose trigger is unknown but may be an infectious agent. This condition is not premalignant, and it may occur in a cutaneous or systemic form. Both forms of Langerhans cell histiocytosis present with lesions in the skin or subcutis, but systemic histiocytosis also involves other tissues. Cutaneous histiocytosis shows no breed predilection, occurs in adult dogs between 3 and 9 years old, and is characterized by the development of nonpainful solitary or multiple nodules in the skin or subcutis. These lesions tend to occur on the head, neck, extremities, perineum, and scrotum. In contrast, systemic histiocytosis tends to occur in large breeds such as Bernese Mountain dogs, Rottweilers, Golden Retrievers and Labradors. Its age of onset is between 4 and 7 years. The lesions develop in the skin, mucus membranes, eyes, nasal cavity, spleen, lung, liver, bone marrow, and spinal cord. Histologically these lesions are characterized by containing a mixture of cells. Phenotyping of both types of lesion shows the following: CD1+, CD11c+, MHC II+, CD4+, CD90+, a phenotype typical of Langerhans cells.

The lesions also contain T cells and neutrophils and may be successfully treated with corticosteroids, cyclosporine, or leflunomide. As many as 30% of cutaneous cases and 10% of systemic cases spontaneously regress.

SOURCES OF ADDITIONAL INFORMATION

Banchereau J, Steinman RM: Dendritic cells and the control of immunity, *Nature* 392:245-252, 1998.

Chan SS, McConnell I, Blacklaws BA: Generation and characterization of ovine dendritic cells derived from peripheral blood monocytes, *Immunology* 107:366-372, 2002.

Cresswell P, Lanzavecchia A: Antigen processing and recognition, *Curr Opin Immunol* 13:11-12, 2001.

Ebner S, Hofer S, Nguyen V, et al: A novel role for IL-3: human monocytes cultured in the presence of IL-3 and IL-4 differentiate into dendritic cells that produce less IL-12 and shift Th cell responses toward a Th2 cytokine pattern, *J Immunol* 168:6199-6207, 2002.

Geijtenbeek TBH, Engering A, van Kooyk Y: DC-SIGN, a C-type lectin on dendritic cells that unveils many aspects of dendritic cell biology, *J Leukocyte Biol* 71:921-923, 2002.

Goldberg AL, Rock KL: Proteolysis, proteasomes and antigen presentation, *Nature* 357:375-379, 1992.

Grusby MJ, Auchincloss H, Lee R, et al: Mice lacking major histocompatibility complex class I and class II molecules, *Proc Natl Acad Sci USA* 90:3913-3917, 1993.

Guagliardi LE, Koppelman B, Blum JS, et al: Co-localization of molecules involved in antigen processing and presentation in an early endocytic compartment, *Nature* 343:133-139, 1990.

Hämmerling GJ, Moreno J: The function of the invariant chain in antigen presentation by MHC class II molecules, *Immunol Today* 11:337-339, 1990.

Hart DNJ: Dendritic cells: unique leukocyte populations which control the primary immune response, *Blood* 90:3245-3287, 1997.

Johansson E, Domeika K, Berg M, et al: Characterization of porcine monocyte-derived dendritic cells according to their cytokine profile, *Vet Immunol Immunopathol* 91:183-197, 2003.

Loss GE, Sant AJ: Invariant chain retains MHC class II molecules in the endocytic pathway, *J Immunol* 150: 3187-3197, 1993.

Monaco JJ: A molecular model of MHC class I-restricted antigen processing, *Immunol Today* 13:173-179, 1992.

Mouritsen S, Meldal M, Werdelin O, et al: MHC molecules protect T cell epitopes against proteolytic destruction, *J Immunol* 149:1987-1993, 1992.

Neefjes JJ, Ploegh HL: Intracellular transport of MHC class II molecules, *Immunol Today* 13:179-183, 1992.

Peters JH, Gieseler B, Thiele B, Steinbach F: Dendritic cells: from ontogenetic orphans to myelomonocytic descendants, *Immunol Today* 17:273-278, 1996.

Porcelli SA, Segelke BW, Sugita M, Wilson IA, et al: The CD1 family of lipid antigen-presenting molecules, *Immunol Today* 19:362-367, 1998.

Rammensee HG: Survival of the fitters, *Nature* 419:443-445, 2002.

Saint-Andre MI, Dezitter-Dambuyant C, Willett BJ, et al: Immunophenotypic characterization of feline Langerhans cells, *Vet Immunol Immunopathol* 58:1-16, 1997.

Shortman K, Caux C: Dendritic cell development: multiple pathways to nature's adjuvants, *Stem Cells* 15:409-419, 1997.

Siedek E, Little S, Mayall S, Edington N, et al: Isolation and characterization of equine dendritic cells, *Vet Immunol Immunopathol* 60:15-31, 1997.

Watts C: Capture and processing of exogenous antigens for presentation on MHC molecules, *Annu Rev Immunol* 15: 821-850, 1997.

Wilkinson KD: Unchaining the condemned, *Nature* 419: 351-353, 2002.

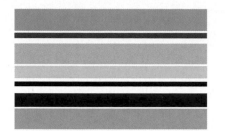

Acquired Immunity: Antigen-Presenting Receptors

CHAPTER 7

In order to trigger an acquired immune response, not only must antigen molecules be broken up inside cells, but the antigen fragments generated must also then be bound to an appropriate antigen-presenting receptor (Figure 7-1). These antigen-presenting receptors are called histocompatibility molecules (or histocompatibility antigens). They are specialized receptor glycoproteins coded for by genes located in a gene cluster called the major histocompatibility complex (MHC). The receptors are therefore called MHC molecules. Antigen fragments can only trigger an immune response if they are bound to MHC molecules. This requirement is called MHC restriction. The genes in the MHC determine which MHC molecules an individual animal can produce. Since the MHC molecules serve as specific antigen receptors, MHC genes also determine which antigens can be presented to the cells of the immune system. Thus the MHC can be considered an organized cluster of genes that control antigen presentation. The MHC genes therefore regulate infectious or autoimmune disease resistance or susceptibility.

MAJOR HISTOCOMPATIBILITY COMPLEX

All vertebrates, from cartilaginous fish to mammals, possess MHC genes, and such genes are almost always maintained in the genome as a linked cluster or gene complex. This gene complex can be very large. For example, the human MHC is about four megabases (mb) in size, which is about the same size as the total genome of the bacterium *Escherichia coli*.

Each MHC consists of three distinct classes of gene loci (Figure 7-2). Class I loci code for MHC molecules found on the surface of most nucleated cells. These class I loci can be classified into those that are highly polymorphic (class Ia loci) and those that show very little polymorphism (class Ib, Ic, or Id loci). (Polymorphism refers to structural variations between proteins.) Class Id loci are located outside the MHC on a different chromosome. Class II loci, on the other hand, code for polymorphic MHC molecules found only on the surface of the professional antigen-presenting cells (dendritic cells, macrophages, and B cells) (Table 7-1). MHC class III loci code for many different proteins with a variety of functions, many of which are linked to innate immunity. For example, the class III loci contain genes coding for complement proteins.

Each MHC contains all three classes of loci, although their number and arrangement vary. The collective name given to the proteins encoded by these MHC genes also depends on the species. In humans these molecules are called human leukocyte antigens (HLA); in dogs they are called DLA; in rabbits, RLA; in cattle (bovines), BoLA; in horses, ELA; in swine, SLA; and so forth. In some species, histocompatibility molecules were identified as blood group antigens before their true function was recognized. In these cases, the nomenclature is anomalous. Thus, in the mouse the MHC is called H-2 and in chickens it is called B. The complete set of alleles found within an animal's MHC is called its MHC haplotype.

MHC CLASS Ia MOLECULES

Class Ia molecules are expressed on the surface of most nucleated cells. They are found in highest concentration on lymphocytes and macrophages. In pigs, for example,

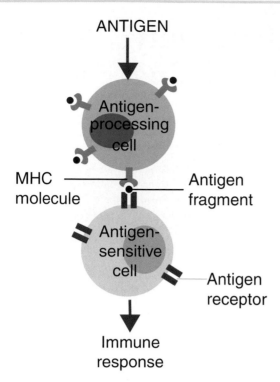

Figure 7-1. The key initial step in any immune response is the presentation of antigens by antigen-processing cells to antigen-sensitive cells. This step is performed by MHC molecules located on the surface of antigen-processing cells.

class I molecules have been detected on lymphocytes, platelets, granulocytes, hepatocytes, kidney cells, and sperm. They are not found on human red blood cells but are present on mouse red blood cells. They are not found on gametes, neurons, or placental trophoblast cells. Some cells, such as myocardium and skeletal muscle, express very few class Ia molecules.

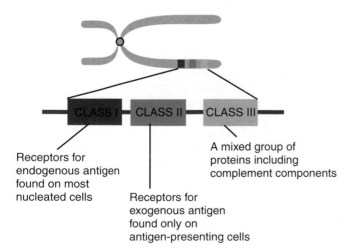

Figure 7-2. The three major classes of genes located within the major histocompatibility complex: distribution and functions.

TABLE 7-1		
A Comparison of MHC Class I and Class II Structure		
	Class I	**Class II**
Loci include	Typically A, B, and C	DP, DQ, and DR
Distribution	Most nucleated cells	B cells, macrophages, and dendritic cells
Function	Present antigen to cytotoxic T cells	Present antigen to T helper cells
Result	T-cell-mediated toxicity	T-cell-mediated help

Structure

All class Ia molecules are heterodimers consisting of two linked glycoprotein chains. An α chain (45 kDa) is associated with a much smaller chain called β_2-microglobulin ($\beta_2 M$) (12 kDa). The α chain is inserted in the lipid bilayer of the cell surface (Figure 7-3). It consists of five domains: three extracellular domains called α_1, α_2, and α_3, each about 100 amino acids long, a transmembrane domain, and a cytoplasmic domain. The antigen-binding site on a class Ia molecule is formed by the folding of the α_1 and α_2 domains. $\beta_2 M$ consists of a single extracellular domain and probably serves to stabilize the structure.

Gene Arrangement

The total number of class I loci varies greatly between mammals. For example, rats have more than 60, mice about 30, humans 20, cattle 13 to 15, and pigs have 11. Despite these numbers, not all of these loci are functional and code for a cell surface protein. For example, in mice, only two or three class Ia genes are expressed. Most of the remainder are clearly pseudogenes (defective genes that cannot be expressed). In humans the functional loci are called *A*, *B*, and *C*. In mice they are called *K* and *D* (and in some strains, *L*) (Figure 7-4). In other species they are usually numbered.

Polymorphism

Some of the class Ia gene loci code have a large number of alleles. These allelic differences cause variations in the amino acid sequences of the α_1 and α_2 domains. This

---

BOX 7–1

Dr. Peter Doherty

Peter Doherty, an Australian veterinarian, won the 1996 Nobel Prize for Medicine for his studies on the function of the MHC. He and his colleague, Rolf Zinkernagel, were the first to show the phenomenon of MHC restriction. They went on to suggest that MHC polymorphism was a device used to enable vertebrates to respond successfully to a vast variety of microbial antigens. This suggestion proved to be correct.

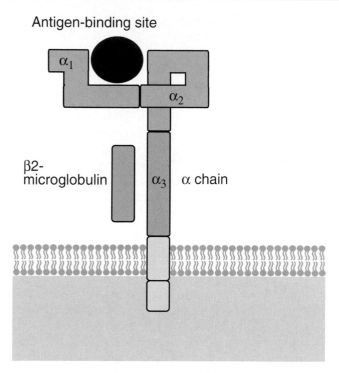

Figure 7-3. Diagram showing the structure of a class Ia MHC molecule on a cell membrane. Its antigen-binding site is formed by the folding of its α_1 and α_2 domains.

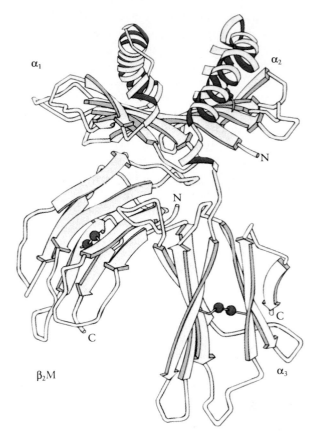

Figure 7-5. Schematic three-dimensional view of the complete structure of HLA-A2 derived by x-ray crystallography. The antigen-binding groove at the top is formed by the α_1 and α_2 domains, whereas the α_3 domain binds to the cell membrane. The β chain (β_2-microglobulin) has no direct role in antigen binding. (From *Nature* 320:506, 1987. Macmillan Magazines Ltd.)

variation is called polymorphism. The polymorphism is restricted to three to four discrete regions within the α_1 and α_2 domains. These are called variable regions. Usually two or three different amino acids may occur at each position and one is usually predominant. The other domains of MHC class Ia molecules are highly conserved and show little sequence variation.

Structural analysis of MHC class Ia molecules has shown that their α_1 and α_2 domains are folded together to form an open-ended groove (Figure 7-5). A flat β sheet forms the floor of this groove, whereas its walls are formed by two α helices (Figure 7-6). This groove is the site where antigen fragments are bound. The variable sequences are located along the walls of this groove and so determine its shape. The shape of the groove determines which fragments can be bound and so determines the ability of an animal to respond to any specific antigen.

The amino acid variability within the α_1 and α_2 domains is a result of nucleotide sequence variability in MHC alleles. The nucleotide variability is a result of

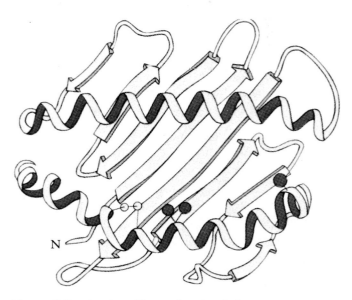

Figure 7-6. A view (from above) of the antigen-binding groove on a MHC class I molecule. The floor of the groove is formed by an extensive β-pleated sheet. The walls of the groove are formed by two parallel α helices. This structure is formed by the folding of the α_1 and α_2 domain of the α chain. (From *Nature* 320:506, 1987. Macmillan Magazines Ltd.)

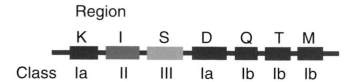

Figure 7-4. Arrangement of genes within the MHC of the mouse; -, a typical mammalian MHC.

point mutations, reciprocal recombination, and gene conversion. Point mutations are simply changes in individual nucleotides. Reciprocal recombination involves crossing over between two chromosomes. In gene conversion, small blocks of genetic material are exchanged between different class I genes in a nonreciprocal fashion. The donated blocks may be derived from nonpolymorphic class I genes or from nonfunctional pseudogenes as well as from other polymorphic class I genes. Because of these processes, MHC genes are unusually variable and have the highest mutation rate of any germ-line genes yet studied (10^{-3} mutations per gene per generation in mice). This high mutation rate does not occur by chance and implies that there must be significant advantages to be gained by having very polymorphic MHC genes.

NONPOLYMORPHIC MHC CLASS I MOLECULES

In addition to the highly polymorphic MHC class Ia molecules, mammalian cells express many nonpolymorphic class I molecules. Some are coded for by genes within the MHC, others by genes located on other chromosomes. Because of their diversity, they have proved difficult to classify. One suggested method is to classify them based on their evolutionary origin.

For example, class Ib molecules show reduced expression and tissue distribution compared to class Ia molecules, but they form part of the MHC complex. They have limited polymorphism and probably originated from class Ia precursors by gene duplication. For example, the class Ib gene loci in mice are found in three clusters called Q, T, and M (see Figure 7-4). They code for proteins found on the surface of regulatory and immature lymphocytes and on hematopoietic cells. These proteins consist of a membrane-bound α chain (44 kDa) associated with β_2-microglobulin. Their shape is similar to that of class Ia molecules and they have an antigen-binding groove. As a result of their lack of polymorphism, MHC class Ib molecules bind to a limited range of peptides or other small molecules. Nevertheless, they act as receptors for specific, commonly encountered, microbial antigens. For example, the mouse MHC class Ib molecule called M3 binds specifically to exogenously processed peptides that have an N-formylmethionine residue at their amino terminus.

Class Ic genes are low-polymorphic MHC molecules found in or close to the MHC but probably originated before the radiation of the placental mammals. This group includes MICA and MICB, specialized molecules that are involved in communicating to T and natural killer cells but do not bind antigenic peptides. They also include genes coding for olfactory receptors.

Class Id genes are class I–related genes not found on the MHC chromosome. They are nonpolymorphic and diverged before the mammalian radiations. In general these show a restricted pattern of tissue expression. Many of these molecules contribute to innate immunity, since they interact with pathogen-associated molecular patterns, including N-formylated peptides and glycolipids. For example, CD1 molecules recognize bacterial lipid antigens including mycolic acids and glycolipids from mycobacteria. FcRn is a class Id MHC molecule that serves as an antibody (Fc) receptor on epithelial cells. It is expressed on mammary gland epithelium and on the enterocytes of newborn mammals (Chapter 19). FcRn binds to antibodies taken in with the mother's milk and transfers them to the bloodstream. It does not have an obvious antigen-binding groove.

MHC CLASS II MOLECULES

Mammals differ in the way they express their MHC class II molecules. In rodents, they are found constitutively on the professional antigen-presenting cells (dendritic cells, macrophages, and B cells) and can be induced on T cells, keratinocytes, and vascular endothelial cells. Resting mouse T cells do not express MHC class II molecules, but in pigs, dogs, cats, mink, and horses the MHC class II products are constitutively expressed on nearly all resting adult T cells. In rabbits, MHC class II molecules are also expressed on granulocytes. In cattle, most MHC class II molecules are expressed only on B cells and activated T cells. However, one unique BoLA class II molecule (H42A) is found on thymic epithelial cells and professional antigen-presenting cells. In pigs, resting T cells express MHC class II molecules at about the same level as macrophages. They are also present on boar sperm in low concentrations. In humans and pigs large amounts of MHC class II molecules are expressed on renal vascular endothelium and glomeruli—a fact of significance in kidney graft rejection. The expression of class II molecules on the cell surface is enhanced in rapidly dividing cells and in cells treated with interferon (Chapter 30).

Structure

MHC Class II molecules consist of two non-covalently linked chains called α (31 to 34 kDa) and β (25 to 29 kDa). Each chain has two extracellular domains, a connecting peptide, a transmembrane domain, and a cytoplasmic domain (Figure 7-7). A third protein chain, called the Ii or γ chain, is associated with intracellular class II molecules and was discussed in Chapter 6.

Gene Arrangement

Within the MHC class II region there are six loci arranged in order: DP, DOA, DM, DOB, DQ, and DR. Within each locus, the genes for the α chains are designated A, whereas the genes for the β chains are called B.

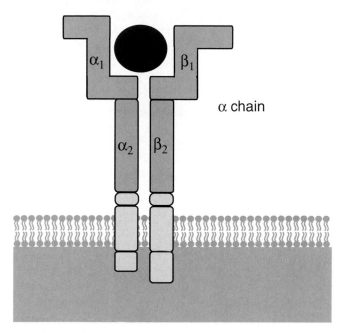

Antigen-binding site

α chain

Figure 7-7. Diagram showing the structure of a MHC class II antigen located on a cell surface. Note that the antigen-binding site is formed by both peptide chains.

Not all loci contain genes for both chains, and some contain many pseudogenes. These pseudogenes may serve as donors of nucleotide sequences that can be used to generate additional class II polymorphisms.

Polymorphism

The classical MHC class II molecules, DP, DQ and DR, have an antigen-binding groove formed by their α_1 and β_1 domains. The groove has a similar structure to that seen in class Ia molecules. Thus its walls are formed by two parallel α helices and its floor consists of a β sheet. Polymorphism results from variations in the amino acid sequences of the α helices at the sides of the groove. These are generated in a similar fashion to those in class Ia molecules. The DO and DM loci code for nonpolymorphic molecules, whose function is to regulate the loading of antigen fragments onto the antigen-binding groove. Some of the other molecules encoded by genes

in the class II region are involved in the antigen-presentation pathway. These include the transporter proteins TAP1 and TAP2 and some proteasesome components. These loci are located between DM and DOB.

MHC CLASS III MOLECULES

The remaining genes located within the major histocompatibility complex are lumped together as class III genes (Figure 7-8). They code for proteins with many different functions. Some of these proteins are involved in the defense of the body. For example, there are at least four genes for complement components: two for C4 and one each for factor B and C2 (Chapter 15). In addition, there are genes that code for the enzyme 21-hydroxylase involved in steroid synthesis, for cytochrome P450, for tumor necrosis factor (TNF-α), for several lymphotoxins, for some NK cell receptors, and for several heat-shock proteins (HSP).

MHC OF DOMESTIC ANIMALS

Every mammal studied has an MHC containing class I, class II, and class III genes. When the MHCs of different mammals are compared, some regions appear to be well conserved whereas others are highly variable. Likewise, the precise arrangement and number of loci varies among species (Figure 7-9). In general the class II and class III genes are orthologous. That is, they are clearly derived from a single ancestor and have not usually been subjected to major rearrangements during evolution (ruminant class II genes are an exception). Class I genes, in contrast, have been reorganized so many different times by deletion and duplication that their amino acid sequences differ widely. As a result, it is very difficult to compare class I genes in different species and they are said to be paralogous. Indeed, class I genes are more closely related within a species than between species. Nevertheless, the overall molecular structure and function of MHC molecules in the domestic mammals does not appear to differ significantly.

In cattle, the BoLA class II region is unique in that inversion of a large chromosome segment has moved several class II genes close to the centromere of bovine

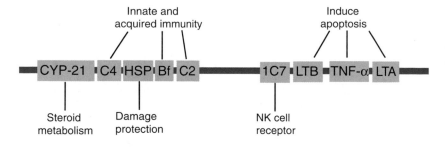

Figure 7-8. The arrangement of selected genes within the MHC class III region. These genes were selected because their functions are related to innate and acquired immunity. There are many other genes in this region that have no apparent role in immunity.

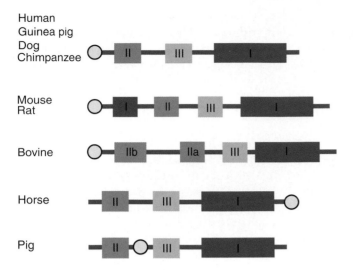

Figure 7-9. Arrangement of gene regions within the MHC in different species of domestic animals.

chromosome 23. Thus the BoLA class II is divided into two distinct regions, IIa and IIb, where the class IIb genes are separated from the classical class I/class IIa genes by a "gap" of 17 centimorgans (cM) (Figure 7-10). Cattle , sheep, and goats possess ruminant-specific class II genes (DY and DI) instead of DP. Another important feature of the BoLA system is that although they possess at least four class Ia loci, none is consistently expressed. Analysis of their haplotypes shows that any combination of one, two, or three class I genes may be expressed. Similar variations in haplotypes occur with *DQ* genes. Sheep and white-tailed deer MHCs are similar to those in cattle.

In the horse, the ELA complex is of conventional structure but its sequence is reversed in relation to the centromere (Figure 7-11). It is located on chromosome 20.

In the pig, the SLA complex (Figure 7-12) is located on chromosome 7 and divided by the centromere. The class I and III regions are located on the short arm, and the class II region is located on the long arm. The SLA class I and class II loci are separated by only 1.1 to 1.5 cm,

which means that the pig MHC is the smallest among mammals that have been examined (about 2 mb). Pigs have 11 class Ia genes, but only three are functional although others may be transcribed, and three are clearly pseudogenes. As in cattle, the number of expressed molecules varies between haplotypes. Of the class II genes, some code for *DR* and *DQ* heterodimers but there is no *DP* product. The arrangement of the class III region is similar to that of humans.

In the dog, the DLA complex is located on chromosome 12. It is likely that there are four transcribed class I genes. These are DLA-12, -79, -64, and -88. Only DLA-88 is polymorphic. About 48 DLA-88 alleles have been identified. In the class II region, DRA, DRB, DQA, and –DQB have been identified. To date, 62 DRB1, 21 DQA1, and 48 DQB1 alleles have been reported. Some class II haplotypes appear to be characteristic of certain breeds whereas variations between breeds is great. This high interbreed and low intrabreed variation may account for the variation in breed susceptibility to infectious and autoimmune diseases.

The cat MHC is intermediate in size between mouse and human and is located on chromosome B2. Its class I region appears to contain only one functional polymorphic locus. Its class II region has no functional *DP* genes and its DQ region has been deleted (a feature seen only in the cat). In compensation, it has a highly polymorphic DR locus with at least two *DRB* genes and 24 alleles and three *DRA* genes.

In humans there are three class Ia loci, A, B, and C, and at least three functional class Ib loci, E, F, and G. Most Old World primates possess all of these except for C, which is found only in humans, gorillas, and chimpanzees, and G, which is found only in humans. In orangutans and rhesus monkeys, the A and B loci are duplicated. In contrast, the New World primates, such as cotton-top tamarins, have MHC class I genes most closely related to HLA-G. They do not possess any genes related to HLA-A, -B, or -C. In view of the lack of class I MHC diversity in cotton-top tamarins it is perhaps not surprising that they are susceptible to fatal infection with a variety of viruses that are not fatal in humans.

Figure 7-10. Arrangement of genes within the human and bovine MHC. The only major difference is the presence of a large inversion in the bovine that leads to the development of a large space within the bovine class II region.

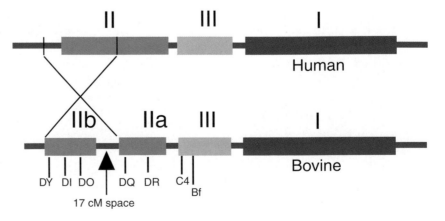

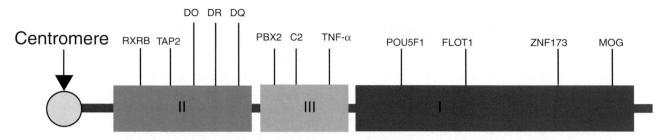

Figure 7-11. Schematic diagram showing the overall structure of the equine MHC (ELA). (Courtesy of Drs. AL Gustafson and L Skow.)

Avian MHC Molecules

The chicken MHC has been fully sequenced. It occupies 92 kb, contains only 19 genes, and so is very much smaller and simpler than mammalian MHCs. It is organized differently with the class III genes located outside the class I and II genes. It is divided into two independent regions designated B and Y. Both are located on microchromosome 16, but they are separated by the nucleolar organizer region (Figure 7-13). The B region contains three gene clusters. The Y region contains two. Each region contains both class I and class II loci. However, these genes differ significantly between birds and mammals. For example, chickens have DM but not DP, DQ, or DR. They also lack most class III region genes. The B region is also organized differently than in mammals. Chickens possess a single dominantly expressed class I gene that determines the immune response to infectious pathogens as a result of its peptide binding specificity. (This is in contrast to most mammals where immune responsiveness is determined by multiple polymorphic genes.) Cluster 1 or the B-F/B-L region contains two class Ia α-chain genes (*B-F*), a *C4* gene, and two class II β-chain genes (*B-L*). There is a single class II α-chain gene located about 5 cM away from the β-chain gene. Two clusters (V and VI) form the *B-G* or class IV region. These encode blood group antigens. The *B-G* gene products are a mixture of membrane proteins with molecular weights ranging from 40 to 48 kDa. These molecules can form monomers, homodimers, and heterodimers and are mainly found on red cells and thrombocytes. Related *B-G* molecules are found at low

levels on lymphocytes and their precursors in the bursa and thymus. Their function is unknown although a mammalian protein found in myelin sheaths called MOG has similarities to *B-G* as does bovine butyrophilin, a protein expressed in the lactating mammary gland. The genes for these two proteins are found close to the MHC in some mammals. There are two gene clusters in the Y region containing two MHC class I and two MHC class II loci. They differ from the B-region loci in that their products are not expressed on red cells. Genes within the Y region also regulate natural killer cell recognition.

MHC MOLECULES AND DISEASE

Class Ia and class II MHC molecules are very polymorphic. As a result, each different MHC molecule will bind a different set of antigenic peptides. The more variety an animal has in its MHC, the more antigens it can respond to. Thus an animal heterozygous at the MHC loci will express more alleles and can bind a greater variety of antigenic peptides than can a homozygous animal (Figure 7-14).

MHC polymorphism is maintained in animal populations by a process called overdominant selection or heterozygote advantage. Simply put, MHC heterozygotes are at an advantage because they can respond to more antigens and so are best fitted to survive infectious diseases. This can be demonstrated by examining the rates of nucleotide substitution in different parts of MHC class Ia and class II genes. In normal proteins the

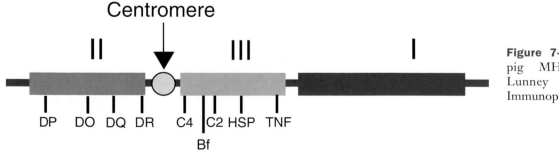

Figure 7-12. Structure of the pig MHC. (Modified from Lunney JK: Vet Immunol Immunopathol 43:19-28, 1994.)

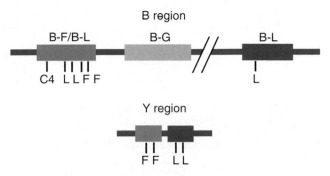

B region

B-F/B-L   B-G   //   B-L

C4 L L F F   L

Y region

F F   L L

Figure 7-13. Structure of the chicken B region (*top*) and the Y region (*bottom*). F genes are class II genes and L genes are class I genes.

rate of silent (or synonymous) substitution greatly exceeds the rates of replacement (or nonsynonymous) substitution. This is because most nonsynonymous substitutions usually have a harmful effect and are eliminated by natural selection. In the polymorphic MHC molecules, however, natural selection has the opposite effect and favors sequence diversity. As a result, in the

Heterozygous

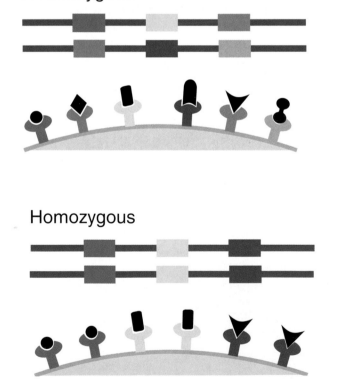

Homozygous

Figure 7-14. Heterozygous animals with two types of MHC molecule coded for at each locus express six different antigen-presenting molecules on the cell surface. Therefore, they generate a more diverse and effective immune response than homozygous animals with only one MHC molecule coded for at each locus. An example of heterozygote advantage.

codons encoding the peptide-binding regions of MHC class Ia and II molecules, the rate of nonsynonymous substitution far exceeds the rate of synonymous substitution. This indicates that MHC polymorphism is maintained by selection processes.

The antigen-binding site of an MHC class Ia or II molecule is also very nonspecific (or degenerate) in that it can bind many different foreign peptides. This is because it binds tightly to the peptide backbone rather than to the amino acid side chains. Nevertheless, structural constraints limit the efficiency of binding of each allele, and one MHC molecule cannot bind all possible peptides. As a result, it is likely that only one or two peptides from an average antigen can bind to any given MHC molecule. The ability of MHC molecules to bind antigens must be a limiting factor in generating acquired immunity and resistance to infectious agents. Increasing the variety of MHC molecules on an individual cell will clearly increase the range of peptides that can be bound and so increase resistance to infections. Because most individuals are MHC heterozygotes, each individual normally expresses at most six different class Ia molecules (in humans, for example, two each are coded for by the HLA-A, -B, and C loci). However, there is a reason why the number of MHC molecules is not larger. Simply put, the presence of more MHC molecules raises the chances that the MHC molecules could bind and present more "self" antigens. This would require the elimination of many more self-reactive T cells during development (Chapter 18). Thus six different MHC class Ia molecules represents a reasonable compromise between maximizing recognition of foreign antigens and minimizing recognition of self-antigens (Figure 7-15).

Some MHC class Ia loci contain highly polymorphic genes that code for very large numbers of alleles. For example, the H-2K locus in the mouse codes for more than 100 alleles. Since there can never be more than two alleles/locus in an individual, it appears that this number of alleles is needed to ensure heterozygosity and maximize polymorphism in a mouse population. One possible reason for this is to protect the population as a whole from disease. Because of MHC polymorphism, most individuals in a population have a unique set of class Ia molecules and each individual can respond to a unique set of antigens. When a new infectious disease strikes, it is likely that at least some individuals in a population will have MHC molecules that can bind the new microbial antigens. These individuals will be able to respond to the agent and become immune. Those that cannot respond will die.

When large populations of humans or mice are examined, no single MHC allele is found to be present at a very high frequency. In other words, no single MHC molecule confers major advantages on an individual. This reflects the futility of the host attempting to match invading organisms in antigenic variability. A microbe will always be able to mutate and evade the immune response

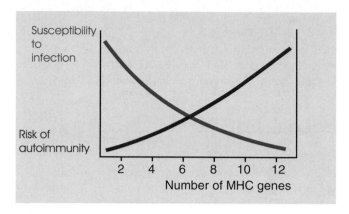

Figure 7-15. The optimal number of MHC genes is a balance between the need to respond to as many different microbial antigens as possible and the need to avoid autoimmune responses. Computer modeling suggests that the optimal number of MHC genes is six.

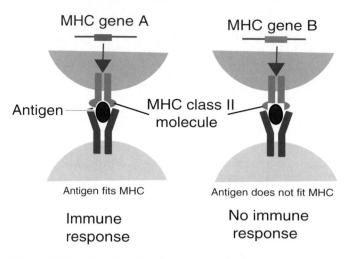

Figure 7-16. MHC molecules regulate the immune response. Only molecules that can bind in the groove of a MHC molecule will trigger an immune response. This is called MHC restriction. Thus the MHC genes that code for these molecules also regulate immune responsiveness.

faster than a mammalian population can develop resistance. Any mutations in an MHC allele, while they may increase resistance to one organism, may at the same time decrease resistance to another. It is more advantageous therefore for each member of a population to possess uniquely different MHC alleles so that any pathogen spreading through a population will have to adapt anew to each individual host.

Highly adaptable social animals, such as humans or mice, with large populations through which disease can spread rapidly, usually show extensive MHC polymorphism. In contrast, low-density solitary species such as the marine mammals (whales and elephant seals), moose, or Asiatic lions, have much less polymorphism. It is also of interest to note the case of the cheetah, which is essentially monomorphic at its class Ia loci as a result of recent population bottlenecks. Because of this lack of MHC diversity, a single lethal infectious disease has the potential to cause the cheetah's extinction. (In fairness, it ought to be pointed out that other investigators claim that the cheetah is not especially genetically impoverished. Indeed, it has been argued that carnivores in general, which live at a low population density, may have less MHC polymorphism than other mammals.)

Since the function of MHC molecules is to present antigens to the cells of the immune system, MHC genes regulate immune responses. A foreign molecule can only stimulate an immune response if it first binds to a MHC molecule. A molecule that cannot bind to the groove of at least one MHC molecule will not stimulate acquired immunity (Figure 7-16). Thus, MHC genes determine susceptibility to diseases in which immune responses have a significant role. These include not only infections but also autoimmune diseases.

There are many examples of relationships between an animal's MHC haplotype and its resistance to infectious disease. For example, in cattle there is an association between possession of certain BoLA alleles and resistance to bovine leukosis, squamous cell eye carcinoma, trypanosomiasis, responsiveness to foot-and-mouth disease virus, and susceptibility to the tick *Boophilus microplus*.

Cows with BoLA-Aw8 are more likely to be seropositive for leukosis, a disease caused by bovine leukemia virus (BLV). Resistance is associated with possession of BoLA-Aw7 and susceptibility is associated with possession of BoLA-Aw12. B-cell proliferation and expression of BLV-induced B-cell tumors are also controlled by BoLA. BoLA-Aw14 seems to influence age at seroconversion whereas BoLA-Aw12 seems to be associated with susceptibility to B-cell proliferation. However, these associations with the BoLA-A locus are relatively weak compared to the association between susceptibility and certain BoLA-DRB alleles such as DRB3. BoLA-DRB3 polymorphism influences resistance or susceptibility to bovine leukemia virus. This resistance is associated with the presence of two amino acids, glutamic acid-arginine, in the antigen-binding site of DRB3 at positions 70 and 71, whereas val-asp-thr-tyr at positions 75 to 78 is associated with susceptibility.

BoLA-A*16 is associated with resistance to mastitis. BoLA-A*6 and BoLA-A*16 are associated with high, and BoLA-A*2 with low, antibody responses to human serum albumin. Disease associations are also seen with class II alleles. Thus possession of BoLA-DRB3.2*23 is associated with an increased incidence of severe coliform mastitis. The DRB3*3 allele is associated with a lower risk of retained placenta, whereas *6 and *22 are associated with a lower risk of cystic ovarian disease. Resistance to *Dermatophilus* has also been mapped to the BoLA DR locus.

In sheep, there is an association of the class I allele SY1 with resistance to *Trichostrongylus colubriformis*. OLA-DRB1 locus affects egg production in *Ostertagia* infection. Resistance to scrapie and to caseous lymphadenitis appears to be associated with possession of certain MHC class I alleles.

In goats, the class I allele Be7 is associated with resistance, and Be1 and Be14 are associated with susceptibility to caprine arthritis-encephalitis (CAE). Genetic resistance or susceptibility to *Ehrlichia ruminantium* infection (heartwater) is associated with class I CLA and Be alleles.

In horses, an allergic response to the bites of *Culicoides* midges is linked to ELA-Aw7. There is also a strong association between ELA-A3, ELA-A15, and ELA-Dw13 and the development of sarcoid tumors (fibroblastic skin tumors likely induced by bovine papilloma viruses).

In pigs, the SLA complex has an influence on major reproduction parameters such as ovulation rate, litter size, and piglet viability. This may be due to the role played by the enzyme 21-hydroxylase whose gene is located in the class III region. Serum antibody levels are also affected in part by SLA haplotype. Even the numbers of larvae of the parasite *Trichinella spiralis* in muscle are regulated by genes in the SLA complex. Quantitative trait loci for backfat thickness, average daily gain, weight, and reproductive traits have been mapped to the SLA complex. For example, low growth performance in large white pigs is associated with possession of SLA class I alleles 4, 5, and 20. High carcass fatness in Landrace pigs is associated with alleles 1, 15, and 18. The precise gene or genes responsible for these traits has not been identified. One possible candidate is the gene that codes for a 17β-hydroxysteroid dehydrogenase called *FABGL* since this enzyme oxidizes estradiol, testosterone, and dihydrotestosterone, and these hormones regulate adipose tissue formation.

In the common chicken haplotypes, only a single class I and a single class II molecule are dominantly expressed. Since viruses contain relatively few proteins, MHC-dependent disease susceptibility may simply depend on the virus antigen binding to the dominant MHC class I molecule. As a result, possession of specific haplotypes determines disease susceptibility. For example, the haplotype B[21] is associated with resistance to Marek's disease whereas the B[19] haplotype is associated with susceptibility to this disease. Chickens homozygous for B[1] generally have high adult mortality, are highly susceptible to Marek's disease, and respond poorly to *Salmonella enterica pullorum* or to human serum albumin. In the OS strain of chickens, homozygous B[1] or B[4] birds are much more susceptible to autoimmune thyroiditis than are B[3] birds. Birds homozygous for B[5] are able to mount a better antibody response and develop less severe lesions in response to infection with *Eimeria tenella* than B[2] homozygous birds.

Selection for specific MHC haplotypes has potential for use in developing disease-resistant strains of domestic animals. However, it must be pointed out that by selecting for a specific gene locus one may also inadvertently select for susceptibility at closely linked loci. This may outweigh the benefits of a resistant allele at one locus. An animal cannot be resistant to all infectious diseases.

MHC AND BODY ODORS

The mammalian MHC contains the genes that code for pheromone olfactory receptors. For example, the class I region of mice, cattle, and pigs contains at least four genes coding for olfactory receptors. As a result, the MHC haplotype affects the recognition of individual odors in an allele-specific fashion and thus influences the mating preferences of mammals. Under controlled conditions, mice (and humans!) prefer to mate with MHC-incompatible individuals. Such matings preferentially produce MHC-heterozygous progeny, which could enjoy enhanced disease resistance. However, this type of mating could also prevent genome-wide inbreeding. Inbreeding avoidance may be the most important function of MHC-based mating preferences and therefore the fundamental selective force diversifying MHC genes in species with such mating patterns.

SOURCES OF ADDITIONAL INFORMATION

Amills M, Ramiya V, Norimine J, Lewin HA: The major histocompatibility complex of ruminants, *Rev Sci Tech Off Int Epiz* 17:108-120, 1998.

Andre P, Biassoni R, Colonna M, et al: New nomenclature for MHC receptors, *Nat Immunol* 2:661, 2001.

Charon P, Renard C, Vaiman M: The major histocompatibility complex in swine, *Immunol Rev* 167:179-192, 1999.

Davies CJ, Andersson L, Ellis SA, et al: Nomenclature for factors of the BoLA system, 1996: report of the ISAG BoLA nomenclature committee, *Anim Genet* 28:159-168, 1997.

Deverson EV, Wright H, Watson S, et al: Class II major histocompatibility complex genes of the sheep, *Anim Genet* 22:211-225, 1991.

Fraser DG, Bailey E: Polymorphism and multiple loci for the horse *DQA* gene, *Immunogenetics* 47:487-490, 1998.

Fremont DH, Matsumura M, Stura EA, et al: Crystal structures of two viral peptides in complex with murine MHC class I H-2K[b], *Science* 257:919-927, 1992.

Geraghty DE, Koller BH, Hansen JA, Orr HT: The HLA class I gene family includes at least six genes and twelve pseudogenes and gene fragments, *J Immunol* 149:1934-1946, 1992.

Hedrick SM: Dawn of the hunt for nonclassical MHC function, *Cell* 70:177-180, 1992.

Hughes AL, Yeager M, Ten Elshof AE, Chorney MJ: A new taxonomy of MHC class I molecules, *Immunol Today* 20:22-26, 1999.

Jacobs K, Mattheeuws M, Van Poucke M, et al: Characterization of the porcine FABGL gene, *Anim Genet* 33:220-227, 2002.

Kaufman J, Milne S, Göbel TWF, et al: The chicken B locus is a minimal essential major histocompatibility complex, *Nature* 401:923-925, 1999.

Kennedy LJ, Barnes A, Happ GM, et al: Extensive interbreed, but minimal intrabreed, variation of DLA class II alleles and haplotypes in dogs, *Tissue Antigens* 59:194-199, 2002.

Kennedy LJ, Barnes A, Happ GM, et al: Evidence for extensive DLA polymorphism in different dog populations, *Tissue Antigens* 60:43-52, 2002.

Lewin HA, Russell GC, Glass EJ: Comparative organization and function of the major histocompatibility complex of domesticated cattle, *Immunol Rev* 167:145-158, 1999.

Madden DR, Gorga JC, Strominger JL, Wiley DC: The three dimensional structure of HLA-B27 at 2.1 Å resolution suggests a general mechanism for tight peptide binding to MHC, *Cell* 70:1035-1048, 1992.

Pamer EG, Bevan MJ, Lindahl KF: Do nonclassical, class Ib MHC molecules present bacterial antigens to T cells, *Trends Microbiol* 1:35-38, 1994.

Pullen JK, Horton RM, Cai Z, Pease LR: Structural diversity of the classical H-2 genes: K,D, and L, *J Immunol* 148:958-967, 1992.

Trowsdale J: "Both man and bird and beast": comparative organization of MHC genes, *Immunogenetics* 41:1-17, 1995.

Vaiman M., Chardon P, Rothschild MF: Porcine major histocompatibility complex, *Rev Sci Tech Off Int Epiz* 17:95-107, 1998.

Van der Zijpp AJ, Egberts E: The major histocompatibility complex and diseases in farm animals, *Immunol Today* 10: 109-111, 1989.

Velten F, Rogel-Gaillard C, Renard C, et al: A first map of the porcine major histocompatibility complex class I region, *Tissue Antigens* 51:183-194, 1998.

Wagner JL, Sarmiento UM, Storb R: Cellular, serological, and molecular polymorphism of the class I and class II loci of the canine major histocompatibility complex, *Tissue Antigens* 59:205-210, 2002.

Yuhki H, Heidecker GF, O'Brien SJ: Characterization of MHC cDNA clones in the domestic cat. Diversity and evolution of class I genes, *J Immunol* 142:3676-3682, 1989.

Xu A, van Eijk MJT, Park C, Lewin HA: Polymorphism in BoLA-DRB3 exon 2 correlates with resistance to persistent lymphocytosis caused by bovine leukemia virus, *J Immunol* 151:6977-6985, 1993.

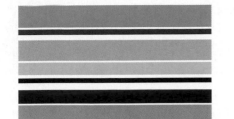

Organs of the Immune System

Although antigens are trapped and processed by dendritic cells, macrophages, and B cells, acquired immune responses are actually mounted by cells called lymphocytes. Lymphocytes are the small round cells that predominate in organs such as the spleen, lymph nodes, and thymus (Figure 8-1). These are called lymphoid organs. Lymphocytes have antigen receptors on their surface and they can therefore recognize and respond to antigens. (For this reason they can be considered "antigen-sensitive" cells.) Lymphocytes are eventually responsible for the production of antibodies and for cell-mediated immune responses. The lymphoid organs must therefore provide an environment for efficient interaction between lymphocytes, antigen-presenting cells, and foreign antigens as well as sites where lymphocytes can respond optimally to processed antigens.

Immune responses must be carefully regulated. Lymphocytes must be selected so that their receptors will only bind foreign antigens, and the response of each lymphocyte must be regulated so that it is sufficient but not excessive for the body's requirements. The lymphoid organs may therefore be classified on the basis of their roles in generating lymphocytes, in regulating the production of lymphocytes, and in providing an environment for trapping foreign antigens, processing them, and maximizing the opportunity for processed antigens to encounter and interact with antigen-sensitive cells (Figure 8-2).

SOURCES OF LYMPHOCYTES

Lymphoid stem cells are first produced in the fetal omentum, liver, and yolk sac. In older fetuses and in adults, these stem cells are mainly found in the bone marrow. The bone marrow has multiple functions in adult mammals. It is a hematopoietic organ containing the stem cells that give rise to all blood cells, including lymphocytes. In some mammals, such as primates, it also acts as a primary lymphoid organ (a site where newly produced lymphocytes can mature). Like the spleen, liver, and lymph nodes, the bone marrow contains many dendritic cells and macrophages and thus removes foreign material from the blood. Finally, it contains large numbers of antibody-producing cells and is therefore a major source of antibodies. Because of these multiple functions, the bone marrow is divided into a hematopoietic compartment and a vascular compartment. These compartments alternate, like slices of cake, in wedge-shaped areas within long bones. The hematopoietic compartment contains stem cells for all the blood cells as well as macrophages, dendritic cells, and lymphocytes and is enclosed by a layer of adventitial cells. In older animals these adventitial cells may become so loaded with fat that the marrow may have a fatty yellow appearance. The vascular compartment, where antigens are mainly trapped, consists of blood sinuses lined by endothelial cells and crossed by reticular cells and macrophages.

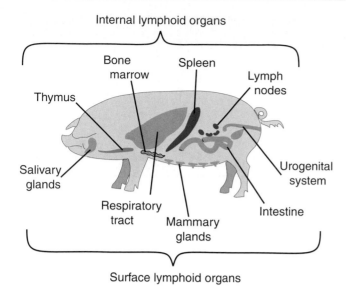

Internal lymphoid organs

Bone marrow   Spleen

Thymus   Lymph nodes

Salivary glands   Urogenital system

Respiratory tract   Mammary glands   Intestine

Surface lymphoid organs

Figure 8-1. The major lymphoid tissues of the pig, a typical mammal.

PRIMARY LYMPHOID ORGANS

The organs that regulate the maturation of lymphocytes are called primary lymphoid organs. Indeed, lymphocytes fall into two major populations called T cells and B cells based on the organ in which they mature. Thus, all T cells mature in the thymus. B cells, in contrast, mature within different organs depending on species. These include the bursa of Fabricius in birds, the bone marrow in primates and rodents, and intestinal lymphoid tissues in rabbits, ruminants, and pigs. The primary lymphoid organs all develop early in fetal life. As animals develop, newly produced, immature lymphocytes migrate from the bone marrow to the primary lymphoid organs where they mature (Table 8-1). The primary lymphoid organs are not sites where lymphocytes encounter antigens and so they do not enlarge in response to antigenic stimulation.

Thymus

The thymus is located in the thoracic cavity in front of and below the heart. In horses, cattle, sheep, pigs, and chickens, it also extends up the neck as far as the thyroid gland. The size of the thymus varies , its relative size being greatest in the newborn animal and its absolute size being greatest at puberty. It may be very small and difficult to find in adult animals.

Structure
The thymus consists of lobules of loosely packed epithelial cells, each covered by a connective tissue capsule. The outer part of each lobule, the cortex, is densely infiltrated with lymphocytes, but the inner medulla contains fewer lymphocytes and the epithelial cells are clearly visible (Figure 8-3). Within the medulla are also found round, layered bodies called thymic or Hassall's corpuscles. These contain keratin, and the remains of a small blood vessel may be found at their center. In cattle these corpuscles may contain immunoglobulin A (Chapter 20). An abnormally thick basement membrane and a continuous layer of epithelial cells surround the capillaries that supply the thymic cortex. This barrier prevents circulating antigens from entering the cortex. No lymphatic vessels leave the thymus. As an animal ages the thymus shrinks and is gradually replaced by fat. However, the aged thymus still contains small amounts of lymphoid tissue and is functionally active.

Function
The functions of the thymus are best demonstrated by studying the effects of its surgical removal in rodents. The effects of this surgery differ, depending on the age of the animal.

Neonatal Thymectomy. Mice thymectomized within a day of birth become susceptible to infections and may fail to grow. These animals have very few circulating lymphocytes and cannot reject foreign organ grafts because they lose the ability to mount cell-mediated

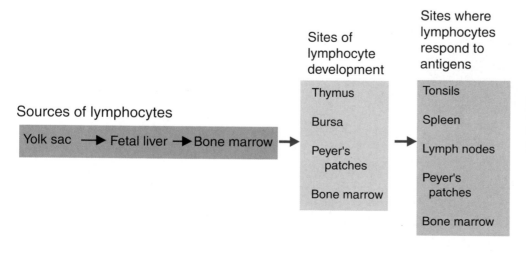

Sources of lymphocytes

Yolk sac → Fetal liver → Bone marrow

Sites of lymphocyte development

Thymus

Bursa

Peyer's patches

Bone marrow

Sites where lymphocytes respond to antigens

Tonsils

Spleen

Lymph nodes

Peyer's patches

Bone marrow

Figure 8-2. Role of lymphoid organs in the development and functioning of lymphocyte populations.

TABLE 8-1
Comparison of Primary and Secondary Lymphoid Organs

	Primary	Secondary
Origin	Ectoendodermal junction or endoderm	Mesoderm
Time of development	Early in embryonic life	Late in fetal life
Persistence	Involutes after puberty	Persists in adults
Effect of removal	Loss of lymphocytes	No or minor effects
Response to antigen	Unresponsive	Fully reactive
Examples	Thymus, bursa, some Peyer's patches	Spleen, lymph nodes

immune responses (Table 8-2). The effect of neonatal thymectomy on antibody production in mice varies. Thus the antibody response to protein antigens, such as bovine serum albumin or sheep red cells, is significantly inhibited (Figure 8-4). On the other hand, the antibody response to polysaccharide antigens may be unaffected. Neonatal thymectomy of domestic animals yields similar but less dramatic results than in mice because the thymus matures earlier in domestic animals and has completed many of its critical functions well before the animal is born (Chapter 19).

Adult Thymectomy. Surgical removal of the thymus from adult mammals has no immediately obvious effect. If, however, these animals are monitored for several months, the number of lymphocytes in their blood and their ability to mount cell-mediated immune responses are gradually reduced. This suggests that the thymus remains functional in adults, but there is a reservoir of long-lived thymus-derived cells that must be exhausted before the effects of adult thymectomy become apparent (Figure 8-5).

The results of thymectomy thus imply that the neonatal thymus is the source of most blood lymphocytes and that these lymphocytes are mainly responsible for mounting cell-mediated immune responses. They are called thymus-derived lymphocytes or T cells. T-cell precursors originate in the bone marrow but then enter the thymus. Once within the thymus, the cells (called thymocytes) divide rapidly. Of the new cells produced, most die by apoptosis, whereas the survivors (about 5% of the total in rodents and about 25% in calves) remain in the thymus for 4 to 5 days before leaving and colonizing the secondary lymphoid organs.

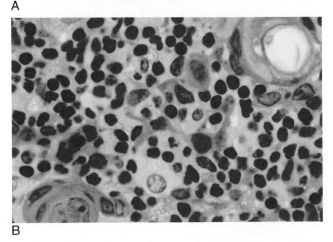

Figure 8-3. **A,** A section of a monkey thymus. Each lobule is divided into a cortex rich in lymphocytes, hence staining darkly, and a paler medulla consisting mainly of epithelial cells. Original magnification ×10. **B,** A high-power view of the medulla of a monkey thymus showing several pale-staining epithelial cells with cytoplasmic processes and many dark-staining, round lymphocytes. Original magnification ×1000.

TABLE 8-2
Effects of Neonatal Thymectomy and Bursectomy

Function	Thymectomy	Bursectomy
Numbers of circulating lymphocytes	↓↓↓	—
Presence of lymphocytes in T-dependent areas	↓↓↓	—
Graft rejection	↓↓↓	—
Presence of lymphocytes in T-independent areas	↓	↓↓↓
Plasma cells in lymphoid tissues	↓	↓↓↓
Serum immunoglobulins	↓	↓↓↓
Antibody formation	↓	↓↓↓

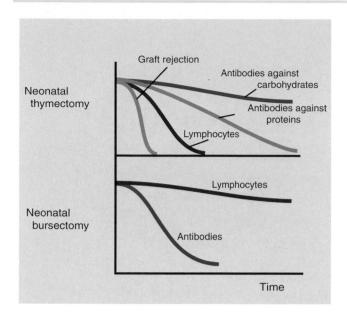

Figure 8-4. Effects of neonatal thymectomy on antibody- and cell-mediated immune responses.

MHC class II-antigen complexes with moderate affinity are stimulated to grow—a process called positive selection. These surviving cells eventually leave the thymus as mature T cells, circulate in the bloodstream, and colonize the secondary lymphoid organs.

Thymic Hormones

Within the thymus, cell functions are regulated by a complex mixture of cytokines and small peptides collectively known as thymic hormones. These include peptides variously called thymosins, thymopoietins, thymic humoral factor, thymulin, and the thymostimulins. Thymulin is especially interesting because it is a zinc-containing peptide secreted by the thymic epithelial cells, and it can partially restore T-cell function in thymectomized animals. Zinc is an essential mineral for the development of T cells. Consequently, zinc-deficient animals have defective cell-mediated immune responses (Chapter 36).

Bursa of Fabricius

The bursa of Fabricius is an organ found only in birds. It is a round sac located just above the cloaca (Figure 8-6). Like the thymus, the bursa reaches its greatest size in the chick about 1 to 2 weeks after hatching and then shrinks as the bird ages. It is very difficult to identify in older birds.

Structure

Like the thymus, the bursa consists of lymphocytes embedded in epithelial tissue. This epithelial tissue lines a hollow sac connected to the cloaca by a duct. Inside the sac folds of epithelium extend into the lumen, and scattered through the folds are round masses of lymphocytes called lymphoid follicles (Figure 8-7). Each follicle is divided into a cortex and a medulla. The cortex contains

T cells that enter the thymus have two conflicting tasks. They must recognize foreign antigens but at the same time must not respond strongly to normal body constituents (self-antigens). This feat is accomplished by a two-stage selection process in the thymic medulla. Thus those thymocytes with receptors that bind self-antigens strongly and that could therefore cause autoimmunity are killed by apoptosis (negative selection) (Box 8-1). Thymocytes with receptors that cannot bind any MHC class II molecules and therefore cannot react to any processed antigen are also killed.

On the other hand, those thymocytes that survive the negative selection process but can still recognize specific

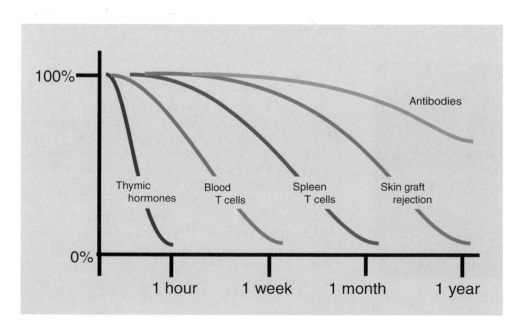

Figure 8-5. Effects of adult thymectomy on immune responses.

BOX 8–1

Apoptosis

Apoptosis is a form of physiological cell death or cell suicide mediated by normal body processes. Apoptotic cells have a characteristic morphology and can be readily recognized in histologic sections (see Figure 17-3).

lymphocytes, plasma cells, and macrophages. At the corticomedullary junction there is a basement membrane and capillary network on the inside of which are epithelial cells. These medullary epithelial cells are replaced by lymphoblasts and lymphocytes in the center of the follicle. Specialized neuroendocrine dendritic cells of unknown function surround each follicle.

Function

The bursa may be removed either surgically or by infecting newborn chicks with a virus that destroys the bursa (infectious bursal disease virus). Since the bursa shrinks when chicks become sexually mature, bursal atrophy can also be provoked by administration of testosterone. Bursectomized birds have very low levels of antibodies in their blood, and antibody-producing cells disappear from lymphoid organs. However, they still possess circulating lymphocytes and can reject foreign skin grafts. Thus, bursectomy has little effect on the cell-mediated immune response. Bursectomized birds are more susceptible than normal to leptospirosis and salmonellosis but not to bacteria against which cell-mediated immunity is important, such as *Mycobacterium avium*.

These results indicate that the bursa is a primary lymphoid organ that functions as a maturation and differentiation site for the cells of the antibody-forming system. Lymphocytes originating in the bursa are therefore called B cells. The bursa acts like the thymus insofar as immature cells produced in the bone marrow migrate

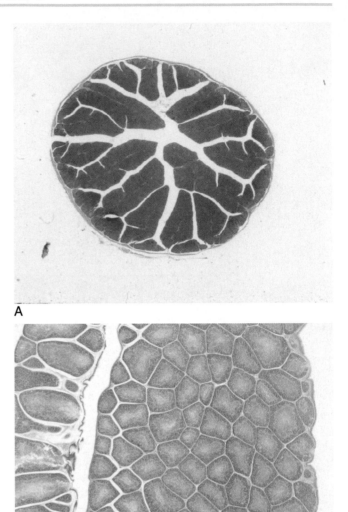

Figure 8-7. Photomicrographs showing the structure of the bursa of Fabricius. **A,** Low-power micrograph showing the bursa of a 13-day-old chick. Original magnification ×5. **B,** A high-power view. Original magnification ×360. (From a specimen provided by Drs. NH McArthur and LC Abbott.)

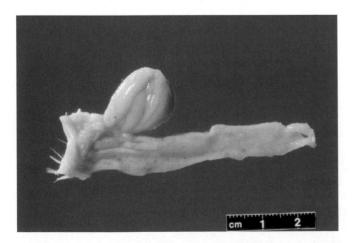

Figure 8-6. The bursa of Fabricius obtained from a 1-week-old chicken. It has been cut open to reveal the folds inside.

to the bursa. These cells then proliferate rapidly but 90% to 95% of these B cells die by apoptosis. This is a result of negative selection of self-reactive B cells. Once their maturation is completed, the surviving B cells emigrate to secondary lymphoid organs.

Close examination shows that the bursa is not a pure primary lymphoid organ because it can also trap antigens and undertake some antibody synthesis. It also contains a small focus of T cells just above the bursal duct opening. Several different hormones have been extracted from the bursa. The most important of these is bursin, a tripeptide (Lys-His-glycylamide). Bursin activates B cells but not T cells.

Peyer's Patches

Structure

Peyer's patches (PPs) are lymphoid organs located in the walls of the small intestine. Their structure and functions vary among species. Thus in ruminants, pigs, horses, dogs, and humans (group I) 80% to 90% of the Peyer's patches are found in the ileum where they form a single continuous structure that extends forward from the ileocecal junction. In young ruminants and pigs the ileal PPs may be as long as 2 m. Ileal PPs consist of densely packed lymphoid follicles, each separated by a connective tissue sheath, and contain only B cells (Figure 8-8).

The ileal PPs reach maximal size and maturity before birth at a time when they are shielded from foreign antigens. The ileal PPs collectively form the largest lymphoid tissue in 6-week-old lambs. (They constitute about 1% of total body weight, like the thymus.) They disappear by 15 months of age and cannot be detected in adult sheep.

These group I species also have a second type of PP that consists of multiple discrete accumulations of follicles in the jejunum. These jejunal PPs persist for the life of the animal. They consist of pear-shaped follicles separated by extensive interfollicular tissue and contain mainly B cells with up to 30% T cells.

In other mammals, such as rabbits and rodents (group II), all the PPs are located at random intervals in the ileum and jejunum. In these mammals, the PPs do not develop until 2 to 4 weeks after birth and persist into old age. The development of the PPs in group II animals seems to depend entirely on antigenic stimulation since they remain small and poorly developed in germ-free mice. The appendix also plays a key role in B-cell development in rabbits.

Function

The behavior of the B cells in sheep ileal PPs resembles that of B cells in the avian bursa. Thus, ileal PPs are sites of rapid B cell proliferation, although most cells then undergo apoptosis (95%) and the survivors are released into the circulation. If their ileal PPs are surgically removed, lambs become B-cell deficient for at least a year and fail to produce antibodies. The bone marrow of lambs contains many fewer lymphocytes than the bone marrow of laboratory rodents, and their ileal PPs are therefore their most significant source of B cells. The group I ileal PPs are therefore primary lymphoid organs that serve a function similar to that of the bursa of Fabricius.

Evidence also exists for similar differences between jejunal and ileal PPs in the pig. Pigs have about 30 jejunal PPs that are of conventional structure and a single, large ileal PP. The ileal PP lacks T cells and has a structure similar to that seen in sheep. It regresses within the first year of life, so it is likely that it is a primary lymphoid organ.

Dogs also have two types of Peyer's patches, including a single ileal PP that shows early involution and contains predominantly immature B cells.

Lymphoglandular Complexes

Lymphoglandular complexes are found in the wall of the large intestine and cecum in horses, ruminants, dogs, and pigs. They consist of submucosal masses of lymphoid tissue penetrated by radially branching extensions of mucosal glands. These glands penetrate both the

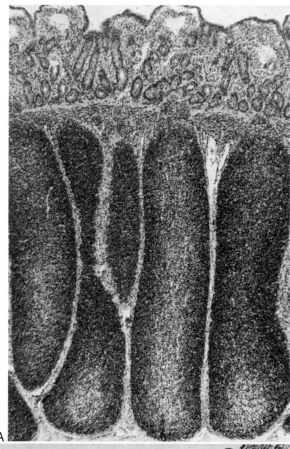
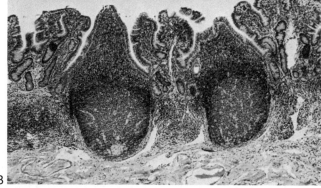

Figure 8-8. Structure of the two different types of Peyer's patch in sheep. **A,** An ileal Peyer's patch at age 8 weeks. **B,** A Peyer's patch from the jejunum, also at 8 weeks. Original magnification ×32. (From Reynolds JD, Morris B: *Eur J Immunol* 13:631, 1983.)

submucosa and the lymphoid nodule. They are lined by intestinal columnar epithelium containing goblet cells, intraepithelial lymphocytes, and M cells (Chapter 20). Their function is unknown, but they contain many plasma cells suggesting that they are sites of antibody production. Because of their structural similarity to the avian bursa and the presence of many M cells, they may be antigen-sampling sites.

Bone Marrow

The specialized ileal Peyer's patch is the primary lymphoid organ for B cells only in group I mammals (ruminants, pigs, and dogs). In group II mammals the bone marrow probably serves this function. There is no exclusive B-cell development site in the bone marrow, although it is suggested that precursor B cells develop at the outer edge of the marrow and migrate to the center as they mature and multiply. Negative selection apparently occurs within the bone marrow so that most of the pre-B cells generated are destroyed.

SECONDARY LYMPHOID ORGANS

In contrast to the primary lymphoid organs, the secondary lymphoid organs arise late in fetal life and persist in adults. Unlike primary lymphoid organs, they enlarge in response to antigenic stimulation. Surgical removal of a secondary lymphoid organ does not significantly reduce immune capability. Examples of secondary lymphoid organs include the spleen, the lymph nodes, the tonsils and other lymphoid tissues in the intestinal, respiratory, and urogenital tracts. These organs contain dendritic cells that trap and process antigens and lymphocytes that mediate the immune responses. The overall anatomical structure of these organs is therefore designed to facilitate antigen trapping and to provide maximal opportunities for processed antigens to be presented to lymphocytes.

Lymph Nodes

Structure

Lymph nodes are round or bean-shaped filters strategically placed on lymphatic vessels in such a way as to trap antigens carried in lymph (Figure 8-9). Lymph nodes consist of a reticular network filled with lymphocytes, macrophages, and dendritic cells through which lymphatic sinuses penetrate (Figure 8-10). A subcapsular sinus is located immediately under the connective tissue capsule of the node. Other sinuses pass through the body of the node but are most prominent in the medulla. Afferent lymphatics enter the node around its circumference, and efferent lymphatics leave from a depression or hilus on one side. The blood vessels supplying a lymph node also enter and leave through the hilus.

The interior of a lymph node is divided into a peripheral cortex, a central medulla, and an ill-defined region

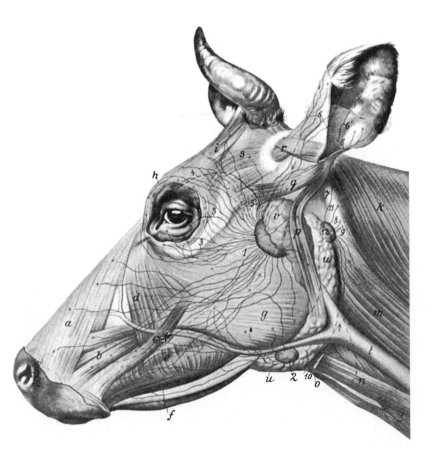

Figure 8-9.   Lateral view of the head of a bovine showing the way in which the lymphatics drain to the parotid lymph node. (From Sisson S [revised by Grossman JD]: *Anatomy of the domestic animals*, ed 4, Philadelphia, 1953, WB Saunders, 1953.)

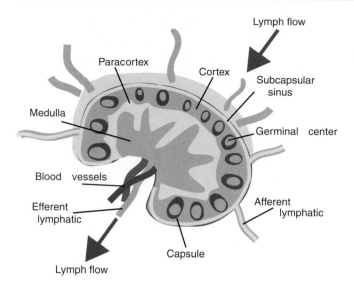

Figure 8-10. Structural features of a typical lymph node.

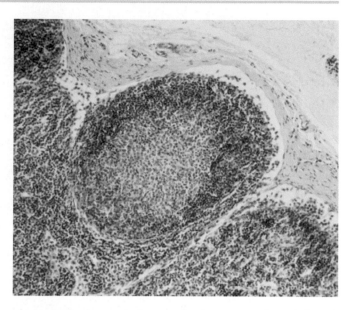

Figure 8-12. A germinal center in the cortex of a cat's lymph node. Note the large, pale area in the center of the germinal center where the cells are dividing. Original magnification ×120. (From a specimen provided by Dr. WE Haensly.)

between these two regions called the paracortex (Figure 8-11). B cells predominate in the cortex where they are arranged in nodules. In lymph nodes that have been stimulated by antigen, some of the cells within these nodules expand to form foci of dividing cells called germinal centers (Figure 8-12). Germinal centers have light and dark zones. The dark zones are sites where B cells proliferate and undergo a process called somatic mutation (Chapter 14). The light zones are sites where immunoglobulin class switching and memory B-cell formation occur (Chapter 11). A few T cells are found in the cortex, in the region immediately surrounding each germinal center.

T cells and dendritic cells predominate in the paracortex. In neonatally thymectomized or congenitally athymic animals this zone loses cells and is said to be a T-dependent region (Figure 8-13). Many different cell types are found in the medulla. They include reticulum cells that generate the fibrillar scaffold, dendritic cells and macrophages that trap antigens, and B cells and plasma cells that produce antibodies. These cells are arranged in cellular cords between the lymphatic sinuses.

Lymphocyte Circulation
T cells constantly circulate around the body in the blood and tissue fluid and are the predominant lymphocytes in blood (Figure 8-14). As they travel, they survey the body for foreign antigens and preferentially home to sites of microbial invasion and inflammation. They also spend time in the secondary lymphoid organs.

Circulating T cells leave the bloodstream by two routes. T cells that have not encountered antigens previously ("naïve" T cells) bind to venules in the paracortex of lymph nodes. These are called high endothelial venules (HEVs) because they are lined with tall, rounded endothelial cells (Figure 8-15) quite unlike the flattened endothelium found in other blood vessels. The high endothelial cells are not joined by tight junctions but are linked by discontinuous "spot-welded" junctions. This means that lymphocytes can pass easily between the high endothelial cells. Circulating lymphocytes can adhere to these high endothelial cells and then migrate into the paracortex. The emigration of lymphocytes from HEVs resembles that of neutrophils in inflamed blood vessels. Thus, the cells first roll along the endothelial surface,

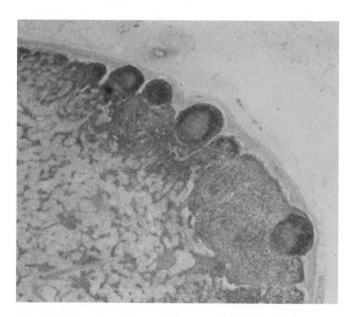

Figure 8-11. A section of bovine lymph node. Original magnification ×12. (From a specimen provided by Dr. WE Haensly.)

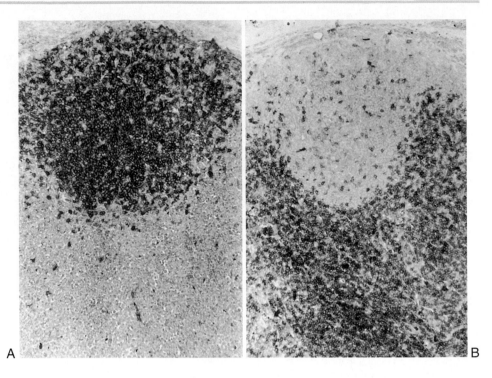

Figure 8-13. Normal bovine lymph node stained by the immunoperoxidase technique (Chapter 16) with **(A)** a monoclonal antibody that identifies B lymphocytes and **(B)** a monoclonal antibody that identifies T lymphocytes. (Courtesy Drs. I Morrison and N MacHugh.)

binding to selectins. For example, L-selectin (CD62L) on lymphocytes binds to receptors such as GlyCAM-1 or CD34 (sialomucin) on the cells lining the high endothelial venules (Figure 8-16). As they roll, the lymphocytes become activated and express integrins. This results in their complete arrest and emigration. The number and length of HEVs are variable and controlled by local

activity. Thus, stimulation of a lymph node by the presence of antigens results in a rapid increase in the length of its HEVs. If, however, a lymph node is protected from antigens, its HEVs shorten. HEVs are not normally found in sheep lymph nodes.

Chemokines control the relocation and recirculation of lymphocytes and ensure that the correct lymphocytes end up in the correct positions. For example, T cells expressing CCR7 are attracted to the perifollicular area of the cortex where the chemokines CCL19 and CCL21 are produced. B cells, on the other hand, express CXCR5 and are attracted to the interior of germinal centers where its ligand, the chemokine CXCL13, is produced.

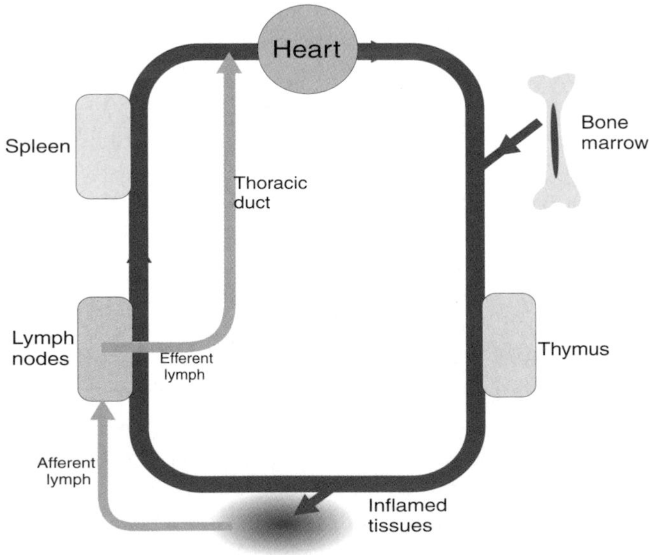

Figure 8-14. Circulation of lymphocytes. Lymphocytes found in blood may be newly formed cells passing from the bone marrow to the primary lymphoid organs or cells passing from the primary to the secondary lymphoid organs. However, the vast majority of these cells are recirculating between the lymph nodes and the bloodstream.

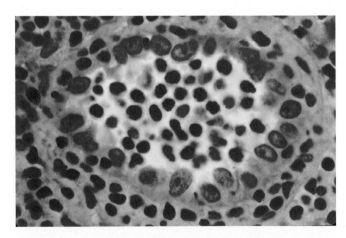

Figure 8-15. A section of human tonsil showing a high endothelial venule with its characteristic high, rounded endothelial cells. Note the lymphocytes emigrating between the endothelial cells.

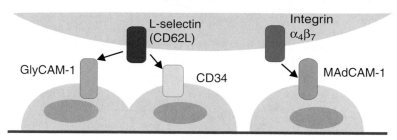

Lymphocyte

High endothelial venule

Figure 8-16. Binding of circulating lymphocytes to ligands on endothelial cells in high endothelial venules is brought about mainly by L-selectin. In the intestine, lymphocytes bearing the integrin $\alpha_4\beta_7$ bind to their ligand on endothelial cells, MAdCAM-1.

When T cells are activated, they too may express CXCR5 and so enter germinal centers where they "help" B cells respond to antigens.

Other lymphoid organs employ other homing receptors. Thus the homing receptor MAdCAM-1 is expressed in blood vessels in intestinal lymphoid tissues such as Peyer's patches. Lymphocytes that recirculate to the intestine tend to express high levels of the integrin $\alpha_4\beta_7$, the ligand for MAdCAM-1.

In contrast to naive T cells, memory T cells leave the bloodstream through conventional blood vessels in tissues and are then carried to lymph nodes by tissue fluid (afferent lymph). Up to 90% of lymphocytes leaving a node are derived from cells entering through HEVs whereas about 10% enter through afferent lymph.

Lymph flows from the tissues to lymph nodes through afferent lymphatics. It leaves the lymph nodes by efferent lymphatics. Typically, afferent lymph in sheep contains 85% T cells, 5% B cells, and 10% dendritic cells. Efferent lymph contains greater than 98% lymphocytes of which 75% are T cells and 25% are B cells. The efferent lymphatics eventually join together to form large lymph vessels. The largest of these lymph vessels is the thoracic duct, which drains the lymph from the lower body and intestine and empties it into the anterior vena cava. If the thoracic duct is cannulated and the lymph removed, blood lymphocyte numbers (essentially all T cells) drop significantly within a few hours. The T cells also disappear from the paracortex of lymph nodes. This rapid depletion of T cells implies that thoracic duct lymphocytes normally circulate back to lymph nodes through the blood.

Species Differences

Domestic pigs and related swine, hippopotamuses, rhinoceroses, and dolphins are different. Their lymph nodes consist of several lymphoid "nodules" oriented so that the cortex of each nodule is located toward the center of the node whereas the medulla is at the periphery (Figure 8-17). Each nodule is served by a single afferent lymphatic that enters the central cortex as a lymph sinus. Thus afferent lymph is carried deep into the node. A cortex surrounds the lymph sinus. Outside this region

are a paracortex and a medulla. This medulla may be shared by adjacent nodules (Figure 8-18). Lymph passes from the cortex at the center of the node to the medulla at the periphery before leaving through the efferent vessels that drain the region between nodules. The cortex and paracortex have a similar structure to that seen in other mammals. The medulla has very few sinuses but consists of a dense mass of cells that is relatively impermeable to cells in the lymph. As a result, few cells migrate through the medulla. T cells in these species enter the lymph node in the conventional way through HEVs. However, they do not leave the lymph node through the lymphatics but migrate directly back to the bloodstream through the HEVs of the paracortex (Figure 8-19). Very few lymphocytes are found in pig lymph.

Response to Antigens

When microbes invade tissues, the resident dendritic cells are activated and migrate to the draining lymph node where they accumulate in the paracortex and cortex. These dendritic cells form a web through which

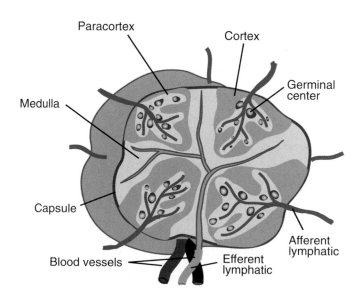

Figure 8-17. Structure of a pig lymph node. Compare this with Figure 8-18.

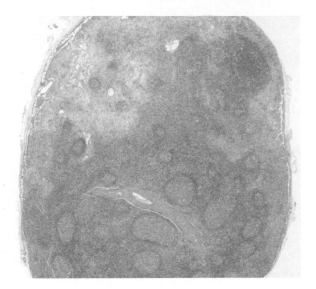

Figure 8-18. A section of a pig lymph node. Note how the germinal centers are located in the interior of the node. Original magnification ×12. (From a specimen provided by Drs. NH McArthur and LC Abbott.)

antigens must pass. Antigens are captured and then presented by these dendritic cells to T cells. The T cells are initially activated in the paracortex whereas the B cells remain randomly dispersed in the primary follicles. Both cell populations then migrate to the edges of the follicles where they interact. Once antibody production is stimulated, the progeny of these B cells move to the medulla and begin to secrete antibodies. Some of these antibody-producing cells may escape into the efferent lymph and colonize downstream lymph nodes. Several days after antibody production is first observed in the medulla, germinal centers appear in the cortex.

Adherence to follicular dendritic cells is the predominant means of antigen trapping once an animal has been sensitized by previous exposure to an antigen. In a secondary response the germinal centers become less obvious as activated memory cells emigrate in the efferent lymph. Once this stage is completed, the germinal centers redevelop.

Antigen-stimulated lymph nodes trap lymphocytes. That is, the passage of lymphocytes through these organs is blocked, the lymphocytes accumulate, and the lymph nodes swell. This trapping concentrates lymphocytes close to sites of antigen accumulation. After about 24 hours the lymph nodes release their trapped cells. As a result, their cellular output is increased for several days.

When responding to antigens that stimulate a cell-mediated rather than an antibody-mediated immune response, such as a skin graft, the T-cell-rich paracortical areas produce large pyroninophilic cells. Pyronin is a stain for RNA; thus, a cell with pyroninophilic cytoplasm is rich in ribosomes and is probably a protein-producing cell. These large pyroninophilic cells give rise, in turn, to the T cells that participate in the cell-mediated immune responses.

Hemolymph Nodes

Hemolymph nodes are structurally similar to lymph nodes found in association with the blood vessels of ruminants and other mammals. Their function is unclear. They differ from conventional lymph nodes in that their lymphatic sinuses contain numerous red cells. They have a cortex containing germinal centers and B cells. T cells predominate at the center in association with lymphatic sinuses. There are some differences, however, in the characteristics of these T cells as compared to conventional lymph nodes (more $\gamma\delta+$,WC1$^+$ T cells, fewer CD8$^+$ T cells) (Chapter 9). Intravenously injected carbon particles are trapped in the sinusoids of hemolymph nodes, suggesting that they may combine features of both the spleen and lymph nodes.

Spleen

Just as lymph nodes filter antigens from lymph, so the spleen filters blood. The filtering process removes both antigenic particles and aged blood cells. The spleen also stores red cells and platelets and undertakes red cell production in the fetus. It is therefore divided into two compartments: one for antigen trapping and for red cell storage, called red pulp, and one rich in lymphocytes where immune responses occur, called white pulp.

Figure 8-19. Comparison between the major route of circulation of T cells in the pig and in other mammals. Note that pig lymphocytes are largely confined to the bloodstream.

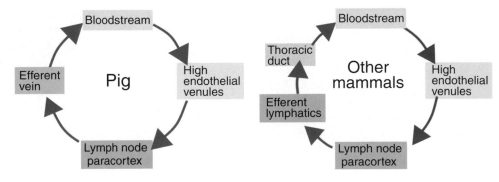

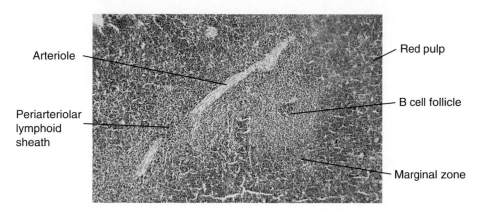

Arteriole

Periarteriolar
lymphoid
sheath

Red pulp

B cell follicle

Marginal zone

Figure 8-20. Histological section and diagram showing the structure of the bovine spleen. Original magnification ×50. (From a specimen provided by Dr. JR Duncan.)

Structure of White Pulp

Vessels entering the spleen travel through muscular trabeculae before entering its functional areas. Immediately on leaving the trabeculae each arteriole is surrounded by a sheath of lymphoid tissue known, naturally enough, as the periarteriolar lymphoid sheath (Figure 8-20). The arteriole eventually leaves this sheath and branches into penicillary arterioles, which possess a characteristically thickened wall forming a structure called an ellipsoid. These arterioles then open, either directly or indirectly, into venous sinuses that drain into the splenic venules. The periarteriolar lymphoid sheath consists largely of T cells. Scattered through the sheath are round primary follicles consisting largely of B cells. Following antigenic stimulation these follicles develop germinal centers. A layer of T cells surrounds each follicle. The white pulp is separated from the red pulp by a marginal sinus, a reticulum sheath, and a marginal zone of cells. This marginal zone is rich in dendritic cells and B cells. Most of the blood that enters the spleen is released into the marginal sinus and flows through the marginal zone

before returning to the circulation through venous sinuses. This ensures that marginal zone dendritic cells and B cells readily encounter any circulating antigens.

Response to Antigen

Intravenously administered antigens trapped in the spleen are taken up by dendritic cells in the marginal zone and in the sinusoids of the red pulp. The dendritic cells carry the antigen to the primary follicles of the white pulp from which, after a few days, antibody-producing cells migrate. These antibody-producing cells colonize the marginal zone and the red pulp, and it is in these regions that antibody production is first detected. Germinal center formation also occurs in the primary follicles. In an animal possessing circulating antibody, trapping by dendritic cells within the follicles becomes significant. As in a primary immune response, the antibody-producing cells migrate from these follicles to the red pulp and the marginal zone, where antibody production occurs, although some antibodies may also be produced within the follicles.

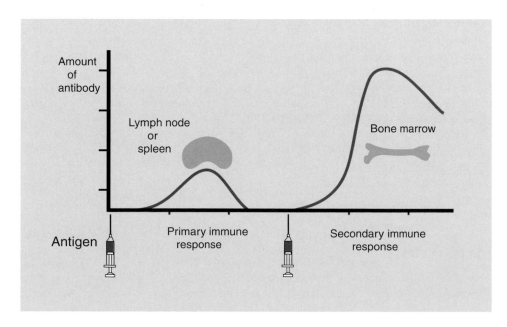

Amount
of
antibody

Lymph node
or
spleen

Bone marrow

Antigen

Primary immune
response

Secondary immune
response

Figure 8-21. Although the primary immune response to intravenously injected antigen takes place in liver or spleen, the antibodies produced in a secondary response are largely produced in the bone marrow.

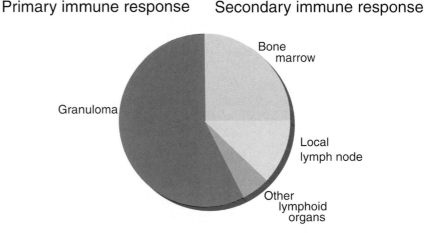

Figure 8-22. Relative contribution of different organs or tissues to antibody production after administration of antigen either intravenously or intramuscularly with Freund's complete adjuvant. The adjuvant (Chapter 21) causes the accumulation of lymphocytes and antigen-processing cells. It thus forms a lymphoid nodule where antibodies are produced.

Other Secondary Lymphoid Organs

Sites where antibodies are produced include not only the spleen and lymph nodes but also the bone marrow, tonsils, and lymphoid tissues scattered throughout the body, most notably in the digestive, respiratory, and urogenital tracts. Although its scattered nature makes it difficult to measure, the bone marrow is the largest mass of secondary lymphoid tissue in an adult. If antigen is given intravenously, much will be trapped not only in the liver and spleen but also in the bone marrow. However, during a primary immune response, antibodies are largely produced in the spleen and lymph nodes (Figure 8-21). Toward the end of that response, memory cells leave the spleen and colonize the bone marrow. When a second dose of an antigen is given, the bone marrow produces very large quantities of antibody and is the major source of immunoglobulin B antibodies in adult rodents. Up to 70% of the antibody to some antigens may be produced by cells in the bone marrow (Figure 8-22).

SOURCES OF ADDITIONAL INFORMATION

Audhya T, Kroon D, Heavner G, et al: Tripeptide structure of bursin, a selective B cell differentiating hormone of the bursa of Fabricius, *Science* 231:997-999, 1986.

Binns RM, Pabst R: Lymphoid tissue structure and lymphocyte trafficking in the pig, *Vet Immunol Immunopathol* 43:79-87, 1994.

Cunningham CP, Kimpton WG, Holder JE, Cahill RN: Thymic export in aged sheep: a continuous role for the thymus throughout pre- and postnatal life, *Eur J Immunol* 31:802-811, 2001.

Duijvestijn A, Hamann A: Mechanisms and regulation of lymphocyte migration, *Immunol Today* 10:23-28, 1989.

Edelson RL, Fink JM: The immunologic function of skin, *Sci Am* 252:46-53, 1985.

Ekino S, Suginohara K, Urano T, et al: The bursa of Fabricius: a trapping site for environmental antigens, *Immunology* 55:405-410, 1985.

Galeotti M., Sarli G, Eleni C, Marcato PS: Identification of cell types present in bovine haemolymph nodes and lymph nodes by immunostaining, *Vet Immunol Immunopathol* 36:319-331, 1993.

Garside P, Ingulli E, Merica RR, et al: Visualization of specific B and T lymphocyte interactions in the lymph node, *Science* 281:96-100, 1998.

Harp JA, Pesch BA, Runnels PL: Extravasation of lymphocytes via paracortical venules in sheep lymph nodes: visualization using an intracellular fluorescent label, *Vet Immunol Immunopathol* 24:159-168, 1990.

Hopkins J, McConnell I: Immunological aspects of lymphocyte recirculation, *Vet Immun Immunopathol* 6:3-33, 1984.

Landsverk T, Halleraker M, Aleksandersen M, et al: The intestinal habitat for organized lymphoid tissues in ruminants; comparative aspects of structure, function and development, *Vet Immunol Immunopathol* 28:1-16, 1991.

Monroe WE, Roth JA: The thymus as part of the endocrine system, *Comp Cont Ed Pract Vet* 8:24-33, 1986.

Motyka B, Reynolds JD: Apoptosis is associated with the extensive B cell death in the sheep ileal Peyer's patch and the chicken bursa of Fabricius: a possible role in B cell selection, *Eur J Immunol* 21:1951-1958, 1991.

Pezzano M, Samms M, Martinez M, Guyden J: Questionable thymic nurse cell, *Microbiol Mol Biol Rev* 65:390-403, 2001.

Ratcliff MJH: The ontogeny and cloning of B cells in the bursa of Fabricius, *Immunol Today* 6:223-227, 1985.

Reynaud C-A, Mackay CR, Müller RG, Weill J-C: Somatic generation of diversity in a mammalian primary lymphoid organ: the sheep ileal Peyer's patches, *Cell* 64:995-1005, 1991.

Reynolds JD: Evidence of extensive lymphocyte death in sheep Peyer's patches. I. A comparison of lymphocyte production and export, *J Immunol* 136:2005-2010, 1986.

Thorp BH, Seneque S, Staute K, Kimpton WG: Characterization and distribution of lymphocyte subsets in sheep hemal nodes, *Dev Comp Immunol* 15:393-400, 1991.

Velinova M, Theilen C, Melot F, et al: New histochemical and ultrastructural observations on normal bovine tonsils, *Vet Rec* 149:613-617, 2001.

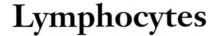

Lymphocytes

Lymphocytes are the cells responsible for mounting the acquired immune responses. Given that there are two forms of immune response, antibody mediated and cell mediated, it is reasonable to infer that there are two major types of lymphocytes, T cells and B cells. However, within these two major types are many diverse subpopulations, each with different characteristics and functions. This chapter reviews the structure and properties of lymphocytes and some important lymphocyte subpopulations.

LYMPHOCYTE STRUCTURE

Lymphocytes are small, round cells, 7 to 15 μm in diameter. Each lymphocyte contains a large, round nucleus that stains intensely and evenly with hematoxylin (Figure 9-1). It is surrounded by a thin rim of cytoplasm containing some mitochondria, free ribosomes, and a small Golgi apparatus (Figure 9-2). Scanning electron microscopy shows that some lymphocytes are smooth surfaced, whereas others are covered by many small projections (Figure 9-3). Their structure provides no clue as to their complex role (Figure 9-4).

LYMPHOCYTE POPULATIONS

Lymphocytes are mainly found in lymphoid organs, in blood, and scattered under mucosal surfaces (Figure 9-5).

Despite their uniform appearance, they are a diverse mixture of cell subpopulations. Although these subpopulations cannot be identified by their structure, they can be identified by their characteristic cell surface molecules and by their behavior (Table 9-1). The pattern of cell surface molecules expressed on a cell is called its immunophenotype. By analyzing cell immunophenotypes it is possible to show the diversity of lymphocyte subpopulations.

Early studies involving neonatal thymectomy demonstrated the existence of T lymphocytes (Figure 9-6). After T cells leave the thymus they accumulate in the paracortex of lymph nodes, the periarteriolar lymphoid sheaths of the spleen, and the interfollicular areas of the Peyer's patches. T cells also account for 40% to 80% of the lymphocytes in blood (Table 9-2).

Similar experiments involving bursectomy in chickens pointed to the existence of B cells. In mammals, B cells originate in the bone marrow but mature within Peyer's patches or in the bone marrow before migrating to the secondary lymphoid organs. They are found in the cortex of lymph nodes, in follicles within the Peyer's patches and spleen, and in the marginal zone of the white pulp of the spleen. B cells account for 10% to 50% of blood lymphocytes (Table 9-2).

A third population of lymphocytes are neither T nor B cells but are natural killer (NK) cells. These NK cells, in most species, are relatively large and contain an extensive cytoplasm and abundant cytoplasmic granules.

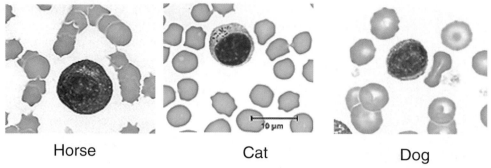

Horse   Cat   Dog

Figure 9-1. Photomicrographs showing lymphocytes in blood smears from horse, cat, and dog. Giemsa stain. (Courtesy of Dr. MC Johnson.)

NK cells probably originate from the same stem cells as T cells but do not undergo thymic processing. They are found in small numbers in the blood and are widely distributed throughout the lymphoid organs.

LYMPHOCYTE SURFACE MOLECULES

It was not until the proteins on the surface of lymphocytes were identified that it became possible to identify subpopulations. Many of these cell surface molecules have now been characterized, especially in humans and mice. Each molecule usually has a functional or chemical name as well as a cluster of differentiation (CD) designation (Figures 9-7 and 9-8). Currently, the CD

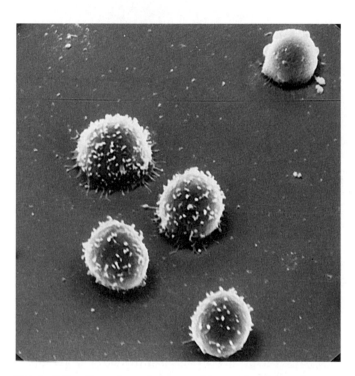

Figure 9-3. Scanning electron micrograph of lymphocytes from a mouse lymph node. Original magnification ×1500.

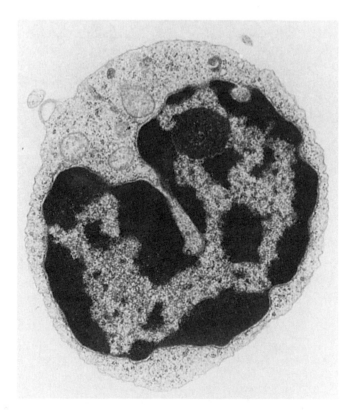

Figure 9-2. A transmission electron micrograph of a blood lymphocyte from a rabbit. (Courtesy of Dr. S Linthicum.)

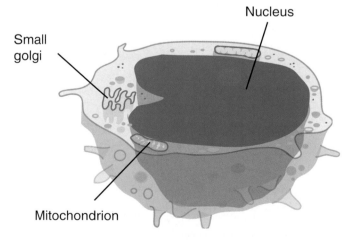

Nucleus

Small golgi

Mitochondrion

Figure 9-4. Essential structural features of a lymphocyte.

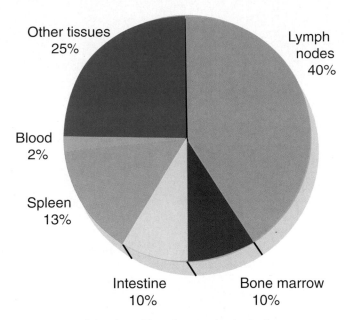

Figure 9-5. Location of lymphocytes in the body.

CD molecules on the cells of the domestic mammals fall into two categories. The great majority of them have homologs in humans and mice and so have the same CD number. There are, however, several cell surface molecules found in these species that have no recognized homolog in man or mouse. These unattributable molecules have been given a species abbreviation and the prefix WC (workshop cluster), such as BoWC1 and BoWC2 found in cattle.

Molecules That Form Part of the Antigen Receptor Complex

The most important structures on the surface of lymphocytes are their antigen receptors. These are abbreviated TCR (T-cell antigen receptor) or BCR (B-cell antigen receptor). Both are complex structures containing many different proteins. Some of these proteins bind antigen whereas others are used for signal transduction. There are two populations of T cells differentiated by the structure of their TCR. One uses α and β peptide chains (TCR α/β) and the other uses γ and δ chains (TCR γ/δ). There are also subpopulations of B cells with different forms of BCR that use five different peptide chains (γ, μ, α, ε, and δ). BCRs also differ from the TCRs in that they are shed from the cell into tissue fluid and the blood where they are called antibodies. Antibodies are simply soluble BCRs.

CD3 is the name given to the set of proteins in the TCR that act as signal transducers. They pass a signal from the receptor to the T cell once antigen is bound. CD3 is therefore found on all T cells. Another protein, CD4, is found only on T cells that recognize processed exogenous antigen, the T helper cells. CD4 is a receptor for major histocompatibility complex (MHC) class II molecules. CD8, in contrast, is only found on T cells that attack and kill abnormal cells—cytotoxic T cells. CD8 is

nomenclature system gives sequential numbers to each molecule: CD4, CD8, CD16, and so on, up to CD247. (A provisional designation, CDw, is given to incompletely characterized molecules.) Since arbitrary numbers are difficult to remember, I have used the basic principle that if the molecule's common name is well accepted or describes its function, then that name will be used. Examples include FcαR (CD89), interleukin-6R (CD126), and L-selectin (CD62L). CD nomenclature will be used for molecules where the designation is well accepted, such as CD8 and CD4. It will also be used for molecules that have an irrational or arbitrary abbreviation or acronym. A complete list of relevant CD molecules and their functions can be found in the Appendix.

TABLE 9-1		
The Identifying Features of T and B Cells		
Property	**B cells**	**T cells**
Develop within	Bone marrow, bursa, Peyer's patches	Thymus
Distribution	Lymph node cortex	Lymph node paracortex
	Splenic follicles	Spleen periarteriolar sheath
Circulate	No	Yes
Antigen receptors	BCR—immunoglobulin	TCR—protein heterodimer
		Associated with CD3, CD4, or CD8
Important surface antigens	Immunoglobulins	CD2, CD3, CD4, or CD8
Mitogens	Pokeweed, lipopolysaccharide	Phytohemagglutinin, concanavalin A, BCG vaccine, pokeweed
Antigens recognized	Free foreign proteins	Processed foreign proteins in MHC antigens
Tolerance induction	Difficult	Easy
Progeny cells	Plasma cells, memory cells	Effector T cells, memory T cells
Secreted products	Immunoglobulins	Cytokines

TCR, T-cell antigen receptor; *BCG,* bacille Calmette–Guerin; *MHC,* major histocompatibility complex.

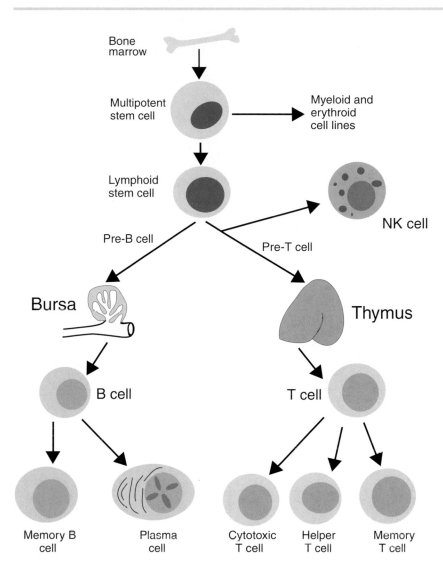

Figure 9-6. Development of T and B lymphocytes. Both arise from bone marrow precursors. B cells develop in the bursa, Peyer's patches, or bone marrow. T cells develop in the thymus. Natural killer cells are a third population of lymphocytes that are distinct from T and B cells.

TABLE 9-2

Major Peripheral Blood Lymphocyte Populations in Domestic Animals and Humans

	T Cells	B cells	CD4+	CD8+	CD4/CD8
Bovine	45–53[a]	16–21[a]	8–31	10–30	1.53[a]
Sheep	56–64[b]	11–50[c]	8–22[c]	4–22[c]	1.55[b]
Pigs	45–57[d]	13–38[e]	23–43	17–39	1.4[f]
Horses	38–66	17–38[g]	56[h]	20–37[g]	4.75[h]
Dogs	46–72	7–30	27–33[i]	17–18[i]	1.7[i]
Cats	31–89[j]	6–50[j]	19–49[j]	6–39[j]	1.9[j]
Human	70–75	10–15	43–48[k]	22–24[k]	1.9-2.4[k]

[a]Park YH et al: *J Dairy Sci* 75:998-1006, 1992.
[b]Thorp BH et al: *Dev Comp Immunol* 15:393-400, 1991.
[c]Smith HE: *Can J Vet Res* 58:152-155, 1994.
[d] Pescovitz MD et al: *Vet Immunol Immunopathol* 43:53-62, 1994.
[e] Saalmüller A et al: *Vet Immunol Immunopathol* 43:45-52, 1994.
[f]Joling P et al: *Vet Immunol Immunopathol* 40:105-118, 1994.
[g]McGorum BC et al: *Vet Immunol Immunopathol* 36:207-222, 1993.
[h]Grunig G et al: *Vet Immunol Immunopathol* 42:61-69, 1994.
[i]Rivas AL et al: *Vet Immunol Immunopathol* 45:55-71, 1995.
[j]Walker R et al: *Aust Vet J* 72:93-97, 1995.
[k]Bleavins MR et al: *Vet Immunol Immunopathol* 37:1-13, 1993.

a receptor for MHC class I molecules and is required for the recognition of processed endogenous antigen.

Most human and mouse T cells express either CD4 or CD8, rarely both. For example, about 65% of human T cells are CD4+CD8− and 30% are CD4−CD8+. The remaining 5% of T cells express neither (CD4−CD8−) and are said to be double negative. The ratio of CD4+ to CD8+ cells in blood may be used to estimate lymphocyte function. An elevated CD4 count implies increased lymphocyte reactivity because helper cells predominate, whereas a high CD8 count implies depressed lymphocyte reactivity. The relative proportions of CD4 and CD8 cells seen in humans are not necessarily seen in other mammals (Tables 9-2 and 9-3). Thus CD4 is not restricted to T helper cells but is also found on monocytes, macrophages, neutrophils, and eosinophils in some species. About 10% of a T-cell surface is covered by CD45 molecules. These regulate signal transduction by the TCR. Several different forms of CD45 have been identified. Thus unprimed T cells have one form of CD45 whereas stimulated and memory T cells have a different form.

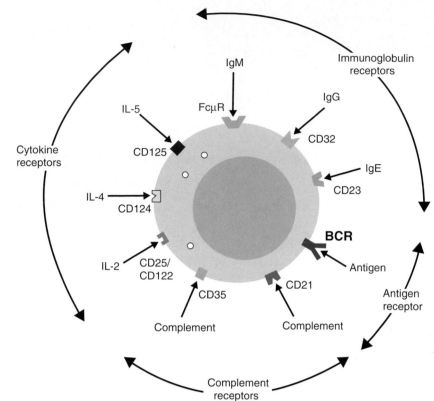

Figure 9-7. Major surface receptors of B cells, their ligands, and their functions.

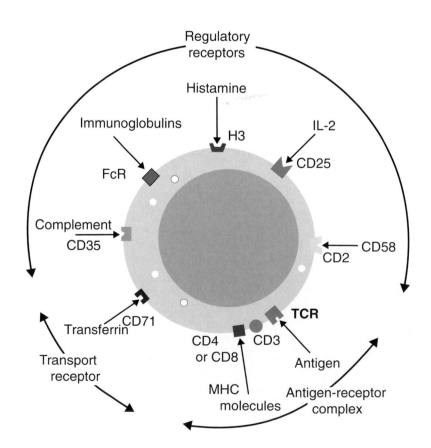

Figure 9-8. Major surface receptors of T cells, their ligands, and their functions.

TABLE 9-3
Surface Molecules on Peripheral Blood T Cells

Marker	Cell percentage			
	Mouse	Bovine	Swine	Sheep
TCRαβ	85–95	5–30	14–34	5–30
TCRγδ	5–15	45–50	31–39	22–68
CD2	95	41–60	58–72	10–36
CD4	24	8–28	23–43	8–22
CD8	11	10–30	17–39	4–22
WC1	—	5–44	40	15–70

The signal-transducing molecules associated with the B-cell antigen receptor are two small peptide heterodimers formed by pairing CD79a (immunoglobulin-α, Ig-α) with CD79b (Ig-β).

Molecules That Regulate Lymphocyte Function

Proteins on cell surfaces serve a physiological function. Some are enzymes, some are transport proteins, and many are receptors. All cells use receptor molecules to communicate with their environment or with other cells. They need receptors for antigen-presenting cells as well as receptors for the many molecules that regulate lymphocyte responses including receptors for cytokines, for antibodies, and for complement components.

Cytokine Receptors

Lymphocytes have receptors for many different cytokines. Examples of CD molecules that are cytokine receptors include CD25, part of the interleukin-2 (IL-2) receptor; CD118, an interferon receptor; CD120, the tumor necrosis factor (TNF) receptor; and CDw210, the IL-10 receptor. (These are discussed in Chapter 12.)

Antibody Receptors

Lymphocytes have receptors for antibodies. Since these receptors bind to the Fc regions of antibody molecules, they are called Fc receptors (FcR). (The meaning of the term Fc can be found in Chapter 13.) The Fc receptors

for IgG are designated FcγR since they bind the γ chain of IgG. Likewise those for IgA are designated FcαR and those for IgE are FcεR. Receptors for IgM and IgD have not been identified.

Three different FcγRs have been described on leukocytes (Table 9-4). They are called FcγRI (CD64), FcγRII (CD32), and FcγRIII (CD16). All these receptors are multichain glycoproteins. One chain usually binds the antibody whereas the other chains are needed for signal transduction. Sometimes these signal-transducing chains are shared with other receptors such as the TCR.

CD64 (FcγRI) is found on dendritic cells, monocytes, and macrophages and to a much lesser extent on neutrophils. (It is not found on lymphocytes but is mentioned here for the sake of completeness.) CD64 binds IgG with high affinity.

CD32 (FcγRII) is found on B cells, dendritic cells, and macrophages. It has a moderate affinity for IgG and will only bind immune complexes (several antibody molecules attached to an antigen). CD32 occurs in two molecular forms (isoforms), called B1 and B2. CD32-B1 is found on B cells where it regulates cell function. CD32-B2 is found on macrophages where it promotes phagocytosis and stimulates the release of cytokines.

CD16 (FcγRIII) binds IgG with low affinity and will therefore only bind immune complexes. It is found on granulocytes, NK cells, and macrophages but not on B cells.

FcεRI is a high-affinity IgE receptor found on mast cells and discussed in Chapter 26. It is a key factor in allergies. CD23 or FcεRII, in contrast, is an IgE receptor expressed on activated B cells, platelets, eosinophils, macrophages, NK cells, dendritic cells, and possibly even T cells. When a B cell is activated it secretes soluble CD23, which then regulates allergic responses.

Complement Receptors

B cells have receptors for several different complement proteins. These include CR1 (CD35), which binds C3b and C4b, and CR2 (CD21), which binds C3d and C3bi. Activated T cells also express CR1. CR2 is closely associated with the BCR and has a role in regulating B-cell responses to antigen.

TABLE 9-4
Receptors for IgG (FcγR)

Property	FcγRI	FcγRII	FcγRIII
CD designation	CD64	CD32	CD16
Molecular weight	75 kDa	39–48 kDa	50–65 kDa
Cells	Monocytes, macrophages	B cells, macrophages granulocytes, eosinophils	NK cells, granulocytes, macrophages
Affinity	High	Moderate	Low
Function	Phagocytosis	B cells: inhibition Macrophages: phagocytosis	NK cells: cytotoxicity Granulocytes: phagocytosis

Adherence Molecules

As discussed in Chapter 3, some cell surface molecules ensure that cells bind together and so interact effectively. They regulate signaling between the cells of the immune system and control the movement of leukocytes in or between tissues. The cell adhesion molecules found on lymphocytes include integrins, selectins, and members of the immunoglobulin superfamily.

Integrins

Integrins are heterodimeric proteins classified according to their β chain use. For example, the β_1 integrins consist of a β_1 chain (CD29) paired with one of several different α chains (CD49). The β_1 integrins bind cells to extracellular matrix proteins such as fibronectin, laminin, and collagen.

The β_2 integrins consist of a β_2 chain (CD18) paired with one of several α chains (CD11). These β_2 integrins control the attachment of leukocytes to vascular endothelium and bind T cells to antigen-presenting cells. For example, CD11a/CD18 on a T cell binds to its ligand, intercellular adhesion molecule-1 (ICAM-1), on the presenting cell. By prolonging and stabilizing cell interactions, this linkage permits successful antigen recognition. Another β_2 integrin, CD11b/CD18, binds the complement component, C3b, while CD11c/CD18 binds fibrinogen (Figure 9-9).

Selectins

The circulation of leukocytes is regulated by binding to vascular endothelium mediated by P-selectin (CD62P), L-selectin (CD62L), and E-selectin (CD62E). P- and E-selectins are found on vascular endothelial cells. When these cells are activated by inflammation, they express selectins that bind neutrophils, activated T cells, and monocytes. L-selectin, in contrast, binds lymphocytes to high endothelial venules in lymphoid organs (Chapter 8).

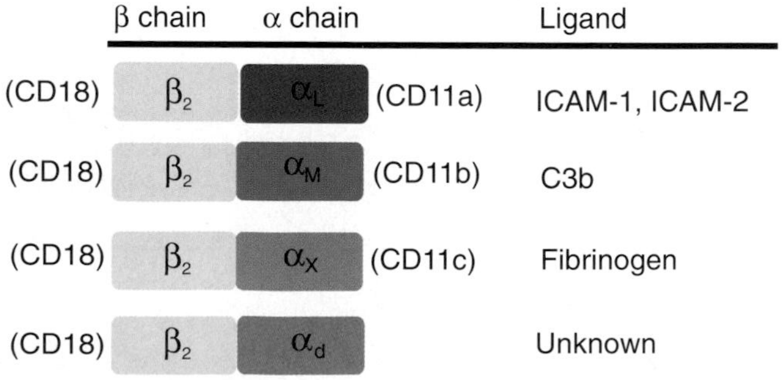

β chain		α chain		Ligand
(CD18)	β_2	α_L	(CD11a)	ICAM-1, ICAM-2
(CD18)	β_2	α_M	(CD11b)	C3b
(CD18)	β_2	α_X	(CD11c)	Fibrinogen
(CD18)	β_2	α_d		Unknown

Figure 9-9. The integrin families are based on the pairing of many different α chains with a limited number of β chains. This example shows the structure of the very important β_2 integrins.

Immunoglobulin Superfamily

Three members of this family are lymphocyte adhesion molecules. For example, ICAM-1 (CD54) is the ligand for CD11a/CD18 and for CD43 (Figure 3-7). It is normally expressed only on dendritic cells and B cells. Inflammation induces ICAM-1 expression on vascular endothelial cells and so permits phagocytic cells to adhere and move into inflamed tissues. ICAM-1 is also responsible for the migration of T cells into areas of inflammation [so-called delayed hypersensitivity reactions (Chapter 29)]. ICAM-2 (CD102) is an adherence protein that also binds CD11a/CD18. Unlike ICAM-1, ICAM-2 is expressed on unstimulated endothelial cells and is not increased during inflammation. ICAM-3 is expressed on resting lymphocytes, monocytes, and neutrophils. Its ligand is also CD11a/CD18. The third adherence molecule that belongs to the immunoglobulin superfamily is called vascular cell adhesion molecule-1 (VCAM-1) or CD106. VCAM-1 is expressed on inflamed vascular endothelial cells. Its ligand is the β_1 integrin, CD49d/CD29, found on lymphocytes and monocytes.

CD58 and CD2

CD58 (also called LFA-3) is the ligand for CD2. CD2 (or LFA-2) is only found on T cells, whereas CD58 is widely distributed on many cell types. Binding of CD2 and CD58 occurs, for example, between cytotoxic T cells and their target cells (Chapter 17). It has been suggested therefore that CD58 facilitates T-cell binding to any cell that is to undergo surveillance. CD58 is also found on antigen-presenting cells such as dendritic cells and macrophages. When it binds T-cell CD2, it enhances the recognition of antigen by the T cell and at the same time stimulates the antigen-presenting cell to secrete cytokines.

Other Major Surface Molecules

B cells, as antigen-presenting cells, express MHC class II molecules on their surface. In contrast, T-cell expression of MHC class II varies between species. Both types of lymphocytes express MHC class Ia and class Ib molecules.

CD1

CD1 molecules are a family of MHC class Id molecules (five in humans, two in mice, and seven in sheep) that present lipid and glycolipid antigens to T cells. There are two separate groups of CD1 molecules. Some CD1 molecules are expressed in large amounts on antigen-presenting cells, especially dendritic cells and B cells. Others are expressed on intestinal epithelium and some thymocytes.

CD90

The expression of CD90 (or Thy-1) varies among species. Thus in mice it is found on both thymocytes and blood T cells. In rats it is found on thymocytes but not blood T cells, whereas in humans it is found on neither. CD90 is also found on the surface of brain cells (astrocytes), epidermal cells, fibroblasts, and blood T lymphocytes. Its function is unknown, but it appears to regulate lymphocyte activation.

WC1

Lymphocytes of the major domestic mammals have several cell surface proteins not found in humans or mice. The best defined of these is WC1. WC1 is a heterodimer with chains of 215 and 300 kDa found on a major subset of γ/δ T cells. In cattle, WC1+ T cells are found in high numbers in the skin and mucous membranes, as well as in hemal nodes and the thymus. WC1 belongs to a multigene family containing at least seven related members in cattle and at least 50 in sheep. Homologs of WC1 have been identified in camels, llamas, deer, and elk. Other members of the family include CD5 and CD6. This family, the scavenger receptor cysteine-rich (SRCR) family, is found in many different mammals, amphibians, and invertebrates. WC1 has no known homologs in humans or mice, although WC1 cDNA probes hybridize with human, rodent, and horse DNA suggesting that related genes do exist but are not expressed. Although its natural ligand is unknown, WC1 is known to bind to ligands on macrophages and dendritic cells and, it is believed, to regulate γ/δ T-cell function.

Changes in Immunophenotype

Lymphocytes do not express the same immunophenotype at all stages in their life cycle. A cell's phenotype depends on its maturity and activation status. For example, immature human T cells carry both CD9 and CD10. As the T cells mature within the thymus, CD9 is lost and the cells gain CD4 and CD8. Mature thymocytes can then split into two subpopulations; one population becomes CD4+CD8−, the other becomes CD4−CD8+. In addition, the phenotype of lymphocytes changes after exposure to antigen. Thus naive T cells express high levels of CD45R and L-selectin and low levels of CD44. Memory T cells show the reverse of this, low levels of CD45R and L-selectin and high levels of CD44.

SPECIES DIFFERENCES

Bovine

Unique Molecules
Cattle lymphocytes express species-specific cell surface molecules named BoWC1 through BoWC15. (Additional studies however, sometimes show that a WC molecule may in fact have a CD homolog. For example, BoWC3 is now known to be CD21 and BoWC10 is CD26.)

α/β and γ/δ T Cells
In adult cattle about 10% to 15% of circulating T cells are γ/δ positive whereas the remainder are α/β positive. In young calves the proportion of γ/δ T cells may rise to 40%. However, this proportion can fluctuate in response to management and stress. The majority of these γ/δ T cells also express WC1. Indeed, these cells can be activated either through their TCR or through WC1. In response they produce TNF-α, IL-1, IL-12, and interferon-γ. This suggests that they may have a role in promoting inflammation while contributing to a Th1 bias in the bovine immune response. They thus provide a link between the innate and acquired immune systems. WC1+ γ/δ T cells have an important role in the early stages of infection by stimulating the rapid influx of lymphocytes and monocytes into granulomas that surround invaders.

CD4/CD8 Cells
Unlike humans, bovine CD4 is not found on macrophages. CD4 is found on 20% to 30% of blood lymphocytes in adult ruminants. Double-negative T cells constitute 15% to 30% of the blood lymphocytes in young ruminants, but this can reach 80% in newborn calves. Most of these double-negative cells are γ/δ^+ and WC1+. Thus the major circulating T cells in ruminants (γ/δ^+, WC1+, CD4−, CD8−) are different from the predominant T cells in the blood of humans and mice (α/β^+, WC1−, CD4+, CD8−).

Sheep

Unique Molecules
Sheep γ/δ T cells express OvWC1 (also called T19). Sheep α/β T cells also express OvWC1, but this is a different isoform from the molecule on γ/δ T cells.

α/β and γ/δ cells
When lambs are born, γ/δ T cells account for 60% of blood T cells, but this drops to 30% by 1 year of age and to 5% by 5 years.

Pigs

Unique Molecules
Pig leukocytes possess nine unique surface proteins (SWC1-SWC9). SWC1 is expressed on resting T cells, monocytes, and granulocytes but not on B cells. SWC3 is found on monocytes/macrophages. SWC9 is expressed only by mature macrophages.

α/β and γ/δ Cells
In adult pigs, γ/δ T cells constitute about 25% to 50% of blood T cells. In young pigs 4 weeks of age, 66% of T cells are γ/δ positive. Pigs have two subpopulations of γ/δ T cells. One is CD2+ and the other is CD2− and has not been identified in other species. A subpopulation

of pig γ/δ T cells can function as professional antigen-presenting cells using MHC class II molecules.

CD4/CD8 Cells

All pig CD4+ cells are α/β cells. Up to 60% of T cells in pig blood are CD4+CD8+. The rest are predominantly double negative (CD4-CD8-). Most memory T cells belong to the double-positive population. Two subpopulations of CD4-CD8+ T cells have been identified: one with a heterodimeric CD8 molecule (CD8α/CD8β), the other with a homodimeric CD8 molecule (CD8α/CD8α). The CD4+CD8-, and CD4+CD8+ cells express CD5 whereas double-negative cells do not. The CD4-CD8+ cells in pig blood fall into two subsets. One does not express CD5 and appears to be a population of NK cells. The other expresses CD5 at high levels and consists of progenitors of cytotoxic T cells.

Horses

Unique Molecules

Horses possess four species-specific proteins EqWC1 through EqWC4. EqWC1 is found on 70% of equine T cells, 30% of B cells, and 50% of granulocytes. It may be a homolog of CD90. EqWC2 is found on granulocytes and most T cells. EqWC3 is CD2. EqWC4 is found on CD4 and CD8 cells, and may be a homolog of CD28.

Dogs and Cats

In dogs, CD4 is expressed on neutrophils and macrophages but not on monocytes, whereas in cats CD4 is found on only a subset of T cells and their precursors.

THE FLOW CYTOMETER

Because of the importance of identifying cell immunophenotypes considerable effort has gone into developing rapid identification methods. Immunophenotypes can now be automatically analyzed in great detail and with high efficiency using a flow cytometer (Figure 9-10). In this instrument a suspension of cells is pumped through a very narrow tube so that the cells pass through in single file. A laser beam is directed through the cell stream, and the effects of each cell on the light beam are measured. Thus the scatter of the light beam in a forward direction can be used to give a measure of a cell's size. The light scattered to the side by a cell gives a measure of a cell's surface roughness and internal complexity. A combination of these two parameters can be used to identify all the leukocytes in a blood sample.

The flow cytometer can, however, be used to measure much more than this. Thus if a cell suspension is mixed with a monoclonal antibody bound to a fluorescent dye, then the labeled antibody will only bind to cells carrying the appropriate antigen. This subpopulation can be characterized and counted (Figures 9-11 and 9-12). By using antibodies labeled with different colored fluorescent dyes, the expression of multiple cell surface antigens can be analyzed simultaneously. It is possible to use the flow cytometer to follow sequential changes in the immunophenotype of mixed-cell populations (Figure 9-13).

CELL SURFACE RECEPTORS AND SIGNAL TRANSDUCTION

Immune responses occur as a result of interactions among many different cell types. Cells need to be able to sense events occurring in their surroundings and react accordingly. For example, neutrophils must be able to detect the presence of nearby bacteria and migrate toward them by chemotaxis. These processes require that cells have many diverse receptors on their surface and that once these receptors bind to their ligands, they transmit signals to the cell to modify its behavior (Figure 9-14). This conversion of an extracellular signal into a series of intracellular events is called signal transduction.

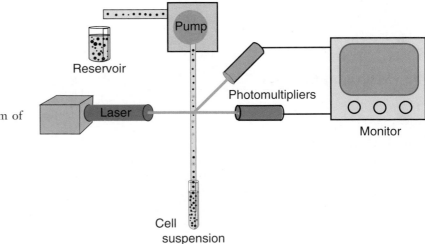

Figure 9-10. Simplified view of the mechanism of action of the flow cytometer.

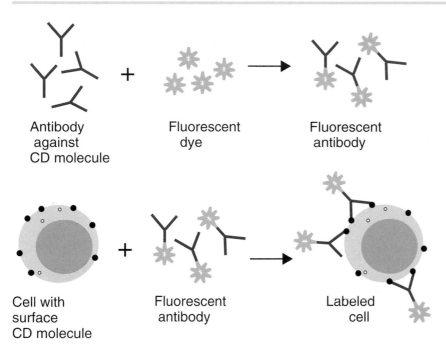

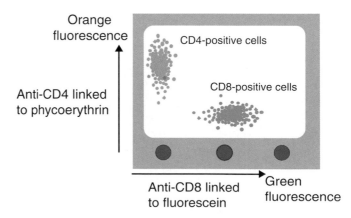

Figure 9-11. How an immunoglobulin bound to a fluorescent dye can be used to identify CD molecules in a flow cytometer.

The key components of signal transduction include binding of an agonist to a receptor, activation of a transducer protein by the receptor, secondary activation of other enzymes, generation of new transcription factors, and gene activation leading to altered cell behavior.

Cell surface receptor proteins belong to one of four classes based on their mode of action (Figure 9-15).

One class of receptor, channel-linked receptors, uses transmitter-gated ion channels. Thus the receptor itself is a channel, and binding of its agonist opens that channel allowing ions to pass through it. Channel-linked receptors are found in inflammatory and immune cells, but their roles are unclear.

A second class of receptor consists of proteins that also act as tyrosine protein kinases (Figure 9-16 and Box 9-1). The receptor site, the membrane-spanning region, and the effector enzyme are usually separate domains of a single protein. Thus when the ligand binds to the extracellular domain, an intracellular kinase domain is activated. These kinases phosphorylate tyrosine residues on other proteins or even the receptor itself (autophosphorylation). The phosphorylation triggers a series of

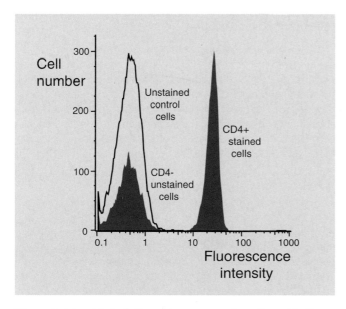

Figure 9-12. Typical flow cytometer readout from labeling a cell population with antiequine CD4. The intensity of fluorescent labeling increases from left to right. Thus unlabeled control cells form the unshaded left peak. When a mixture of CD4+ and CD4− cells is examined it forms two distinct peaks (*shaded area*). The left peak consists of unlabeled (CD4−) cells. The right peak consists of labeled (CD4+) cells. The area under each peak is a measure of the size of each cell subpopulation. (Courtesy of Dr. RR Smith III.)

Figure 9-13. The pattern seen on a flow cytometer screen when analyzing lymphocyte populations stained with two different fluorescence-conjugated antibodies. It is usual to label one population with a green dye and the second population with a red or orange dye.

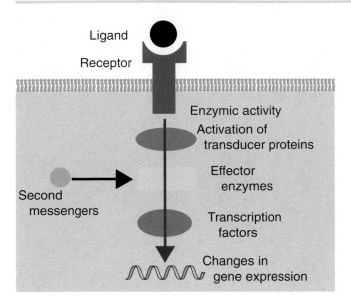

Figure 9-14. Generic view of signal transduction. Although receptor signaling varies in its details, the overall process of signal transduction has some consistent features shown here.

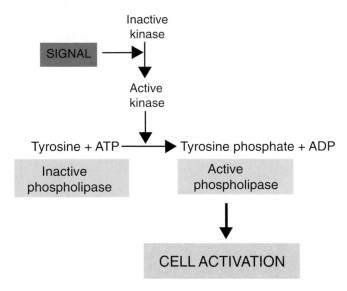

Figure 9-16. Phosphorylation of tyrosine by a protein kinase results in phospholipase activation, which leads eventually to cell activation.

changes in cellular activities. Many reactions of the immune system operate through this type of receptor (especially through protein kinases of the src family). A related type of receptor consists of proteins that are not themselves tyrosine kinases but can activate tyrosine kinases associated with the receptors. This type of receptor is also widely employed in the cells of the immune system. Examples of tyrosine kinase–linked receptors include the TCR and the BCR.

The JAK-STAT signal transduction pathway is a variant of the above. In this pathway the receptor and the effector enzyme are on separate proteins. Ligand binding to the receptor activates the tyrosine kinase activity of the tightly associated JAK (Janus family tyrosine kinases). STAT proteins (signal transducers and activators of transcription) associate with the JAK enzyme and so become phosphorylated. The phosphorylated STAT proteins then dissociate from JAK and translocate to

the nucleus where they act as transcription factors and modulate the expression of target genes. These pathways are commonly used by cytokines and interferons.

A third class of receptors is associated with membrane-bound guanosine triphosphate (GTP)-binding proteins,

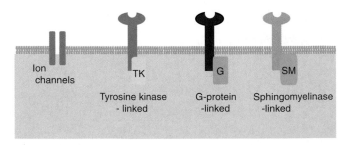

Figure 9-15. The four different classes of protein receptors found on cell surfaces. There are two forms of tyrosine kinase–linked receptor. In some the tyrosine kinase activity is an integral part of the receptor protein. In others, as shown here, the enzyme may be on a linked protein. All the receptors of immunological importance fall into one of these categories.

BOX 9–1

Protein Phosphorylation

Phosphorylation is the most important form of reversible modification of proteins. All the signal transduction systems involve the use of a high-energy compound (e.g., guanosine triphosphate) to modify a protein and send a signal to a cell. Cell growth, cell division, as well as other critical processes are all regulated by protein phosphorylation. Protein kinases enzymatically phosphorylate the amino acids serine, threonine, and tyrosine (Figure 9-18).

Protein kinase
$$\text{Protein} + \text{ATP} \longrightarrow \text{protein P} + \text{ADP}$$

In some proteins only one amino acid is phosphorylated; in others, multiple amino acids are phosphorylated. Phosphorylated and nonphosphorylated proteins have different functional properties. For example, the phosphorylation of serine or threonine activates some enzymes, whereas dephosphorylation has the opposite effect. Phosphorylation of the three key amino acids (serine, threonine, and tyrosine) plays a critical role in the regulation of many cellular functions. When phosphorylated proteins are examined, about 90% of the phosphate is attached to serine and about 10% to threonine. Only about 1/2000 of the phosphate is linked to tyrosine. Thus tyrosine phosphorylation is a rare event despite its being a key mechanism in almost all the signal transduction pathways described in this book.

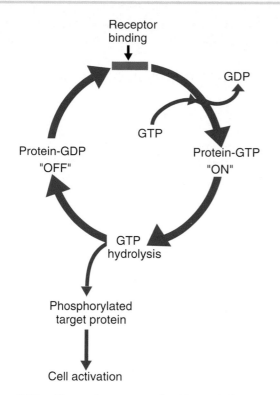

Figure 9-17. G proteins act as a signaling switch to turn cell functions on and off.

called G proteins. G proteins act as chemical switches. When inactive, they bind guanosine diphosphate (GDP). When active, they bind GTP. Thus once these receptors bind their ligand, a change in the receptor/G-protein complex results in a loss of GDP and a gain of GTP (Figure 9-17). The activated G protein then activates other substrates. The GTP is rapidly hydrolyzed to GDP by the G-protein's own GTPase so that the G protein is then turned off. More than 20 different G proteins have been identified and some play key roles in the immune response. The targets of G proteins can include ion channels, enzymes such as adenylate cyclase, phospholipase C, and some protein kinases. When activated by a G protein, phospholipase C splits the membrane-bound lipid, phosphatidylinositol 4,5-bisphosphate (PIP_2), into two messenger molecules, inositol triphosphate and diacylglycerol (Figure 9-18). Inositol triphosphate binds to intracellular receptors releasing Ca^{2+} from internal stores and so increases the concentration of intracellular Ca^{2+}. These calcium ions can activate many different proteins. The diacylglycerol remains in the plasma membrane and along with calcium activates an enzyme called protein kinase C.

A fourth class of receptor activates a neutral sphingomyelinase which then hydrolyzes sphingomyelin in the cell membrane to ceramide. The ceramide then stimulates a ceramide-activated serine-threonine protein kinase that phosphorylates cellular proteins. This mechanism of signal transduction is used by the receptors for IL-1 and TNF-α.

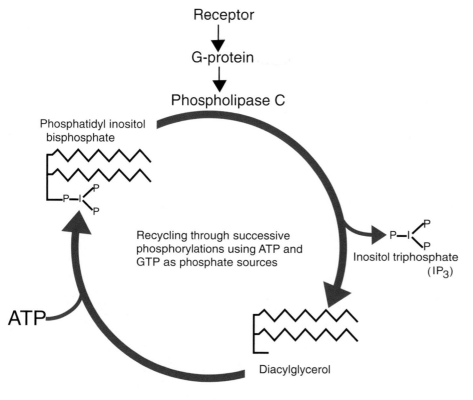

Figure 9-18. Activation of cell membrane phospholipase C generates inositol triphosphate and diacylgycerol. These two molecules are messengers that initiate cell activation.

You can read about signal transduction in B cells in Chapter 11, in T cells in Chapter 10, and in mast cells in Chapter 26.

LYMPHOCYTE MITOGENS

In addition to their surface proteins, lymphocytes can be characterized by the stimulants that make them divide. The most important of these are proteins called lectins that bind to cell surface glycoproteins and so trigger cell division (Box 9-2). These lectins are commonly isolated from plants. Examples include phytohemagglutinin (PHA) obtained from the red kidney bean (*Phaseolus vulgaris*), concanavalin A (Con A) obtained from the jack bean (*Canavalis ensiformis*), and pokeweed mitogen (PWM) obtained from the pokeweed plant (*Phytolacca americana*). Lectins specifically bind sugar residues on glycoprotein side chains. For example, PHA binds *N*-acetylgalactosamine, and Con A binds α-mannose and α-glucose. Not all lymphocytes respond equally well to all lectins. Thus PHA primarily stimulates T-cell division, although it has a slight effect on B cells. Con A is also a T-cell mitogen, whereas PWM acts on both T and B cells.

Although the plant lectins are the most efficient lymphocyte mitogens, mitogenic activity is also found in other unexpected sources. For example, an extract from the snail *Helix pomata* stimulates T cells whereas lipopolysaccharide from gram-negative bacteria stimulates B cells. Other important B-cell mitogens include neutral proteases, such as trypsin, and Fc fragments of immunoglobulins. Bacille Calmette–Guerin (BCG) vaccine, an avirulent strain of *Mycobacterium bovis* that is used as a vaccine against tuberculosis, is a T-cell mitogen. These mitogens can assist in the differentiation of T and B cells and, by measurement of the response provoked, quantitate the ability of T and B cells to respond to stimuli.

BOX 9–2

How to Measure Mitogenicity

To measure the effect of mitogens, lymphocytes are grown in tissue culture. Lymphocytes can be obtained directly from blood. The lymphocytes are cultured for at least 34 hours before the mitogen is added. Once this is done they begin to divide, synthesize new DNA, and take up any available nucleotides from the medium. It is usual to incorporate a small quantity of thymidine labeled with the radioactive isotope of hydrogen, tritium (^{3}H), in the tissue culture fluid. The thymidine is only incorporated into the DNA of cells that are dividing. After about 24 hours, the cultured cells are separated from the tissue culture fluid, either by centrifugation or filtration, and their radioactivity is counted. The amount of radioactivity in the mitogen-treated cells may be compared with that in an untreated lymphocyte culture. This ratio is called the stimulation index. As an alternative to the use of tritiated thymidine, a radiolabeled amino acid such as ^{14}C-leucine can be used. Uptake of this compound indicates increased protein synthesis by the cells.

SOURCES OF ADDITIONAL INFORMATION

Albelda SM, Buck CA: Integrins and other cell adhesion molecules, *FASEB J* 4:2868-2880, 1990.

Antczak DF, Kydd J, eds: Equine leukocyte antigens, *Vet Immunol Immunopathol* 42:1-116, 1994.

Appleyard GD, Wilkie BN: Characterization of porcine CD5 and CD5+ B cells, *Clin Exp Immunol* 111:225-230, 1998.

Becker BA, Misfeldt ML: Evaluation of the mitogen-induced proliferation and cell surface differentiation antigens of lymphocytes from pigs 1 to 30 days of age, *J Anim Sci* 71:2073-2078, 1993.

Binns RM: The null/γδ+ T cell family in the pig, *Vet Immunol Immunopathol* 43:69-77, 1994.

Carr MM, Howard CJ, Sopp P, et al: Expression on porcine γδ lymphocytes of a phylogenetically conserved surface antigen previously restricted in expression to ruminant γδ T lymphocytes, *Immunology* 81:36-40, 1994.

Elangbam CS, Qualls CW Jr, Dahlgren RR: Cell adhesion molecules: update, *Vet Pathol* 34:61-73, 1997.

Evans CW, Lund BT, McConnell I, Bujdoso R: Antigen recognition and activation of ovine γδ T cells, *Immunology* 82:229-237, 1994.

Hein WR, Mackay CR: Prominence of γδ T cells in the ruminant immune system, *Immunol Today* 12:30-34, 1991.

Howard CJ, Morrison WI, eds: Leukocyte antigens in cattle, sheep and goats, *Vet Immunol Immunopathol* 27:1-276, 1991.

Jungi TW, Francey T, Brcic M, et al: Sheep macrophages express at least two distinct receptors for IgG which have similar affinity for homologous IgG$_1$ and IgG$_2$, *Vet Immunol Immunopathol* 33:321-337, 1992.

Mackay CR, Marston WL, Dudler L, Hein WR: Expression of the T19 and "null cell" markers on γ/δ T cells of the sheep, *Vet Immunol Immunopathol* 27:183-188, 1991.

Martin KH, Slack JK, Boerner SA, et al: Integrin connections map: to infinity and beyond, *Science* 296:1652-1653, 2002.

O'Keeffe MA, Metcalfe SA, Cunningham CP, Walker ID: Sheep CD4+ αβ T cells express novel members of the T19 multigene family, *Immunogenetics* 49:45-55, 1999.

Otani I, Niwa T, Tajima M, Ishikawa A, et al: CD56 is expressed exclusively on CD3+ T lymphocytes in canine peripheral blood, *J Vet Med Sci* 64:441-444, 2002.

Saalmüller A, Bryant J: Characteristics of porcine T lymphocytes and T-cell lines, *Vet Immunol Immunopathol* 43:45-52, 1994.

Saalmüller A, Hirt W, Maurer S, Weiland E: Discrimination between two subsets of porcine CD8+ cytolytic T lymphocytes by the expression of CD5 antigen, *Immunology* 81: 578-583, 1994.

Smith HE, Jacobs RM, Smith C: Flow cytometric analysis of ovine peripheral blood lymphocytes, *Can J Vet Res* 58: 152-155, 1994.

Walker ID, Glew MD, O'Keefe MA, et al: A novel multi-gene family of sheep γ/δ T cells, *Immunology* 83:517-523, 1994.

Wijngaard PLJ, Metzelaar MJ, MacHugh ND, et al: Molecular characterization of the WC1 antigen expressed specifically on bovine CD4−CD8− γ/δ T lymphocytes, *J Immunol* 149:3273-3277, 1992.

Yang H, Parkhouse RME: Phenotypic classification of porcine lymphocyte subpopulations in blood and lymphoid tissues. *Immunology* 89:76-83, 1996.

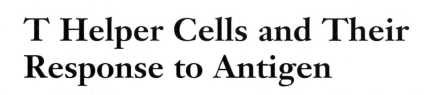

T Helper Cells and Their Response to Antigen

CHAPTER

10

Unlike the innate immune responses that respond to a limited number of molecules restricted to the major groups of pathogenic microorganisms, the lymphocytes of the acquired immune system must be able to recognize and respond to a large number of very diverse foreign antigens. These lymphocytes have cell surface receptors that are specific for antigen. When exposed to an antigen that binds their receptors, under the right conditions, these lymphocytes will mediate either a cell-mediated or an antibody-mediated immune response.

There are three major populations of antigen-sensitive lymphocytes. These are the T helper cells that regulate immune responses; the effector or cytotoxic T cells that destroy endogenous antigens, and the B cells that produce antibodies to destroy exogenous antigens. The cells in each of these populations are selected so that only antigens that bind to their specific receptors will trigger an immune response. This chapter discusses the first of these lymphocyte populations, the T helper cells.

Exogenous antigen trapped and processed by dendritic cells is presented to T helper cells in secondary lymphoid organs. Each T helper cell has several thousand identical antigen receptors on its surface. If these receptors bind their specific antigen in the correct manner, a T helper cell will initiate an immune response by proliferating and differentiating. As you will see later, the other antigen-sensitive cell populations, the B cells and the cytotoxic T cells, cannot respond optimally to antigens unless they too are stimulated by T helper cells. Because of the central role of T helper cells they must be carefully regulated. T helper cells are controlled through cell–cell interactions and by the activities of many different cytokines.

It is important to point out at this stage that the antigen receptors on T cells are not designed to react with any specific foreign antigen or microbe. On the contrary, antigen receptors are generated randomly. However, the universe of receptors on all T cells in the body forms a vast repertoire. As a result, it can be expected that any foreign antigen will bind to the receptors on at least one T cell. Because each T cell can have only one receptor specificity, the repertoire of receptors is, in effect, the repertoire of the T cells. Given the random nature of receptor binding, the strength of binding (or affinity) between an antigen and its receptors will vary. Thus an antigen may be bound strongly by some receptors and weakly by others. If the affinity falls below a specific threshold, the encounter between an antigen and its receptor may be insufficient to activate the T cell.

In a newborn animal that has never encountered antigens previously, the number of T cells that can bind any specific antigen may be very low. In order to increase the probability of an antigen encountering a T cell with the appropriate receptor, T cells are concentrated at sites such as lymph nodes where the chances of a successful interaction with antigen-bearing dendritic cells are maximized. In primed animals where mature T cells are plentiful, they migrate from lymphoid organs into the tissues where they can encounter the other antigen-presenting cells, macrophages, and B cells. Thus during a secondary immune response, mature T cells can circulate through the tissues and seek out encounters with processed antigen.

A T helper cell can respond to a foreign antigen only when the antigen is presented in association with an appropriate MHC molecule. Only when the binding site of a dendritic cell MHC class II molecule is filled by an antigenic peptide can the complex be recognized by its corresponding T cell antigen receptor.

THE IMMUNOGLOBULIN SUPERFAMILY

Proteins are constructed by linking together multiple peptide modules or domains. Each domain usually has a well-defined function. For example, in proteins located on a cell surface, the membrane-binding domain contains hydrophobic amino acids so that it can penetrate the plasma membrane. Other domains may be responsible for the structural stability of a protein or for its biological activities. In antibody (immunoglobulin) molecules, one domain is used to bind antigen and other domains are responsible for cell binding. The presence of similar domains in dissimilar proteins suggests that they have a common origin and proteins may be assigned to families or superfamilies based on their domain structure.

Proteins belonging to the immunoglobulin superfamily play key roles in the immune system. The members of this superfamily all contain at least one immunoglobulin domain. In a typical immunoglobulin domain the peptide chains weave back and forth to form a pleated sheet that folds into a sandwich-like structure. Immunoglobulin domains were first identified in antibody molecules (immunoglobulins). They have since been found in many other proteins, and collectively these proteins form the immunoglobulin superfamily. The superfamily includes some proteins with multiple immunoglobulin domains and some with only a single domain. The proteins with multiple domains include the B-cell antigen receptors (BCRs), the T-cell antigen receptors (TCRs), and the MHC class I and II molecules (Figure 10-1). All of the members of this superfamily are receptors; most are found on cell surfaces; and none have enzymatic activity. Many cellular interactions are mediated by linkage between two different members of the superfamily as, for example, between TCR and MHC molecules.

THE T-CELL ANTIGEN RECEPTOR

The Antigen-Binding Component

Each T cell has about 30,000 antigen receptors (TCRs) on its surface. Because all the TCRs expressed on an individual cell are identical, a T cell can only respond to peptides that bind that receptor. Each TCR is a complex

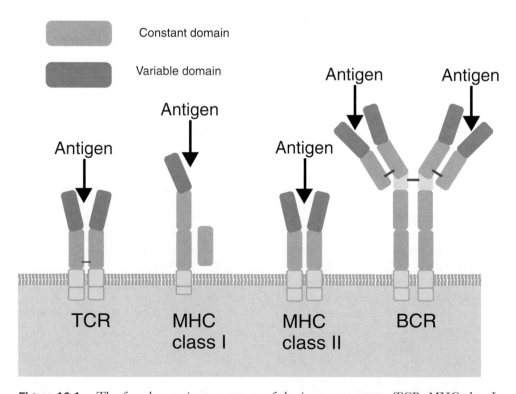

Figure 10-1.   The four key antigen receptors of the immune system—TCR, MHC class I, MHC class II, BCR—are constructed using immunoglobulin domains as building blocks. Each binds antigen through the use of variable domains. All are members of the immunoglobulin superfamily.

structure consisting of six glycoproteins. Two of the glycoproteins bind antigen; the other four amplify the signal generated by antigen binding and transmit it to the cell. Two different types of TCR have been identified based on the antigen-binding chains used (Figure 10-2). One type employs two protein chains called γ and δ (γ/δ). The other employs two different chains called α and β (α/β). In humans, mice and probably most non-ruminants, between 90% and 99% of T cells have α/β receptors. The remaining T cells in these species carry γ/δ receptors. In calves and lambs, in contrast, as many as 60% of T cells may have γ/δ TCRs.

The four antigen-binding chains (α, β, γ, δ) are similar in structure being members of the immunoglobulin superfamily, although they differ in size. Thus the α chain is 43 to 49 kDa, the β chain is 38 to 44 kDa, the γ chain is 36 to 46 kDa, and the δ chain is 40 kDa. The ranges are due to variations in glycosylation. Each TCR chain is formed from four domains (Figure 10-3). The N-terminal domain contains about 100 amino acids whose sequence varies greatly among cells. This is therefore called the variable (V) domain. The second domain contains about 150 amino acids. Its amino acid sequence does not vary and so it is called the constant (C) domain. The third, very small domain consists of 20 hydrophobic amino acids passing through the T-cell membrane. The C-terminal domain within the cytoplasm of the T cell is only 5 to 15 amino acids long. The two chains are joined by a disulfide bond between their constant domains to form a stable heterodimer. Because each TCR consists of paired chains, the two V domains form a groove in which antigenic peptides bind. The precise shape of this antigen-binding groove varies among different TCRs because of the variable amino acid sequences in the V domains. The specificity of the binding between a TCR and an

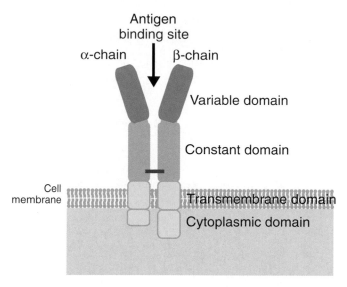

Figure 10-3. Schematic diagram showing the domain structure of the two peptide chains that make up the antigen-binding component of an α/β TCR.

antigenic peptide is determined by the receptor shape generated by the paired V domains.

When the V domains are examined closely, it is found that within each V domain is an area of the chain where the amino acid sequence is especially highly variable. This is the region that actually comes into contact with the antigen. For this reason it is called the hypervariable or the complementarity-determining region (CDR). The antigen-binding site of the TCR is formed by the paired CDRs that line the groove on the molecule's surface. The rest of the V domain outside the CDRs has a constant sequence and is called the framework region.

The Signal Transduction Component

CD3

The binding of antigen to the TCR must send a signal to the T cell in order to trigger its response. The two antigen-binding chains of each TCR are therefore associated with a cluster of proteins called the CD3 complex (Figure 10-4). The CD3 complex consists of five different protein chains (γ, δ, ε, ζ (zeta)(or CD247), and η (eta)) (Table 10-1) arranged as three dimers γ–ε, δ–ε, and ζ–ζ or ζ–η. The TCR β chain is directly linked to the γ-ε dimer, and the TCR α chain is linked to the δ–ε dimer. About 80% of α/β TCRs contain a ζ–ζ homodimer, so that the complete complex consists of αβ-γε-δε-ζζ. The remaining 20% contain ζ–η heterodimers (they therefore consist of αβ-γε–δε-ζη).

CD4 and CD8

Two other proteins closely associated with the TCR are CD4 and CD8. CD4 is a single-chain glycoprotein of 55 kDa and CD8 is a dimer of 68 kDa. (One chain is called CD8α, whereas the other is called CD8β.) Both

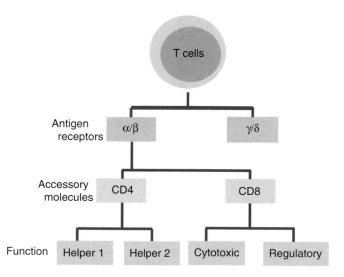

Figure 10-2. T cells can be divided into many different subpopulations based on the antigen receptors they employ, on the accessory molecules that support their activity, and ultimately on their functions.

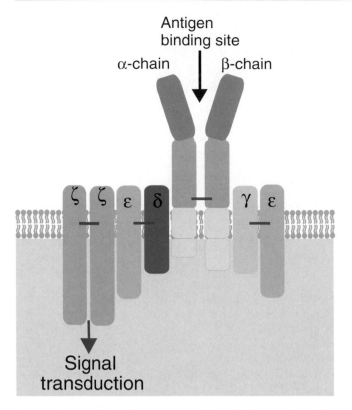

Antigen binding site

α-chain   β-chain

ζ ζ ε δ — γ ε

Signal transduction

Figure 10-4. Overall structure of the TCR complex. The signal transduction proteins are collectively classified as CD3. Approximately 80% of α/β TCRs use ζζ dimers. The remaining 20% use ηζ heterodimers. Most γ/δ TCRs probably use a completely different signal transduction complex.

CD4 and CD8 are members of the immunoglobulin superfamily. The presence of CD4 or CD8 determines the class of MHC molecule recognized by a T cell (Figure 10-5). For example, CD4, found only on T helper cells, binds MHC class II molecules on antigen-processing cells. CD8, in contrast, is found only on cytotoxic T cells and binds MHC class Ia molecules.

TABLE 10-1
The TCR–CD3 Receptor Complex

Peptide Chain	Function	Molecular Weight (kDa)
TCR α	Recognition of antigen and MHC	45–60
TCR β	Recognition of antigen and MHC	40–55
TCR γ	Recognition of antigen	36–46
TCR δ	Recognition of antigen	40–60
CD3 γ	Signal transducer	21–28
CD3 δ	Signal transducer	20–28
CD3 ε	Signal transducer	20–25
CD3 ζ	Signal transducer	16
CD3 η	Signal transducer	22
CD4	MHC II receptor	55
CD8	MHC I receptor	34

In humans, pigs, mice, and cats, CD8 is expressed on T cells as an α-β heterodimer or, much less commonly, as an α-α homodimer. CD4 and CD8 stimulate TCR signal transduction 100-fold when they bind to an MHC molecule on an antigen-presenting cell.

COSTIMULATORS

The binding of a TCR to a peptide–MHC complex is usually insufficient to trigger a T helper cell response. Several other costimulatory signals are needed to induce an optimal T-cell response. These costimulatory signals fall into three major groups. First, several ligands, such as CD40, are expressed on antigen-presenting cells and these bind to receptors on T cells. Their role is to amplify responses once initial T-cell activation is achieved. Second, additional costimulation is provided by cytokines secreted by the antigen-presenting cells. These determine the way in which a T cell responds to antigen. Finally, maximal costimulation requires cell surface adhesion molecules to bind the T cells and antigen-presenting cells firmly together.

Costimulatory Receptors

CD40 is a cell surface receptor that belongs to the tumor necrosis factor (TNF) receptor family. It is expressed constitutively on dendritic cells and on B cells and induced on macrophages. Its ligand, CD154 (CD40L), is a cell surface molecule expressed by T helper cells several hours after their TCR has bound to its antigen (Figure 10-6). Once expressed, CD154 binds to its receptor, CD40. This CD40–CD154 interaction is important because it results in signals being sent in both directions. The T cell sends signals to the antigen-presenting cell and the antigen-presenting cell signals the T cell. The signal to the T cell stimulates it to express a surface molecule called CD28. The signal to the antigen-presenting cell stimulates it to express CD80 or CD86 or both. The binding of CD40 to CD154 also stimulates the antigen-presenting cell to secrete cytokines, including interleukin-1 (IL-1), IL-6, IL-8, IL-12, CCL3 and TNF-α. This signal also prolongs dendritic cell survival, permits B cells to respond to antigen, and activates macrophages.

CD28 is a receptor induced on the T-cell surface by signals from interacting CD40 and CD154. Its ligands are CD80 on dendritic cells, macrophages or activated B cells, or CD86 on B cells. The binding of CD28 to CD80/86 stimulates the T cell in turn, to express another receptor, CD152 (CTLA-4). CD152 also binds to CD80 or CD86. The binding of CD80/86 to CD28 is required for complete T helper cell activation since the engagement of CD28 amplifies the signal to the T cell 100-fold. The T cells are now primed for optimal proliferation and cytokine production. On the other hand, when CD80 or

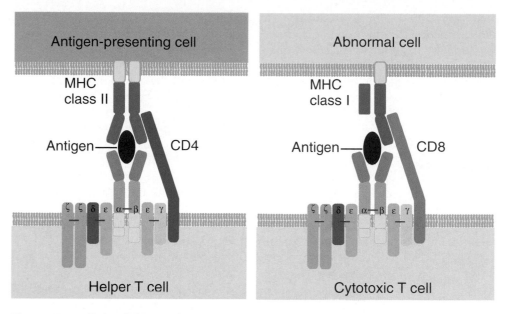

Figure 10-5. Role of CD4 and CD8 in promoting T-cell responses. These molecules link the T cell to the antigen-presenting cell, binding the two cells together and ensuring that an effective signal is transmitted between them. This interaction is seen in Figure 6-7, *A*.

CD86 binds to CD152, T-cell activation is suppressed. Thus the opposing signals delivered to T cells through these two receptors, CD28 and CD152, effectively regulate the intensity of T-cell responses.

Resting antigen-presenting cells do not express either CD80 or CD86. It takes 48 to 72 hours after T cell

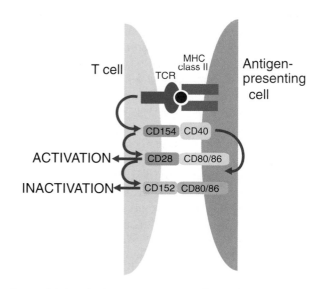

Figure 10-6. Antigen-presenting cells and T helper cells engage in a dialogue. Thus binding of antigen to the TCR causes the T cell to express CD40 ligand (CD154). This engages CD40 on the antigen-presenting cell. As a result, CD28 and CD152 are expressed on the T cell and CD80 or CD86 is expressed on the antigen-presenting cell. Depending on which receptors are engaged, the T cell may be stimulated or suppressed.

CD154 binds to CD40 before antigen-presenting cells can express CD80/86 and T cells can express CD152. Both CD80 and CD86 can bind to either CD28 or CD152. However, because CD152 binds these molecules with a higher affinity than does CD28, the inhibitory effect of this molecule gradually predominates. When CD152 binds to CD80 on dendritic cells, it induces the production of indoleamine dioxygenase, an enzyme that destroys tryptophan. In the absence of this amino acid, T cells are unresponsive to antigen and the T-cell response is terminated. In the absence of CD28, T cells cannot be activated. In the absence of CD152, the T cells undergo uncontrolled activation.

Costimulatory Cytokines

Cytokines, as described previously, are short-range signaling proteins. Cytokine secretion by antigen-presenting cells is triggered by many different stimuli including phagocytosis of bacteria, parasites, and other foreign particles. This secretion can also be induced by T cells signaling through CD40 and CD154. As described in the chapter on dendritic cells, different dendritic cell populations secrete different cytokine mixtures. These mixtures in turn determine the nature of the induced T helper cell response. For example, the development of a subpopulation of T helper cells called Th1 cells is stimulated by IL-12 from dendritic cells or macrophages. This cytokine stimulates Th1 cells to produce interferon-γ (IFN-γ), which together with IL-12 further stimulates the Th1 cells. Finally, complete activation, cell proliferation, and maximal IFN-γ production is achieved by additional stimulation with IL-18 and IL-23. On the other hand, dendritic cells that secrete IL-1 or IL-4 preferentially stimulate a subset of T helper cells called Th2 cells. Once produced by antigen-presenting cells, IL-1 may either be secreted into the tissue fluid (IL-1β) or remain bound to the cell surface (IL-1α). Cell-bound IL-1α, together with properly presented antigen, will stimulate adherent T cells.

Adherence Molecules

In addition to the dialogue mediated by costimulatory molecules, T cells and antigen-presenting cells stimulate each other most effectively if they are held in close contact by adherence molecules such as the integrins. Thus, CD2 and CD11a/CD18 on T cells bind to their ligands CD58 and CD54 on antigen-presenting cells and lock them in place.

IMMUNOLOGICAL SYNAPSE FORMATION

All the molecules described above must interact in the correct manner and in the correct order if a T cell is to respond appropriately to an antigen. Thus when a T cell and an antigen-presenting cell come into contact, the TCR–peptide–MHC complexes and the costimulatory molecules cluster together into a specialized structure called an immunological synapse (Figure 10-7). The TCRs and costimulatory molecules such as CD28 are clustered into supramolecular activation clusters (SMACs). The synapse forms a characteristic "bull's eye" consisting of a

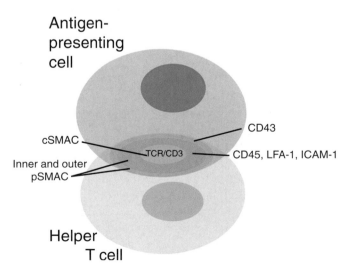

Figure 10-7. Interaction between a T cell and an antigen-presenting cell generated the supramolecular structure called an immunological synapse. Thus a series of concentric rings form around the interacting TCR–MHC complex. These rings contain different costimulating molecules.

central area (the cSMAC), surrounded by an outer peripheral ring (the pSMAC). The cSMAC contains MHC and TCR molecules as well as CD4, CD3, CD2, CD28, CD80/86, and CD40/154. The pSMAC contains CD45, and the adhesion molecules ICAM-1 and LFA-1. A third, outer ring contains proteins excluded from the synapse such as CD43. CD43 is a very large molecule that could interfere with the functioning of the synapse.

The cytoplasmic membranes of T cells contain regions (or domains) where the membrane is enriched in specific lipids and cholesterol called lipid rafts. In order to form an immunological synapse, these lipid rafts move within the cell membrane. Small rafts are distributed evenly over the surface of resting T cells but aggregate within the synapse after TCRs and CD28 engage. Synapses form within minutes after TCR engagement and are very stable. However, it is important to note that T cells are always ready to shift from one antigen-presenting cell to another if the new cell can offer a higher level of stimulation. Thus in effect, the T cell seeks the antigen that binds most strongly to its TCR. Eventually, key components of immunological synapses are endocytosed and degraded, so terminating T cell signaling.

In the absence of effective costimulation, the T cell undergoes abortive activation. It does not divide or produce cytokines. It either becomes unresponsive to antigen (is anergic) for several weeks or undergoes apoptosis and dies.

SIGNAL TRANSDUCTION

Once a TCR binds to antigen on a presenting cell, the receptor signals to the cell. The first signal is transmitted from the antigen-binding TCR α and β chains to the peptide chains of the CD3 complex (Figure 10-8). This is probably the result of the clustering of several TCRs together. The CD3 proteins and their associated ζ and η chains have specific amino acid sequences on their cytoplasmic domains called "immunoreceptor tyrosine-based, activation motifs" (ITAMs). When the ITAMs are clustered, they in turn activate several protein tyrosine kinases (PTKs). The first activated PTK, called lck, phosphorylates the ITAMs. As a result these can bind a second PTK, called zeta-associated protein-70 (ZAP-70). The bound ZAP-70 is phosphorylated in turn and then can follow three possible signaling pathways. One pathway leads via the second messengers diacylglycerol and inositol triphosphate to the activation of the transcriptional activator nuclear factor of activated T cells (NF-AT). The inositol triphosphate also releases calcium ions from intracellular organelles and opens transmembrane channels allowing Ca^{2+} to enter the cell and raising intracellular calcium. A second pathway leads to the activation of protein kinase C, which in turn induces the transcription factor NF-κB (Box 10-1). The third pathway involves activation of ras, a GTP-binding protein, and leads in turn to activation of fos. At the same

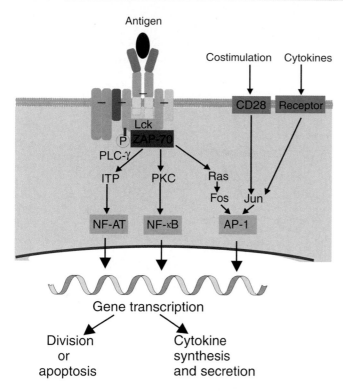

Figure 10-8.   Biomechanical basis of TCR signal transduction. Once TCRs cluster they activate several protein kinases. The most important of these is called ZAP-70. This in turn triggers three signaling pathways and, with appropriate costimulation, generates multiple transduction factors. The jun-fos heterodimer (AP-1) is required to stimulate the genes for cytokines and their receptors. The final results of the stimulus include cell division or apoptosis as well as cytokine production. *DAG*, Diacylglycerol; *ITP*, inositol triphosphate; *PKC*, protein kinase C.

time, costimulatory signals initiated by CD28 lead to the activation of jun.

The net effect of these reactions is that multiple transcription factors are activated and turn on many new genes. These factors include NF-κB, fos, and jun. The fos and jun proteins bind together to form a heterodimer called activator protein-1 (AP-1). AP-1 is a transcription factor that activates a second wave of genes coding for the cytokines, IL-2, IL-2R, IL-3, IL-4, IL-5, IL-6, and IFN-γ (Figure 10-9).

The net result of all this signaling is that T cells are driven to enlarge, enter the cell cycle, and secrete cytokines (Figure 10-10). It is these cytokines that trigger the next stages of the immune responses.

OVERALL CONSIDERATIONS

When antigen engages the TCR, an immunological synapse forms and TCRs and costimulatory molecules generate signals to the T cell. However, the TCR does not function as a binary (on/off) switch. Instead differences in

BOX 10–1

NF-κB

The NF-κB family of transcription factors are activated by signaling, not only through antigen receptors, but also through cytokine receptors, cell death receptors, and stress signals. They play a key role in both inflammation and immunity. In a resting cell, NF-κB is bound to its inhibitor IκB so that it cannot move to the nucleus and activate genes. When a lymphocyte is stimulated, the two molecules dissociate, the IκB is destroyed, and the released NF-κB moves to the nucleus and switches on the genes for various cytokines and chemokines that serve as inflammatory mediators. Molecules or organisms that block the destruction of IκB will have antiinflammatory and immunosuppressive effects. Thus corticosteroids stimulate the production of excess IκB whereas some bacteria can block its degradation. Either way, the activation of cells and the development of inflammation and immune responses will be blocked.

the strength of binding, in the amount of costimulation, and in the duration of the stimulus result in markedly different T cell responses.

T-cell recognition of antigen by T cells must be exquisitely sensitive. Because MHC molecules can bind a large variety of antigenic peptides, any individual peptide will usually only be displayed in small amounts. T cells must also be able to recognize these few specific peptide–MHC complexes among a vast excess of MHC molecules carrying irrelevant self-peptides. Thus recognition by T cells must be highly specific. Finally, T cells must be able to recognize that they are binding an endogenous or exogenous antigen in order to mount an appropriate form of immune response.

The number of MHC–peptide complexes signaling to the T cell is important since the stimulus needed to trigger a response varies among T-cell populations. For example, only one MHC–peptide complex is needed to trigger a CD8+ T cell response whereas about 1000 such

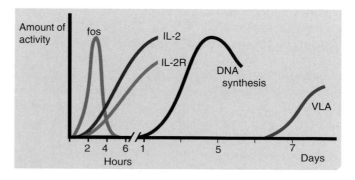

Figure 10-9.   The time–course of events following the stimulation of a T cell by antigen and IL-1. *fos*, a transcription factor; *VLA*, very late activation antigen. (From Krensky AM: *N Engl J Med* 322:515, 1991.)

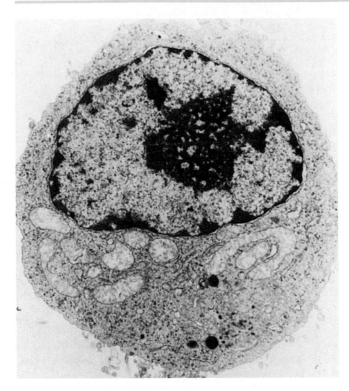

Figure 10-10. Transmission electron micrograph of a lymphoblast. Compare this with an unstimulated lymphocyte in Figure 9-2. Note the extensive cytoplasm, ribosomes, and large mitochondria. (Courtesy Dr. S Linthicum.)

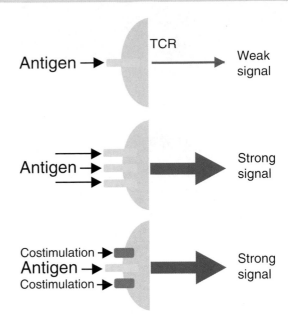

Figure 10-11. Successful stimulation of a T cell requires multiple signals. Depending on the antigen, the T cell may be activated by signals from multiple TCRs or by appropriate costimulation.

complexes are required to trigger a CD4+ T cell. T-cell activation, in general, appears to involve tunable thresholds. Each threshold for signaling depends on the level of costimulation (Figure 10-11). For example, for a CD4+ T cell that expresses 30,000 TCRs, the number of TCRs that must bind antigen in order for the cell to become activated has been estimated to be about 8000 in the absence of CD28-mediated costimulation and about 1000 in its presence. The duration of signaling is also a key factor that determines a T cell's fate. Sustained signaling is required for T-cell activation and is maintained by serial triggering of its TCRs. Thus, during the prolonged cell interaction process, each MHC–peptide complex triggers many TCRs. (Typically, one complex can trigger up to 200 TCRs.) This serial triggering depends on the kinetics of TCR–ligand interaction. The costimulator CD28 increases signal transduction by reducing the time needed to trigger a T cell and lowers the threshold for TCR triggering. Adhesion molecules stabilize the paired T-cell antigen-processing cell and so allow the signal to be sustained for hours.

The fate of a T helper cell is determined by the type of antigen-presenting cell used and by the nature of the signal received from it. Thus naive T cells have strict requirements for activation. They must receive a sustained signal for at least 10 hours in the presence of costimulation or for up to 30 hours in its absence. This level of costimulation can only be provided by dendritic cells,

which can supply high levels of costimulatory and adhesion molecules. In contrast, other antigen-presenting cells act only transiently. Thus, although macrophages and B cells can briefly trigger a TCR, they are unable to complete the process and so fail to induce activation of naive T cells. Once primed, T cells require about an hour to reach commitment. Only then can they be activated by macrophages and B cells.

SUPERANTIGENS

When animals are exposed to a foreign antigen, usually only a small proportion of their T cells, perhaps less than 1 in 10,000 cells, have TCRs that can bind the antigen and respond to it. However, some microbial molecules are unique in that they can stimulate as many as one in five T cells to divide. It was originally thought that these proteins were simply nonspecific mitogens. This is not the case. Superantigens only activate T cells whose TCR β chains contain certain V domains. These powerful antigens have been called superantigens. All superantigens come from microbial sources such as streptococci, staphylococci, and mycoplasmas, and from viruses such as rabies virus and possibly human immunodeficiency virus (HIV). Concentrations of less than 0.1 pg/ml of a bacterial superantigen may be sufficient to uncontrollably stimulate T cells resulting in fever, shock and death. In mice some cell surface molecules, called minor lymphocyte-stimulating antigens, can also act as superantigens. These antigens have been shown to be endogenous superantigens, the products of integrated retroviral

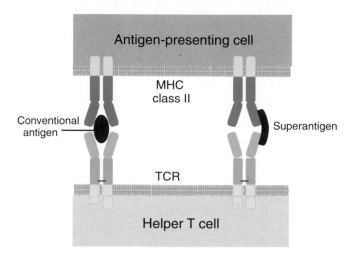

Figure 10-12.   Differences in binding to a TCR between a conventional antigenic peptide that fills the groove between the α and β chains as opposed to a superantigen that binds only to the β chain.

genes. (The mouse genome may contain more than 1000 of these endogenous retroviral sequences.) The responses to superantigens are not MHC restricted (i.e., they don't depend on specific MHC haplotypes), but the presence of MHC antigens is required for an effective response.

Unlike conventional antigens that must bind inside the grooves of both an MHC molecule and a TCR, superantigens bind to both a TCR V_β domain and an MHC class II molecule on the antigen-presenting cell. As a result, they tightly link the T cell and the antigen-presenting cell and trigger T cell activation. Superantigens do not bind to the antigen-binding groove of the MHC class II molecule but attach elsewhere on its surface (Figure 10-12). Because of their strong binding, superantigens trigger a powerful T-cell response. This may be a conventional response associated with the secretion of unusually large amounts of cytokines or it may be expressed as tolerance. Indeed, because of the large proportion of T cells stimulated by superantigens, this tolerance can be much less specific than tolerance induced by conventional antigens. Thus the superantigen staphylococcal enterotoxin B can inactivate most T cells carrying the $V_\beta 8$ domain. Some superantigens may stimulate the secretion of large amounts of cytokines to produce the disease called toxic shock syndrome (Chapter 4).

T HELPER CELL SUBPOPULATIONS

Two major subpopulations of $CD4^+$ T helper cells have been identified. They are called helper 1 (Th1) and helper 2 (Th2) T cells and they can be distinguished by the mixture of cytokines that they secrete (Figure 10-13). As always, many of the details of their function have been investigated in mice and humans, and it must not be assumed that they function in an identical manner in other mammals. The two helper cell subpopulations are activated by antigen and costimulators presented by different antigen-presenting cells. Thus DC1 cells preferentially stimulate a Th1 response whereas DC2 cells trigger a Th2 response.

Th1 Cells

Th1 cells respond optimally to antigen presented by myeloid dendritic cells (DC1) and by B cells using the costimulatory molecule CD80. The DC1 myeloid

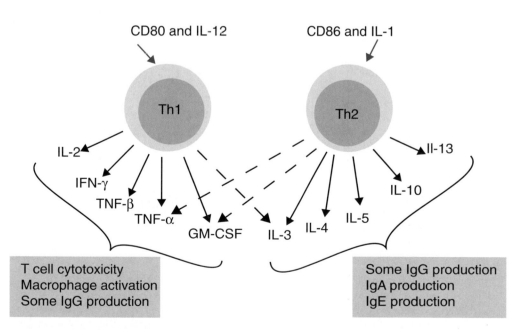

Figure 10-13.   Major differences between T helper cell subpopulations. Note that the costimuli that trigger them are different as are the set of cytokines they secrete.

dendritic cells induce Th1 responses by secreting IL-12. Th1 cells secrete IL-2, IFN-γ, and lymphotoxin (TNF-β) within a few hours after stimulation by antigen, and costimulation by IL-12 and IL-18. These Th1 cells promote cell-mediated immune responses such as the delayed hypersensitivity reaction and macrophage activation. They thus generate resistance to intracellular organisms such as the mycobacteria and to viruses (Figure 10-14). Th1 cells lack IL-1 receptors and do not respond to IL-1. In the absence of IL-12, the helper T cell response switches automatically from Th1 to Th2.

Th2 Cells

Th2 cells respond optimally to antigen presented by lymphoid or plasmacytoid dendritic cells (DC2) (Fig. 6-4) and macrophages, and less well to antigen presented by B cells. DC2 cells preferentially induce Th2 responses by secreting IL-4 and providing costimulation through the costimulatory molecule CD86. Th2 cells also have IL-1 receptors and may also require costimulation by IL-1 from macrophages or dendritic cells. Once activated, Th2 cells secrete IL-4, IL-5, IL-10, and IL-13 for several days. The cytokines from Th2 cells stimulate B-cell proliferation and immunoglobulin secretion but have no effect on delayed hypersensitivity or other cell-mediated reactions. The cytokines from Th2 cells enhance B-cell production of IgG1 and IgA up to 20-fold and production of IgE up to 1000-fold. Th2 responses are associated with enhanced immunity to some helminth parasites such as *Toxocara canis* but with decreased resistance to mycobacteria and other intracellular organisms.

Th1 and Th2 cells may migrate preferentially into different types of inflamed tissue as a result of differential expression of receptors for P- and E-selectin and the chemokine CCL11 (eotaxin). This may be important in ensuring that the correct T-cell subpopulation is employed against a specific invader.

Th0 Cells

Although the T-cell subpopulations described above are usually considered to be discrete subsets, it can be argued that T-cell cytokine profiles form a continuous spectrum with Th1 and Th2 cells as the extreme phenotypes. Thus a third T helper cell phenotype secretes a cytokine mixture that is representative of both Th1 and Th2. These cells, called Th0 cells, may be precursors of Th1 and Th2 or cells that are in transition between the two populations. They secrete IL-2, IL-4, IL-5, and IFN-γ. Some IL-2-secreting T cells may become IL-4-secreting cells after exposure to antigen, implying the existence of an interleukin switch and a change in phenotype from Th1 to Th2. The principal molecules that control this switch are IL-4 and IL-12. When cultured in the presence of IL-4, Th0 cells become Th2 cells. When cultured in the presence of IL-12, they become Th1 cells. Mixed (Th0) cell populations are most obvious

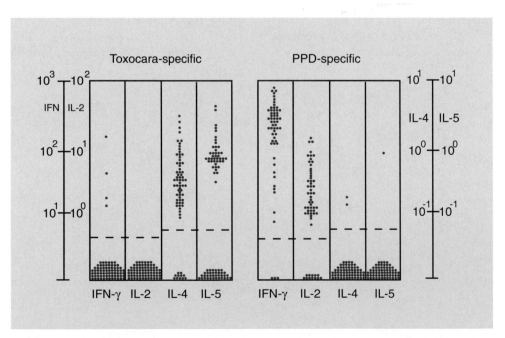

Figure 10-14. Different antigens can trigger distinctly different Th cell subpopulations. For example, T cells exposed to a parasite antigen from the roundworm *Toxocara canis* mount a Th2 response and secrete primarily IL-4 and IL-5. In contrast, T cells exposed to PPD, an antigen from *Mycobacterium tuberculosis*, mount a Th1 response characterized by secretion of IFN-γ and IL-2. (From Del Prete G, De Carli M, Mastromauro C, et al: *J Clin Invest* 88:346-350, 1991.)

early after initiation of the immune response, whereas Th1 and Th2 subsets are more obvious in chronic diseases where the antigens are persistent and cannot be easily removed. This is also observed in vitro where repeated antigenic stimulation of T cells leads to increasing polarization of T-cell populations into Th1 and Th2 subpopulations.

Species Differences

The details of T helper cell subpopulation function described above have largely been derived from studies in laboratory mice. Cattle most certainly possess Th1 and Th2 cells and can mount polarized immune responses. Bovine IgG1 expression is positively regulated by IL-4 and IgG2 expression by IFN-γ. A large proportion of bovine CD4$^+$ cells produce multiple cytokines, including IL-2, IL-4, IL-10, and IFN-γ, and thus are like Th0 cells.

γ/δ T CELLS

The function of T cells bearing γ/δ TCRs remains an enigma. One reason is a result of major species differences. Thus 5% to 15% of blood lymphocytes in humans and mice and up to 60% in ruminants have γ/δ TCRs, and it is probable that these cells have different functions in the two groups of mammals. Another reason is that even within a single species, they may have different functions depending on their location and state of maturity.

In humans and mice where γ/δ T cells are a minor lymphocyte subpopulation, they can be subdivided into subsets based on the expression of different types of γ/δ antigen receptors. One subset has very limited γ/δ receptor diversity and is mainly found in the epidermis of the skin and genital tract. The other subset has extensive receptor diversity and is mainly found in secondary lymphoid organs and in the gut mucosa. The skin T cells thus express a γ/δ receptor with very limited diversity. These cells preferentially bind to widely distributed microbial molecules, especially heat-shock proteins and phospholigands (carbohydrates or nucleotides with a phosphate group). Other γ/δ T cells preferentially respond to two class Ib MHC molecules, MICA and MICB, both of which are produced by stressed cells, including cancer cells and virus-infected cells. When stimulated, some of these γ/δ T cells secrete molecules such as fibroblast growth factor and appear to play a key role in promoting wound healing. The functions of these skin γ/δ cells may differ according to the stages of infection. Thus, early in infection, the cells with restricted antigen binding may serve an innate immune function and help resist organisms, especially intracellular bacteria such as *Mycobacterium* or *Listeria*. Later in infections, they may serve an anti-inflammatory or wound healing role.

In contrast, the antigen-binding site on the other γ/δ T cell subset binds to a diverse array of antigens, and these cells can recognize antigens directly without the need for a MHC molecule. These γ/δ T cells with diverse antigen-binding receptors form at least two populations. One population produces cytokines and chemokines and can be divided into Th1 and Th2 subsets based on their secreted cytokines. The other population is cytotoxic and can destroy various target cells, such as cells infected with mycobacteria and some leukemic cells. Since the vast majority of these cells are located on body surfaces, they almost certainly serve their major defensive functions on surfaces.

In immature ruminants and pigs γ/δ T cells are a major circulating lymphocyte population. They can bind a wide variety of antigens, suggesting that they have a role in acquired immunity in these species. These cells colonize the skin, the mammary gland, the reproductive organs, and the intestinal wall where they form the major T-cell population. In pigs, γ/δ T cells are polyclonal at birth, but this declines and their T-cell diversity becomes increasingly restricted with age. In addition, γ/δ T cells located in different organs or even different parts of the gastrointestinal tract have different repertoires.

A subset of ruminant γ/δ T cells also express the surface molecule WC1 whose function is unknown but these cells appear to have an important role in immunity to intracellular organisms. Thus in mycobacterial and schistosomal infections, granulomas form around the invading organisms. In both cases the initial T-cell infiltration is dominated by γ/δ T cells and is followed later by α/β T cells. A second wave of γ/δ T cells may terminate the response. These WC1$^+$ γ/δ T cells secrete IL-12 and IFN-γ and may thus promote a Th1 bias in the immune response.

The role of γ/δ T cells on mucosal surfaces is discussed further in Chapter 20.

MEMORY T CELLS

When naive T cells are stimulated by antigen under conditions that give rise to Th1 cells, two subpopulations develop. One population secretes IFN-γ and serves as effector cells. The other subpopulation does not secrete IFN-γ. The IFN-γ-secreting cells are short lived because they are eliminated either by autocrine IFN-γ and IL-2 that trigger fas-mediated apoptosis or by nitric oxide production by macrophages. The IFN-γ^- cells, on the other hand, are resistant to apoptosis and develop into long-lived memory cells. Because repeated stimulation drives all Th1 cells into the IFN-γ-secreting group, it may be that the nonsecreting population is a precursor population. Interestingly, this dichotomy does not occur with Th2 cells where IL-4$^+$ and IL-4$^-$ cells have similar life spans.

SOURCES OF ADDITIONAL INFORMATION

Abbas AK, Murphy KM, Sher A: Functional diversity of helper T lymphocytes, *Nature* 383:787-793, 1996.

Brown WC, Woods VM, Chitko-McKown CG, et al: Interleukin 10 is expressed by bovine type 1 helper, type 2 helper and unrestricted parasite-specific T-cell clones and inhibits proliferation of all three subsets in an accessory-cell-dependent manner, *Infect Immun* 62: 4697-4708, 1994.

Clarke SRM: The critical role of CD40/CD40L in the CD4-dependent generation of CD8+ T cell immunity, *J Leukocyte Biol* 67:607-613, 2000.

Davis WC, Hamilton MJ: Comparison of the unique characteristics of the immune system in different species of mammals, *Vet Immunol Immunopathol* 63:7-13, 1998.

Dustin ML, Chan AC: Signaling takes shape in the immune system. *Cell* 103:283-294, 2000.

Heath WR: γδ T cells: have we been looking in the wrong direction? *Trends Mol Med* 8:368, 2002.

Holtmeier W, Käller J, Geisel W, et al: Development and compartmentalization of the porcine TCR delta repertoire at mucosal and extraintestinal sites: the pig as a model for analyzing the effects of age and microbial factors, *J Immunol* 169:1993-2002, 2002.

Janes PW, Ley SC, Magee AI, Kabouridis PS: The role of lipid rafts in T cell antigen receptor (TCR) signaling, *Immunology* 12:23-34, 2000.

Kabelitz D: Do CD2 and CD3-TCR T-cell activation pathways function independently? *Immunol Today* 11:44-46, 1990.

Kuchroo VK, Das MP, Brown JA, et al: B7-1 and B7-2 costimulatory molecules activate differentially the Th1/Th2 developmental pathways: application to autoimmune disease therapy, *Cell* 80:707-718, 1995.

Matis LA: The molecular basis of T cell specificity, *Annu Rev Immunol* 8:65-82, 1990.

Miller-Edge M, Worley M: In vitro mitogen responses and lymphocyte subpopulations in cheetahs, *Vet Immunol Immunopathol* 28:337-349, 1991.

Morrison WI, Howard CJ, Hinson CJ, et al: Identification of three distinct allelic forms of bovine CD4, *Immunology* 83: 589-594, 1994.

Nel AE: T-cell activation through the antigen receptor. 1: Signaling components, signaling pathways, and signal integration at the T-cell antigen receptor synapse, *J Allergy Clin Immunol* 109:758-770, 2002.

Nel AE, Slaughter N: T-cell activation through the antigen receptor. 2: Role of signaling cascades in T-cell differentiation, anergy, immune senescence, and development of immunotherapy, *J Allergy Clin Immunol* 109:901-915, 2002.

Noelle RJ: CD40 and its ligand in host defense, *Immunity* 4:415-419, 1996.

Rissoan M-C, Soumelis V, Kadowaki N, et al: Reciprocal control of T helper and dendritic cell differentiation, *Science* 283:1183-1186, 1999.

Seder RA, Le Gros GG: The functional role of CD8+ helper type 2 cells, *J Exp Med* 181:5-7, 1995.

Sprent J, Tough DF: T cell death and memory, *Science* 293: 245-247, 2001.

Thome M, Hirt W, Pfaff E, et al: Porcine T-cell receptors: molecular and biochemical characterization, *Vet Immunol Immunopathol* 43:13-18, 1994.

Van der Merwe PA, Davis SJ, Shaw AS, Dustin ML: Cytoskeletal polarization and redistribution of cell-surface molecules during T cell antigen recognition, *Immunology* 12:5-21, 2000.

Weaver CT, Unanue ER: The costimulatory function of antigen-presenting cells, *Immunol Today* 11:49-55, 1990.

Wilson E, Hedges JF, Butcher EC, et al: Bovine γδ T cell subsets express distinct patterns of chemokine responsiveness and adhesion molecules: a mechanism for tissue-specific γδ T cell subset accumulation, *J Immunol* 169:4970-4975, 2002.

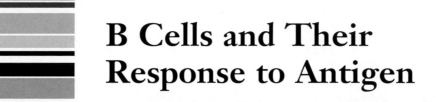

B Cells and Their Response to Antigen

The division of the acquired immune system into two major components is based on the need to recognize two distinctly different forms of foreign invaders. Some invaders enter the body openly and grow in extracellular fluids. These exogenous antigens are destroyed by antibodies. Other invaders grow inside cells, where antibodies cannot reach. They are destroyed by T cell–mediated responses. Antibodies are produced by the lymphocytes called B cells. This chapter discusses B cells and their response to antigens.

B cells are found in the cortex of lymph nodes, in the marginal zone in the spleen, in the bone marrow, and in Peyer's patches. Few B cells circulate in the blood. Like T cells, each B cell has a large number of identical antigen receptors on its surface. Each B cell, therefore, can only bind and respond to a single antigen. Antigen receptors are generated at random during B cell development in a process described in Chapter 14. If a B cell encounters an antigen that can be bound by its receptors, it will, with appropriate costimulation, respond by secreting receptor molecules into body fluids, where they act as antibodies. Each B cell thus makes antibodies of the same binding specificity as its receptors. This specificity is the result of a series of ordered gene rearrangements, all of which must be successfully performed if the B cell is to survive. In addition, a second selection process occurs during the course of an immune response, in which the B cell repertoire is progressively modified by somatic mutation or gene conversion. Only B cells with receptors

that can bind an antigen with a high affinity will survive to become memory cells.

THE B CELL ANTIGEN RECEPTOR

Each B cell is covered with about 200,000 to 500,000 identical antigen receptors (BCRs)—many more than the 30,000 TCR expressed on each T cell. Each BCR is constructed from multiple glycoproteins and, like the TCR, can be divided into antigen-binding and signaling components. Unlike the TCR, however, the BCR can also bind antigens when released from the B cell surface. Antibodies are simply soluble forms of BCR secreted into body fluids; they all belong to the class of proteins called immunoglobulins (Chapter 13).

The Antigen-Binding Component

The antigen-binding component of the BCR (or immunoglobulin) is a glycoprotein of 160 to 180 kDa consisting of four peptide chains. These four chains consist of two identical pairs—a pair of heavy chains, each 60 kDa in size, and a pair of smaller chains (about 25 kDa each) called light chains (Figure 11-1). The light chains are linked by disulfide bonds to the heavy chains so that the complete molecule is shaped like the letter Y. The tail of the Y (called the Fc region) is formed from paired heavy chains and is attached to the B cell surface.

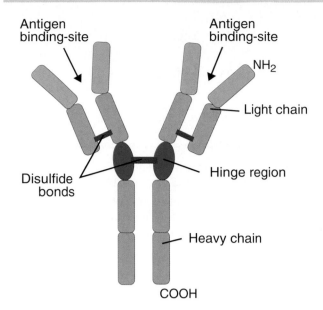

Figure 11-1. The overall structure of an immunoglobulin molecule. When bound to a B cell surface, this molecule acts as an antigen receptor (BCR). When released by the B cell and free in the circulation, it acts as an antibody. Note that unlike a TCR, it has two antigen-binding sites.

The C-terminal domains of the heavy chains are inserted into the lipid bilayer of the B cell surface. The arms of the Y (called the Fab regions) are formed by paired light and heavy chains and bind antigen (Figure 11-2). Each antigen-binding site is formed by the groove between a light and a heavy chain. Thus each BCR has two identical antigen-binding sites.

Light Chains

Light chains are constructed from two domains each containing about 110 amino acids. The amino-acid sequences in the C-terminal domain of light chains are identical and so form a constant domain (C_L). In contrast, the sequences in the N-terminal domain differ in each light chain examined and so form a variable domain (V_L).

Mammals make two distinct types of light chains, called κ (kappa) and λ (lambda). Although their amino-acid sequences are different, they are functionally identical. The ratio of κ to λ chains in BCRs varies among mammals, ranging from mice and rats, which have more than 95% κ chains, to cattle and horses, which have 95% λ chains. Primates such as the rhesus monkey or the baboon have 50% of each, whereas humans have 70% κ chains. Carnivores such as cats and dogs have 90% λ chains.

Heavy Chains

The heavy chains of a typical immunoglobulin contain 400 to 500 amino acids. They consist of four or five domains each of about 110 amino acids. The N-terminal domain has a highly variable sequence and is therefore called the variable (V_H) domain. The remaining three or four domains show few sequence differences and so form constant (C_H) domains.

B cells can make five different sorts (classes) of heavy chain. These differ in their amino acid sequence and in their domain structure. Most important, each immunoglobulin class has a different biological activity. The five distinct immunoglobulin heavy chains are called α, γ, δ, ε, and μ. These heavy chains determine the immunoglobulin class (or isotype). Thus immunoglobulin molecules that use α heavy chains are called immunoglobulin A (IgA), and those that use γ chains are called IgG; μ chains are used in IgM, δ chains in IgD, and ε chains in IgE.

Variable Regions

When the amino-acid sequences of a large number of immunoglobulin V domains from light and heavy chains are examined in detail, two features become apparent. First, their sequence variation is largely confined to three small regions, each consisting of six to ten amino acids, within the variable domain (Figure 11-3). These regions are said to be hypervariable. Situated between the three hypervariable regions are relatively constant sequences of amino acids called framework regions. The three hypervariable regions on each chain determine the overall shape of the antigen-binding site and so determine the

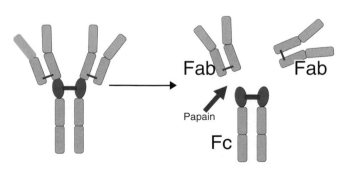

Figure 11-2. The effect of treating an immunoglobulin molecule with the proteolytic enzyme papain. Papain cleaves the molecule into three large fragments. The names of these fragments denote the nomenclature of different regions of an immunoglobulin molecule.

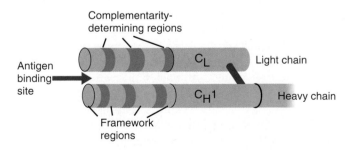

Figure 11-3. The variable regions of the light and heavy chains of an immunoglobulin molecule are divided into three highly variable complementarity-determining regions separated by relatively constant framework regions.

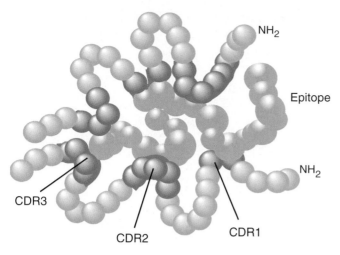

Figure 11-4. The way in which the complementarity-determining regions are folded to form the antigen binding site on an immunoglobulin molecule. A similar folding occurs in the peptide chains of the TCR.

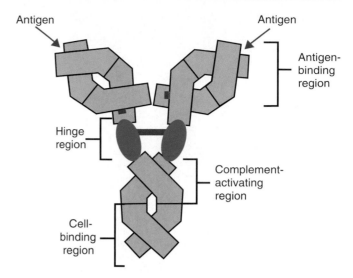

Figure 11-5. A diagram of an IgG molecule, showing how the light and heavy chains intertwine to form clearly defined regions of the molecule. Each region has defined biological functions.

specificity of antigen binding. Since the shape of the anti-body-binding site is complementary to the conformation of the antigenic determinant, the hypervariable sequences are also called complementarity-determining regions (CDRs). Each V-domain is folded in such a way that its three CDRs come into close contact with the antigen (Figure 11-4).

Constant Regions

The number of constant domains differs between immunoglobulin classes. For example, there are three constant domains in a γ heavy chain: they are labeled, from the N-terminal end, as C_H1, C_H2, and C_H3. A similar arrangement is found in α and most δ chains, whereas μ and ε chains have an additional constant domain called C_H4.

Since heavy chains are paired, the domains in each chain come together to form structures by which anti-body molecules can exert their biological functions. Thus V_H and V_L form a paired domain that binds antigen, and C_H1 and C_L together stabilize the antigen-binding site. The paired C_H2 domains of IgG contain a site that activates the classical pathway of the complement system (Chapter 15) and a site that binds to Fc receptors on phagocytic cells (Figure 11-5). The heavy chain also regulates placental transfer of IgG and antibody-mediated cellular cytotoxicity (Chapter 17), although these are probably caused by the combined activities of several domains.

When immunoglobulin molecules serve as BCRs, part of their Fc region is embedded in the B cell surface membrane. These cell-bound immunoglobulins differ from the secreted form in that they have a small transmembrane domain located at their C-terminus. This contains hydrophobic amino acids that associate with the cell-membrane lipids.

Hinge Region

One important feature of the immunoglobulins is that the Fab regions, which contain the antigen-binding sites, are mobile and can swing freely around the center of the molecule as if they are hinged. This hinge consists of a small domain of about 12 amino acids located between the C_H1 and C_H2 domains. The hinge region contains many hydrophilic and proline residues. The hydrophilic residues cause the peptide chain to unfold and make this region readily accessible to proteases. This region also contains all the interchain disulfide bonds. Proline, because of its configuration, produces a 90-degree bend when inserted in a polypeptide chain. Because amino acids can rotate around peptide bonds, the effect of closely spaced proline residues is to produce a universal joint around which the immunoglobulin chains can swing freely. The μ chains of IgM do not possess a hinge region.

The Signal-Transducing Component

B cell receptor immunoglobulins cannot signal directly to their B cell since their cytoplasmic domains contain only three amino acids. However, their C_H4 and trans-membrane domains associate with glycoprotein het-erodimers formed by pairing CD79a (Ig-α) (47 kDa) and CD79b (Ig-β) (37kDa). These act as signal transducers (Figure 11-6). The CD79b chains are identical in all BCRs. The CD79a chains differ depending on their associated heavy chains and so employ different signaling pathways.

BCR signaling is initiated by antigen binding. This leads to receptor aggregation and subsequent phos-phorylation of the immunoreceptor tyrosine-based acti-vation motifs (ITAMs) on the cytoplasmic domains of

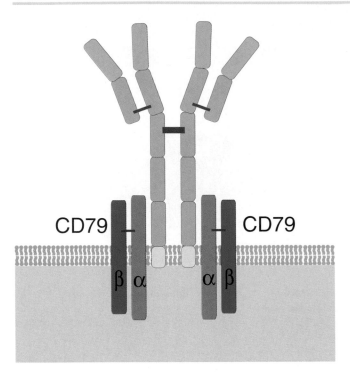

Figure 11-6. The structure of a complete BCR, showing both the antigen-binding component (immunoglobulin) and the signal transducing components (CD79). Note the small transmembrane domain at the end of each heavy chain.

CD79a and CD79b. Phosphorylation of the tyrosines in these motifs by the Src family kinases lyn, fyn, or blk results in recruitment of another kinase called syk. Syk initiates several downstream signaling cascades. Another key signaling pathway activated through BCRs involves the production of a lipid kinase that mediates production of PIP3 (Chapter 10).

COSTIMULATION OF B CELLS

As in the T cell response, B cells require many different signals if they are to be fully activated (Figure 11-7). Thus although the binding of antigen to a BCR is an essential first step in triggering a B cell response, this is usually insufficient to trigger antibody formation. Complete activation of a B cell also requires costimulation from helper T cells. In order to be effective, however, the helper T cell must itself be presented with antigen. This antigen presentation can come from one of the professional antigen-presenting cells, a dendritic cell, a macrophage, or even from a B cell. Thus a B cell can capture and process antigen, present it to a T cell, and then receive costimulation from the same T cell. B cells thus play two simultaneous roles. They respond to antigen by making antibodies while at the same acting as antigen-processing cells. The signals from the BCR thus pass to two overlapping pathways. The helper T cells

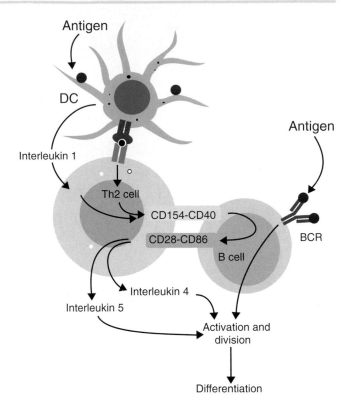

Figure 11-7. The sequence of events that must occur for a B cell to respond to antigen. Not only must the B cell be stimulated by antigen, but it must also receive costimulation from helper T cells and their cytokines. This complex interaction can be seen in Figure 6-7, *D*.

provide the B cell with costimulatory signals from cytokines, as well as from interacting receptor pairs.

Antigen Presentation by B Cells

B cells are effective antigen-presenting cells. They can bind antigen through the BCR and then endocytose and fragment this antigen before linking it to MHC class II molecules. Subsequently, they present it to helper T cells while at the same time expressing CD40 and CD86 and secreting IL-1 and IL-12 (Figure 11-8). Following antigen binding, the BCR may be internalized and degraded or transported to an intracellular compartment called the MIIC, where newly synthesized MHC class II molecules and antigen fragments are bound together to form complexes. These peptide-MHC class II complexes are carried to the B cell surface, where they are recognized by the TCR of a helper T cell. This activates the T cell so that the activated T cell provides costimulation to the B cell and permits its full activation through secreted cytokines and cell interactions via an immunological synapse. The synapse that forms between a B cell and a helper T cell contains the BCR, several tyrosine phosphorylated proteins, actin, and phospholipase C.

Since all the receptors on a single B cell are identical, each B cell can bind only one antigen. This makes them

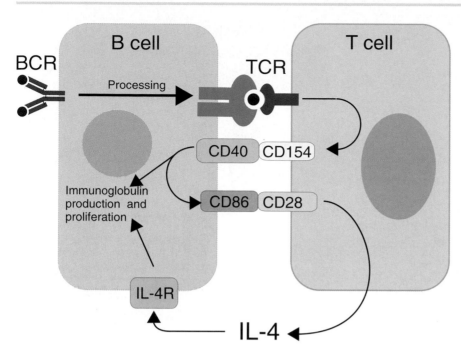

Figure 11-8. The sequence of events that occurs when an antigen-processing B cell interacts with a helper T cell. The costimulators, such as CD154 and CD28, engage serially to trigger IL-4 secretion by the T cell and IL-4R production by the B cell.

much more efficient antigen-presenting cells than macrophages that must ingest any foreign material that comes their way. This is especially true in a primed animal, in which large numbers of B cells may be available to bind a specific antigen. B cells can thus activate Th cells with 1/1000 of the antigen concentration of nonspecific antigen-processing cells such as macrophages.

Cytokine Secretion

Helper T cells secrete a mixture of many different cytokines. Most of these act on B cells to either initiate their activation or promote their differentiation. The most important are IL-4 and IL-5.

Interleukin 4

IL-4 from Th2 cells stimulates the growth and differentiation of activated B cells. IL-4 also enhances their expression of MHC class II and Fc receptors and induces mouse B cells to switch classes to IgG1 or IgE production while suppressing IgG3 and IgG2b production. The actions of IL-4 are inhibited by the Th1-derived cytokine interferon-γ (IFN-γ).

Interleukin 5

IL-5 from Th2 cells acts on activated B cells to enhance their differentiation into plasma cells. It stimulates IgG and IgM production and enhances IL-4–induced IgE production. IL-5 selectively enhances IgA production in B cells from the intestine.

Other Interleukins

B cells can be further stimulated by many different cytokines derived from helper T cells such as IL-3, IL-6,

and IL-13. IL-13 shares part of its receptor with IL-4 and has very similar B cell-stimulating properties. IL-6 is needed for the final differentiation of activated B cells into plasma cells. It acts together with IL-5 to promote IgA production and with IL-1 to promote IgM production.

Cytokines alone are not sufficient to fully activate B cells. Further costimulation also requires cell-cell interactions mediated by receptor pairs such as CD40 and CD154.

CD40 and CD154

The costimulatory molecule CD40 is found on resting B cells, whereas its ligand, CD154, is found on activated helper T cells. The interaction of CD40 with CD154 is required for B cells to begin the cell cycle and upregulates IL-4, as well as IL-5 receptors and costimulatory ligands (Figures 11-8 and 11-9). It is believed that signals from CD40 synergize with IL-4 and IL-5 to drive B cell activation. In addition, interactions between CD40 and CD154 are essential for the formation of germinal centers, for the development of memory B cells, and for immunoglobulin class switching. (This is in addition to the role of these molecules in the activation of helper T cells by antigen-presenting cells). CD154 has been found on bovine Th1 and Th2 cells and at a low level on bovine γ/δ T cells. CD40 is expressed on activated but not resting bovine B cells. Unlike in humans, CD40 is also expressed on bovine T cells.

The interaction between CD40 on the B cell and CD154 on the T cell is not able to fully activate B cells. CD28 on a helper T cell must also interact with CD86 on the B cell. CD86 is absent from resting cells but is induced on activated B cells. The dual signal makes T cells competent to activate B cells.

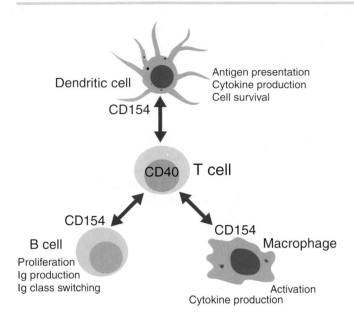

Figure 11-9. CD40 and CD154 participate in a dialogue between T cells and the professional antigen-presenting cells. As a result, both cell types are stimulated. In the case of B cells, T cell stimulation permits B cell proliferation and immunoglobulin production and class switching.

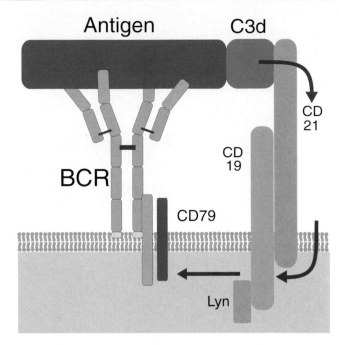

Figure 11-10.   The stimulation of B cells by the CD21/CD19 complex. CD21 binds to C3d on the antigen. Signaling through CD19, it generates a potent costimulatory signal to enhance B cell responses.

The CD21/CD19 Complex

In order to fully respond to antigen, B cells must also receive signals transmitted through a complex consisting of CD21 and CD19 on the B cell surface. CD21 is a complement receptor (CR2) that can bind to its ligand, C3d. CD19 is its accompanying signaling component. If an antigen molecule has C3d attached to it, this binds to CD21 and a signal is transmitted via CD19 to the BCR (Figure 11-10). The signals generated by each receptor synergize so that the dual binding of BCR with CD19/CD21 lowers the threshold for B cell activation by about 100-fold. The additional signal provided by CD19 enhances the recruitment of tyrosine kinases to the BCR. The importance of complement in providing a signal to B cells is emphasized by the observation that mice deficient in some complement components (C3, C4, or CR2) cannot mount an effective antibody response to T-dependent antigens. In addition to CD19 and CD21, the complex also contains CD81. CD81, or TAPA-1, is a widely expressed cell surface protein that is also found on T cells. It is believed to be a costimulatory molecule, facilitating the interaction of B cells with nearby T cells.

The B cell Fc receptor, FcγRIIB is a negative regulator of B cell function. When an IgG molecule binds to it and cross-links to a BCR through antigen, it inhibits antibody formation. This has important practical consequences when vaccinating young animals (Chapter 19).

THE B CELL RESPONSE

Binding of antigen to the BCR, especially if two receptors are cross-linked, exposes ITAMS, triggers activation of several different tyrosine kinases, and results in phosphorylation of a phospholipase C and possibly a G-protein (Figure 11-11). As with the TCR, these reactions are dynamically regulated by CD45 tyrosine phosphatases. Subsequent hydrolysis of phosphatidylinositol and calcium mobilization leads to activation of a protein kinase C and calcineurin and activation of transcription factors such as fos and myc.

Differential Signaling

Like the TCR, the BCR probably produces a tunable signal. As a result, it triggers biological responses that differ depending on the properties of the antigen and the costimulation received. Thus receptor affinity can influence responses such as B cell proliferation and antibody secretion. On the other hand, receptor occupancy influences MHC class II expression and signal transduction. The precise direction of the immunoglobulin class switch will depend on whether the B cell is exposed to Th1 or Th2 cytokines. Differential BCR signaling by antigen also determines whether an antibody response will be T-independent or T-dependent.

Certain antigens can provoke antibody formation in the absence of helper T cells. These so-called T-independent

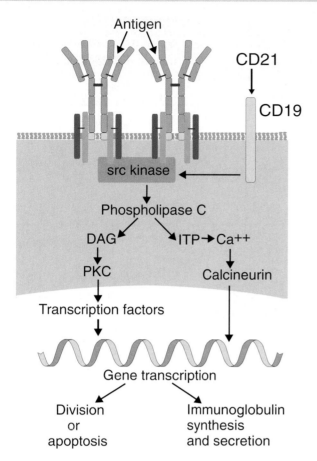

Figure 11-11. Signal transduction by two cross-linked BCRs activates B cells triggering cell division, differentiation, and immunoglobulin synthesis. *DAG*, Diacylglycerol; *ITP*, inositol triphosphate; *PKC*, protein kinase C.

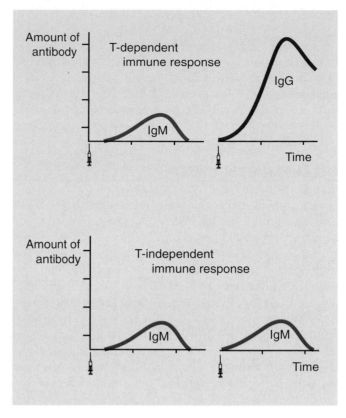

Figure 11-12. The differences in the time course of a T-dependent and T-independent antibody response. T-independent antigens cannot induce an immunoglobulin switch or immunological memory, as demonstrated by a secondary antibody response.

antigens are usually simple repeating polymers, such as *Escherichia coli* lipopolysaccharide, polymerized salmonella flagellin, and pneumococcal polysaccharide. T-independent antigens bind directly to B cells. Because they are repeating polymers, they cross-link several BCRs and so provide a sufficient signal for B cell proliferation. (This is similar to the situation observed in T cells. Signaling through multiple antigen receptors can reduce or eliminate the need for costimulation.) Characteristically, T-independent antigens only trigger IgM responses in B cells and fail to generate memory cells (Figure 11-12). This is because they do not induce secretion of cytokines from helper T cells and so cannot trigger the class switch.

It is appropriate to emphasize at this stage that the B cell receptor for antigen has the same antigen-binding ability as do antibody molecules. Thus, they can bind to free intact antigenic molecules in solution. This is very different from the α/β TCR that can bind and respond only to processed antigen fragments bound to an MHC molecule (Figure 11-13). This difference in the antigen-recognizing ability of B and T cells is significant in that B cells can respond to a greater variety of antigens than T cells. Likewise, antibodies are directed, not against

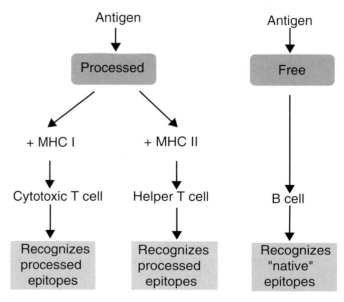

Figure 11-13. TCRs and BCRs recognize antigen in a very different fashion. Thus a BCR can bind to free, soluble antigen. A TCR, in contrast, can recognize only antigen processed and presented on a MHC molecule.

breakdown products of antigens, but against determinants on intact antigen molecules. As a result, antigen-antibody interactions usually depend on maintenance of the three-dimensional conformation of the antigen. A good example of this is seen with tetanus toxoid. Antibodies raised against the intact molecule will bind only to the intact molecule and are unable to bind to proteolytic fragments such as those produced by macrophage processing.

CELLULAR RESPONSES

When antigen enters the body, it can stimulate a B cell only through its specific receptors. The term *clonotype* is used to describe a clone of B cells with a BCR capable of responding to a single epitope. A newborn animal has only a small number of different clonotypes, but this number increases as the animal matures as a result of increased use of alternative sets of V genes and somatic hypermutation in these V genes (Chapter 14). In an adult animal the number of B cells within a given clonotype varies as a result of exposure to different antigens over the animal's lifetime. Thus, as an individual ages, the most used clonotypes will grow. For some rarely encountered antigens, there may be as few as 10 responsive cells in the spleen or bone marrow; for other, commonly encountered antigens, there may be as many as 10^4 cells.

In mice and probably most other mammals, each resting B cell carries both IgM and IgD BCRs on its surface with about ten times as many IgD molecules as IgM. These unstimulated B cells may spontaneously secrete a small quantity of monomeric IgM. When antigen binds to BCR in the presence of helper T cells and IL-4, signals are transmitted to the cell. This signal eventually leads to increased expression of IgM BCR, MHC class II, IL-4, IL-5, IL-6, TNF-α, and TGF-β receptors and starts the process that leads to B cell division.

It is unclear why immature B cells should express both IgM and IgD BCR since animals that fail to express IgD appear to suffer no ill effects.

An appropriately stimulated B cell will enlarge and divide repeatedly. Some of its progeny cells develop a rough endoplasmic reticulum, increase their rate of synthesis, and start to secrete large quantities of immunoglobulins. Within a few days, the cell switches to synthesizing another immunoglobulin class. This switch occurs while a B cell is in the germinal center and results in a change from IgM to IgG, IgA, or IgE. This class switch is a result of deletion of unwanted heavy-chain gene segments and the joining of variable-region genes to the next available constant-region genes (Chapter 14). The specificity of the antibody produced remains unchanged. Class switching is controlled by IL-4, IFN-γ, and TGF-β. Thus IL-4 directs mouse B cells to produce IgG1 and IgE, whereas it directs human B cells to produce IgG4 and IgE. However IL-4 alone is insufficient for class switching, and additional signals are

required to complete the process. In humans, the additional signal is provided by T cells through CD40 and its ligand CD154 (p. 121). IFN-γ stimulates a switch to IgG2a and IgG3 in mouse B cells and effectively suppresses the effects of IL-4. As an immune response progresses, there is a gradual increase in antibody affinity for antigen. This increase is due to progressive somatic mutation and selection within responding B cell populations.

The two subpopulations of helper T cells, Th1 and Th2, respond in different ways to cytokines and, more important, secrete different mixtures of cytokines. Thus Th2 cells are optimized to help antibody formation by B cells by promoting the synthesis of certain immunoglobulin classes or subclasses (Table 11-1). Th1 cells secrete IL-2 and IFN-γ that do not stimulate specific antibody formation. Th2 cells, in contrast, secrete IL-4, IL-5, IL-6, IL-10, and IL-13 that strongly enhance B cell production of IgG, IgA, and IgE.

PLASMA CELLS

Plasma cells develop from antigen-stimulated B cells (Figure 11-14). Cells that are structurally intermediate among lymphocytes and plasma cells (plasmablasts) can be identified in areas where T cell and B cell cooperation occurs. Plasmablasts are found, therefore, between the lymph-node cortex and paracortex and in the marginal zone in the spleen. Fully developed plasma cells migrate away from these areas and can be found distributed throughout the body. Plasma cells are found in greatest numbers in the spleen, the medulla of lymph nodes, and in the bone marrow.

Plasma cells are ovoid cells, eight to 9 μm in diameter (Figure 11-15). They have a round, eccentrically placed nucleus with unevenly distributed chromatin. As a result, the nucleus may resemble a clock face or cartwheel. Plasma cells have an extensive cytoplasm that is rich in rough endoplasmic reticulum and stains strongly with basic dyes and pyronin. They have a large, pale-staining

TABLE 11-1

Immunoglobulin Class Distribution of the Polyclonal Response of Normal B Cells to Antigen-Specific Helper T-Cell Clones in Mice

Class	Th1 Cell (ng/ml)	Th2 Cell (ng/ml)
IgG1	<8	21,600
IgG2a	14	39
IgG2b	<8	189
IgG3	<8	354
IgM	248	98,000
IgA	<1	484
IgE	<1	187

Adapted from Coffmann RL et al: *Immunol Rev* 102:5, 1988.

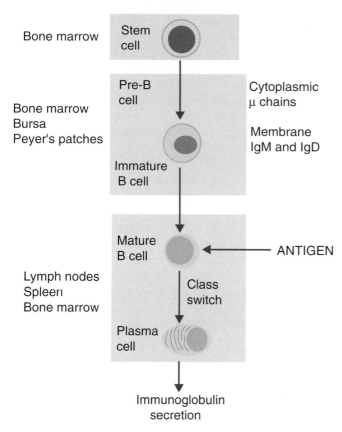

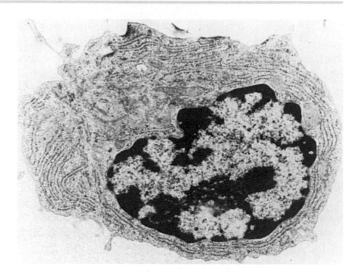

Figure 11-16. A transmission electron micrograph of a plasma cell from a rabbit. (Courtesy of Dr S Linthicum.)

months, although most die within a few days. This death does not immediately result in decreased serum-antibody levels, since the immunoglobulins, once secreted, decline slowly through catabolism. It is likely that some plasma cells may survive for longer than one year in the bone marrow and continue to secrete antibodies during this time.

MEMORY CELLS

One reason why the primary immune response terminates is because many responding B cells and plasma cells are simply removed by apoptosis. If all these cells died, however, immunological memory could not develop.

Figure 11-14. B cells originate in the bone marrow and proceed through a series of differentiation stages before becoming able to respond to antigen. When B cells respond to antigen, they respond by division and differentiation of their progeny into plasma cells.

Golgi apparatus (Figures 11-16 and 11-17). Plasma cells can make and secrete up to 10,000 molecules of immunoglobulin per second. The immunoglobulin produced by a plasma cell is of identical antigen-binding specificity to the original BCRs on its parent B cell. Most plasma cells are probably terminally differentiated and do not divide. Their life spans vary from a few days to many

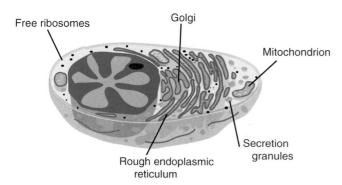

Figure 11-15. The structure of a typical plasma cell. The possession of an extensive rough endoplasmic reticulum is typical of a cell dedicated to the rapid production of large amounts of immunoglobulin.

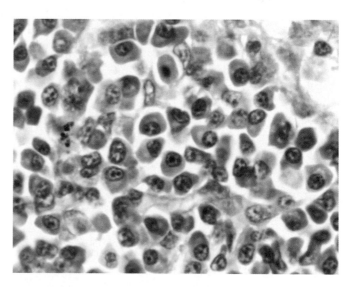

Figure 11-17. Plasma cells in the medulla of a dog lymph node. Their cytoplasm is rich in ribosomes and so stains intensely with pyronin, giving a dark red appearance. Original magnification ×450. (From a specimen kindly provided by Drs N McArthur and LC Abbott.)

Clearly some B cells must survive to become memory cells. In fact, when B cells are stimulated by antigen in association with helper T cells, the B cell activation takes place in the T cell rich zones (paracortex) of lymph nodes. Most of these B cells differentiate into plasma cells and migrate to the bone marrow, but some memory precursors remain in the cortex, begin to proliferate, and form germinal centers. These cells persist in the germinal center under the influence of programming and rescue signals. Thus, memory cells are first screened for their ability to bind antigen. This induces CD154 on nearby T cells, which in turn facilitates memory B cell survival by promoting expression of a gene called *bcl-2*. *Bcl-2* is expressed in memory cells but not in short-lived B cells and plasma cells. Activation of the *bcl-2* gene allows a cell to avoid death by apoptosis and to differentiate into a memory cell.

Memory cells form a reserve of antigen-sensitive cells to be called on subsequent exposure to an antigen. There are probably two types of memory cells. One population consists of small, long-lived resting cells with IgG BCR. These cells, unlike plasma cells, do not have a characteristic morphology but resemble other lymphocytes. Their prolonged survival does not depend on antigen contact. On exposure to antigen they proliferate and differentiate into plasma cells without undergoing further mutation. It has been calculated that in response to secondary antigenic stimulation, the clonal expansion of memory B cells results in 8- to 10-fold more plasma cells than does a primary immune response. A second type of memory cell population consists of large, dividing cells with IgM BCR. These cells persist within germinal centers where their continued survival depends on exposure to antigen on follicular dendritic cells.

One feature of B cell memory is the prolonged production of antibodies over many months or years after immunization. Thus cats immunized with killed panleukopenia virus will continue to produce antibodies at low levels for many years. The source of these antibodies is believed to be memory B cells stimulated to secrete antibodies by exposure to common polyclonal stimulants such as CpG DNA and to bystander T cell help.

If a second dose of antigen is given to a primed animal, it will encounter large numbers of memory B cells, which respond in the manner described previously for antigen-sensitive B cells (Figure 11-18). As a result, a secondary immune response is much greater than a primary immune response. The lag period is shorter since more antibodies are produced and they can be detected earlier. IgG is also produced in preference to the IgM that is characteristic of the primary response.

GERMINAL CENTERS

As described in Chapter 8, the development of germinal centers in the secondary lymphoid tissues such as lymph nodes and spleen parallels the development of memory B cells. These germinal centers are sites where many critical events in the life of B cells occur (Figure 11-19), such as antigen-driven cell proliferation, somatic hypermutation, and positive and negative selection of B cell

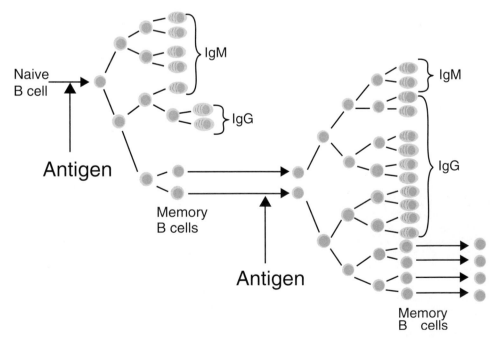

Figure 11-18. The cellular events in a primary and secondary B cell response. Note how some IgG is made in the primary immune response, whereas a small amount of IgM is made in a secondary immune response.

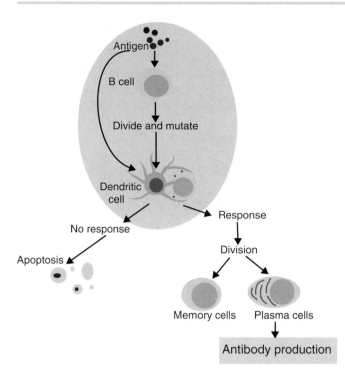

Figure 11-19. B cells in the germinal center undergo somatic mutation as they respond to antigen presented by dendritic cells. If the mutation enables them to bind antigen more strongly, they will be stimulated to grow still further. If, on the other hand, the mutation reduces their antigen-binding ability, they will undergo apoptosis.

populations. B cells stimulated by antigen and helper T cells migrate to a germinal center about 6 days after the response begins. There they divide rapidly. These large dividing cells give a germinal center its pale appearance in histological sections. During this stage of rapid B cell division, the BCR V region genes mutate at a rate of about one mutation per division. This somatic mutation generates large numbers of B cells whose BCRs differ from those of the parent cell. Once these cells have been clonally expanded, a process that takes 10 to 20 days, they then migrate to the periphery of the germinal center, where they encounter antigen on dendritic cells. Dendritic follicular cells in germinal centers trap antigen. Because of mutation, some of the germinal center B cells bind this antigen with greater affinity, but many, perhaps the great majority, bind the antigen less strongly. If mutation has resulted in greater affinity of the BCR for the antigen, then B cells with these receptors will divide further and leave the center to form either plasma cells or memory cells. However, the majority of mutated BCRs will show reduced antigen binding. The cells with these receptors undergo apoptosis, and their remains are removed by macrophages. Thus the B cell population that emerges from a germinal center is very different from the population of cells that entered it. In addition to mutation of BCR V genes, BCRs undergo the immunoglobulin class switch within germinal centers.

B Cell Subpopulations

B cells can be divided into two major subpopulations. The B cells that develop earliest in life are called B1 cells. Those that develop later are called B2 cells and are the conventional B cells discussed in this chapter. Most B1 cells express CD5, an adhesion and receptor molecule. (CD5 is the receptor for CD72.) B1 cells are the source of so-called natural antibodies—IgM antibodies directed against widespread antigens, especially carbohydrates—and thus play an important role in innate immunity. They recognize common bacterial molecules such as phosphoryl-choline, as well as self antigens such as phosphatidyl choline, immunoglobulins, and DNA. They produce antibodies in a T-independent manner. B1 cells also differ from conventional B2 cells in that they are found in the peritoneal and pleural cavities of rodents and have the potential to renew themselves. It is possible that B1 cells are a distinct B cell lineage originating from precursors in the fetal liver or omentum rather than the bone marrow. Alternatively, they may be in a long-lived self-renewing state as a result of the way in which they contact antigen. B1 cells may play an important role in some autoimmune diseases such as rheumatoid arthritis. Many of the IgA-producing cells in the intestine originate from B1 cells. B1 cells have been identified in humans, mice, rabbits, guinea pigs, sheep, and cattle. Up to 30% of pig blood B cells are CD5+, with the highest proportion in neonates.

MYELOMAS

Malignant transformation of a single B cell may give rise to the development of a clone of immunoglobulin-producing tumor cells. The structure of these cells may vary, but they are usually recognizable as plasma cells (Figure 11-20). Plasma cell tumors are called myelomas or plasmacytomas. Because myelomas arise from a single precursor cell or clone, they secrete a homogeneous immunoglobulin called a myeloma protein. On serum electrophoresis, this homogeneous myeloma protein will appear as a sharp, well-defined peak. This is called a monoclonal gammopathy (Figure 11-21).

Myeloma proteins may belong to any immunoglobulin class. For example, IgG, IgA, and IgM myelomas have been reported in the dog. In humans, in addition to myelomas of the major immunoglobulin classes, rare cases of IgD and IgE myelomas have also been described. The prevalence of the various immunoglobulin classes in myeloma proteins correlates well with their relative quantities in normal serum, indicating that the tumor arises as a result of a random mutation in a single B cell. Light chain disease is a myeloma in which light chains alone are produced or the production of light chains is greatly in excess of the production of heavy chains. Similarly, there is a very rare form of myeloma in which

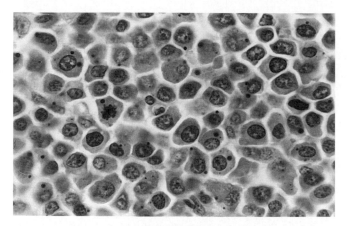

Figure 11-20. A section of myeloma tumor mass in a dog. Original magnification ×900. The cells are clearly plasma cells. (From a specimen kindly provided by Dr. RG Thompson.)

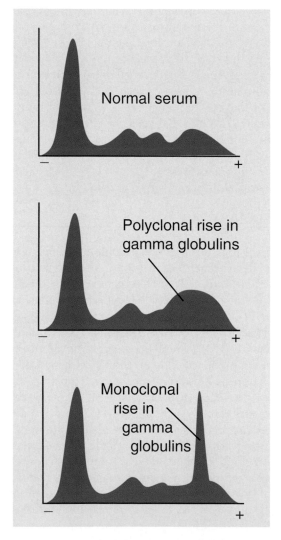

Figure 11-21. Serum electrophoretic patterns showing the normal pattern and the characteristic features of monoclonal and polyclonal gammopathies. The monoclonal antibody spike reflects the production of large amounts of homogeneous immunoglobulins. Monoclonal gammopathies commonly result from the presence of a myeloma.

Fc fragments alone are produced. This condition is erroneously termed heavy chain disease.

Myelomas have been described in humans, mice, dogs, cats, horses, cows, pigs, ferrets, and rabbits. They account for less than 1% of all canine tumors, and they are considerably rarer in the other domestic species. The clinical presentation of myelomas is highly variable. There are, however, several key manifestations, including bleeding disorders, hyperviscosity, renal failure, and hypercalcemia. Other symptoms include lethargy, recurrent infections, anemia, lameness, bone fracture, and neurological signs including dementia and peripheral neuropathy. The most common clinical manifestation in dogs is excessive bleeding as a result of a thrombocytopenia and a loss of clotting components as they bind to myeloma proteins. The presence in serum of abnormally large quantities of immunoglobulins results in a hyperviscosity syndrome, which is especially severe in animals with IgM myelomas (macroglobulinemia). As a result of the increase in blood viscosity, the heart must work harder and congestive heart failure, retinopathy, and neurological signs may result. Because myeloma cells stimulate osteoclast activity, the presence of tumor masses in bone marrow may lead to severe bone destruction. Multiple radiolucent osteolytic lesions and diffuse osteoporosis develop and are readily seen by radiography (Figure 11-22). These lesions result in pathological fractures. Light chains, being relatively small, are excreted in the urine. Unfortunately, they are toxic for renal tubular cells and, as a result, may cause renal failure. The light chains may be detected by

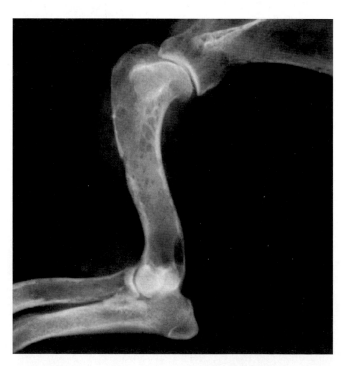

Figure 11-22. A radiograph of a dog leg, showing the round, radiolucent areas where bone has been eroded by the presence of a myeloma. (Courtesy of Dr Claudia Barton.)

electrophoresis of concentrated urine or, in some cases, by heating the urine. Light chains precipitate when heated to 60° C but redissolve as the temperature is raised to 80° C. Proteins possessing this curious property are called Bence-Jones proteins, and their presence in urine suggests a myeloma. They are seen in about 40% of canine cases. Nonsecretory myelomas are occasionally diagnosed in dogs.

Because of the overwhelming commitment of the body's immune resources to the production of neoplastic plasma cells, as well as the replacement of normal marrow tissue by tumor cells and the negative feedback induced by elevated serum immunoglobulins, animals with myelomas are immunosuppressed and anemic. In humans, renal failure and overwhelming infection are the most common causes of death in myeloma patients.

Animals with myelomas characteristically have a monoclonal gammopathy that can be identified by serum electrophoresis. The class of immunoglobulin involved can be identified by immunoelectrophoresis (Figure 11-23), and it may be measured by radial immunodiffusion (Chapter 16).

Affected animals should receive supportive therapy to relieve their immediate clinical problems. Antibiotics can be used to control secondary infections, and fluid therapy should be administered to combat the dehydration resulting from renal failure. Steroids and diuretics may assist in promoting calcium excretion. The serum hyperviscosity may be reduced by plasmapheresis to remove the myeloma protein. The tumor itself can be treated with specific chemotherapy. The drug of choice is melphalan, an alkylating agent. Prednisone may be used in association with melphalan. In unresponsive cases cyclophosphamide or thalidomide may be employed.

Sometimes, in clinically normal humans, dogs, and horses, a benign monoclonal gammopathy may develop that is not due to a myeloma. These monoclonal antibodies are usually an inadvertent finding on serum electrophoresis, and their origin is unclear. They may disappear spontaneously within a short period, or they may persist for many years. Affected animals may show abnormally large numbers of plasma cells in their internal organs on necropsy.

Polyclonal Gammopathies

In contrast to monoclonal gammopathies, which are usually due to a myeloma, polyclonal gammopathies are observed in a wide variety of pathological conditions. (Polyclonal gammopathies are characterized by an increase in all immunoglobulins as a result of excessive activity of many different clones of plasma cells.) The condition that most resembles a myeloma is Aleutian disease in mink (Chapter 24). Animals infected by the Aleutian disease virus show, in the progressive form of the disease, marked plasmacytosis and lymphocyte infiltration of many organs and tissue, as well as polyclonal (occasionally monoclonal) gammopathy. As a result of the elevated immunoglobulin levels, affected mink experience a hyperviscosity syndrome and are severely immunosuppressed.

Other causes of polyclonal gammopathy include autoimmune diseases such as systemic lupus erythematosus, rheumatoid arthritis, and myasthenia gravis (Chapter 34), as well as certain infections such as tropical pancytopenia of dogs (*Ehrlichia canis*), African trypanosomiasis, and chronic bacterial infections such as pyometra and pyoderma. In horses heavily parasitized with *Strongylus vulgaris*, polyclonal IgG3 levels rise significantly. Polyclonal gammopathy also occurs in virus infections such as feline infectious peritonitis and African swine fever and in conditions in which there is extensive liver damage.

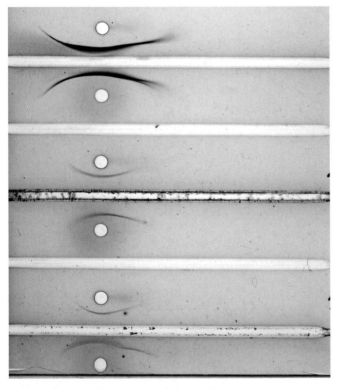

Figure 11-23. Immunoelectrophoresis of serum from a cat with an IgM myeloma. Note that the line of precipitate formed by the reaction between anti-cat IgM and the myeloma serum is distorted (*bottom*). The line is much thicker than the control, and it forms two distinct joined arcs as a result of the presence of the IgM myeloma protein. (Details of this technique can be found in Chapter 16.) (Courtesy of Dr G Elissalde.)

HYBRIDOMAS

The plasma cells in myelomas become neoplastic in an entirely random manner, so that the immunoglobulins that they secrete are not usually directed against any antigen of practical importance. Nevertheless, myeloma cells can be grown in tissue culture, where they survive indefinitely. It would be highly desirable to be able to set up a system to obtain large quantities of absolutely pure, specific immunoglobulins directed against an antigen of interest. This can be done by fusing a normal plasma cell, making the antibody of interest, with a myeloma cell able to grow in tissue culture. The resulting mixed cell is called a hybridoma.

The first stage in making a hybridoma is to generate antibody-producing plasma cells (Figure 11-24). This is done by immunizing a mouse against the antigen of interest and repeating the process several times to ensure that a good antibody response is mounted. Two to four days after the antigen is administered, its spleen is removed and broken up to form a cell suspension. These spleen cells are suspended in culture medium, together with cultured mouse myeloma-cells. Generally, myeloma cells that do not secrete immunoglobulins are used, since this simplifies purification later on. Polyethylene glycol is added to the mixture. This compound induces many of the cells to fuse (although it takes about 200,000 spleen cells on average to form a viable hybrid with one myeloma cell). If the fused cell mixture is cultured for several days, any unfused spleen cells will die. The

myeloma cells would normally survive, but they are eliminated by a simple trick.

There are three biosynthetic pathways by which cells can synthesize nucleotides and therefore nucleic acids. The myeloma cells are selected so that they lack two enzymes: hypoxanthine phosphoribosyl transferase and thymidine kinase. As a result, they cannot use either thymidine or hypoxanthine and are obliged to use an alternative biosynthetic pathway to convert uridine to nucleotides. The fused cell mixture is therefore grown in a culture containing three compounds: hypoxanthine, aminopterin, and thymidine (known as HAT medium). Aminopterin is a drug that prevents cells from making their own nucleotides from uridine. Since the myeloma cells cannot use hypoxanthine or thymidine and the aminopterin stops them from using the alternative synthetic pathway, they cannot make nucleic acids and soon die (Figure 11-25). Hybrids made from a myeloma and a normal cell will grow, since they possess the critical enzymes and can therefore utilize the hypoxanthine and thymidine in the culture medium and survive. The hybridomas divide rapidly in the HAT medium, doubling their numbers every 24 to 48 hours. On average, about 300 to 500 different hybrids can be isolated from a mouse spleen, although not all will make antibodies of interest.

Figure 11-24.   A schematic diagram showing the method of production of monoclonal antibodies.

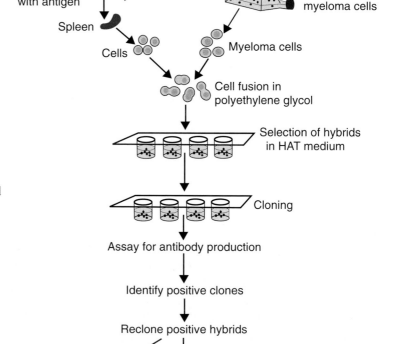

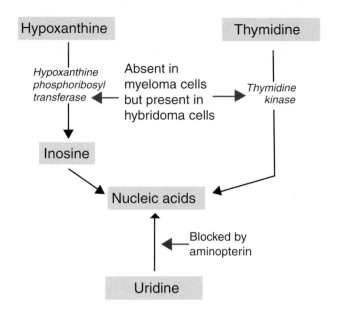

Figure 11-25. The pathways of purine synthesis and the mechanism of action of HAT medium.

If a mixture of cells from a fusion experiment is cultured in wells on a plate with about 50,000 myeloma cells per well, it is usual to obtain about one hybrid in every three wells. After culturing for 2 to 4 weeks, the growing cells can be seen and the supernatant fluid can be screened for the presence of antibodies. It is essential to use a sensitive assay at this time. Radioimmunoassays or enzyme-linked immunosorbent assays (ELISAs) are preferred (Chapter 16). Clones that produce the desired antibody are grown in mass culture and recloned to eliminate nonantibody-producing hybrids.

Unfortunately, antibody-producing clones tend to lose this ability after being cultured for several months. Thus it is usual to make large stocks of hybridoma cells and store them frozen in small aliquots. These can then be thawed as required and grown up in bulk culture. Alternatively, the hybridoma cells can be injected intraperitoneally into mice. Since they are tumor cells, the hybridomas grow rapidly and provoke the effusion of a large volume of fluid into the mouse peritoneal cavity. This fluid is rich in monoclonal antibody and can be readily harvested.

Although the classical methods of making hybridomas produce only mouse immunoglobulins, it is possible to

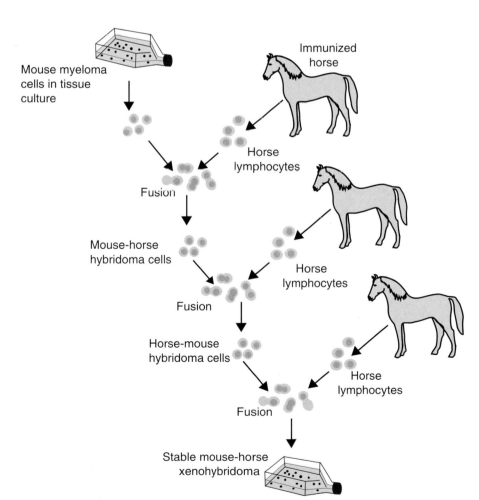

Figure 11-26. A schematic diagram showing one method of making xenohybridomas, in this case using horse cells.

produce monoclonal antibodies from cells of other mammalian species. For example, it is possible to make bovine hybridomas by fusing bovine B cells with a cultured bovine lymphoblastoid cell line. It is generally easier, however, to make hybridomas by fusing B cells from the species under study with mouse myeloma cells. These xenohybridomas or heterohybridomas are made as described previously, but the source of the antibody-producing cells is a species other than a mouse. Thus equine xenohybridomas can be produced by fusing antibody-producing equine spleen cells with mouse myeloma cells. The resulting interspecific hybridomas may secrete equine monoclonal antibodies. Unfortunately, these xenohybridoma cells are unstable and tend to lose the non-murine chromosomes as they divide. As a result, they may cease immunoglobulin synthesis prematurely. Improved stability can be achieved by first growing the xenohybridoma cells in the presence of 8-azaguanine to select for aminopterin sensitivity. These xenohybridomas are then used as fusion partners with lymphocytes from immunized animals of the correct species (Figure 11-26). The resulting secondary xenohybridomas may be further selected and used as fusion partners to produce tertiary xenohybridomas.

Monoclonal antibodies have become the preferred source of antibodies for much immunological research. They are absolutely specific for single epitopes and are available in large numbers. Because of their purity, they can function as standard chemical reagents. Monoclonal antibodies are rapidly being incorporated into clinical diagnostic techniques in which large quantities of antibodies of consistent quality are required. Although mouse cells have been the preferred source, recent experimental studies have shown that cattle and goats can be genetically engineered to produce monoclonal antibodies in their milk. It has even proved possible to incorporate antibody genes into plants such as soy, corn, or tobacco. These "plantibodies" are produced in very large quantities, and although heavily glycosylated, they appear to be functional.

SOURCES OF ADDITIONAL INFORMATION

Armitage RJ, Maliszewski CR, Alderson MR, et al: CD40L: a multifunctional ligand, *Semin Immunol* 5:401-412, 1993.

Berek C: The development of B cells and the B-cell repertoire in the microenvironment of the germinal center, *Immunol Rev* 126:5-19, 1992.

Berek C, Ziegner M: The maturation of the immune response, *Immunol Today* 14:400-404, 1993.

Bernasconi NL, Traggiai E, Lanzavecchia A: Maintenance of serological memory by polyclonal activation of human memory B cells, *Science* 298:2199-2202, 2002.

Cambier JC, Campbell KS: Membrane immunoglobulin and its accomplices: new lessons from an old receptor, *FASEB J* 6:3207-3217, 1992.

Carter RH, Fearon DT: CD19: lowering the threshold for antigen receptor stimulation of B lymphocytes, *Science* 256:105-107, 1992.

Clark MR, Campbell KS, Kazlauskas A, et al: The B cell antigen receptor complex: association of Ig-α and Ig-β with distinct cytoplasmic effectors, *Science* 258:123-125, 1992.

Durie FH, Foy TM, Masters SR, et al: The role of CD40 in the regulation of humoral and cell-mediated immunity, *Immunol Today* 15:406-411, 1994.

Esser C, Radbruch A: Immunoglobulin class switching: molecular and cellular analysis, *Annu Rev Immunol* 8:717-735, 1990.

Finkelman FD, Holmes J, Katona IM, et al: Lymphokine control of *in vivo* immunoglobulin isotype selection, *Annu Rev Immunol* 8:303-333, 1990.

Finkelman FD, Lees A, Morris SC: Antigen presentation by B lymphocytes to CD4+ T lymphocytes in vivo: importance for B lymphocyte and T lymphocyte activation, *Semin Immunol* 4:247-255, 1992.

Gauld SB, Dal Porto JM, Cambier JC: B cell antigen receptor signaling: roles in cell development and disease, *Science* 296:1641-1642, 2002.

Gearhart PJ: The roots of antibody diversity, *Nature* 419:29-31, 2002.

Gold MR: To make antibodies or not: signaling by the B-cell antigen receptor, *Trends Pharm Sci* 23:316-324, 2002.

Greenlee AR, Magnuson NS, Smith C, et al: Characterization of heteromyeloma fusion partners which promote the outgrowth of porcine hybridomas, *Vet Immunol Immunopathol* 26:267-284, 1990.

Lutje V, Black SJ: Cellular interactions regulating the in vitro response of bovine lymphocytes to ovalbumin, *Vet Immunol Immunopathol* 28:275-288, 1991.

Nossal GJV: The molecular and cellular basis of affinity maturation in the antibody response, *Cell* 68:1-2, 1992.

Pleiman CM, D'Ambrosio D, Cambier JC: The B-cell antigen receptor complex: structure and signal transduction, *Immunol Today* 15:393-399, 1994.

Reth M, Hombach J, Weiser P, Weinands J: Structure and signalling function of B cell antigen receptors of different classes. In *Molecular mechanisms of immunological self-recognition*, New York, 1993, Academic Press, pp 69-75.

Tedder TF, Zhou L-J, Engel P: The CD19/CD21 signal transduction complex of B lymphocytes, *Immunol Today* 15:437-442, 1994.

Wakabayashi C, Adachi T, Wienands J, Tsubata T: A distinct signaling pathway used by the IgG-containing B cell antigen receptor, *Science* 298:2392-2395, 2002.

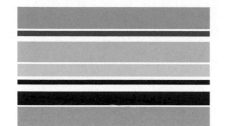

Cytokines and the Immune System

CHAPTER 12

The cells of the immune system secrete a bewildering variety of proteins whose function is to regulate the immune responses by communicating among cells. These proteins are called cytokines. Cytokines differ from conventional hormones in several important respects (Table 12-1). For example, unlike classical hormones, which tend to affect a single target organ, cytokines affect a wide variety of cells and organs. Second, cells rarely secrete only one cytokine at a time. For instance, macrophages secrete at least five: IL-1, IL-6, IL-12, IL-18, and TNF-α. Third, cytokines appear to be "redundant" in their biological activities in that many different cytokines may have similar effects. For example, IL-1, TNF-α, TNF-β, IL-6, HMGP-1, and the chemokine CCL3 all cause fever. This complexity has given rise to the concept of a cytokine network, a web of signals among all the cell types of the immune system mediated by complex mixtures of cytokines.

CYTOKINE NOMENCLATURE

The nomenclature of cytokines is not based on any systematic relationship among these proteins. However, many were originally named after their cell of origin or the bioassay used to identify them.

Interleukins are cytokines that regulate the interactions between lymphocytes and other leukocytes (Table 12-2). They are numbered sequentially in the order of their discovery. Because their definition is so broad, the interleukins are a heterogeneous mixture of proteins with little in common except their name.

Interferons are antiviral cytokines that are produced in response to virus infection or immune stimulation. Their name is derived from the fact that they interfere with viral RNA and protein synthesis (Table 12-3). The two most important type I interferons are interferon alpha (IFN-α), and interferon-beta (IFN-β). There is a single type II interferon, called interferon-gamma (IFN-γ).

TABLE 12-1
A Comparison of Cytokines and Hormones

Property	Hormones	Cytokines
Sources	Specific endocrine glands	Many different cell types
Targets	Specific cell targets	Many different cell types
Functional redundancy	Very low	Very high
Effect	Endocrine	Autocrine Paracrine Endocrine
Function	Homeostasis	Tissue repair Resistance to infection

TABLE 12-2
The Interleukins

Name	Produced Mainly by	Major Targets
IL-1	Macrophages (many)	Th2 cells, B cells (many)
IL-2	Th1 cells, NK cells	T cells, B cells, other
IL-3	T cells	Hematopoietic cells, stem cells
IL-4	Th2 cells	T cells, B cells, mast cells
IL-5	Th2 cells	B cells, T cells
IL-6	Fibroblasts, T cells	B cells (many)
IL-7	Stromal cells	Immature lymphocytes
IL-8 (CXCL8)	Macrophages	T cells, neutrophils
IL-9	Th2 cells	T cells
IL-10	Th2 cells, B cells	Th1 cells
IL-11	Bone marrow stroma	B cells, stem cells
IL-12	Macrophages, B cells	Th1 cells, NK cells
IL-13	Th2 cells	B cells
IL-14	CD4+ T cells	B cells
IL-15	Macrophages	T cells
IL-16	CD8 T cells	CD4+ T cells, eosinophils, macrophages
IL-17	CD4+ T cells	T cells, fibroblasts
IL-18	Macrophages	Th1 cells, NK cells
IL-19	B cells and monocytes	Monocytes, T cells
IL-20	Skin	Keratinocytes
IL-21	T cells, mast cells	Hepatocytes
IL-22	T cells	Hepatocytes
IL-23	Dendritic cells	T cells
IL-24	Mononuclear cells	Tumor cells
IL-26	Memory cells	T cells
IL-28	Virus-infected cells	Virus-infected cells
IL-29	Virus-infected cells	Virus-infected cells
IL-30	Dendritic cells	Naïve CD4+ T cells

TABLE 12-3
The Different Forms of Interferons

Class	Interferon	Source	Function
Type I	α	Dendritic cells	Antiviral
	β	Fibroblasts	Antiviral
	δ	Trophoblast	Pregnancy signaling
	ω	Trophoblast	Pregnancy signaling
	τ	Trophoblast	Pregnancy signaling
Type II	γ	Th1 cells	Immune activation

TABLE 12-4
The Tumor Necrosis Factors

Name	Produced Mainly by	Major Targets
TNF-β	T cells, other	Tumor cells
TNF-α	Macrophages, other	Endothelium

TABLE 12-5
Some Selected Growth Factors

Name	Produced Mainly by	Major Targets
G-CSF	Fibroblasts, macrophages	Hematopoietic cells
GM-CSF	Fibroblasts, macrophages	Monocytes, stem cells
GM-CSF	T cells, others	Hematopoietic cells
TGF-β	Platelets, nucleated cells	Many targets

Many interferons also play a role in the maintenance of pregnancy.

Tumor necrosis factors (TNFs) are cytokines derived from macrophages and T cells. As their name suggests, they can kill tumor cells, although this is not their primary function (Table 12-4). Thus TNF-α is the key mediator of acute inflammation. TNFs are members of a family of related proteins, the TNF superfamily, which is involved in immune regulation and inflammation. Other important members of the TNF superfamily include CD178 (also called CD95L or fas ligand; see Chapter 17), and CD154 (CD40 ligand).

Many cytokines serve as growth factors (or colony-stimulating factors) and control leukocyte production by regulating stem cell growth (Table 12-5). They thereby ensure that the body is supplied with sufficient cells to defend itself.

Chemokines are a family of cytokines that play an important role in leukocyte circulation and migration, especially in inflammation. They act primarily as chemotactic factors and leukocyte activators. A typical example of a chemokine is CXCL8 (also known as interleukin 8).

CYTOKINE FUNCTIONS

Cytokines are produced in response to many different stimuli. The most important of these are antigens acting through the TCR or BCR, antigen-antibody complexes acting through Fc receptors, superantigens acting

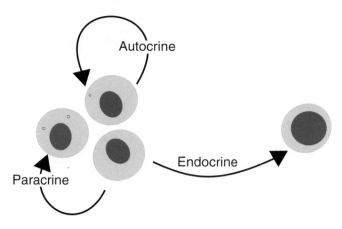

Figure 12-1. The distinction among autocrine, paracrine, and endocrine effects. Cytokines differ from hormones in that most of their effects are autocrine or paracrine, whereas hormones act on distant cells in an endocrine fashion.

TABLE 12-6		
A Molecular Classification of the Cytokines		
Group 1	IL-2 subfamily	IL-2, 3, 4, 5, 6, 7, 9, 11, 13, 15, and 30; G-CSF, GM-CSF, M-CSF, growth hormone, leptin
	Interferon subfamily	IFN-α, IFN-β
	IL-10 subfamily	IL-10, 19, 20, 22, 24, 26
Group 2		TNFs, IL-1 family, TGF-β
Group 3		Chemokines
Group 4		IL-12
Unique molecules		IL-17 family, IL-14, IL-16

through the TCR, and PAMPs such as lipopolysaccharides acting through TLRs.

Cytokines act on many different cellular targets. They may, for example, bind to receptors on the cell that produced them and thus have an autocrine effect. Alternatively, they may bind only to receptors on cells in close proximity to the cell of origin and thereby have a paracrine effect. They may spread throughout the body, affecting cells in distant locations, and thus have an endocrine effect (Figure 12-1).

When cytokines bind to target cells, they affect cell behavior. They may induce the target cell to divide or differentiate, or they may stimulate the production of new proteins. Alternatively they may inhibit these effects—preventing division, differentiation, or new protein synthesis. Most cytokines act on many different target cell types, perhaps inducing different responses in each one, a feature that is called pleiotropy. Conversely, many different cytokines may act on a single target, a feature known as redundancy. Thus IL-3, IL-4, IL-5, and IL-6 all affect B cell function. Some cytokines work best in association with other cytokines in a process called synergy. For example, the combination of IL-4 and IL-5 stimulates B cell switching to IgE production. Synergy can also occur in sequence when one cytokine induces the receptor for another cytokine. Finally, some cytokines may antagonize the effects of others. The best example of this is the mutual antagonism of IL-4 and IFN-γ.

CYTOKINE STRUCTURE

Cytokine molecules can be arranged into structural families (Table 12-6). The largest family, the group 1 cytokines (or hematopoietins), includes many different interleukins: IL-2, IL-3, IL-4, IL-5, IL-6, IL-7, IL-9, IL-11, IL-13, IL-15, IL-23, and IL-30. This group also

includes many molecules not called interleukins, such as G-CSF, M-CSF, and GM-CSF. Hormones such as growth hormone and leptin also belong to this family. Within group 1 are two subfamilies, the interferon subfamily and the IL-10 subfamily. All these protein molecules consist of four α-helices bundled together.

Group 2 cytokines are characterized by having long chain β-sheet structures. They include the tumor necrosis factors, the IL-1 family, and TGF-β. Group 3 cytokines are small proteins with both α-helices and β-sheets. These include the chemokines and related molecules (Chapter 2). Group 4 cytokines have mixtures of different structural motifs and include IL-12. The interleukin 17 family, IL-14, and IL-16 are structurally unique and do not therefore belong to any of the major families.

When cytokines are classified according to their structure, patterns can also be seen in their biological activities. Thus the group 1 cytokines are all involved in immune regulation or hematopoiesis. The group 2 cytokines are mainly involved in the growth and regulation of cells, cell death, and inflammation. The group 3 cytokines are involved in inflammation. The activities of the group 4 cytokines depend on their subcomponents. For example, IL-12 is a mosaic of a group 1 structure and a hematopoietin receptor, but it acts like a group 1 cytokine.

CYTOKINE RECEPTORS

Cells sense the presence of cytokines through specific receptors. These receptors are membrane glycoproteins consisting of at least two functional units, one for ligand binding and one for signal transduction. These may or may not be on the same protein. Cytokine receptors can also be classified into families based on their structure and activities.

The IL-1/toll-like receptor family consists of molecules that participate in host responses to injury and infection. They include the receptors for IL-1 and IL-18, as well as the TLRs. The family can be split into the molecules that are IL-1R–like (IL-1R1, IL-18R) and the molecules that are toll-like (TLR). Ligation of these receptors triggers signal cascades that activate innate immune responses.

The class I cytokine receptor family is large and includes the receptors for IL-2, IL-3, IL-4, IL-5, IL-6, IL-7, IL-9, IL-11, IL-12, IL-13, IL-15, IL-21, G-CSFR, GM-CSFR, IFN-α/βR, IFN-γR, and IL-10R. It also includes the common β chain of IL-3, IL-5, and GM-CSF receptors and the common γ chain of IL-2, IL-4, IL-7, IL-9, and IL-15 receptors. These receptors usually bind only one ligand, and many exist in high- and low-affinity forms.

The class II receptor family binds the type I and type II interferons, IL-10, and related proteins including IL-28 and IL-29.

The receptor kinase family shares common intracellular domains. In many cases they are monomers that dimerize on activation. TGF-βR belongs to this family.

The TNF receptor superfamily (TNFRSF) consists of at least 18 related transmembrane proteins whose cytoplasmic domains have little structural homology. As a result, the biological activities of their ligands are diverse. They bind not only TNF-α and TNF-β, but also related cytotoxic molecules such as CD95 (Chapter 17) and CD154 (CD40L; Chapter 10). Binding to these receptors may trigger apoptosis.

The serpentine receptor family has, as its name implies, a structure that winds in and out through the cell membrane. It includes the receptors for the chemokines, as well as the receptors for C5a (Chapter 15) and platelet-activating factor.

CYTOKINE REGULATION

Cytokine activities are regulated in many different ways—by alteration of receptor expression, by specific binding proteins, and by other cytokines that exert opposite effects. For example, IL-2 receptor expression largely determines the response of T cells to IL-2. Resting T cells express few receptors for IL-2 but express many more when activated. In contrast, the actions of interleukin 1 are regulated by a receptor antagonist (IL-1RA). IL-1RA is a form of IL-1 that binds to the IL-1 receptor but does not stimulate signal transduction. It therefore blocks the activities of active IL-1 (Figure 12-2). Some cytokines bind to specific binding proteins found in body fluids. These binding proteins are mainly soluble receptors. Examples include soluble receptors for IL-1, IL-2, IL-4, IL-5, IL-6, IL-7, IL-9, TNF-α, and M-CSF. In most cases these soluble receptors reduce cytokine binding to cell surface receptors. In other cases the soluble cytokine-receptor complex may be biologically active. For example, soluble IL-6R α chains complex with IL-6 to form a biologically active structure.

Cytokines such as IL-1, IL-12, and TGF-β may bind to glycosaminoglycans such as heparin or CD44 in

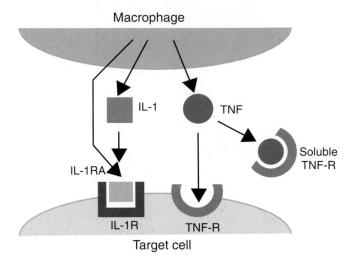

Figure 12-2. The control of cytokine activities as exemplified by IL-1 and TNF-α. IL-1 activity is regulated by the presence of IL-1RA, an inert isoform that binds and blocks the IL-1R, preventing signal transduction. Soluble TNF-αR, in contrast, competes for TNF-α with the cell-membrane receptor.

connective tissue, where they form a reservoir of readily available molecules. Alternatively, the adsorbed cytokine molecules may be aligned in such a way that their biological activity is enhanced.

Perhaps the most important way by which cytokine function is regulated is through the opposing effects of different cytokines. For example, IL-4 stimulates B cells to switch to IgE production, whereas IFN-γ suppresses IgE production (Chapter 26). Similarly, IFN-γ antagonizes TGF-β in stimulating collagen synthesis.

CYTOKINES PRODUCED MAINLY BY MACROPHAGES OR DENDRITIC CELLS

Macrophages and dendritic cells produce many different cytokines (Figure 12-3). Their production is triggered by diverse stimuli, including bacteria, endotoxins, leukotrienes, activated complement components, immune complexes, T cell signals, and other cytokines.

Interleukin 1

Although it plays a critical role in inflammation (Chapter 2), the activities of IL-1 are not restricted to inflammation. It plays a key role in fever, hematopoiesis, appetite control, bone metabolism, and acquired immunity. Active IL-1 is a mixture of two molecules, IL-1α and IL-1β. They are members of a family of ten closely related proteins. The four major members of the family—IL-1α (IL-1F1), IL-1β (IL-1F2), IL-1RA (IL-1F3), and IL-18 (IL-1F4)— have well-defined functions. As a result of genomic studies, six additional family members (IL-1F5 through IL-1F10) have been identified, but their functions are

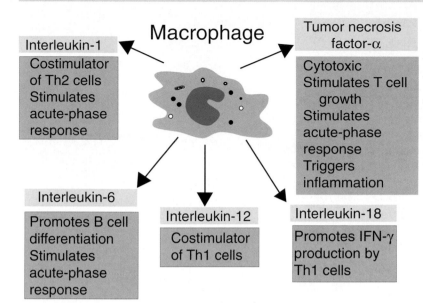

Figure 12-3. The major cytokines secreted by macrophages and their principal functions.

unclear. Most of these newly identified molecules are expressed in macrophages and monocytes.

Although its major source is the macrophage, IL-1 is also produced by dendritic cells, T cells, B cells, NK cells, vascular endothelium, fibroblasts, and keratinocytes. IL-1 acts on T cells, B cells, NK cells, neutrophils, eosinophils, dendritic cells, fibroblasts, endothelial cells, and hepatocytes. IL-1β is produced as a large protein that must be cleaved by IL-1β–converting enzyme (also called caspase 1) to form the active molecule. IL-1α and IL-1β, as described previously, are costimulators of Th2 cells. They also promote inflammation and stimulate the acute phase response.

There are nine members of the IL-1 receptor family, but the most significant are CD121a and CD121b. CD121a is a signaling receptor, whereas CD121b is not. CD121b inhibits IL-1 functions. Soluble CD121b can bind IL-1 and acts as an IL-1 antagonist.

Interleukin 1RA

IL-1 receptor antagonist binds to CD121a. Its only known function is to block active IL-1 binding. IL-1RA is an important regulator of IL-1 activity and inflammation. It reduces mortality in septic shock and graft-versus-host disease (Chapter 4) and has anti-inflammatory effects. Encouraging results have been obtained in treating experimental equine osteoarthritis by gene therapy, employing adenoviruses expressing the interleukin-1RA gene. This resulted in increased expression of IL-1RA within joints and decreased disease activity.

IL-18 is produced, like IL-1β, by cleavage of a larger precursor by IL-1β converting enzyme. IL-18 acts on Th1 cells to promote the production of IFN-γ, TNF-α, IL-1, CD95L, and several chemokines. Because of the effects of IFN-γ on macrophages, this can lead to positive feedback where the IL-18 and IFN-γ reinforce each other.

Interleukin 6

IL-6 is produced not only by activated macrophages but also by T and B cells, mast cells, vascular endothelial cells, fibroblasts, keratinocytes, and mesangial cells. It is also produced by muscle cells during exercise. IL-6 acts on T cells, B cells, hepatocytes, and bone marrow stromal cells. It promotes IL-2 and IL-2R production and T cell differentiation; it synergizes with IL-4 to promote Th2 cell differentiation, and it is required for the final maturation of B cells into plasma cells. IL-6 acts as a cofactor with IL-1 in IgM synthesis and with IL-5 in IgA synthesis. It is a major stimulator of the acute-phase response.

Interleukin 12

IL-12 is a heterodimeric 70 kDa glycoprotein, consisting of 35 and 40 kDa subunits. It is produced by monocytes and macrophages, dendritic cells, B cells, and keratinocytes. In the dog, horse, and mouse, the p35 subunit is constitutively induced, whereas the p40 subunit is inducible following macrophage activation. IL-12 may be stored preformed in macrophages and rapidly released in large quantities on activation. IL-12 promotes Th1 cell activity by inducing secretion of IL-2 and IFN-γ and enhances T and NK cell proliferation and cytotoxicity. TNF-α and IL-12 synergize in promoting IFN-γ production. As a secondary effect it reduces IgE production by suppressing IL-4 synthesis. Its receptor, IL-12R, is classified as CD212 and is expressed on mononuclear cells. The p40 subunit of IL-12 can link to a protein called p19 to form interleukin-23. A dimer of p40 can act as an IL-12 antagonist.

Tumor Necrosis Factor-α

The tumor necrosis factor superfamily (TNFSF) contains at least 18 related proteins that regulate cellular activation, viability, and proliferation through the transcription factor, NF-kB. Its most important member is TNF-α, a 25kDa trimeric protein produced by macrophages, mast cells, T cells, endothelial cells, B cells, and fibroblasts. It can occur in soluble or membrane-bound forms. The membrane-bound form is cleaved from the cell surface by a protease called TNF-α convertase. TNF-α mediates many immune and inflammatory functions and regulates the growth of many cell types. It is a potent proinflammatory molecule and many of its activities are shared with IL-1. Of major importance are its effects on vascular epithelium at sites of microbial invasion. Thus TNF-α enhances their expression of adhesive molecules and triggers procoagulant activity. It promotes fibroblast proliferation and collagen production, a feature of importance in chronic inflammation. TNF-α activates macrophages to increase its own synthesis together with that of IL-1, IL-6, M-CSF, and GM-CSF. As its name implies, TNF-α can trigger killing of some tumor cells and virus-infected cells. It does so by activating caspases, the proteases that are the major mediators of apoptosis. In high doses, TNF-α can cause septic shock. Other members of this superfamily include TNF-β (TNFSF1), CD40L (TNFSF5), and CD95L (TNFSF6). TNF-α receptors are found on almost all nucleated cells. They are of two types (CD120a and CD120b).

CYTOKINES PRODUCED MAINLY BY T CELLS

Helper T cells produce many different cytokines. These fall into two major groups—those produced by Th1 cells and those produced by Th2 cells. In general, the Th1-derived cytokines tend to have biological activities that counteract the activities of the Th2-derived cytokines. Thus the balance between these two groups determines the nature of the immune response to a specific antigen.

Cytokines Produced by Th1 cells

IL-12 and IL-18 produced by dendritic cells, macrophages, and B cells specifically stimulate Th1 cell activity. As a result, Th1 cells produce IL-2 and IFN-γ (Figure 12-4). Th1 cells also secrete TNF-β.

Interleukin 2
Only Th1 cells produce IL-2. Its targets include other T cells, B cells, and NK cells. IL-2 receptors are trimers consisting of α (CD25), β (CD122), and γ (CD132) chains. Different combinations of these chains give rise to different forms of IL-2 receptors (Figure 12-5). For example, a combination of β and γ chains binds IL-2 with low affinity. The presence of the α chain is required for high-affinity binding. B cells have about 1000 high-affinity receptors and 10,000 low-affinity receptors. T cells have only high affinity receptors. Monocytes constitutively express β and γ chains and thus can be stimulated by

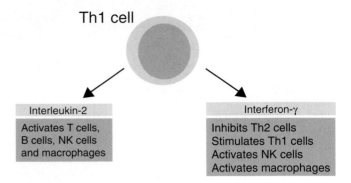

Figure 12-4. The major cytokines secreted by Th1 cells and their principal functions.

IL-2 even when resting. In dogs, mutations in the IL-2Rγ gene cause X-linked severe combined immunodeficiency disease (Chapter 35).

IL-2 activates helper and cytotoxic T cells and NK cells but in order to be responsive to IL-2, antigen and IL-12 must first activate T cells and induce expression of both IL-2 and its receptor. The IL-2 then triggers the T cell to proliferate. Acting on Th1 cells, IL-2 stimulates their proliferation and cytotoxicity (Chapter 17). IL-2 also induces production of IFN-γ and IL-5 and regulates

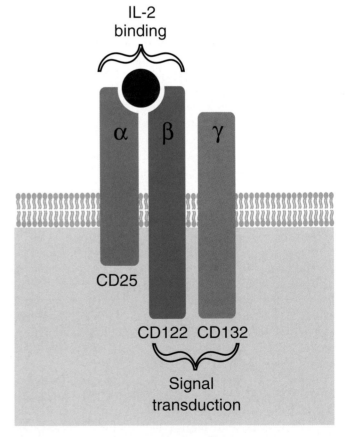

Figure 12-5. The structure of the IL-2 receptor complex. The complete trimer serves as a high-affinity receptor. A β-γ dimer serves as a low-affinity receptor.

TNF-α receptor expression. Recombinant IL-2 in low doses causes fever, malaise, chills, and diarrhea. In high doses it causes thrombocytopenia, hypotension, pulmonary edema, and death. This has proved to be the major impediment to its clinical use.

Interferon-γ

IFN-γ is unrelated to the other interferons and is only so named because of its antiviral activity. It is produced by Th1 cells, by some CD8+ T cells, and by NK cells; it acts on B cells, T cells, NK cells, and macrophages. IFN-γ stimulates B cell production of IgG2a but lowers production of the other immunoglobulin subclasses in mice. It enhances T cell production of MHC class I molecules but not production of MHC class II molecules. It stimulates Th1 cells to produce both IL-2 and IL-2R. IFN-γ inhibits the production of IL-4 by Th2 cells and as a result, blocks IgE production *in vitro*. It enhances the activities of NK cells and is thus a potent stimulator of innate immunity. NK cells respond to activation by producing IFN-γ so that a positive loop exists whereby activation of some NK cells results in interferon secretion and activation of other NK cells. IFN-γ activates macrophages and induces the production of NOS2, so increasing their ability to destroy ingested microorganisms. It also promotes antibody-mediated phagocytosis, as well as antibody-dependent cell-mediated cytotoxicity (ADCC) reactions.

IFN-γ increases MHC class I expression on tumor cells. It induces the appearance of MHC class II molecules on endothelial cells, keratinocytes, myeloid cells, some dendritic cells, and fibroblasts, as well as on macrophages. It upregulates the expression of both MHC class I and II molecules on virus-infected cells. Thus when T cells secrete IFN-γ during graft rejection, MHC class II molecules are induced on the cells of the graft so enhancing the rejection process (Chapter 30).

Tumor Necrosis Factor-β

TNF-β (lymphotoxin-α), another member of the TNF superfamily, is produced by Th1 cells and activated CD8+ T cells. It is either secreted in a soluble form or forms a complex with lymphotoxin-β in the T cell membrane. TNF-β kills tumor cells and activates neutrophils, macrophages, endothelial cells, and B cells.

Cytokines Produced by Th2 cells

Th2 cells secrete a complex mixture of cytokines, including IL-4, IL-5, IL-9, IL-10, and IL-13, and generally provide helper activity for B cell immunoglobulin production (Figure 12-6). They are stimulated to produce these cytokines by IL-1 (or possibly by the absence of IL-12).

Interleukin 4

IL-4 is produced by activated Th2 cells, mast cells, and activated basophils. It acts on B cells, T cells, macrophages, endothelial cells, fibroblasts, and mast cells. IL-4 stimulates the growth and differentiation of B cells. It induces B cells to switch to IgE production and is therefore of major importance in the development of allergic reactions. IL-4 enhances the development of cytotoxic T cells from resting T cells and can make helper T cells grow in the absence of IL-2. IL-4 has complex effects on macrophages. It down-regulates IL-1, IL-6, and TNF-α secretion but increases their MHC class II expression, their antigen presenting ability, and their cytotoxic activity.

The actions of IL-4 are neutralized by IFN-γ. As a result, IFN-γ inhibits IgE synthesis and B cell proliferation. IFN-γ enhances macrophage secretion of IL-1, IL-6, and TNF-α, all of which are inhibited by IL-4. It is interesting to note, however, that both IL-4 and IFN-γ enhance MHC class II expression in macrophages.

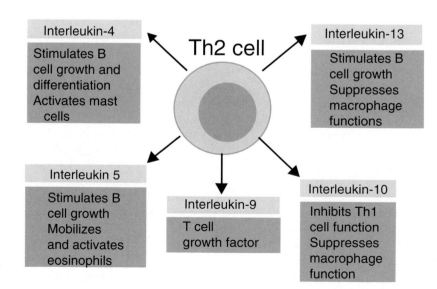

Figure 12-6. The major cytokines secreted by Th2 cells and their principal functions.

Interleukin 5

Activated Th2 cells, mast cells, and eosinophils produce IL-5. In humans its main activity is the control of eosinophil production by stimulating growth and differentiation of eosinophil precursors in the bone marrow. In mice it also enhances B cell growth, IL-4–induced IgE synthesis and FcεRII (CD23) expression.

Interleukin 9

IL-9 is a stem cell growth factor produced only by Th2 cells. It promotes the growth of helper T cells and mast cells. It also potentiates the effects of IL-4 on IgE production and so contributes to the development of allergic diseases.

The Interleukin 10 Family

The IL-10 family includes IL-19, IL-20, IL-22, IL-24, and IL-26. They are all α-helical proteins related to IL-10. None share its immunoregulatory functions, but they have strong antitumor and some proinflammatory properties.

IL-10 is an immunosuppressive and antiinflammatory cytokine that regulates inflammation as well as T cell, NK cell, and macrophage function. It is mainly produced by Th2 cells but may also come from activated macrophages. Its targets are Th1 cells, B cells, macrophages, NK cells, and mast cells. IL-10 selectively inhibits costimulation of T cells by blocking CD28 phosphorylation. As a result it inhibits the synthesis of the Th1 cytokines, IL-2, IFN-γ and TNF-β. IL-10 suppresses the secretion of IL-1, IL-6, TNF-α, and oxidants by macrophages. It down-regulates MHC class II expression and stimulates production of IL-1RA. Its receptor is CDw210.

The other members of the IL-10 family include IL-19, produced by B cells and activated monocytes. It acts on monocytes to induce production of IL-6 and TNF-α and induces their apoptosis. Interleukin 20 is produced by monocytes and keratinocytes and regulates their participation in inflammation. Interleukin 22 is produced by activated Th1 cells and mast cells. It induces acute-phase protein production in the liver. IL-22 also inhibits some Th2 cytokine production. Interleukin 24 is produced by monocytes and Th2 cells. It is involved in antitumor activity and stimulates acute phase responses in hepatocytes. Interleukin 26 is produced by memory T cells (especially Th1 cells) and induces the proliferation of keratinocytes and T cells.

Interleukin 13

IL-13 is produced by Th2 cells, cytotoxic T cells, mast cells, and dendritic cells. It has structural and biological characteristics similar to those of IL-4, because it acts through a receptor (CD213) that shares a common α chain with the IL-4R. It has no effect on T cells since they do not express functional IL-13R. Unlike IL-4, therefore, IL-13 cannot induce differentiation of Th cells. It has similar effects to IL-4 on B cells, stimulating

their proliferation and increasing immunoglobulin secretion. IL-13 is required for optimal induction of IgE, especially if IL-4 is low or absent. It enhances macrophage expression of integrins and is a chemoattractant for monocytes. However, it also acts as a macrophage suppressor by inhibiting FcγR expression and reducing their production of IL-1, IL-6, IL-12, and nitric oxide. It induces giant cell formation by stimulating macrophage fusion. IL-13 also stimulates neutrophils to produce IL-1RA and so has an antiinflammatory effect.

The Interleukin 17 Family

Activated memory T cells produce IL-17, a family of cytokines involved in regulating immune responses. The family contains several related proteins—IL-17, IL-17B, IL-17C, IL-17D (also called IL-27), IL-17E (once called IL-25), and IL-17F—that have similar but not identical biological properties. They induce the production of cytokines by cells such as fibroblasts, keratinocytes, and epithelial and endothelial cells. IL-17 can induce proliferation of T cells and myeloid stem cells.

IL-17 is proinflammatory since it can recruit and activate neutrophils by stimulating T cell chemokine release. Thus IL-17 is a link between T cell activation and the mobilization of neutrophils via chemokines.

IL-17D (IL-27) is produced by dendritic cells and macrophages and activates Th1 cells. IL-17E enhances production of IL-4, IL-5, and IL-13 and so amplifies Th2 responses, eosinophil infiltration, and IgE formation.

Other Interleukins

IL-16 is produced by CD8+ T cells, eosinophils, dendritic cells, and mast cells, as well as by some nonimmune cells such as fibroblasts. Its receptor is CD4. IL-16 thus regulates CD4+ T cell recruitment and activation. When it binds to T cells, it stimulates chemotaxis and cell adhesion, it induces IL-2R and MHC class II expression, and it suppresses antigen-induced proliferation and the replication of the human, feline, and simian immunodeficiency viruses. IL-16 is also a potent chemoattractant for CD4+T cells, eosinophils, dendritic cells, and macrophages. The production of IL-16 directly correlates with the number of infiltrating CD4+ T cells in asthmatic lungs. Since its production by mast cells is stimulated by histamine, IL-16 attracts eosinophils and plays an important role in the development of allergies.

Interleukin 21 is produced by activated T cells and regulates NK, B, and T cell function. It upregulates production of IL-18R and IFN-γ, induces acute phase protein production, and blocks the maturation and proliferation of NK cells while at the same time stimulating the proliferation of mature B and T cells. Thus it aids in the transition from innate to acquired immunity.

Interleukin 23 is a member of the IL-12 family produced by activated dendritic cells. It has similar properties to IL-12, with which it shares a receptor, and stimulates Th1 responses and IFN-γ production. However, whereas

BOX 12–1

Cytokine Nomenclature

The naming of cytokines is the responsibility of the Interleukin Nomenclature Subcommittee of the International Union of Immunological societies. This naming has been based on the each cytokine's origin and structure, as well as the demonstration of functional effects on leukocytes. Unfortunately, the gene nomenclature committee of the Human Genome Organization has recently assigned interleukin names to molecules based only on sequence similarity to other interleukins. The result has been a rash of duplications and mislabelings! For example, several different proteins have been called IL-25. This has caused such confusion that name IL-25 is no longer in use. The number of "interleukins" has grown rapidly, while their biological significance remains quite unclear.

IL-12 stimulates naive Th1 cells, IL-23 stimulates Th1 memory cells (Box 12-1).

Interleukins 28, 29, and 30 are related to the type 1 interferons and the IL-10 family. Their classification is unclear, and they have also been called λ-interferons. Like other interferons, they show antiviral activity.

Interleukin 30 is a protein secreted by antigen-presenting cells that acts on naive CD4 T cells. It synergizes strongly with IL-12 to promote IFN-γ production by Th1 cells.

CYTOKINES PRODUCED BY NEUTROPHILS

Although much less effective in this respect than macrophages or lymphocytes, neutrophils have a limited ability to produce cytokines. Under the influence of bacterial products such as lipopolysaccharides, they can secrete IL-1α, IL-1β, IL-1RA, TNF-α, IL-6, CXCL8 (IL-8), IL-10, and TGF-β. Although they produce only small quantities of these cytokines, neutrophils are present in inflammatory sites in large numbers, so their total contribution may be significant. Chemokines probably also regulate lymphocyte trafficking. Different tissues produce different chemokines, and different lymphocyte populations express different chemokine receptors. T cells express different receptors from B cells; effector cells express different receptors from naive T cells; and Th1 cells express different receptors from Th2 cells. Together these actions regulate the migration and location of these cells within tissues.

CYTOKINES PRODUCED BY MAST CELLS

Mast cells secrete IL-4, IL-5, IL-6, IL-13, IL-16, TNF-α, and the chemokine CCL3. These cytokines either are proinflammatory or promote Th2 responses, or both.

High levels of these cytokines may be found in tissue fluids in allergic reactions.

ANTIVIRAL CYTOKINES

The type I interferons are glycoproteins secreted by virus-infected cells that protect other cells against viral, bacterial, and protozoan invasion. IFN-α is produced in large quantities by lymphoid dendritic cells (DC1) and in much smaller amounts by lymphocytes, monocytes, and macrophages. In cattle IFN-α is encoded for by a multigene family with 10 to 12 members. IFN-β is produced by fibroblasts. Its gene family contains at least five members. IFN-ω is produced by lymphocytes, monocytes, and human, horse, and dog trophoblast cells. IFN-τ is produced by ruminant trophoblast cells, and IFN-δ is produced by pig trophoblast cells. As mentioned previously, IFN-λ has recently been identified. In most cases these molecules probably act on virus-infected cells to inhibit viral growth. The trophoblast interferons also regulate a mother's immune responses to her fetus. The receptor complex for both IFN-α and IFN-β consists of a heterodimer of IFNAR1 and IFNAR2. Signals are transcribed through jak and stat proteins to activate antiviral genes (Figure 12-7).

Interferon-α is a potent stimulator of both innate and adaptive immunity. It is produced in large amounts by plasmacytic dendritic cells. It activates NK cell-mediated cytotoxic activity, and it stimulates the differentiation of monocytes into dendritic cells, as well as the maturation and activity of dendritic cells. INF-α also participates in the transition from innate to acquired immunity and drives certain γ/δ T cell responses. It stimulates memory T cell proliferation, it activates naive T cells, and it enhances antigen specific T cell priming. INF-α also promotes antibody production and alters class switching.

GROWTH FACTORS

Many cytokines control the proliferation and maturation of stem cells in the bone marrow (see Table 12-5). Each of these cytokines is produced by multiple cell types and may affect several different cellular targets.

Interleukin 3

IL-3 is derived from activated Th1 and Th2 cells, NK cells, eosinophils, and mast cells. It stimulates the growth and maturation of bone marrow stem cells for eosinophils, neutrophils, and monocytes. It stimulates mast cell and basophil differentiation and activation, activates eosinophils, promotes macrophage cytotoxicity and phagocytosis, and promotes immunoglobulin secretion by B cells.

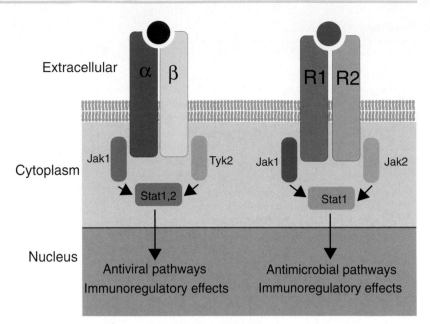

Figure 12-7. The receptors for the two types of interferon. *Left*, Type I IFN receptor. *Right*, INF-γ receptor.

Interleukin 7

IL-7 is produced by bone marrow and thymic stromal cells. It acts on thymocytes, T cells, B cells, monocytes and lymphoid stem cells. It regulates the activity of lymphoid stem cells. Its major role, however, is to control lymphocyte function by regulating V(D)J recombination in both B and T cells (Chapter 14). IL-7 is necessary for lymphocytes to produce functioning antigen receptors.

Interleukin 11

Bone marrow stromal cells, epithelial cells, and fibroblasts produce IL-11, which stimulates B cell growth in association with IL-6. IL-11 also stimulates megakaryocyte colony formation in association with IL-3 and promotes the production of acute-phase proteins. Its physiologic role is unknown.

Interleukin 14

IL-14 is produced by T cells and some malignant B cells. It inhibits immunoglobulin secretion and selectively expands some B cell subpopulations.

Interleukin 15

IL-15 is derived from activated macrophages, dendritic cells, endothelial cells, and fibroblasts. It shares many biological activities with IL-2 because the β and γ peptides of the IL-15 receptor are shared by the IL-2 receptor. IL-15 acts as a T cell, B cell, and NK cell growth factor. It induces the expression of chemokines and their receptors on T cells. It enhances proliferation of both cytotoxic and helper T cells and recruits neutrophils, NK cells, and lymphocytes to sites of inflammation. IL-15 is essential for the prolonged survival of memory cells.

Granulocyte Colony-Stimulating Factor

G-CSF is produced by macrophages, endothelial cells, and fibroblasts and regulates the maturation of granulocyte progenitors into mature neutrophils. The term *colony-stimulating factor* refers to its ability to promote the growth of bone marrow stem cell "colonies" in tissue culture.

Macrophage Colony-Stimulating Factors

M-CSF includes two glycoproteins from lymphocytes, macrophages, fibroblasts, epithelial cells, and endothelial cells. These act on monocyte progenitors to induce their proliferation and differentiation and promote macrophage cytotoxicity.

Granulocyte-Macrophage Colony-Stimulating Factor

GM-CSF is derived from T cells, macrophages, fibroblasts, and endothelial cells. It is the major regulator of granulocyte and macrophage stem cells. It induces phagocytosis, superoxide production, and ADCC by neutrophils. It acts on eosinophils to enhance superoxide production and leukotriene C_4 synthesis. GM-CSF activates macrophages, enhancing superoxide production, phagocytosis, cytotoxic activity, and the expression of MHC class II molecules.

The Transforming Growth Factor β Family

TGF-βs are a family of five glycoproteins, three of which (TGF-β1, TGF-β2, and TGF-β3) are found in mammals, whereas two others (TGF-β4 and TGF-β5) have been described in chickens and *Xenopus* toads. They are secreted as an inactive or latent molecule and subsequently activated. They are produced by platelets, activated macrophages, neutrophils, B cells, and T cells and act on most cell types, including T and B cells, dendritic cells, macrophages, neutrophils, and fibroblasts. The TGF-βs have three fundamental activities: they regulate cell division, they enhance the deposition of extracellular matrix proteins, and most important, they are immunosuppressive.

TGF-β regulates the growth, differentiation, and function of all classes of lymphocytes, dendritic cells, and macrophages. In general, TGF-β inhibits T and B cell proliferation and stimulates their apoptosis, effectively acting as an immunosuppressive molecule. Apoptotic T cells release TGF-β, thus contributing to the suppressive environment. A subset of activated CD4+ T cells can act as regulatory cells by secreting large amounts of TGF-β. These have been called Th3 cells and probably play an important role in some forms of tolerance. TGF-β influences the differentiation of Th subsets. It tends to promote Th1 responses and the production of IL-2 in naive T cells, but it also antagonize the effects of IFN-γ and IL-12 on memory cells.

TGF-β is required for optimal dendritic cell development and regulates the interaction between follicular dendritic cells and B cells. It also controls the development and differentiation of B cells, inhibiting their proliferation and inducing apoptosis. It also regulates the switching of B cells to IgA production.

TGF-β is produced by macrophages and regulates their activities. It can be either inhibitory or stimulatory, depending on the presence of other cytokines. Thus it can activate integrin expression, as well as phagocytosis by blood monocytes. On the other hand, it suppresses the respiratory burst and nitric oxide production by phagocytic cells. It blocks monocyte differentiation and the cytotoxic effects of activated macrophages. Some protozoan parasites such as *Trypanosoma cruzi* and *Leishmania* can induce infected cells to secrete TGF-β and so evade intracellular killing.

VIRAL CYTOKINES

Some viruses can produce proteins that are closely related to, or may affect, mammalian cytokines. These are called virokines. Many of the virokines tend to be suppressive molecules that inhibit antiviral immune responses. For example, vaccinia and cowpox viruses make an IL-1β–binding protein. Cowpox virus also inhibits the IL-1β convertase required for the production of active IL-1β. Both these mechanisms can effectively reduce the amount of IL-1β available to promote an immune response. The human herpesvirus, Epstein-Barr virus, makes a protein closely related to IL-10 called vIL-10. Since IL-10 is an inhibitory cytokine, this effectively reduces the T cell–mediated response to this virus. Another example is the production of a protein related to

the IFN-γR by myxoma and pox viruses. Presumably, by binding IFN-γ, this prevents the interferon from binding to cell receptors and inhibiting viral replication.

SOURCES OF ADDITIONAL INFORMATION

Aggarwal S, Gurney AL: IL-17: prototype member of an emerging cytokine family, *J Leukoc Biol* 71:1-8, 2002.

Casatella MA: The production of cytokines by polymorphonuclear neutrophils, *Immunol Today* 16:21-27, 1995.

Dinarello CA: IL-18: a Th1-inducing, proinflammatory cytokine and a new member of the IL-1 family, *J Allergy Clin Immunol* 103:11-24, 1999.

Febbraio MA, Pedersen BK: Muscle-derived interleukin-6: mechanisms for activation and possible biological roles, *FASEB J* 16:1335-1247, 2002.

Fickenscher H, Hor S, Kupers H, et al: The interleukin-10 family of cytokines, *Trends in Immunol* 23:89-96, 2002.

Fort MM, Cheung J, Yen D, et al: IL-25 induces IL-4, IL-5, and IL-13 and Th2-associated pathologies in vivo, *Immunity* 15:985-995, 2001.

Frisbee DD, Ghivizzani SC, Robbins PD, et al: Treatment of experimental equine osteoarthritis by in vivo delivery of the equine interleukin-1 receptor antagonist gene, *Gene Ther* 9:12-20, 2002.

Heaney ML, Golde DW: Soluble cytokine receptors, *Blood* 87:847-857, 1996.

Hurst S, Muchamuel T, Gorman D, et al: New IL-17 family members promote Th1 or Th2 responses in the lung: in vivo function of the novel cytokine IL-25, *J Immunol* 169:443-453, 2002.

Lankford CSR, Frucht DM: A unique role for IL-23 in promoting cellular immunity, *J Leukoc Biol* 73:49-56, 2003.

Liao Y, Liang W, Chen F, et al: IL-19 induces production of IL-6 and TNF-α and results in cell apoptosis through TNF-α, *J Immunol* 169:4288-4297, 2002.

Metcalf D: The hemopoietic regulators—an embarrassment of riches, Bioessays 14:799-805, 1992.

Myers MJ, Murtaugh MP, eds: *Cytokines in animal health and disease*, New York, 1995, Marcel Dekker.

Nardelli B, Zaritskaya L, Semenuk M, et al: Regulatory effects of IFN-kappa, a novel type I IFN, on cytokine production by cells of the innate immune system, *J Immunol* 169:4822-4830, 2002.

Okano F, Satoh M, Ido T, Yamada K: Cloning of cDNA for canine interleukin-18 and canine interleukin-1β converting enzyme and expression of canine interleukin-18, *J Interferon Cytokine Res* 19:27-32, 1999.

Ozaki K, Spolski R, Feng C, et al: A critical role for IL-21 in regulating immunoglobulin production, *Science* 298:1630-1631, 2002.

Parham C, Chirica M, Timans J, et al: A receptor for the heterodimeric cytokine IL-23 is composed of IL-12β1 and a novel cytokine receptor subunit, IL-23R, *J Immunol* 168:5699-5708, 2002.

Parrish-Novak J, Foster DC, Holly RD, Clegg CH: Interleukin-21 and the IL-21 receptor: novel effectors of NK and T cell responses, *J Leukoc Biol* 72:856-863, 2002.

Pflanz S, Timans JC, Cheung J, et. al: IL-27, a heterodimeric cytokine composed of EB13 and p28 protein, induces proliferation of naive CD4+ T cells, *Immunity* 16:779-790, 2002.

Scheerlink J-P, Chaplin PJ, Wood PR: Ovine cytokines and their role in the immune response, *Vet Res* 29:369-383, 1998.

Sheppard P, Kindsvogel W, Xu W, et al: IL-28, IL-29, and their class II cytokine receptor IL-28R, *Nature Immunol* 4:63-68, 2002.

Starnes T, Broxmeyer H, Robertson J, Hromas R: IL-17D, a novel member of the IL-17 family, stimulates cytokine production and inhibits hemopoiesis, *J Immunol* 169: 642-646, 2002.

Strengell M, Sareneva T, Foster D, et al: IL-21 up-regulates the expression of genes associated with innate immunity and Th1 response, *J Immunol* 169:3600-3605, 2002.

Vilcek J: Novel interferons, *Nature Immunol* 4:8-9, 2003.

Wolf SF, Sieburth D, Sypek J: Interleukin 12: a key modulator of immune function, *Stem Cells* 12:154-168, 1994.

Wolk K, Kunz S, Asadullah K, Sabat R: Immune cells as sources and targets of the IL-10 family members, *J Immunol* 168: 5397-5402, 2002.

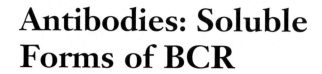

Antibodies: Soluble Forms of BCR

CHAPTER 13

Some of the properties of the B cell antigen receptors (BCRs) were discussed in Chapter 11. These receptors are, of course, not restricted to the B cell surface. Once a B cell response is triggered, the receptors are shed into the surrounding fluid, where they act as antibodies. These antibodies bind to specific antigens and hasten their destruction or elimination. Antibodies are found in many body fluids but are present in highest concentrations and are most easily obtained from blood serum. Antibodies have to defend an animal against a variety of microbes, including bacteria, viruses, and protozoa. They also must act in several different environments, for example, in blood, milk, and body surfaces. It is not surprising, therefore, that several different immunoglobulin classes exist. Each class is optimized for action in a specific environment; for instance, IgA protects body surfaces. Immunoglobulins may also be optimized for activity against a specific group of pathogens. For example, IgE is especially effective against parasitic worms.

IMMUNOGLOBULINS

Antibody molecules are glycoproteins called immunoglobulins (abbreviated as Ig). The term *immunoglobulin* is used to describe all soluble BCRs. There are five different classes (or isotypes) of immunoglobulins, which differ in their use of heavy chains. The class found in highest concentrations in serum is called immunoglobulin G

(abbreviated IgG). The class with the second highest serum concentration (in most mammals) is immunoglobulin M (IgM). The third highest concentration in most mammals is immunoglobulin A (IgA). IgA is, however, the predominant immunoglobulin in secretions such as saliva, milk, or intestinal fluid. Immunoglobulin D (IgD) is primarily a BCR and so is rarely encountered in body fluids. Immunoglobulin E (IgE) is found in very low concentrations in serum and mediates allergic reactions. The characteristics of each of these classes are shown in Table 13-1.

When serum is subjected to electrophoresis, its proteins separate into four major fractions (Figure 13-1). The most negatively charged fraction consists of a single, but homogeneous protein called serum albumin. The other three major fractions contain protein mixtures classified as α, β, and γ globulins, according to their electrophoretic mobility (Figure 13-2). Most immunoglobulins are found in the γ globulins, although IgM migrates among the β globulins.

IMMUNOGLOBULIN CLASSES

Immunoglobulin G

IgG is made and secreted by plasma cells in the spleen, lymph nodes, and bone marrow. It is the immunoglobulin found in highest concentration in the blood

TABLE 13-1
Major Immunoglobulin Classes in the Domestic Mammals

Property	Immunoglobulin Class				
	IgM	IgG	IgA	IgE	IgD
Molecular weight	900,000	180,000	360,000	200,000	180,000
Subunits	5	1	2	1	1
Heavy chain	μ	γ	α	ε	δ
Largely synthesized in:	Spleen and lymph nodes	Spleen and lymph nodes	Intestinal and respiratory tracts	Intestinal and respiratory tracts	Spleen and lymph nodes

(Table 13-2) and for this reason plays the major role in antibody-mediated defense mechanisms. It has a molecular weight of 180 kDa and a typical BCR structure with two identical light chains and two identical γ heavy chains (Figure 13-3). The light chains may be of the κ or λ type. Because it is the smallest of the immunoglobulin molecules, IgG can escape from blood vessels more easily than can the others. This is especially important in inflamed tissues, in which an increase in vascular permeability readily permits IgG to participate in the defense of tissues and body surfaces. IgG binds to specific antigens such as those found on bacterial surfaces. The presence of these antibody molecules on a bacterial surface can cause clumping (agglutination) and lead to opsonization. IgG antibodies can activate the classical complement pathway only when sufficient molecules have accumulated in a correct configuration on the antigenic surface (Chapter 15).

Immunoglobulin M

IgM is also produced by plasma cells in the spleen, lymph nodes, and bone marrow. It occurs in the second highest concentration after IgG in most mammalian serum.

While on the B cell surface and acting as a BCR, IgM is a 180-kda immunoglobulin monomer. However, the secreted form of IgM consists of five (occasionally six) 180 kDa subunits linked by disulfide bonds in a circular fashion. Its total molecular weight is then 900 kDa (Figure 13-4). A small polypeptide called the J chain (15 kDa) joins two of the units to complete the circle.

Each IgM monomer is of conventional immunoglobulin structure and so consists of two λ or two κ light chains and two μ heavy chains; μ chains differ from γ chains in that they have an additional, fourth constant domain (C_H4), as well as an additional 20–amino acid segment on their C terminus but do not contain a hinge region. The complement activation site on IgM is located on the C_H4 domain.

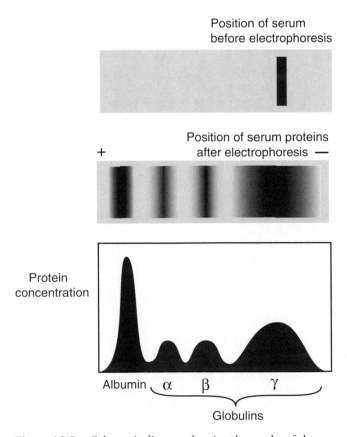

Position of serum before electrophoresis

Position of serum proteins after electrophoresis —

+

Protein concentration

Albumin   α   β   γ

Globulins

Figure 13-2. Schematic diagram showing the results of electrophoresis of whole serum.

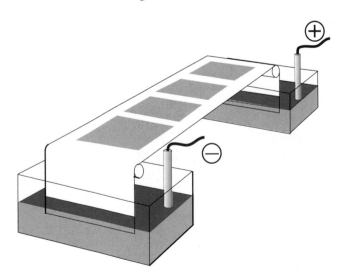

Figure 13-1. The electrophoresis of a protein mixture on a strip of paper or other support. The support bridges two buffer baths, and an electrical potential is applied across them.

TABLE   **13-2**
Serum Immunoglobulin Levels in the Domestic Animals and Humans

Species	Immunoglobulin Levels (mg/dl)			
	IgG	IgM	IgA	IgE
Horse	1000-1500	100-200	60-350	8.4±9.09
Cattle*	1700-2700	250-400	10-50	
Sheep	1700-2000	150-250	10-50	
Pig	1700-2900	100-500	50-500	
Dog	1000-2000	70-270	20-150	2.3-4.2
Cat†	400-2000	30-150	30-150	
Chicken	300-700	120-250	30-60	
Human	800-1600	50-200	150-400	0.002-0.05

*Cattle show significant seasonal differences in serum immunoglobulin levels.

†Immunoglobulin levels in SPF cats are approximately half those in pet cats.

IgM is the major immunoglobulin produced during a primary immune response (Figure 13-5). It is also produced in a secondary response, but this tends to be masked by the predominance of IgG. Although produced in small amounts, IgM is considerably more efficient (on a molar basis) than IgG at complement activation, opsonization, neutralization of viruses, and agglutination. Because of their very large size, IgM molecules rarely enter tissue fluids even at sites of acute inflammation.

Immunoglobulin A

IgA is secreted by plasma cells located under body surfaces. Thus it is made in the walls of the intestine, respiratory tract, urinary system, skin, and mammary gland. Its serum concentration in most mammals is usually lower than that of IgM. IgA monomers have a molecular weight of 150 kDa, but they are normally secreted as dimers. Each IgA monomer consists of two light chains and two α heavy chains containing three constant domains. In dimeric IgA, the molecules are joined by a J chain (Figure 13-6). Higher polymers of IgA are occasionally found in serum.

IgA produced in body surfaces passes through epithelial cells into external secretions. For example, most of the IgA made in the intestinal wall is carried into the intestinal fluid. This IgA is transported through intestinal

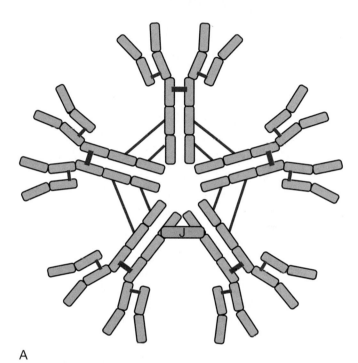

A

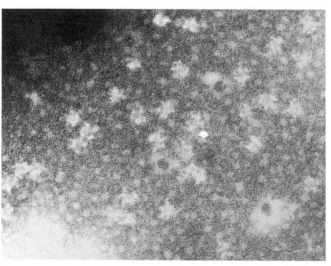

B

Figure 13-4.   The structure of IgM and an electron micrograph of this immunoglobulin from bovine serum (×240,000). Note that some of the molecules are five-pointed and others are six-pointed stars.(Courtesy of Drs K Neilsen and B Stemshorn.)

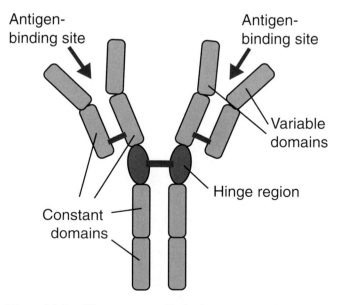

Figure 13-3.   The structure of IgG, the prototypical immunoglobulin molecule. Compare this with Figure 11-6, a typical BCR.

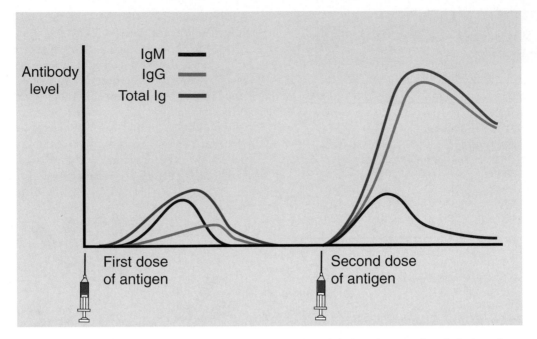

Figure 13-5. The relative amounts of each immunoglobulin class produced during the primary and secondary immune responses. Note that IgM predominates in a primary immune response, whereas IgG predominates in a later response.

epithelial cells bound to a protein of 71 kDa called the polymeric immunoglobulin receptor (pIgR) or secretory component. Secretory component binds IgA dimers to form a complex molecule called secretory IgA (SIgA). It protects the IgA from digestion by intestinal proteases.

Secretory IgA is the major immunoglobulin in the external secretions of nonruminants. As such, it is of critical importance in protecting the intestinal, respiratory, and urogenital tracts, the mammary gland, and the eyes against microbial invasion. IgA does not activate the classical complement pathway, nor can it act as an opsonin. It can, however, agglutinate particulate antigens and neutralize viruses. IgA prevents the adherence of invading microbes to body surfaces. IgA is also unique in that it can act inside cells. Because of its importance, IgA is examined in more detail in Chapter 20.

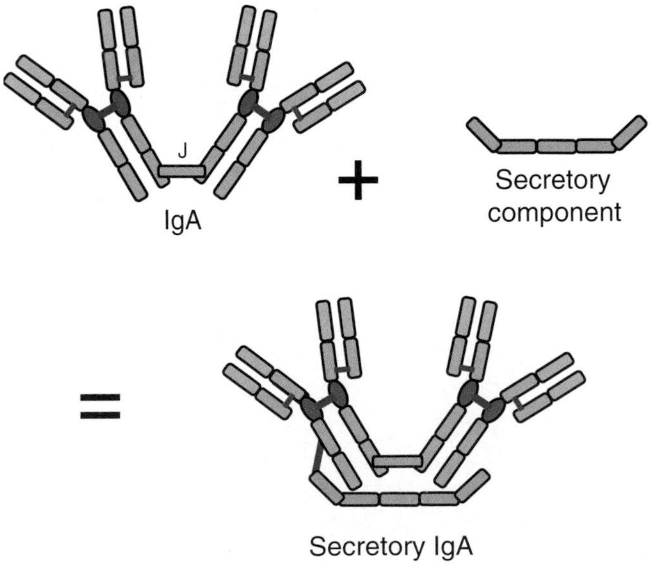

Immunoglobulin E

IgE, like IgA, is made by plasma cells located beneath body surfaces. It is a typical Y-shaped, four-chain immunoglobulin with four constant domains in its ε heavy chains and a molecular weight of 190 kDa (Figure 13-7). IgE

Figure 13-6. The structure of IgA and secretory IgA. Secretory component consists of five linked immunoglobulin domains. It is found on the surface of certain epithelial cells, where it acts as a receptor for polymeric immunoglobulins (pIgR). It can also bind to IgM.

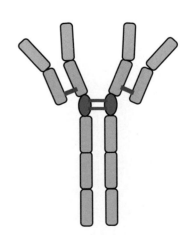

Figure 13-7. The structure of IgE. Note the presence of four constant domains in addition to a hinge in the heavy chain.

is, however, present in extremely low concentrations in serum. Because of this, it cannot act simply by binding and coating antigens, as the other immunoglobulins do. IgE triggers acute inflammation by acting as a signal transducing molecule. Thus IgE molecules bind tightly to receptors (FcεRI) on mast cells and basophils. When antigen binds to this IgE, it triggers the rapid release of inflammatory molecules from the mast cells. The resulting acute inflammation enhances local defenses and helps eliminate the invader. IgE mediates Type I hypersensitivity reactions and is largely responsible for immunity to parasitic worms. IgE has the shortest half-life of all immunoglobulins (2 to 3 days) and is readily destroyed by mild heat treatment. IgE is described in more detail in Chapter 26.

Immunoglobulin D

IgD is unique among the major immunoglobulin classes in that it has not been detected in all mammals. It has been found in primates, rodents, cattle, sheep, and pigs and is probably present in dogs. It has not been detected in horses or rabbits. It has been identified in certain fish (catfish, salmon, and cod) but has not been found in chickens. IgD is a BCR mainly found attached to B cells. Very little of this IgD is secreted into the blood. IgD molecules consist of two δ heavy chains and two light chains. Mouse IgD lacks a Cδ2 domain and thus has only two constant domains in its heavy chains. It has a molecular weight of about 170 kDa (Figure 13-8). Human, cow, sheep, and pig IgD, in contrast, have three heavy chain constant domains and a hinge region. In cattle, sheep and pigs, the Cδ1 domain is almost identical to the Cμ1 domain of IgM, whereas the other constant domains are distinctly different. In mice, the two constant region domains (Cδ1 and Cδ3) are separated by a very long exposed hinge region. Because of this long hinge region and the fact that it has no interchain disulfide bonds, IgD is unusually susceptible to destruction by proteases. Since proteases are generated when the blood clots, IgD is not found in serum but may be detected in plasma. Like IgE, IgD is destroyed by mild heat treatment.

THREE-DIMENSIONAL STRUCTURE OF IMMUNOGLOBULINS

Like other proteins, immunoglobulin peptide chains fold in a very complex manner. Thus an IgG molecule consists of three globular regions (two Fab regions and one Fc region) linked by a flexible hinge (Figure 13-9). Each of these globular regions is made up of paired domains. Thus, the Fab regions each consist of two interacting domains (V_H-V_L and C_H1-C_L), while the Fc region contains either two or three paired domains, depending on the immunoglobulin class (i.e., C_H2-C_H2, C_H3-C_H3, and in IgE or IgM, C_H4-C_H4). The peptide chains within each domain are closely intertwined. In the Fab globular regions a groove is located between the two variable-domains, V_H and V_L. The amino acids of the CDRs line this groove, and as a result, the surface of the groove has a highly variable shape. This groove forms the antigen-binding site. The CDRs from both light and heavy chains contribute to the binding of an antigen, although the heavy chain usually contributes most to the process. Because immunoglobulins are bilaterally identical, the CDRs on each of the Fab regions are also identical. Thus, the molecule has two identical antigen-binding sites and binds two identical epitopes.

The presence of a hinge region in the middle of their heavy chains gives immunoglobulins such as IgG great flexibility. Since the two antigen-binding sites on each Fab region are identical, immunoglobulins are able to cross-link two antigens at the same time. Thus bacteria may be clumped together by antibody molecules in a process called agglutination. If sufficient soluble protein molecules or viruses are cross-linked by antibody, they may precipitate out of solution.

IMMUNOGLOBULIN VARIANTS

Subclasses

All immunoglobulin molecules are made of two heavy and two light chains. Several different heavy chains are

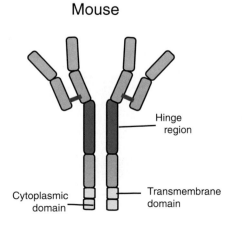

Mouse

Hinge region

Cytoplasmic domain

Transmembrane domain

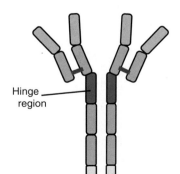

Other mammals

Hinge region

Figure 13-8. The structure of IgD in mice and other mammals. Note the long exposed hinge region in mouse IgD that makes this molecule very unstable.

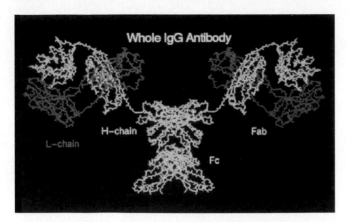

Figure 13-9. A computer-generated molecular model of IgG. It is instructive to compare this with the diagrams of IgG structure seen earlier in Figure 13-3. (Courtesy of Dr. S Linthicum.)

employed in making these molecules. Thus when γ chains are used, the resulting immunoglobulin is IgG. IgM contains μ chains, IgA contains α chains and so on. However, closer examination shows that these immunoglobulin classes consist of a mixture of molecules with structurally different heavy chains known as subclasses.

Immunoglobulin subclasses have arisen as a result of gene duplication. Thus during the course of evolution, heavy chain (*IGH*) genes have been duplicated and the new gene then gradually changed through mutation. The amino acid sequences coded by these new genes may differ from the original in only minor respects. For example, bovine IgG is a mixture of three subclasses—IgG1, IgG2, and IgG3, coded for by the genes *IGHG1, IGHG2,* and *IGHG3*, respectively. They differ in amino acid sequence and in physical properties such as electrophoretic

mobility. These immunoglobulin subclasses may also have different biological activities; for example, bovine IgG2 agglutinates antigenic particles, whereas IgG1 does not. All animals of a species will possess all these subclasses.

The number and properties of immunoglobulin subclasses vary greatly among species. For example, whereas most mammals have only one or two IgA subclasses, rabbits have as many as 13. These variations among species are probably not of major biological significance; they simply reflect the number of immunoglobulin gene duplications a species has undergone.

Allotypes

In addition to subclass differences, individual animals show inherited variations in immunoglobulin amino acid sequences. Thus the immunoglobulins of one individual may differ from those of another individual of the same species (Figure 13-10). These inherited sequence variations in heavy chain genes are called allotypes. Homozygous individuals have the same allotypes on all immunoglobulins in a class. In heterozygous individuals, half of their immunoglobulin molecules will be of one allotype and half will be the other.

Idiotypes

The third group of structural variants found in immunoglobulins results from the variations in the amino acid sequences within the variable domains on light and heavy chains. These variants are called idiotopes. The collection of idiotopes on an immunoglobulin is called its idiotype. Some idiotopes may be located within the antigen-binding site. Others are located on nonantigen binding areas of the V domain.

All cattle possess a complete set of classes and subclasses (ISOTYPES)

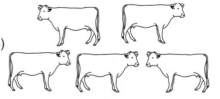

Figure 13-10. A schematic diagram showing the differences among the inheritance of the major immunoglobulin variants.

Within a population individual cattle possess different ALLOTYPES. For example, some possess IgG2(A1), others possess IgG2(A2)

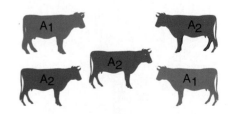

Each individual animal has a very large number of different IDIOTYPES

PRODUCTION OF IMMUNOGLOBULIN HEAVY CHAINS

Each immunoglobulin class has its own characteristic heavy chain. Each heavy chain is coded for by two different genes. One gene codes for the variable domain (and thus the antigen-binding site), whereas a different gene codes for the constant domains. The way in which genes can code for the variable domains is discussed in Chapter 14. The genes that code for the constant region of immunoglobulin heavy chains (*IGH* genes) each consist of several exons (expressed sequences). One exon codes for each constant domain, and one codes for the hinge region (Figure 13-11). A complete IgM constant region gene (*IGHM*) therefore consists of five exons, whereas an IgA constant region gene (*IGHA*) contains four exons. All the heavy chain constant region genes are located together on one chromosome. They are generally arranged in the order *5'-IGHV-IGHM-IGHD-IGHG-IGHE-IGHA-3'*. Thus all the genes for μ chains are followed by the genes for δ chains, which are in turn followed by the γ chain genes and so on.

During their life span, B cells undergo two entirely different DNA recombination events. The first, called V(D)J recombination, creates the genes that code for the antigen binding site of the B cells as they develop within the bone marrow in the absence of antigens. Later in life when the B cells are activated by antigens, a second DNA recombination event occurs. This second event changes genes and hence the class of antibody produced by a B cell. This class switch recombination does not affect the antigen-binding specificity of a cell but results in the expression of a different heavy chain constant region.

Class Switch Recombination

During the course of an antibody response, the class of an immunoglobulin changes, although its antigen-binding ability does not. This "class switch" can be explained by the way in which heavy chain genes are constructed and used.

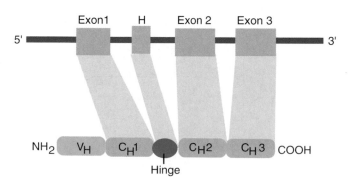

Figure 13-11. A peptide chain such as an immunoglobulin heavy chain is coded for by a series of exons separated by intervening sequences or introns. Usually each exon codes for a single domain.

During an antibody response, the immunoglobulin classes are synthesized in a standard sequence. Thus, a B cell first uses the *IGHM* genes to make IgM BCRs. The remaining genes located 3' to *IGHM* are ignored. In species that make IgD, the B cell also transcribes the *IGHD* genes and then expresses both IgM and IgD. Eventually, however, as the immune response progresses, a responding B cell switches to using *IGHG*, *IGHA*, or *IGHE* genes and becomes committed to synthesizing BCRs and immunoglobulins of one of the other major classes—namely, IgG, IgA, or IgE. The unwanted, unused IGH genes are excised as a DNA circle and lost from the cell while the required IGH gene is spliced directly to the IGHV genes.

For example, if IgM is to be synthesized, the IGHV genes are spliced directly to the IGHM genes (Figure 13-12). On the other hand, if IgA is to be synthesized, the genes coding for Cμ to Cε inclusive are deleted and the IGHV genes are then spliced directly to the IGHA genes. There are several ways by which the intervening genes can be excised. The simplest is called looping out–deletion. In this case the V region and C gene segments come together by looping out and then excising the intervening DNA using an enzyme called a recombinase. Two signals are needed to initiate class switching in a B cell. First, the B cell must receive an activation signal.

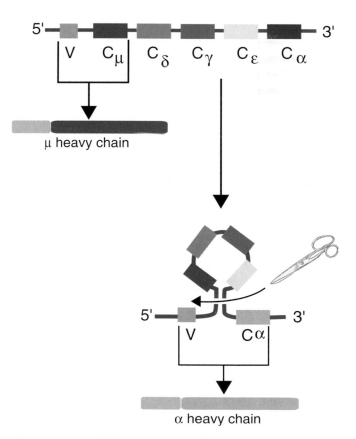

Figure 13-12. The mechanism of class switching. In this example a switch is made from IgM production to IgA production.

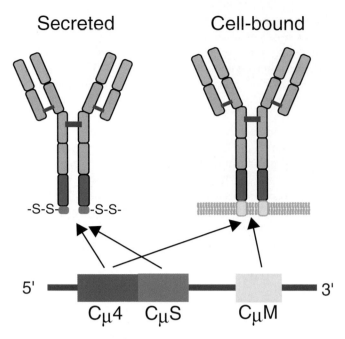

Secreted **Cell-bound**

-S-S- -S-S-

5' 3'

Cμ4 CμS CμM

Figure 13-13. Immunoglobulins serving as BCRs have a hydrophobic transmembrane C-terminus. In contrast, the secreted form lacks this sequence. The difference between the two forms is determined by RNA splicing following transcription.

This comes from cross-linking CD40 on the B cell surface with CD154 on a helper T cell. Second, the specific class switch must be determined. This choice is regulated by cytokines, especially by IL-4, TGF-β and IFN-γ. Signals from the CD40 and antigen activate the recombinase in the B cell while the cytokines, by activating specific promoter regions, target the recombinase to a specific site on a gene.

BCRs and Soluble Immunoglobulins

Immunoglobulins can exist either as BCRs or as secreted antibodies. The heavy chain of a BCR contains a hydrophobic transmembrane C-terminal domain that attaches it to a B cell. This domain is absent from the secreted antibody. The switch between the two forms depends on the differential splicing of exons. For example, in the *IGHM* gene, there are two short exons, CμS and CμM located 3′ to Cμ4 (Figure 13-13). CμS codes for the C-terminal domain of the secreted form, whereas CμM codes for the hydrophobic domain of the cell-bound form. When IgM is made, all the Cμ exons are first transcribed to mRNA. To produce cell-bound IgM, the mRNA is then cleaved so that the CμS exon is deleted and the Cμ4 exon is spliced directly to the CμM exon. To produce secreted IgM, the exon coding for the CμM domain is deleted and translation is stopped after Cμ4 and CμS are read.

IMMUNOGLOBULINS OF DOMESTIC MAMMALS

All mammals possess genes for and express four or five major immunoglobulin classes (IgG, IgM, IgA, IgE, IgD), although these may not have been formally identified in all species (Table 13-3). The basic characteristics of each of these classes are as described previously. However, during the course of evolution, as pointed out above, the immunoglobulin heavy chain (*IGH*) genes have duplicated, sometimes several times. These duplicated genes can then mutate so that mammals may produce several different subclasses of a specific immunoglobulin. If a duplicated gene mutates in such a way that it is no longer functional, then it becomes a pseudogene. The number of duplications and hence the number of immunoglobulin subclasses and pseudogenes varies greatly among species. In looking at these species differences, the reader might gain additional insight by examining the phylogeny of domestic animal species (Figures 38-11 and 38-12).

Horses

The horse has six *IGHG* genes, and all six are expressed. Thus there are six IgG subclasses: IgG1 (IgGa), IgG2

TABLE 13-3
Immunoglobulin Classes and Subclasses in Domestic Animals and Humans

	Immunoglobulin Classes				
Species	**IgG**	**IgA**	**IgM**	**IgE**	**IgD**
Horse	G1, G2, G3, G4, G5, G6	A	M	E	?
Cattle	G1, G2, G3	A	M	E	D
Sheep	G1, G2, G3	A1, A2	M	E	D
Pig	G1, G2a, G2b, G3, G4	A	M	E	D
Dog	G1, G2, G3, G4	A	M	E1, E2	D
Cat	G1, G2, G3, (G4?)	(A2?)	M	(E1, E2?)	?
Chimpanzee	G1, G2, G3,	A1, A2	M	E	D
Mouse	G1, G2a, G2b, G3	A1, A2	M	E	D
Human	G1, G2, G3, G4	A1, A2	M	E	D

(IgGc), IgG3 (IgG[T]), IgG4 (IgGb), IgG5, and IgG6 (IgG[B]). (The previously used designation for IgG3—IgG[T]—was originally derived from the observation that this subclass predominates in the serum of horses used for tetanus immune globulin production). IgG3 does not activate guinea pig complement and reacts in a precipitation reaction by a rather characteristic flocculation. Horses also possess and express IgM, IgA, and IgE. Horses have two IgG4 allotypes (IgG4^a and IgG4^b) and four IgE allotypes (IgE$^{1-4}$).

Cattle

Cattle have three *IGHG* genes and thus three subclasses: IgG1, IgG2, and IgG3. IgG1 constitutes about 50% of the serum IgG and is remarkable for being the predominant immunoglobulin in cows' milk rather than IgA. IgG2 levels are highly heritable; thus concentrations vary greatly among cattle. Cattle possess a unique Fc receptor on their macrophages and neutrophils that is structurally unlike any other Fc receptor and binds only IgG2. Since bovine IgG2 has a very small hinge region, this receptor might represent a special adaptation to the structure of this immunoglobulin. Two heavy chain allotypes (a and b) have been identified in all three classes. Allotype B1 is found on light chains of some cattle but is relatively uncommon. IgA, IgM, and IgE also occur in cattle. Cattle have functional *IGHD* genes, and IgD may be expressed on the B cell surface. Cattle are also unique in that they have two *IGHM* genes. One, the *IGHML*-gene, is a pseudogene located on chromosome 9. The functional *IGHM* gene is located on chromosome 21 together with the other heavy chain genes.

Sheep

The immunoglobulin subclasses of sheep are similar to those of cattle with three *IGHG* genes coding for IgG1, IgG2, and IgG3. Some sheep have an IgG1a allotype. An *IGHD* gene has been detected in sheep. They have two IgA subclasses and a single IgE.

Pigs

Pigs have at least five IgG subclasses—named IgG1, IgG2a, IgG2b, IgG3, and IgG4. Whether all deserve to be called subclasses is unclear. For example, IgG2a and IgG2b differ by only three amino acids. However, DNA analysis has indicated that pigs may have 8 to 12 distinct *IGHG* genes. IgG is the predominant serum immunoglobulin accounting for about 85% of the total. IgM accounts for about 12%, and dimeric IgA for about 3% of serum immunoglobulins. Pigs have a single *IGHA* gene that occurs in two codominant allelic variants. One form, *IGHAa*, has a normal hinge region with six amino acids. The other allele, *IGHAb*, has a deletion mutation so that its hinge contains only two

---

> ### BOX 13–1
>
> #### The Curious Case of the Camel
>
> Members of the camel family from both the old and new worlds (camels and llamas) have three IgG subclasses: IgG1, IgG2, and IgG3. IgG1 has a conventional four-chain structure and therefore has a molecular weight of 170 kDa. In contrast, IgG2 and IgG3, which together account for 75% of camel immunoglobulins, are 100-kDa heavy chain dimers that have no light chains! In addition, camel IgG2 heavy chains lack a CH1 domain but compensate for this by having a very long hinge region. Despite lacking light chains, these molecules can still bind to many antigens. A similar truncated molecule has been reported to occur in some sharks.

amino acids. The biological consequences of this are unclear. Swine IgE and IgD have also been identified. Four IgG allotypes and one IgM allotype have been reported (Box 13-1).

Dogs and Cats

Dogs have four *IGHG* genes and hence four IgG subclasses, named IgG1, IgG2, IgG3, and IgG4 in order of abundance. (These were previously called IgG-A, -B, -C, and -D). In addition, dogs have IgA, IgM, and IgE. Preliminary evidence also suggests that they may have two IgE subclasses, IgE1 and IgE2. An IgM allotype has been described in the dog.

Cats have at least three, and possibly four, *IGHG* genes (IgG1, IgG2, IgG3, IgG4), one IgM subclass, and possibly two IgA subclasses (IgA1 and IgA2), as well as two possible IgE subclasses.

Primates

Humans have four *IGHG* genes coding for IgG1 to IgG4. Chimpanzees and rhesus macaques possess three *IGHG* genes coding for IgG1, IgG2, and IgG3. The chimpanzee IgG2 molecule contains epitopes also found on both human IgG2 and IgG4, suggesting that the *IGHG2* and *IGHG4* genes split after humans separated from chimpanzees. Baboons (*Papio cynocephalus*) have four *IGHG* genes but they differ significantly from human IgG in their hinge region. Rhesus macaques may have two IgM subclasses. All the great apes, with the exception of the orangutan, have two IgA subclasses.

Other Species

Rats and mice have four or five functional *IGHG* genes. In contrast, rabbits have only one *IGHG* gene despite having 13 *IGHA* genes, at least 12 of which are functional! The expression of these IgA subclasses varies among different tissues.

SOURCES OF ADDITIONAL INFORMATION

Baldwin CI, Denham DA: Isolation and characterization of three subpopulations of IgG in the common cat (*Felis catus*), *Immunology* 81:155-160, 1994.

Burton DR: Antibody: the flexible adaptor molecule, *Trends Biochim Sci* 15:64-69, 1990.

Butler JE, Brown WR: The immunoglobulins and immunoglobulin genes of swine, *Vet Immunol Immunopathol* 43:5-12, 1994.

Conrath KE, Wernery U, Muyldermans S, Nguyen VK: Emergence and evolution of functional heavy-chain antibodies in *Camelidae*, *Dev Comp Immunol* 27:87-103, 2003.

Foster AP, Duffus WPH, Shaw SE, Gruffydd-Jones TJ: Studies on the isolation and characterization of a reaginic antibody in a cat, *Res Vet Sci* 58:70-74, 1995.

Grant CK: Purification and characterization of feline IgM and IgA isotypes and three subclasses of IgG. In Willett BJ, Jarrett O, eds: *Feline immunology and immunodeficiency*, Oxford, 1995, Oxford University Press.

Hamers-Casterman C, Atarhouch T, Muyldermans S, et al: Naturally occurring antibodies devoid of light chains, *Nature* 363:446-448, 1993.

Kacsovics I, Sun J, Butler JE: Five putative subclasses of swine IgG identified from the cDNA sequence of a single animal, *J Immunol* 153:3565-3574, 1994.

Naessens J, Newson J, Williams DJL, Lutie V: Identification of classes and allotypes of bovine immunoglobulin M with monoclonal antibodies, *Immunology* 63:569-574, 1988.

Overesch G, Wagner B, Radbruch A, and Leibold W: Organization of the equine immunoglobulin constant heavy chain genes II. Equine Cγ genes, *Vet Immunol Immunopathol* 66:273-287, 1998.

Purkerson J, Isakson P: A two-signal model for regulation of immunoglobulin isotype switching, *FASEB J* 6:3245-3252, 1992.

Roe JM, Patel D, Morgan KL: Isolation of porcine IgE and preparation of polyclonal antisera, *Vet Immunol Immunopathol* 37:83-97, 1993.

Tang L, Sampson C, Dreitz MJ, McCall C: Cloning and characterization of cDNAs encoding four different canine immunoglobulin gamma chains. *Vet Immunol Immunopathol* 80:259-270, 2001.

Yang M, Becker AB, Simons ER, Peng Z: Identification of a dog IgD-like molecule by a monoclonal antibody, *Vet Immunol Immunopathol* 47:215-224, 1995.

Zhang G, Young JR, Tregaskes CA, et al: Identification of a novel class of mammalian Fcγ receptor, *J Immunol* 155:1534-1541, 1995.

Zhao Y, Kacskovics I, Pan Q, et al: Artiodactyl IgD: the missing link, *J Immunol* 169:4408-4416, 2002.

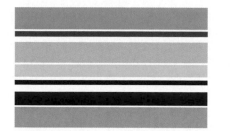

Generation of Antigen-Binding Receptors

CHAPTER 14

One of the central problems encountered in understanding the acquired immune response is how lymphocytes can recognize each of the enormous variety of infectious agents that may invade the body. Given that microorganisms evolve and change rapidly, the immune system must be able to respond not only to existing organisms but also, within reason, to newly evolved organisms. This implies that any animal can produce a huge variety of different B-cell antigen receptors. Any explanation of antibody production must account for this. Similar considerations apply to the T-cell–mediated responses. The ability of the acquired immune responses to respond specifically to an enormous number of foreign antigens implies the existence of an enormous number of different lymphocytes each with its own antigen-specific T-cell receptors (TCRs) or B-cell receptors (BCRs).

The ability of a BCR or TCR to bind an antigen is determined by the shape of its antigen-binding site. The shape of this binding site depends on the folding of its peptide chains, which is governed, in turn, by their amino acid sequence. Each amino acid in a peptide chain exerts an influence on its neighboring amino acids, which determines their relative orientation. The shape of a peptide chain therefore represents the total effect of all amino acids in the chain as the peptide assumes its most energetically favorable conformation. The shape of a protein is determined only by its amino acid sequence, and that sequence is determined by the sequence of bases in the DNA coding for that protein.

The antigen receptors on T and B cells have not evolved to deal with specific microbial antigens; that is the role of innate immunity. On the contrary, the repertoire of TCRs and BCRs is so diverse that at least some of these receptors will bind to any individual antigen.

RECEPTOR–ANTIGEN BINDING

When an antigen and its receptor combine, they interact through the chemical groups on the surface of the antigen and on the complementarity-determining regions (CDRs) of the receptor. In classical chemical reactions, molecules are assembled through the establishment of firm, covalent bonds. These bonds can be broken only by the input of a large amount of energy—energy that is not readily available in the body. In contrast, the formation of noncovalent bonds provides a rapid and reversible way of forming complexes and permits reuse of molecules in a way that covalent bonding would not allow. However, noncovalent bonds act over short intermolecular distances and, as a result, form only when two molecules approach each other very closely. The binding of an antigen to a BCR or TCR is exclusively noncovalent, so the strongest binding occurs when the two components are closely approximated and when the shape of the antigen and the shape of the receptor conform to each other. This requirement for a close conformational fit has been likened to the specificity of a key for its lock.

The major bonds formed between an antigen and its receptor are hydrophobic (Figure 14-1). When antigen and antibody molecules come together, they exclude water molecules from the area of contact. This exclusion frees some water molecules from constraints imposed by the proteins, and is therefore energetically stable. (The bond can be likened to two wet glass microscope slides stuck together. Anyone who has tried to separate wet slides can confirm the effectiveness of this type of bonding.)

A second type of binding between an antigen and its receptor is mediated by hydrogen bonds. When a hydrogen atom covalently bound to one electronegative atom (e.g., an –OH group) approaches another electronegative atom (e.g., an O=C– group), the hydrogen is shared between the two electronegative atoms. This situation is energetically favorable and is called a hydrogen bond. The major hydrogen bonds formed in antigen–receptor interaction are O-H-O, N-H-N, and O-H-N. Hydrogen bonds are normally present between proteins and water molecules in aqueous solution, so the binding of an antigen to its receptor by hydrogen bonds requires relatively little net energy change.

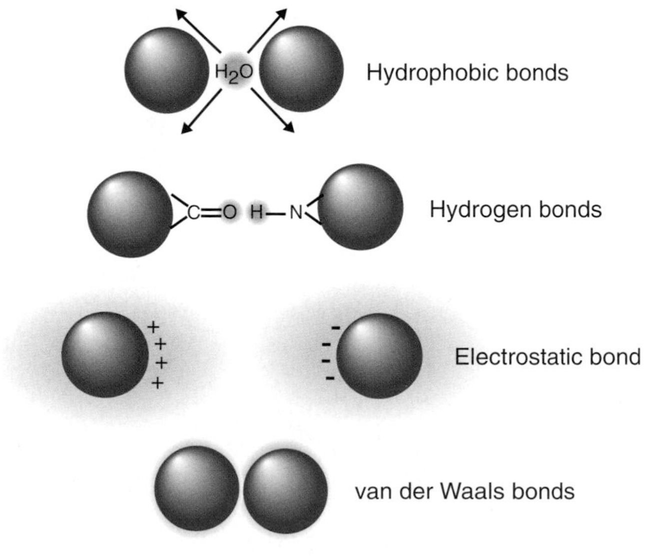

Electrostatic bonds formed between oppositely charged amino acids may contribute to antigen–receptor binding, but the charge on many protein groups is commonly neutralized by electrolytes in solution. As a result, the relative importance of electrostatic bonds is unclear.

When two atoms approach very closely, a nonspecific attractive force, called a van der Waals force, becomes operative. It occurs as a result of a minor asymmetry in the charge of an atom because of the position of its electrons. This force, though very weak, may become collectively important when two large molecules come into contact. It can therefore contribute to antigen–receptor binding.

The binding of a receptor to its antigen is therefore mediated by multiple noncovalent bonds. Each bond is relatively weak in itself but collectively the bonds may have a significant binding strength. All these bonds act only across short distances and weaken rapidly as that distance increases. Electrostatic bond and hydrogen bond strengths are inversely proportional to the square of the distance between the interacting molecules; the van der Waals forces and hydrophobic forces are inversely proportional to the seventh power of that distance. Thus the strongest binding between an antigen and its receptors occurs when their shapes match perfectly and multiple noncovalent bonds form. Nevertheless, antigens can bind to receptors when they fit less than perfectly, although the strength of binding will be reduced.

Figure 14-1. Noncovalent bonds that link an antigen with its receptor arranged in order of relative importance. All these bonds are effective only over a very short distance. It is therefore essential that the shape of the antigen and its receptor site match very well if strong binding is to be achieved.

ANTIGEN RECEPTOR GENES

The information needed to make all proteins, including both immunoglobulins and TCRs, is stored in an animal's genome. Likewise the information needed to make the antigen-binding sites is also encoded in DNA. Thus all that is required for the production of these molecules is that the necessary genes be turned on. Once the appropriate genes are activated, they can be transcribed into RNA and translated into the appropriate receptor protein on B or T cells. It has been estimated that mammals can produce up to 10^{15} different antigen receptors to be expressed on B and T cells but that in order to produce this enormous diversity they use fewer than 500 genes! In B cells this feat is achieved by mechanisms that differ among species. In T cells, in contrast, the generation of antigen receptor diversity is similar in all species examined.

The key to generating receptor diversity lies in that fact that multiple genes are required to code for each receptor peptide chain. Several code for each variable region whereas one codes for the constant region. As a result, a single constant-region gene can be combined with any one of a large number of different variable-region genes to make a complete receptor peptide chain. Thus, instead of having to store information about all possible receptor chains, it is only necessary to store the information (genes) for all the variable domains and to match these, when required, with the appropriate constant-region gene to produce a complete range of receptors. Following this, light and heavy chains may be paired in different combinations, a process called combinatorial association.

IMMUNOGLOBULIN/B-CELL RECEPTOR DIVERSITY

In order to make as many different antibodies as possible, it is necessary to generate great diversity in the amino acid sequence of the variable domains in both light and heavy chains. Since the amino acid sequences are determined by the nucleotide sequences in the genes coding for the variable regions, mechanisms must exist for generating this nucleotide sequence diversity. In practice, antigen receptor diversity is mediated through three distinct mechanisms: gene recombination, somatic mutation, and gene conversion. All three mechanisms alter and diversify germ line genes in such a way that an incredibly diverse array of antigen receptors is generated. The relative importance of each of these mechanisms differs between species. Thus the diversity mechanisms that operate in humans and mice are not the same as those that operate in domestic animals.

GENE RECOMBINATION

The process of gene recombination relies on random selection of one gene from each of several groups of genes followed by combination to generate sequence diversity. It is best explained by examining the genes that code for immunoglobulins.

Three gene clusters code for immunoglobulin peptide chains and each is found on a different chromosome (Figure 14-2). One cluster, called *IGK*, codes for κ light chains; one, called *IGL*, codes for λ light chains; and one, called *IGH*, codes for heavy chains. Each of these three gene clusters contains a large number of genes coding for

variable regions (*V* genes), one or more genes coding for constant regions (*C* genes), and a variable number of small genes called *J* (joining) or *D* (diversity) genes. Antibody diversity arises as a result of randomly combining some of these genes during lymphocyte development.

The IGL Cluster

Each λ light chain is coded for by three genes from the *IGL* cluster. The *IGLV* gene codes for most of the V region up to the amino acid located at position 95 from the N terminus. The *IGLC* gene codes for the C region starting at position 110. The intervening 15 amino acids in the V region are coded for by a short gene called *IGLJ*. In humans each *IGL* cluster consists of about 100 different *IGLV*, six *IGLJ*, and three *IGLC* genes. (The three *IGLC* genes code for three λ chain subtypes). The *IGL* cluster in cattle contains about 20 *IGLV* genes but 14 of these are pseudogenes. These *IGLV* genes are closely spaced, and many of the pseudogenes are fused to *IGLJ* in the germ line suggesting that they are probably not expressed. There is more than one *IGLJ* gene but only one is expressed. There are 90 to 100 *IGLV* genes in sheep but only one *IGLJ* gene.

The IGK Cluster

κ light chains are also coded for by three genes. In the human *IGK* cluster, for example, there are 40 different *IGKV* genes, five different *IGKJ* genes, and a single *IGLC* gene. Horse *IGK* contains up to 30 *IGKV* genes, three *IGKJ* genes, and a single *IGKC* gene.

The IGH Cluster

In humans, the *IGH* cluster contains about 90 different *IGHV* genes. Mouse *IGH* may have as many as 1500 different *IGHV* genes but up to 40% of them may be pseudogenes. The *IGH* cluster also contains several *IGHJ* genes (four in mice, six in humans) situated 3′ to the *IGHV* genes. In addition, several additional short genes, called *IGHD* genes (D for diversity), are located between the *IGHV* and *IGHJ* genes (Figure 14-2). In mice there are about 12 *IGHD* genes, and in humans there are at least 30.

IGK and *IGL* gene clusters

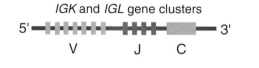

IGH gene cluster

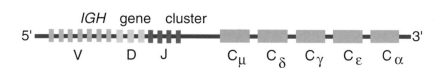

Figure 14-2. Genes coding for immunoglobulin light chains and heavy chains. Note that there are two distinct clusters of light chain genes, one coding for kappa chains and one coding for lambda chains. These are located on different chromosomes. The precise number of V, D, and J genes varies among species.

A large noncoding intron separates the *IGHJ* genes from the *IGHC* genes. The *IGHC* genes consist of a series of constant-region genes, one for each heavy chain class, arranged in the order -Cμ-Cδ-Cγ-Cε-Cα– along the chromosome.

GENERATION OF JUNCTIONAL DIVERSITY

Gene Rearrangement

The most obvious way to generate V-region diversity is to randomly select one V gene from the available pool and join it to one randomly selected J gene —a process called recombination. Since multiple V and J genes are available, the number of possible combinations can be very large. For example, if there are 100 V genes and 10 J genes, then $100 \times 10 = 1000$ different V regions can be constructed.

Light chain assembly requires recombination of one V, one J, and one C gene. During B cell development, they first loop out, excise, and discard the intervening sequences (introns). The V and J genes have special sites at each end that guide the cutting enzymes (Figure 14-3). The looped-out intron is chopped off and the free ends of the DNA are rejoined so that the genes form a continuous sequence that leaves a V gene attached directly to a J gene. Two sets of enzymes are used in this process. Recombinases cut the germ line DNA at two points so excising unwanted gene segments. Following this, DNA repair enzymes join the two free ends to form a continuous sequence. If these enzymes are defective, then antibodies (and TCRs) cannot be made. In foals with severe combined immunodeficiency, for example, there is a defect in the DNA repair enzyme that joins the cut ends. As a result, these foals cannot make either TCR or BCR and so have no functional B or T cells (Chapter 35).

Gene recombination occurs in two stages. Randomly selected V and J genes are first joined to form a complete V-region gene. The joined V-J genes remain separated from the C gene until messenger RNA is generated. The complete V-J-C mRNA is then translated to form a light chain (Figure 14-4).

When a heavy chain V region is assembled, the situation is complicated by the presence of a cluster of D genes between the V and J genes. Thus construction of this V region requires the splicing together of *IGHV*, *IGHD*, and *IGHJ* genes (Figure 14-5). This use of three randomly selected genes enormously increases the amount of variability possible. For example, if one combines genes from a pool of 100 V, 10 J, and 10 D genes, then $100 \times 10 \times 10 = 10,000$ different V regions can be constructed. The joining of these genes also occurs in a specific order. Thus *IGHD* is first joined to *IGHJ* and *IGHV* is added last. After transcription, enzymes delete any remaining introns and the complete V-D-J-C mRNA is translated to form a heavy chain.

Although the random selection of genes from two or three different pools generates a large number of different V-region combinations, not all of these combinations of genes will necessarily provide usable antibodies. Some combinations may result in a nucleotide sequence that cannot be translated into protein. These are called nonproductive rearrangements. For example, nucleotides are read as triplets called codons, each of which codes for a specific amino acid. If the codons are to be read correctly, then the sequence must be in the correct reading frame. If additional bases are inserted or deleted so that the codon reading frame is changed, the resulting gene may code for a totally different amino acid sequence. If this frameshift results in inappropriate splicing, out-of-phase rearrangements are transcribed into full-length mRNA but translation of these is prematurely terminated. It is probable that nonproductive rearrangements are produced two out of three times during B-cell development. When this happens, the B cell has several additional opportunities to produce a functional antibody. For example, in mice, pre-B cells

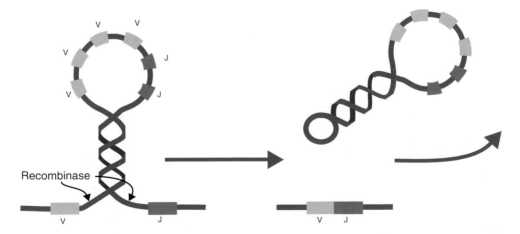

Figure 14-3.   One of the most important mechanisms of deleting unwanted genes is by looping out. In this case, unwanted V genes form a loop that is then cut off and the cut ends joined together. As a result, the desired V gene is linked directly to a J gene.

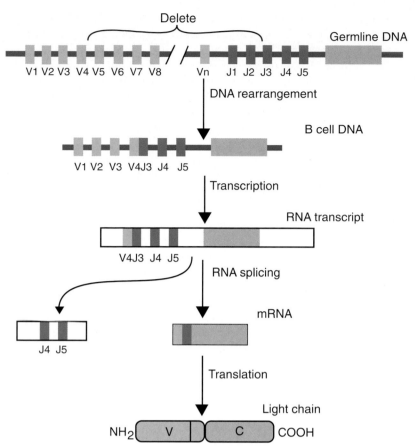

Figure 14-4.   Construction of an immunoglobulin light chain. V and J genes are first joined. The VJ and C genes remain separated until RNA splicing occurs. DNA rearrangement occurs during early B-cell development so that each individual B cell is committed to making a single form of light chain for its antigen receptor.

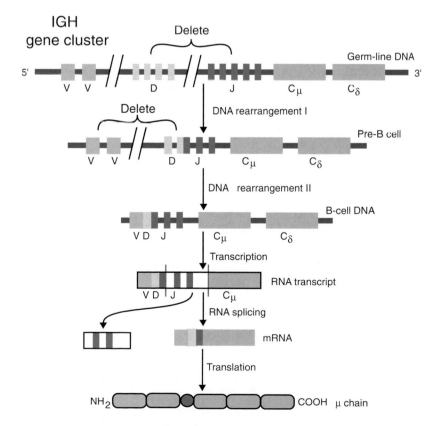

Figure 14-5.   Production of a complete immunoglobulin heavy chain gene. Two DNA rearrangement events are required to link V, D, and J genes together.

initially use one of the *IGK* genes (Figure 14-6). If this fails to produce a functional light chain, they switch to the other *IGK* allele for a second attempt. If this doesn't work, the B cell will use one of the *IGL* alleles, and if this fails, the second *IGL* allele represents the last resort. If all these efforts fail to produce a functional light chain, the B cell cannot make a functional immunoglobulin. This cell cannot be stimulated by antigen and will die without participating in an immune response.

The sequence of events described above has been worked out in mice and humans and may not apply to domestic mammals. One obvious difference lies in the use of κ and λ light chains. In mice, rabbits, pigs, and humans, κ chains are preferentially used (95% in mice, 90% in rabbits, 60% in pigs, 60% in humans). In the other domestic species, λ light chains predominate (98% in ruminants, 60% to 90% in horses). The reasons for these differences are unknown.

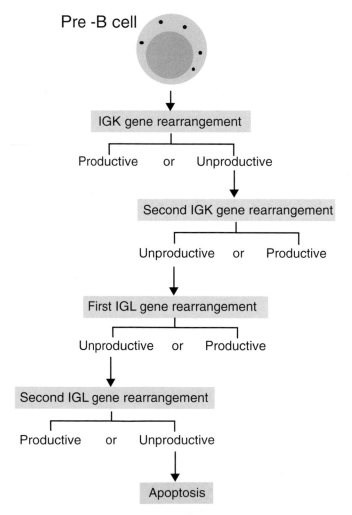

Figure 14-6. The B cell has four attempts to make a functional immunoglobulin. In these attempts it must make not only a functional antibody, but also one that does not bind to "self" antigens (this is known as receptor editing). If it fails in all four attempts, the cell undergoes apoptosis.

Despite the discussion above, it should be pointed out that immunoglobulin gene rearrangement is not entirely random. For example, in rabbits, mice, and humans the most 3′ *IGHV* genes tend to be used most often. This preferential use is the result of a combination of several factors including the recombination signal sequences, the accessibility of the genes to the recombinase enzyme, sequences at the splicing sites, and, of course, cellular selection by antigen.

Base Deletion

Although random recombination of genes generates much V-region diversity, additional mechanisms can increase this diversity still further. For example, endonucleases can remove bases from the cut ends of the genes being spliced together. Thus, the actual nucleotide at which V and J genes join can vary, and changes in the base sequence will occur at the splice site. This, of course, leads to changes in the amino acid sequence in the V region.

Base Insertion

In immunoglobulin heavy chain gene processing, additional bases may be inserted at the V-D and D-J splice sites. Some nucleotides (N nucleotides) are added randomly by an enzyme called terminal deoxynucleotidyltransferase (TdT). TdT adds bases to the exposed 3′ ends of genes. Between one and ten N-nucleotides may be inserted between V and D and between D and J. Alternatively, short palindromic sequences (P-nucleotides) may be inserted at each end of the gap.

Receptor Editing

Although each new B cell expresses a distinct antigen receptor, developing B cells can continue to rearrange their V, D, and J genes even after exposure to antigens. Thus, a B cell expressing a specific κ chain may reinitiate V-gene rearrangement by switching to the other *IGKV* genes or even switching to either of the *IGLV* genes. It can continue to rearrange upstream, non-rearranged V genes or downstream non-rearranged J genes. This receptor editing, which occurs within germinal centers, may be a device to eliminate receptors that bind to self-antigens. Alternatively, this may simply be a device to generate additional diversity in antigen-binding sites.

SOMATIC MUTATION

Although gene recombination can generate many different antigen receptors, antibodies produced early in an immune response can only bind antigens relatively weakly and gene recombination cannot account for all the variability that occurs within immunoglobulin V regions. For example,

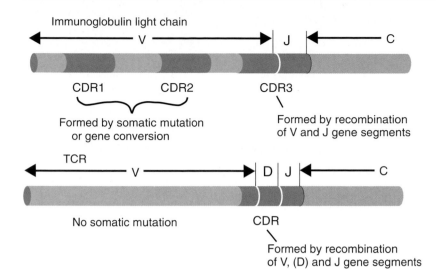

Figure 14-7. The major difference between the variable regions of the T-cell receptor (TCR) and immunoglobulins is in the formation of complementarity-determining regions (CDRs). Immunoglobulins have three CDRs. CDR1 and CDR2 are generated by somatic mutation. CDR2 is generated by gene conversion. This option is not available to the TCR where somatic mutation is stringently avoided.

there are three CDRs within the V regions (Figure 14-7). One of these, CDR3, is found around position 96 and can be readily explained by gene recombination. However, CDR1 and CDR2 are located far from V-J or V-D-J splice sites. Other mechanisms of antibody variability generation must exist (Table 14-1). In fact, gene recombination is only the first step in generating antibody diversity. It must be followed by additional mechanisms that can generate antibodies that bind very strongly and specifically to an antigen. Thus the antibody response must be "fine tuned," and this is driven by somatic mutation.

Following initial exposure to an antigen, B cells form germinal centers. The B cells proliferate in the dark zones of germinal centers and then undergo antigen-driven selection in the light zones. If antibodies are isolated at intervals after immunization and the sequence of their V regions studied, progressive changes are seen as the immune response progresses. These changes are due to mutations within the recombined *IGHV* genes and are examples of somatic mutation.

Somatic mutation is mediated by a B-cell enzyme called cytosine deaminase. It deaminates the cytosines in the DNA coding for V regions and so converts them to uracils. These uracils are seen as mistakes (After all, uracil is not normally found in DNA.), and their presence triggers repair processes. One repair mechanism employs a DNA polymerase that mistakenly reads uracil as

thymine during transcription. Other mechanisms delete the uracils and leave a gap that is repaired by an error-prone DNA polymerase (DNA polymerase iota) using randomly selected nucleotides. Thus, the gaps can be "patched" by short nucleotide sequences. In any case, the result of this "repair" is that V-region gene sequences change randomly as the B cells respond to antigens.

Those B cells whose newly modified BCRs fail to bind an antigen will no longer be stimulated by antigen and so will die. In contrast, those B cells whose modified receptors can bind antigens with a higher affinity will be preferentially stimulated. They will survive and proliferate (Figure 14-8). The better the fit, the greater will be the stimulus to divide. On average, one mutation occurs each time a B cell divides. Thus while responding to an antigen, successive cycles of mutation and selection lead to the generation of populations of B cells producing very-high-affinity antibodies.

When immunoglobulin sequences are analyzed in mice it is found that somatic mutation does not begin until after B cells have switched from making IgM to making either IgG or IgA. This suggests that the mutation mechanism is not activated until after a responding B cell had become committed to utilizing a specific heavy chain V gene. This may explain why the affinity of IgM antibodies does not increase during an immune response whereas the affinity of IgG antibodies does.

TABLE **14-1**
Methods of Generating Antibody Diversity

VJ and VDJ gene recombination
Base deletion
Base insertion
Somatic mutation
Combinatorial association
Gene conversion
Receptor editing

GENE CONVERSION

In species other than the human and mouse, there may be very little diversity among the V genes or there may be very few of them. As a result, gene recombination can generate very little additional diversity. In these species, V-region diversity is generated by a process called gene conversion (Figure 14-9). Species that employ gene conversion have available either multiple V genes or pseudogenes. (Pseudogenes are segments of DNA that

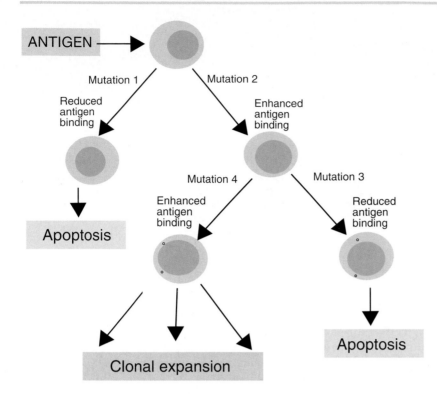

Figure 14-8. Selection of somatic mutants. Spontaneous mutation during the expansion of a B-cell clone results in the development of cells with B-cell receptors that differ in their ability to bind antigen. Cells that bind antigen strongly will be more intensely stimulated than cells that bind it weakly.

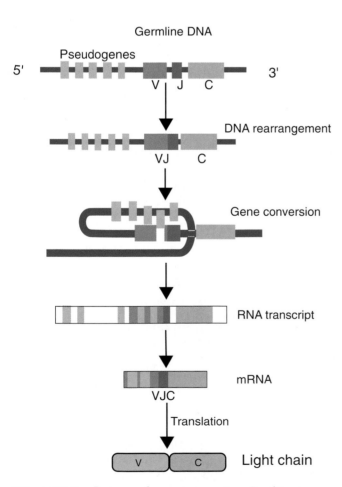

Figure 14-9. Process of gene conversion. In this process, segments of pseudogenes are inserted into a single V region to generate sequence diversity.

cannot be transcribed by conventional means.) During this process a cut is made in the most 3′ V gene (the one nearest the C genes). Once cut, the gap is repaired by insertion of randomly selected short segments from one or more of the upstream V-region genes or pseudogenes. The "repaired" V gene will therefore have a very different sequence than its precursor. Some of these gene conversions will result in an "inactive" V gene that cannot make a functional V region. In these cases, such B cells are eliminated. Active V genes, on the other hand, are transcribed and expressed.

Potential Immunoglobulin Diversity

The processes of gene rearrangement described above can generate V-region diversity and antigenic specificity in several ways. First, as occurs in the case of the human *IGKV* family, only one of a possible 80 V genes is selected for transcription, as is only one of the five *IGKJ* genes. This random joining of segments will provide significant variability since there are 400 (80 × 5) possible *IGKV-IGKJ* combinations. The use of a third randomly selected gene segment will increase sequence diversity still further. Thus with 300 *IGHV*, 5 *IGHD*, and 2 *IGHJ* segments employed, as many as 3000 (300 × 5 × 2) different heavy chain V regions can be generated in humans. Since both heavy and light chains are used to form the antigen-binding site, the total number of possible combinations in humans is 1.2 million (3000 × 400). In addition, the presence of two splice sites multiplies the potential for diversity arising as a result of base deletion and insertion. However, as pointed out above, many of the combinations so formed may be of little functional use.

Taking all possible mechanisms into account, the number of potential combinations and hence binding specificities generated is about 1.8×10^{16} without accounting for somatic mutation. (This figure may be compared with the estimated 1×10^7 different antigens that the immune system can recognize.)

SPECIES DIFFERENCES

Mechanisms of antigen receptor diversity generation tend to fall into two distinct patterns depending on species. Thus, some species rely on gene recombination followed by somatic mutation. In these species, immunoglobulin diversity is continuously generated from B-cell precursors throughout an animal's life. Other species, in contrast, use gene conversion for a short period early in life. After initial B-cell diversity is generated, this pool of B cells expands by a self-renewing mechanism with little somatic mutation.

Humans and Mice

Humans and mice with many *IGHV* genes use multiple gene segment rearrangements to generate much of their antibody diversity (Table 14-2). Additional diversity is generated at junctions by base deletion and insertion. The final layer of diversity is generated in these species by somatic mutation. In these species B cells with diverse antigen receptors are produced throughout an animal's life.

Chickens

The chicken has only a single functional V gene at its heavy and light chain loci, but it does have a large number of V pseudogenes. Thus it relies entirely on gene conversion. Immature precursor B cells first join their V (D) and J segments to form a complete V-region gene. There is no combinatorial diversity and very little junctional diversity involved in this process. The immature B cells then migrate to the bursa of Fabricius in ovo. Here they form follicles and diversify their V-region genes by gene conversion. They remain in the bursa for a few weeks before emigrating to the secondary lymphoid organs. After the bursa degenerates at puberty, the chicken must largely make do with the B-cell diversity generated in early life. However, once a mature chicken B cell is stimulated by exposure to an antigen it can generate additional V-region diversity by further gene conversion. If gene conversion is blocked in a chicken, then somatic mutation can occur. Indeed, species that undertake gene conversion also show limited somatic mutation although the reverse is not true.

Rabbits

Rabbits generate antibody diversity by gene conversion like the chicken, but in this case they do it within their appendix rather than in a bursa. Thus immature rabbit B cells first join their V (D) and J genes and then migrate to the appendix. The V genes are subsequently diversified by gene conversion and somatic mutation within the appendix germinal centers. The presence of a gut flora is necessary for this diversification to occur. Perhaps microbial antigens, endotoxins, or a superantigen from within the intestine are required to provoke antibody diversification and B-cell growth. Rabbits actually have more than 200 *IGHV* genes but almost 90% of V-region rearrangements employ the V gene closest to the D segment. The other V genes presumably serve as donors in the gene conversion process.

Sheep

The pattern of B cell development in the sheep resembles that seen in chickens and rabbits with some important differences. Thus sheep immature B cells first diversify their V (D) and J genes in lymphoid tissues such as the spleen or bone marrow. The immature cells then migrate to follicles within the ileal Peyer's patches where most diversification occurs as a result of somatic mutation (Figure 14-10). The initial diversification step is mediated by a mixture of mechanisms. Thus, sheep light chain genes have more than 90 *IGLV* genes and a single *IGLJ* gene. Many of these V genes have been found in rearranged DNA, suggesting that light chains are diversified through gene recombination. On the other hand, sheep have only a limited number of *IGHV* genes and therefore rely on gene conversion to diversify their heavy chains. They have six *IGHJ* genes, two of which are pseudogenes. One of the active genes, *IGHJ1*, is used in

TABLE **14-2**
Examples of Different Gene Usages in Mammals

Species	IGKV	IGKJ	IGKV × IGKJ	IGLV	IGLJ	IGLV × IGLJ
Human	80	5	400	100	6	600
Mouse	250	5	1250	2	4	8
Sheep	10	3	30	100	1	100

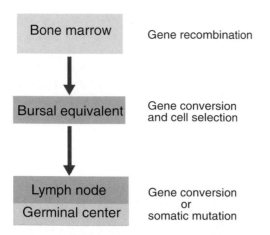

Figure 14-10. Lymphoid organs where gene recombination, gene conversion, and somatic mutation occur.

90% of heavy chains suggesting that gene recombination is minimal. More than 98% of all rearrangement events are in frame, and there are few N- or P- nucleotides. This is in marked contrast to the mouse where more than 60% of all rearrangements are nonproductive despite extensive use of combinatorial rearrangement. Unlike rabbit, human, or mouse, a gut flora or antigenic stimulation is not absolutely necessary for V-gene diversification in sheep.

Cattle

Cattle likely use a two-stage process similar to that seen in sheep. That is, initial diversification occurs in lymphoid organs followed by somatic mutation in ileal Peyer's patches. Cattle may have as few as 10 closely related *IGHV* genes, all of which belong to a single family (Table 14-3). Cattle also have many V pseudogenes. Cattle may have both very long and short *IGHD* genes. As a result, their CDR3 regions are highly variable in size and in extreme cases may contain as many as 61 amino acids.

Pigs

Pigs probably employ the same two step process as cattle and sheep, although the precise details of their light and heavy chain rearrangements differ somewhat. Pigs have a single germ line *IGHJ* gene, two *IGHD* genes, and about 20 *IGHV* genes. At least one of these, *IGHV1*, the most 3′ *IGHV* gene, is a pseudogene. Early in fetal life the pig uses only four or five *IGHV* genes and their early repertoire consists of only 8 to 10 combinations. Later in fetal life this restricted repertoire is compensated for by early TdT activity and extensive, in frame, N-region addition leading to significant junctional diversity. There are, however, differences between lymphoid organs in the frequency of in-frame rearrangements. Pig B cells do not undergo receptor editing because they have only one *IGHJ* gene. As a result, piglets are born with relatively limited B cell receptor diversity. The presence of gut flora significantly assists the development of pig B cells whose numbers increase greatly during the first 2 weeks of age. Receptor diversity may not increase significantly until 4 to 6 weeks of age. Germ-free pigs have serum immunoglobulin levels 20- to 100-fold less than conventional pigs. In addition, conventional pigs exhibit greater diversity in mucosal IgM and IgA V genes (but not splenic IgG V genes) than germ-free pigs. It is believed that the developing B cells require either direct stimulation by bacterial products or stimulation by bacteria-activated antigen-presenting cells in order to fully mature.

T-CELL RECEPTOR DIVERSITY

TCR and immunoglobulin gene rearrangements are specific in that immunoglobulin genes are not rearranged in T cells and TCR genes are not rearranged in B cells. Like immunoglobulins, the four peptide chains, α, β, γ, and δ, that make up the two types of TCR can bind specific antigens. They are able to do this because they each consist of a variable region attached to a constant region.

TABLE 14-3										
Immunoglobulin Diversity Among Mammals										
	C_H genes					CL genes		V_H and V_L families		
Species	**IgM**	**IgD**	**IgG**	**IgE**	**IgA**	λ	κ	**H**	λ	κ
Mouse	1	1	4	1	1	3	1	14	3	4
Human	1	1	4	1	2	7	1	7	7	7
Bovine	2	1	3	1	1	4	1	1	2	?
Sheep	1	1	3	1	2	1?	1?	1	6	3
Rabbit	1	0	1	1	13	8	2	1	?	?
Pig	1	1	8-12	1	1	1?	1?	1	?	?
Horse	1	0	6	1	1	4?	1	7	1	?
Dog	1	1	4	2?	1					

From Butler JE: *Scand J Immunol* 45:455-462, 1997.

The diversity of the TCR V region is generated by gene recombination and combinatorial association in all species examined to date unlike the diverse mechanisms employed by B cells.

T-Cell Receptor Gene Structure

The four T-cell receptor peptide chains are coded for by three gene clusters. The *TRA/D* cluster codes for both α and δ chains, the *TRB* cluster codes for β chains, and the *TRG* cluster codes for γ chains. All three clusters contain V, J, and C genes, and the *TRB* and *TRD* cluster also contain D genes (Figure 14-11). Each TCR cluster contains two or more C genes. In the *TRA/D* cluster the two C genes are functionally and structurally different, so that one codes for *TRAC* and the other for *TRDC*. The number of *TRGC* genes varies among species. Thus there are two different *TRGC* genes in humans, three in mice, four in pigs, and five in cattle and sheep. There are two identical *TRBC* genes in humans and mice. Some helper and cytotoxic T cells rearrange and express *TRA* and *TRB* genes (α/β T cells), whereas others use *TRG* and *TRD* genes (γ/δ T cells). As pointed out in earlier chapters, the relative size and significance of these two T-cell populations vary among species.

α *and* δ *Chains*

The *TRA/D* cluster is unusual in that the *TRD* genes are embedded in the *TRA* cluster. When T cells are immature, they use δ chains for their antigen receptors. As the T cells mature, they switch and begin to use the α chain. To do this, the *TRD* genes are looped out and deleted. Some V genes in the α/δ cluster are bifunctional and can participate in the assembly of both α and δ TCR chains.

The *TRA* cluster contains V, J, and C genes separated into two regions by the embedded *TRD* genes. There are about 100 *TRAV* genes, about 75 *TRAJ* genes, and a single *TRAC* gene in humans. Thus there are many more J genes here than are found in the immunoglobulin gene clusters. The *TRD* cluster contains V, D, J, and C genes. In mice there are about 10 *TRDV* genes, 2 *TRDD* genes, 2 *TRDJ* genes, and 1 *TRDC* gene. Both the *TRDD* genes may contribute to the final product so that a complete Vδ sequence may be coded for by *TRDV*, *TRDD1*, *TRDD2*, and *TRDJ* genes. This arrangement can generate much greater diversity than the other receptor chains. In pigs there are 61 *TRAJ* genes, 31 *TRDV* genes, 3 *TRDD* genes, and 4 *TRDJ* genes. There are 24 *TRDV* genes in sheep and 12 in cattle. Both have 3 *TRDJ* genes but *TRDD* genes have not been described in these species.

β *Chain*

The *TRB* cluster contains a large number of V genes located upstream of two nearly identical D-J-C clusters each containing about six functional J genes. The D genes are all similar in sequence and length and their use is optional. Any of the *TRBV* genes may be joined to either of the two D-J-C genes and the V gene may join to either a D or a J gene. The bovine β cluster appears to have a third constant region. Dogs have about 20 *TRBV* genes, but about one third of these make up 90% of the T-cell repertoire. TCR V-gene usage may in fact be restricted to a single V-gene family in the dog.

γ *Chain*

The *TRG* cluster in humans contains about 50 V genes, 5 J genes, and 2 C genes. Horses also possess 2, mice, pigs, and cattle 4, and sheep 5 *TRGC* genes. There is no *TRGD* gene, so that *TRGV* genes combine directly with *TRGJ* genes.

TRB cluster

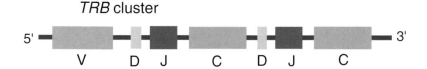

5'　V　　D　J　　C　　D　J　　C　3'

TRA/D cluster

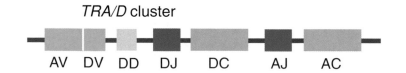

AV　DV　DD　DJ　DC　AJ　AC

Figure 14-11. Basic structure of the three gene clusters that code for the four different T-cell receptor polypeptide chains. The genes for δ chains are embedded within the α-chain genes to form a single cluster.

TRG cluster

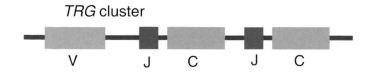

V　　J　C　J　C

Generation of T-Cell Receptor V-Region Diversity

There are three hypervariable regions (CDRs) in each TCR V region. The first two, located within the V genes, have probably arisen through selection of V genes. The third is encoded in the region where V, D, and J genes recombine. The greatest diversity in amino acid sequences seen in the TCR chains is generated by the recombination of multiple V, J, and D genes (Table 14-4). Neither somatic mutation nor gene conversion occurs in the TCR genes. Thus the various genes that are separate in the germ line are brought together by DNA rearrangement, combinatorial association, and base insertion or deletion as T cells differentiate (Figure 14-12).

Gene Rearrangement

TCR α and γ chains use V and J genes to form their V regions. TCR β and δ chains use V, D, and J genes to form their V regions. Mouse δ chains can use both of their D genes and, as a result, V-D-D-J constructs can be formed. In β and δ chains the reading frame of the D genes is commonly changed and can yield productive rearrangements. This is a rare event in immunoglobulins. Looping out and deletion account for more than 75% of TCR rearrangements. The remainder of the rearrangements are due to either unequal sister chromatid exchange or inversion, i.e., moving an inverted segment of gene into a position beside a segment in the opposite orientation. Looping out and deletion of TCR genes are mediated by signals identical to those of immunoglobulins. Thus the same joining enzyme (a recombinase) probably acts on both immunoglobulin and TCR genes.

Base Insertion and Deletion

Although in general TCRs are constructed from fewer V-, D-, and J-region genes than immunoglobulins, their potential diversity is greater as a result of junctional diversity. Thus random bases may be inserted at the V, D, and J junctions as a result of the action of terminal TdT. As many as five nucleotides can be added between V and D and four between D and J genes. Likewise random nucleotides may be removed by the actions of nucleases. This N-region addition and base deletion is much more extensive than that seen in immunoglobulin genes and is probably the most significant component of TCR junctional diversity.

Somatic Mutation

Somatic mutation does not occur in TCR V genes. Although T cells must be able to recognize a foreign

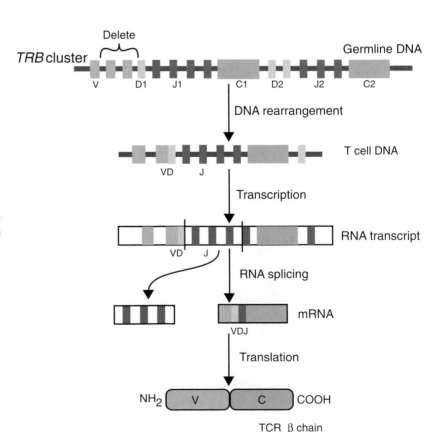

Figure 14-12. The production of a complete T-cell receptor peptide chain. Note the similarities between this and Figure 14-5.

antigen in association with the presenting major histocompatibility complex (MHC) molecule, it is essential that they recognize self-MHC molecules while not responding to self-antigens. If random somatic mutation were to occur, it would carry the unacceptable risk of altering MHC restriction and so rendering the foreign antigen unrecognizable. It might also lead to generation of TCRs capable of binding self-antigens and thus trigger autoimmunity.

Where Does This Happen?

TCR genes are rearranged and expressed in the developing thymus. The developing T cell first attempts to rearrange the genes for γ and δ and, if this is not productive, proceeds to rearrange those for α and β chains. (Alternatively, it has been suggested that γ/δ and α/β belong to two different cell lines and express these receptors independently.) Rearrangement in the *TRD* cluster appears to be the earliest event in T-cell development. Because of the geometry of the *TRA/D* cluster, joining of a *TRAV* gene to a *TRAJ* gene inevitably deletes the D genes on that allele. Thus α-chain rearrangements eliminate any possibility of δ-chain expression.

Potential T-Cell Receptor Diversity

In the human *TRA* locus there are 75 *TRAJ* genes and 100 *TRAV* genes, giving $75 \times 100 = 75 \times 10^2$ possible combinations. There is, in addition, N-region addition and base deletion resulting in great junctional diversity. After correction for codon redundancy and correct reading frame, the number of potentially different TCR α chains is about 10^6. In the human *TRB* locus there are about 75 *TRBV* genes, 2 *TRBD* genes, and 12 *TRBJ* genes giving $75 \times 2 \times 12 = 1800$ possible combinations. In addition, there is junctional diversity and the use of perhaps 110 possible different *TRBD* combinations. After corrections there are about 5×10^9 possible *VDJβ* sequences. Thus, the number of possible different TCR α/β combinations is $5 \times 10^9 \times 10^6 = 5 \times 10^{15}$. (A somewhat similar figure can be arrived at for the mouse. However, a mouse has only 5×10^7 T cells, so this is much more potential diversity than a mouse would ever be able to use.)

In the human *TRD* cluster, a combination of V-region diversity, two *TRDD* genes, three sites where N addition and deletion can occur, and diversity in V-J joining position can generate about 10^{14} possible amino acid sequences, whereas in *TRGV* 7×10^6 different sequences are possible. There is no difficulty, therefore, in accounting for the enormous diversity seen in the TCRs.

γ/δ T-CELL DIVERSITY

The function of γ/δ T cells appears to differ among mammalian species. For example, in humans and mice there are few V genes in the *TRD* and *TRG* loci and the combinational repertoire is relatively small. In addition, the γ/δ TCR repertoire is severely restricted since the cells bearing these receptors use only a few V-gene combinations. For example, in humans, 70% to 90% of γ/δ T cells in blood express the *TRGV9* and *TRDV2* gene products. In contrast, human α/β T cells show a wide range of binding specificities. Thus, in humans and mice there is a marked difference between the size of the α/β and γ/δ TCR repertoires. The α/β T cells recognize and respond to a wide variety of processed antigens. In contrast, the function of γ/δ T cells is still in dispute, and it is still unclear how they respond to antigens. γ/δ T cells probably have a limited role in defense and recognize a limited number of antigens in humans and mice.

The situation in artiodactyls is different. In these mammals, γ/δ T cells form a much larger proportion of total T cells. For example, in young lambs or calves, they account for up to 60% of T cells. In addition, ruminant γ/δ T cells show a considerably greater receptor diversity. Thus in the sheep, γ/δ V-region diversity results from the use of 40 to 50 *TRDV* genes and 15 to 20 *TRGV* genes that contain two distinct hypervariable segments similar to the CDRs seen in immunoglobulin V genes. In addition, the sheep γ/δ heterodimer occurs in at least five forms made by the association of one Cδ chain with one of five Cγ chains. All this suggests that the sheep γ/δ T cells may have a major functional role and recognize a wide variety of antigens.

SOURCES OF ADDITIONAL INFORMATION

Baltimore D: Somatic mutation gains its place among the generators of diversity, *Cell* 26:295-296, 1981.

Butler JE: Immunoglobulin gene organization and the mechanism of repertoire development, *Scand J Immunol* 45: 455-462, 1997.

Butler JE: Immunoglobulin diversity, B-cell and antibody repertoire development in large farm animals, *Rev Sci Tech* 17:43-70, 1998.

Butler JE, Sun J, Weber P, et al: Antibody repertoire development in fetal and newborn piglets, III. Colonization of the gastrointestinal tract selectively diversifies the preimmune repertoire in mucosal lymphoid tissues, *Immunology* 100: 119-130, 2000.

Calame KL: Immunoglobulin gene transcription: molecular mechanisms, *Trends Genet* 5: 395-399, 1989

Conrad ML, Pettman R, Whitehead J, et al: Genomic sequencing of the bovine T cell receptor beta locus, *Vet Immunol Immunopathol* 87:439-441, 2002.

Davis MM: Molecular genetics of T-cell antigen receptors, *Hosp Pract* 23: 157-170, 1988.

Davis MM, Bjorkman PJ: T-cell antigen receptor genes and T-cell recognition, *Nature* 334: 395-402, 1988.

Diaz M, Flajnik MF: Evolution of somatic hypermutation and gene conversion in adaptive immunity, *Immunol Rev* 162: 13-24, 1998.

Eckhardt LA: Immunoglobulin gene expression only in the right cells at the right time, *FASEB J* 6:2553-2560, 1992.

Faili A, Aoufouchi S, Flatter E, et al: Induction of somatic hypermutation in immunoglobulin genes is dependent on DNA polymerase iota, *Nature* 419:944-946, 2002.

Gearhart PJ, Bogenhagen DF: Clusters of point mutations are found exclusively around rearranged antibody variable genes, *Proc Natl Acad Sci U S A* 80: 3439-3443, 1983.

Glusman G, Rowen L, Lee I, et al: Comparative genomics of the human and mouse T cell receptor loci, *Immunity* 15: 337-349, 2001

Jenne CN, Kennedy LJ, McCullagh P, Reynolds JD: A new model of sheep Ig diversification: shifting the emphasis toward combinatorial mechanisms and away from hypermutation, *J Immunol* 170:3739-3750, 2003.

Kallenbach S, Doyen N, D'Andon MF, Rougeon F: Three lymphoid-specific factors account for all junctional diversity characteristic of somatic assembly of T-cell receptor and immunoglobulin genes, *Proc Natl Acad Sci USA* 89: 2799-2803, 1992.

Lai E, Wilson RK, Hood LE: Physical maps of the mouse and human immunoglobulin-like loci, *Adv Immunol* 46: 1-59, 1989.

Moss PA, Rosenberg WMC, Bell JI: The human T cell receptor in health and disease, *Annu Rev Immunol* 10: 71-96, 1992.

Niku M, Pessa-Morikawa T, Andersson L, Iivanainen A: Oligoclonal Peyer's patch follicles in the terminal small intestine of cattle, *Dev Comp Immunol* 26:689-695, 2002.

Papavasiliou FN, Schatz DG: Somatic hypermutation of immunoglobulin genes: merging mechanisms for genetic diversity, *Cell* 109:S35-S44, 2002.

Reynaud C-A, Mackay CR, Müller RG, Weill J-C: Somatic generation of diversity in a mammalian primary lymphoid organ: the sheep ileal Peyer's patches, *Cell* 64: 995-1005, 1991.

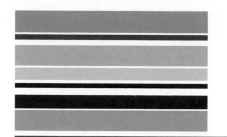

Innate and Acquired Immunity: The Complement System

Although we have treated innate and acquired immune responses as distinctly different entities, they are in fact closely linked. This linkage is typified by the complement system. The complement system is a defense mechanism that can be activated by both innate and acquired immune mechanisms. It consists of a set of enzymic pathways that cause specific proteins to bind covalently to the surface of invading microbes. Once bound, these proteins can destroy the invaders. In healthy uninfected animals these pathways are inactive. However, they are activated by either antibodies attached to the surface of an organism or simply by the complex carbohydrates found on the surface of infectious agents. Because the complement system is so potentially destructive, it must be carefully regulated and controlled. This in turn makes for significant complexity.

The complement system is inactive in healthy, uninfected animals. It can be activated by at least three different mechanisms, referred to as the classical, the alternative, and the lectin pathways (Figure 15-1). The classical pathway is activated by antibodies bound to antigens and thus works only in association with acquired immunity. The alternative and lectin pathways, in contrast, are activated directly by microbial carbohydrates, typical examples of the pathogen-associated molecular patterns that trigger innate immunity.

COMPLEMENT COMPONENTS

The proteins that form the complement system are either labeled numerically with the prefix C (e.g., C1, C2, C3) or designated by letters of the alphabet (B, D, P, and

so forth). There are at least 30 such proteins. Some are found free in serum whereas others are cell-bound receptors. Complement components account for about 15% of the globulin fraction of serum. The molecular weights of complement components vary from 24 kDa for factor D to 460 kDa for C1q. Their serum concentrations in humans vary between 20 μg/mL for C2 and 1300 μg/mL for C3 (Table 15-1). Complement components are synthesized at various sites throughout the body. Most C3, C6, C8, and B are made in the liver whereas C2, C3, C4, C5, B, D, P, and I are made by macrophages. Neutrophils can store large quantities of C6 and C7. As a result, these components are readily available for defense at sites where macrophages and neutrophils accumulate.

ACTIVATION PATHWAYS

The Alternative Pathway

The alternative pathway of complement activation is triggered by contact between microbial cell walls and complement components. It is activated immediately when an invading organism comes into contact with blood and thus is a key component of innate immunity.

The most important complement protein is called C3. C3 is a disulfide-linked heterodimer with α and β chains. It is synthesized by liver cells and macrophages and is the complement component of highest concentration in serum.

In healthy normal animals, C3 breaks down slowly but spontaneously into two breakdown products, C3a and

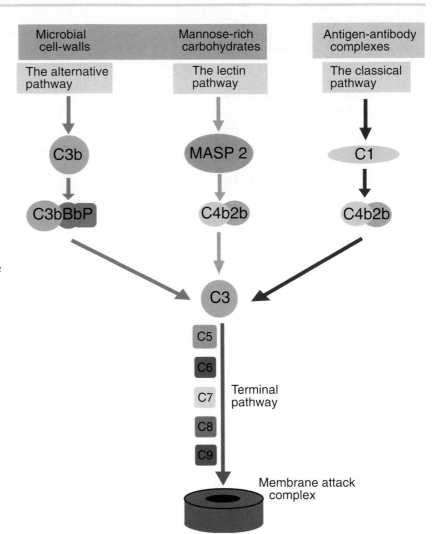

Figure 15-1. The three pathways by which the complement system may be activated.

C3b (Figure 15-2). This breakdown activates an exposed thioester bond on the C3b fragment, which then generates a reactive carbonyl group. The highly reactive carbonyl group covalently and irreversibly attaches the C3b to nearby surfaces (Figure 15-3). However, under normal circumstances this surface-bound C3b also binds a protein called factor H and as a result is promptly destroyed by a protease called factor I (Figure 15-4). Thus surface-bound C3b is normally destroyed soon after being deposited. This destruction depends on the activity of factor H, which depends in turn on the nature of the target surface. When factor H interacts with normal cell surfaces, glycoproteins rich in sialic acid and other neutral or anionic polysaccharides enhance its binding to C3b, factor I is activated, and the C3b is destroyed. Thus in a healthy individual, factors H and I destroy C3b as fast as it is generated. On the other hand, on bacterial cell walls, lipopolysaccharides and other carbohydrates lack sialic acid. As a result, factor H cannot bind to C3b, factor I is inactivated, and the C3b persists. This bound C3b then binds another complement protein called factor B to form a complex called C3bB. The bound

factor B is then cleaved by a protease called factor D, releasing a soluble fragment called Ba and leaving C3bBb on the bacterial wall. This bound C3bBb is a potent protease whose preferred substrate is C3. (It is therefore called the alternative C3 convertase.) Factor D can act only on factor B after it is bound to C3b but not before. This constraint is called substrate modulation, and it occurs at several points in the complement pathways. It presumably ensures that the activities of enzymes such as factor D are confined to the correct target molecules.

The alternative C3 convertase, C3bBb, can split C3 and so generate more C3b. However C3bBb has a half-life of only 5 minutes. If another protein called factor P (or properdin) binds to the complex to form C3bBbP, its half-life is extended to 30 minutes. Since C3b thus serves to generate more C3bBbP, the net effect of all this is that a positive loop is generated where increasing amounts of C3b are irreversibly bound to the surface of the invading organism.

Bound C3b also binds another protein called C5 (Figure 15-5). Once C5 is bound to C3b, substrate modulation occurs and the C5 can also be cleaved by C3bBb (Figure 15-6). This enzyme splits off a small

TABLE 15-1
Complement Components

Name	MW (kDa)	Serum conc. (μg/mL)
CLASSICAL PATHWAY		
C1q	460	80
C1r	83	50
C1s	83	50
C4	200	600
C2	102	20
C3	185	1300
ALTERNATE PATHWAY		
D	24	1
B	90	210
TERMINAL COMPONENTS		
C5	204	70
C6	120	65
C7	120	55
C8	160	55
C9	70	60
CONTROL PROTEINS		
C1-INH	105	200
C4BP	550	250
H	150	480
I	88	35
Ana INH	310	35
P	4×56	20
S	83	500

peptide called C5a, leaving a large fragment C5b attached to the C3b. This cleavage also exposes a site on C5b that can bind two new proteins, C6 and C7, to form a multimolecular complex called C5b67 (Figure 15-7). The C5b67 complex can then insert itself into the

microbial cell membrane. Once inserted in the surface of an organism, the complex will bind one C8 and multiple C9 molecules. Twelve to eighteen C9 molecules aggregate with the C5b678 complex to form a tubular structure called the membrane attack complex (MAC). The MAC inserts itself into a microbial cell membrane and effectively punches a hole in the invader. If sufficient MACs are formed on an organism it will be killed by osmotic lysis. These MACs can be seen by electron microscopy as ring-shaped structures on the microbial surface with a central electron-dense area surrounded by a lighter ring of poly C9 (Figure 15-8).

The Lectin Pathway

The second method of activating the complement system involves recognition of microbial carbohydrates by serum proteins. Like the alternative pathway, this is an innate defense mechanism triggered simply by the presence of bacterial cell wall carbohydrates in the bloodstream.

The serum protein mannose-binding lectin (MBL) can bind to mannose or *N*-acetylglucosamine on microbial cell walls. (Carbohydrates such as galactose or sialic acid found on mammalian glycoproteins do not bind MBL.) Thus MBL can bind to the surface of bacteria, fungi, parasitic protozoa, and viruses. MBL is a C-type lectin that belongs to the collectin family (Chapter 2).

Once it has bound to microbial surfaces, the MBL will form complexes with and then activate the serum protease MASP-2. It is believed that binding of MBL to sugar groups on the microbial surface results in conformational changes that activate MASP-2. (MASP stands for MBL-associated serine protease.) Activated MASP-2, in turn, acts on the protein C4, splitting it into C4a and C4b. Removal of C4a activates an exposed thioester bond on the C4b and generates a reactive

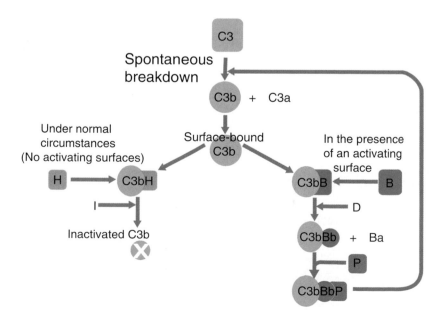

Figure 15-2. The alternative complement pathway. Surface-bound C3b may either be destroyed, as normally happens, or be activated by the presence of an activating surface.

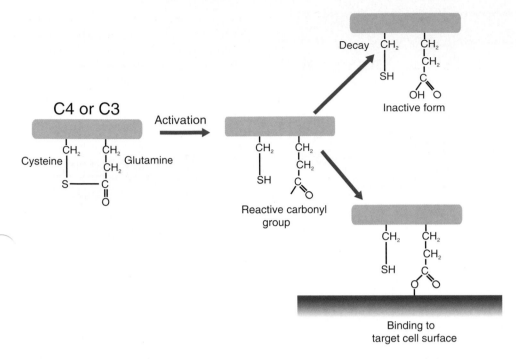

Figure 15-3.   Activation of C3 or C4 not only involves cleavage of a peptide off these proteins but also cleavage of a thioester bond between a cysteine and a glutamine. This enables the molecule to bind covalently (and hence irreversibly) to target cell surfaces.

carbonyl group that covalently attaches the C4b to the microbial surface (Figure 15-9). C2 is a glycoprotein that binds to C4b to form a complex, C4b2. C2 is then also cleaved by MASP-2 to generate C4b2b.

Cell-bound C4b2b next acts on the α chain of C3 to generate C3a and C3b. As in the activation of C4, C3 has an exposed thioester bond that is activated when C3a is split off. As a result, C3b molecules also bind covalently

to surfaces carrying C4b2b. The activation of C3b by C4b2b is a major step because each C4b2b complex can activate as many as 200 C3 molecules, which are then irreversibly attached to nearby surfaces. Since the reactions of the complement system are usually confined to the microenvironment close to microbial surfaces, C3 will bind to these organisms. The bound C3b can bind C5 and cleave it to C5a and C5b. The complement

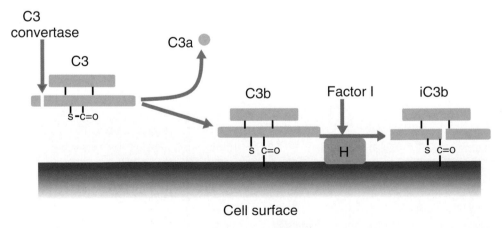

Figure 15-4.   C3 is activated by the action of the C3 convertases. These cleave off a small peptide (C3a) and enable the active component of the molecule (C3b) to bind to cell surfaces. This C3b is normally inactivated by the actions of factors H and I. However, factor H must first be activated by binding to the surface. In the absence of factor H, factor I will not work. In this case C3b persists and activates the terminal complement pathway.

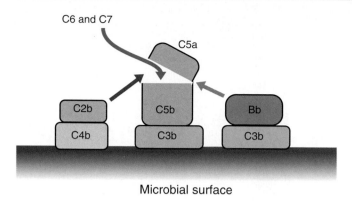

Figure 15-5. The two C3 convertases, C3b2b and C3bBb, act on C5 when it is linked to C3b and cleave off a small peptide called C5a. In so doing they reveal a site that binds C6 and C7.

pathway then can proceed to completion and the killing of the organism by membrane attack complexes as described above.

The MBL-MASP-2 pathway is ancient, having existed for at least 300 million years. Although in many ways it duplicates the alternative pathway, it provides yet another example of duplication of mechanisms to "guarantee" protection.

The Classical Pathway

The classical complement pathway (Figure 15-10) is triggered by antibodies bound to antigens on the surface of a foreign organism. It is thus part of the acquired immune system. Because of this, it cannot be triggered until antibodies are made, which may occur as late as 7 to 10 days after infection. Nevertheless, once activated it is a very efficient complement activating pathway.

When antibody molecules bind to an antigen they change their molecular shape and expose active sites on their Fc regions. In addition, if several antibody

molecules are bound to an organism, multiple active sites will be exposed within a small area. It is these active sites that trigger classical complement pathway activation.

The first component of the classical complement pathway is a multimolecular protein complex called C1. C1 consists of three proteins (C1q, C1r, C1s) bound together by calcium. C1q looks like a six-stranded whip when viewed by electron microscopy (Figure 15-11). Two molecules of C1r and two of C1s form a figure-of-eight structure located between the C1q strands. C1q is activated when the tips of at least two strands bind to complement-activating sites on immunoglobulin Fc regions. Binding to the immunoglobulin causes a conformational change in C1q that is transmitted to C1r. As a result, C1r changes to reveal an active proteolytic site that cleaves a peptide bond in C1s to convert that molecule to an enzymatically active form.

Single, antigen-bound molecules of IgM or paired, antigen-bound molecules of IgG are needed to activate C1. The polymeric IgM structure readily provides two closely spaced complement-activating sites. In contrast, two IgG molecules must be located very close together in order to have the same effect. As a result IgG is much less efficient than IgM in activating the classical pathway. C1 may also be activated directly by some viruses, or by bacteria such as *Escherichia coli* and *Klebsiella pneumoniae*.

Activated C1s cleaves C4 into C4a and C4b. C2 then binds to C4b to form C4b2. Activated C1s then splits the bound C2 generating a small peptide C2a and C4b2b. C1s cannot act on soluble C2; the C2 must first be bound to C4b before it can be cleaved (another example of substrate modulation). The C4b2b complex, as described above, is a potent protease that cleaves C3. C4b2b is therefore called classical C3 convertase. C3b generated in this way binds and activates C5. Subsequent reactions

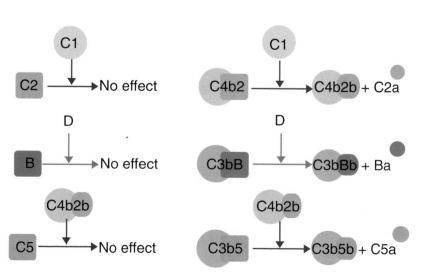

Figure 15-6. Substrate modulation is one way in which the complement system is regulated. The target for a protease is not susceptible to cleavage unless it is first bound to another protein.

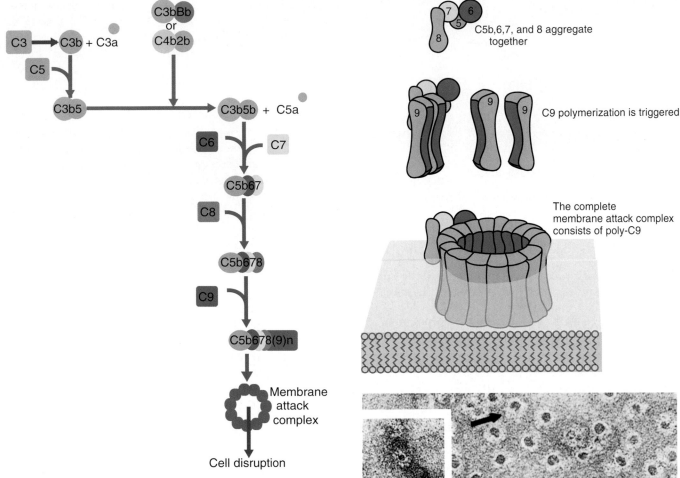

Figure 15-7. The terminal complement pathway. This eventually leads to the formation of a membrane attack complex.

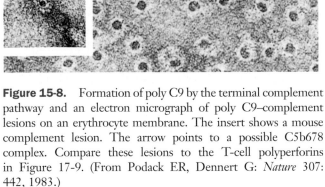

Figure 15-8. Formation of poly C9 by the terminal complement pathway and an electron micrograph of poly C9–complement lesions on an erythrocyte membrane. The insert shows a mouse complement lesion. The arrow points to a possible C5b678 complex. Compare these lesions to the T-cell polyperforins in Figure 17-9. (From Podack ER, Dennert G: *Nature* 307: 442, 1983.)

lead to formation of the membrane attack complex and microbial killing.

REGULATION OF COMPLEMENT

The consequences of complement activation are so significant and potentially dangerous that all of the activation pathways must be carefully regulated. This regulation is mediated by regulatory proteins (Figure 15-12).

The most important regulator of the classical pathway is C1 inactivator (C1-INH). C1-INH controls the assembly of C4b2b by blocking the activities of active C1r and C1s. Many other regulatory proteins control the activities of the C3 and C5 convertases. For example, CD55, or decay accelerating factor, is a glycoprotein expressed on the surface of red blood cells, neutrophils, lymphocytes, monocytes, platelets, and endothelial cells. CD55 binds to the convertases and accelerates their decay. Its function is to protect normal body cells from complement attack. Other proteins that accelerate

degradation of the convertases include factor H and C4-binding protein (C4BP) found in plasma and CD35 (CR1) and CD46 found on cell membranes. Control of the C56789 complex is mediated by three glycoproteins: vitronectin, clusterin, and, most importantly, CD59 (protectin). They all inhibit C5b678 insertion and C9 polymerization in cell membranes.

Complement Receptors

Four cell surface receptors for C3 or its fragments have been identified. These are called CR1 (CD35), CR2 (CD21), CR3 (CD11a/CD18), and CR4 (CD11c/CD18).

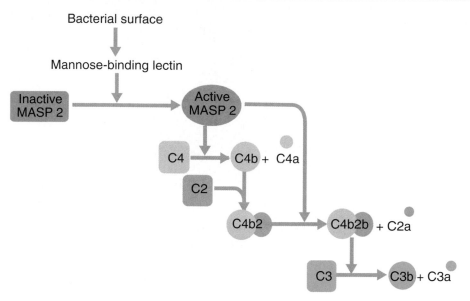

Figure 15-9. Complement activation by the lectin pathway.

CR1 binds C3b and C4b as well as a C3b breakdown product called iC3b. CR1 is found on primate red cells, neutrophils, eosinophils, monocytes, macrophages, B cells, and some T cells. Red cell CR1 accounts for 90% of all CR1 in the blood. In primates, CR1 removes immune complexes from the circulation. [Immune complexes bind to CR1 on red cells and the coated red cells are then removed in the liver and spleen (Chapter 28)]. Deficiencies of complement components or their receptors may allow circulating immune complexes to accumulate in organs such as kidney and cause tissue damage. For example, some patients with the autoimmune disease systemic lupus erythematosus have a CR1 deficiency and are thus unable to remove these immune complexes effectively. C3-deficient dogs develop immune complex–mediated kidney lesions for the same reason.

CR2 (CD21) is found on most B cells. It binds a breakdown fragment of C3 called C3d. CR2 forms a complex with CD19. This acts as a B-cell costimulator (see Figure 11-10). B cells require costimulation from C3d through CR2 in order to respond optimally to antigens.

CR3 (CD11a/CD18) is an integrin that binds the breakdown fragment of C3 called iC3b. It is found on macrophages, neutrophils, and natural killer cells. A genetic deficiency of CR3 (leukocyte adherence deficiency, LAD) has been described in humans, cattle, and dogs in which affected individuals experience severe recurrent infections (Chapter 35).

CR4 (CD11c/CD18) is another integrin found on neutrophils, T cells, natural killer cells, platelets, and macrophages. It binds breakdown fragments of C3.

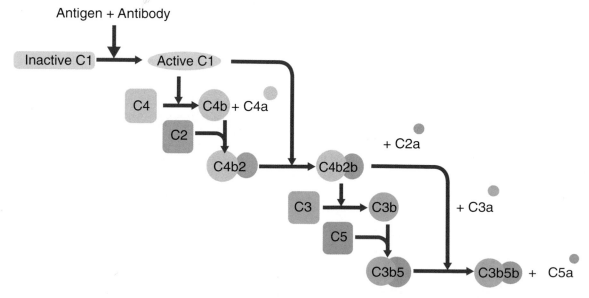

Figure 15-10. Basic features of the classical complement pathway.

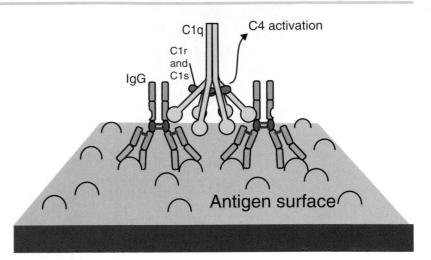

Figure 15-11. The structure of C1 and its role in interacting with antibodies to initiate the classical complement pathway.

OTHER CONSEQUENCES OF COMPLEMENT ACTIVATION

While microbial killing due to lysis mediated by MACs is the most obvious activity of the complement system, its protective effects go far beyond this, and complement contributes to the body's defenses in many ways.

Opsonization

C3b bound to a microbial surface is a very potent and effective opsonin since phagocytic cells possess CR1. Thus, C3b-coated organisms will bind strongly to these cells and undergo type II phagocytosis (Chapter 3). If for some reason these organisms cannot be ingested, then neutrophils may secrete their lysosomal enzymes and oxidants into the surrounding tissue fluid. These molecules will cause inflammation and tissue

damage—a reaction classified as type III hypersensitivity (Chapter 28).

Chemotaxis

The complement system is a major contributor to acute inflammation. For example, activation of the complement system by any of its pathways generates several potent chemotactic peptides, including C5a and C5b67 (Table 15-2). C5b67 is chemotactic for neutrophils and eosinophils, whereas C5a attracts not only neutrophils and eosinophils but also macrophages and basophils. When C5a attracts neutrophils, it stimulates their respiratory burst, aggregates them, and up-regulates CR1 and integrin expression.

Inflammation

The small peptides C3a and C5a cause acute inflammation when injected into the skin. These molecules have been called anaphylatoxins because they degranulate mast cells and stimulate platelets to release the vasoactive molecules histamine and serotonin. They increase vascular permeability, causing lysosomal enzyme release from neutrophils and thromboxane release from macrophages (Figure15-13).

Immune Regulation

Complement regulates antibody formation through C3d bound to antigen. When an antigen molecule binds to a

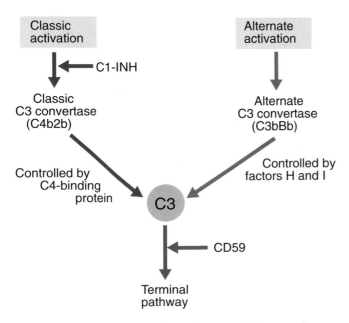

Figure 15-12. Basic control mechanisms of the complement system.

TABLE 15-2	
Complement-Derived Chemotactic Factors	
Factor	**Target**
C3a	Eosinophils
C5a	Neutrophils, eosinophils, macrophages
C567	Neutrophils, eosinophils
Bb	Neutrophils
C3e	Promotes leukocytosis

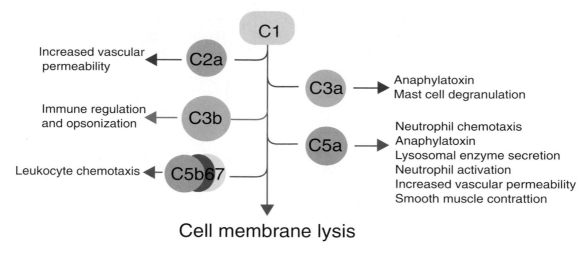

Figure 15-13. Some of the biological consequences of complement activation.

B-cell receptor, any attached C3d will bind to CD21/CD19 complexes on the B-cell surface. (Remember that several hundred C3 molecules may attach to an antigen as a result of C3 convertase activity.) Activation of the CD21/CD19 complex sends a signal that significantly enhances B-cell receptor signaling and is an important costimulatory pathway for mature B cells. Thus depletion of C3 is associated with reduced primary antibody responses.

Coating of antigens with C3d also permits antigens to bind to CR2 on dendritic cells and so influences antigen processing. Absence of C3 means that immune complexes will not localize on follicular dendritic cells in germinal centers.

COMPLEMENT GENES

The genes coding for complement proteins are mainly scattered throughout the genome. However, two major gene clusters have been identified. Thus the genes coding for C4, C2, and factor B are clustered within the major histocompatibility complex class III region. Likewise the genes for C4BP, CD55, CD35, CD21, CD46, and factor H are linked in the RCA (regulation of complement activation) cluster.

Complement components, like other proteins, may occur in different allelic forms. The precise number varies between components and species. For example, bovine factor H has three allotypes encoded by two codominant alleles at a single autosomal locus. Equine C3 exists in six allotypes inherited at three codominant alleles at a single autosomal locus. Two allotypes of canine C3 have been identified at a single locus. Canine C6 occurs as seven allotypes inherited as autosomal codominants. Porcine C6 occurs as 14 allotypes controlled by five autosomal codominant alleles. Eleven allotypes of canine C7 have been identified. They are inherited at two loci and a null allele has been identified.

Canine C4 is encoded at a single locus with at least five allotypes. There is an association among the C4-4 allotype, low serum C4 levels, and the development of autoimmune polyarthritis in dogs. Feline and equine C4 have at least four different allotypes.

COMPLEMENT DEFICIENCIES

Canine C3 Deficiency

Because the complement system is an essential protective mechanism, complement deficiencies increase susceptibility to infections. The most severe of these diseases occurs in individuals deficient in C3. For example, a colony of Brittany spaniels with an autosomal recessive C3 deficiency has been described (Figure 15-14). Dogs that are homozygous for this trait have no detectable C3, whereas heterozygous animals have C3 levels that are approximately half normal. Heterozygous animals are clinically normal. The homozygous-deficient animals have lower IgG levels than normal, and their ability to make antibodies against defined antigens is reduced. The dogs tend to make more IgM and less IgG. They experience recurrent sepsis, pneumonia, pyometra, and wound infections. The organisms involved include *Clostridium*, *Pseudomonas*, *E. coli*, and *Klebsiella*. Some affected dogs develop amyloidosis and many develop an immune complex–mediated kidney disease (Chapter 28). The mutation responsible for this deficiency (deletion of a cytosine residue) shortens the C3 chain as a result of a frameshift and the generation of a premature stop codon (Figure 15-15).

Porcine Factor H Deficiency

Factor H is a critical component of the alternative complement pathway. It normally inactivates C3b as soon as it is generated and so prevents excessive alternative

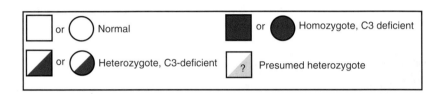

Figure 15-14. Inheritance of a C3 deficiency in a colony of Brittany spaniels. The number below each circle or square represents the animal's C3 level as a percentage of a standard reference serum. The mean level in healthy spaniels was 126. (From Winkelstein JA, Cork LC, Griffin DE, et al: *Science* 212:1169-1170, 1981.)

pathway activation. If an animal fails to make factor H, then C3b will be generated in an uncontrolled fashion. Factor H deficiency has been identified as an autosomal recessive trait in Yorkshire pigs. Affected piglets are healthy at birth and develop normally for a few weeks. However, eventually they fail to thrive, stop growing, become anemic, and die of renal failure.

On autopsy multiple petechial hemorrhages are seen on the surface of the kidneys accompanied by atrophy of the renal papillae. On light microscopy, alterations are seen in the renal glomeruli, i.e., mesangial cell proliferation and capillary basement membrane thickening (Figure 15-16). On electron microscopy, extensive intramembranous electron-dense deposits are found within the glomerular basement membranes (Figure 15-17). This is typical of type II membranoproliferative glomerulonephritis or dense-deposit disease (Chapter 28). Indirect immunofluorescence demonstrates massive deposits of C3 but no immunoglobulins in the basement membranes. C3 can be found in the glomeruli before birth, but the morphological changes (mesangial proliferation and intramembranous dense deposits) are never seen before 5 days of age. These pigs have no plasma C3.

Nephritic piglets are almost totally deficient in factor H (2% of normal levels), whereas heterozygotes have half the normal levels. If factor H is replaced by plasma

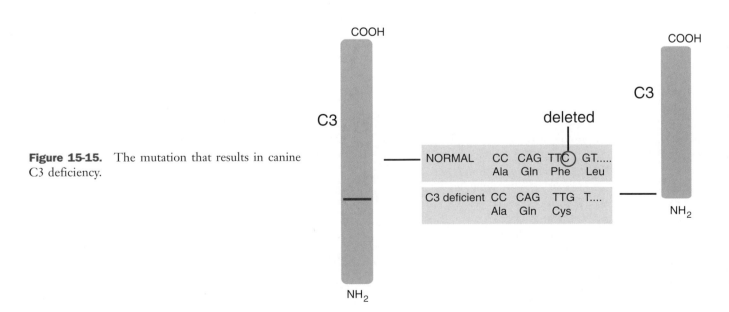

Figure 15-15. The mutation that results in canine C3 deficiency.

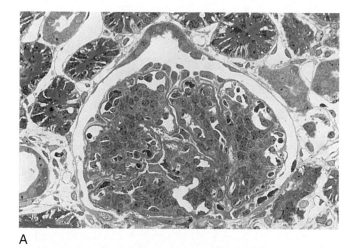

A

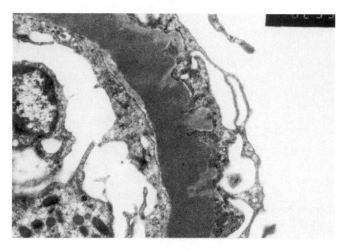

Figure 15-17. Electron micrograph showing dense intramembranous deposits in the glomerulus of a piglet with factor H deficiency. (From Jansen JH: *APMIS* 101:281-289, 1993.)

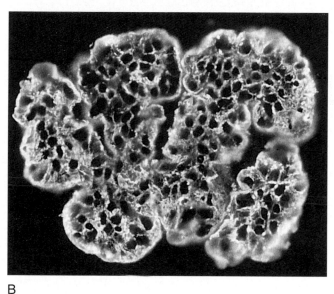

B

Figure 15-16. **A,** A thin section of the glomerulus of a piglet with factor H deficiency. Note the thickened basement membrane and increased numbers of mesangial cells (*arrows*), hence the name membranoproliferative glomerulonephritis. **B,** An immunofluorescence photomicrograph of another glomerulus from a factor H-deficient piglet. This is stained with fluorescent anti-C3. The bright fluorescence indicates the presence of C3 deposited in this glomerulus. Compare this figure with Figure 28-10. (**A** courtesy of Johan H. Jansen; **B** from Jansen JH, Hogasen K, Mollnes TE: *Am J Pathol* 143:1356-1365, 1993.)

transfusions the progress of the disease can be slowed and piglet survival enhanced. Since heterozygotes can be readily detected by measurement of plasma C3, this disease can be eradicated from affected herds.

Other Complement Deficiencies

MBL deficiency has been described in children where it results in increased susceptibility to infection. It has not yet been described in domestic animals. In contrast to the severe effects of a C3 deficiency, congenital deficiencies of other complement components in laboratory animals or humans are not necessarily lethal. Thus, individuals with C6 or C7 deficiencies have been described who are quite healthy. Apparently healthy C6-deficient pigs have been described. The lack of discernible effect of these deficiencies suggests that the terminal portion of the complement pathway leading to lysis may not be biologically essential.

SOURCES OF ADDITIONAL INFORMATION

Ameratunga R, Winkelstein JA, Brody L, et al: Molecular analysis of the third component of canine complement (C3) and identification of the mutation responsible for hereditary canine C3 deficiency, *J Immunol* 160:2824-2830, 1998.

Carroll MC: The role of complement and complement receptors in induction and regulation of immunity, *Annu Rev Immunol* 16:545-568, 1998.

Day MJ, Kay PM, Clark WT, et al: Complement C4 allotype association with and serum C4 concentration in an autoimmune disease in a dog, *Clin Immunol Immunopathol* 35:85-91, 1985.

DiScipio R: The relationship between polymerization of complement component C9 and membrane channel formation, *J Immunol* 147:4239-4247, 1991.

Fujita T: Evolution of the lectin-complement pathway and its role in innate immunity, *Nat Rev Immunol* 2:346-386, 2002.

Høgåsen K, Jansen JH, Molines T, et al: Hereditary porcine membranoproliferative glomerulonephritis type II is caused by factor H deficiency, *J Clin Invest* 95:1054-1061, 1995.

Hourcade D, Holers VM, Atkinson JP: The regulators of complement activation (RCA) gene cluster, *Adv Immunol* 45:381-416, 1989.

Jansen JH, Høgåsen K, Grøndahl AM: Porcine membranoproliferative glomerulonephritis type II: an autosomal recessive deficiency of factor H, *Vet Rec* 137:240-244, 1995.

Jansen JH, Høgåsen K, Molines TE: Extensive complement activation in hereditary porcine membranoproliferative glomerulonephritis type II (porcine dense deposit disease), *Am J Pathol* 143:1356-1365, 1993.

Lublin DM, Atkinson JP: Decay-accelerating factor: biochemistry, molecular biology, and functions, *Annu Rev Immunol* 7:35-58, 1989.

Matsushita M, Fujita T: Activation of the classical complement pathway by mannose-binding protein in association with a novel C1s-like serine protease, *J Exp Med* 176:1497-1502, 1992.

Menger M, Aston WP: Isolation and characterization of the third component of bovine complement, *Vet Immunol Immunopathol* 10:317-331, 1985.

Molina H, Kinoshita T, Inoue K, et al: A molecular and immunological characterization of mouse CR2: evidence for a single gene model of mouse complement receptors 1 and 2, *J Immunol* 145: 2974-2983, 1990.

Morgan BP: *Complement: clinical aspects and relevance to disease*, London, 1990, Academic Press.

Muller-Eberhard HJ: The membrane attack complex of complement, *Annu Rev Immunol* 4:503-528, 1986.

Nielsen CH, Fischer EM, Leslie RGQ: The role of complement in the acquired immune response *Immunology* 100: 4-12, 2000.

O'Neil KM, Ochs HD, Heller SR, et al: Role of C3 in humoral immunity: defective antibody formation in C3-deficient dogs, *J Immunol* 140:1939-1945, 1988.

Sahu A, Lambris JD: Structure and biology of complement protein C3, a connecting link between innate and acquired immunity, *Immunol Rev* 180:35-48, 2001.

Shibata T, Akita T, Abe T: Genetic polymorphism of the sixth component of complement (C6) in the pig, *Anim Genet* 24:97-100, 1993.

Van den Berg CW, Harrison RA, Morgan BP: The sheep analogue of human CD59: purification and characterization of its complement inhibitory activity, *Immunology* 78: 349-357, 1993.

Walport MJ: Complement, *N Engl J Med* 344:1140-1144, 2001.

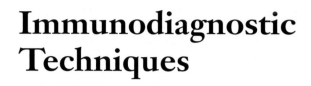

Immunodiagnostic Techniques

CHAPTER 16

The immune responses of animals can be used in two general ways in the diagnostic laboratory. First, specific antibody may be used to detect or identify an antigen. This antigen can be associated with an infectious agent, or simply be a molecule that needs to be located or measured. Second, by detecting the presence of specific antibody in serum, it is possible to determine whether an animal has been previously exposed to a specific organism. This will assist in establishing a diagnosis or determining the degree of exposure of the population to that organism. The measurement of antigen–antibody interactions for diagnostic purposes is called serology.

Serological techniques can be classified into three broad categories. Primary binding tests that directly measure the binding of antigen to antibody (Table 16-1). Secondary binding tests that measure the results of antigen–antibody interaction in vitro. These tests are usually less sensitive than the primary binding tests, but may be simpler to perform or require simpler technology.

The most complex tests, in vivo tests, measure the actual protective effect of antibodies in an animal.

REAGENTS USED IN SEROLOGICAL TESTS

Serum

The most common source of antibody for testing is serum obtained by allowing a blood sample to clot and the clot to retract. Serum may be stored frozen and tested when convenient. If necessary the serum can be depleted of complement activity, by heating to 56° C for 30 minutes.

Complement

Complement is a normal constituent of all fresh serum, but the complement in fresh, unheated guinea pig serum is the most efficient in hemolytic tests. Serum used as a source of complement for serological applications should

TABLE 16-1
Smallest Amount of Antibody Protein Detectable by Selected Immunological Tests

Tests	Protein (μg/mL)
PRIMARY BINDING TESTS	
ELISA	0.0005
Competitive radioimmunoassay	0.00005
SECONDARY BINDING TESTS	
Gel precipitation	30
Ring precipitation	18
Bacterial agglutination	0.05
Passive hemagglutination	0.01
Hemagglutination inhibition	0.005
Complement fixation	0.05
Virus neutralization	0.00005
Bactericidal activity	0.00005
Antitoxin neutralization	0.06
IN VIVO TEST	
Passive cutaneous anaphylaxis	0.02

be stored frozen in small volumes. Once thawed, it should be used promptly. It should not be repeatedly frozen and thawed.

Antiglobulins

Because immunoglobulins are complex proteins they are antigenic when injected into an animal of a different species. For example, purified dog immunoglobulins can be injected into rabbits. The rabbits respond by making specific antibodies called antiglobulins. Depending on the purity of the injected immunoglobulin, it is possible to make nonspecific antiglobulins against immunoglobulins of all classes; or very specific antiglobulins directed against single classes. Antiglobulins are essential reagents in many immunological tests.

Monoclonal Antibodies

Hybridoma-derived monoclonal antibodies are pure and specific, can be used as standard chemical reagents, and can be obtained in almost unlimited amounts (Chapter 11). As a result, monoclonal antibodies frequently replace conventional antiserum as reagents in immunodiagnostic tests.

PRIMARY BINDING TESTS

Primary binding tests are performed by allowing antigen and antibody to combine and then measuring the amount of immune complex formed. Radioisotopes, fluorescent dyes, colloidal metals, and enzymes are used as labels to identify one of the reactants.

RADIOIMMUNOASSAYS

Assays involving the use of radioisotopes as labels have the advantage of being exquisitely sensitive. On the other hand, such detection systems are expensive. The expense factor combined with the hazards of radioactivity and the need to dispose of radioactive material in a safe manner has ensured that radioimmunoassays are only used when very high sensitivity is required.

Radioimmunoassays for Antibody

The radioallergosorbent test (RAST) is used to measure levels of specific IgE in allergic animals. In this technique, antigen-impregnated cellulose disks are immersed in test serum so that any antibody binds to the antigen. After washing to remove unbound antibody, the disk is immersed in a solution containing radiolabeled antiglobulin (e.g., anti-IgE). The antiglobulin binds to the disk only if antibodies have already bound to the antigen. The amount of radioactivity bound to the disk is a measure of the level of antibody activity in the serum.

Radioimmunoassays for Antigen

Competitive immunoassays are based on the principle that unlabeled antigen will displace radiolabeled antigen from immune complexes (Figure 16-1). These tests are exquisitely sensitive and so are commonly used to detect trace amounts of drugs. The antigen (or drug) is labeled with an isotope such as tritium (H^3), carbon 14, or iodine 125. When radiolabeled antigen is mixed with its specific antibody, it combines to form immune complexes that may be precipitated out of solution. The radioactivity of the supernatant fluid is a measure of the amount of

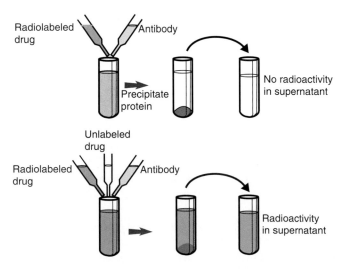

Figure 16-1. Principle of competitive radioimmunoassay. Unlabeled antigen displaces labeled antigen from immune complexes. The amount of labeled antigen released is proportional to the amount of unlabeled antigen added.

unbound antigen. If unlabeled antigen is added to the mixture, it will compete with the labeled antigen for antibody-binding sites. As a result, some labeled antigen will be unable to bind, and the amount of radioactivity in the supernatant will increase. If a standard curve is first constructed based on the use of known amounts of unlabeled antigen, then the amount of antigen in a test sample may be measured by reference to this standard curve.

IMMUNOFLUORESCENCE ASSAYS

Fluorescent dyes are commonly employed as labels in primary binding tests, the most important being fluorescein isothiocyanate (FITC). FITC is a yellow compound that can be bound to antibodies without affecting their reactivity. When irradiated with invisible ultraviolet or blue light at 290 and 145 μm, FITC re-emits visible green light at 525 μm. FITC-labeled antibodies are used in the direct and indirect fluorescent antibody tests.

Direct Fluorescent Antibody Tests

Direct fluorescent antibody tests are used to identify the presence of antigen. Antibody directed against a specific antigen such as a bacterium or virus is first labeled with FITC. A tissue or smear containing the organism is fixed to a glass slide, incubated with a labeled antiserum, and washed to remove unbound antibody (Figure 16-2). When examined by darkfield illumination under a microscope with an ultraviolet light source, the organisms that bind the labeled antibody fluoresce brightly. This test can identify bacteria when their numbers are very low. For example, it can be used when examining the feces of animals suspected of shedding *M. avium* ssp. *paratuberculosis* or when examining smears from lesions for the presence of *Fusobacterium necrophorum*, *Listeria monocytogenes*, or the clostridial organisms (Figure 16-3). It may also be employed to detect viruses growing in tissue culture or in tissues from infected animals such as rabies

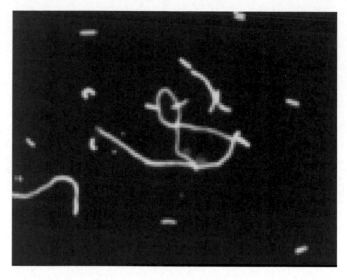

Figure 16-3. Direct immunofluorescence of a smear of *Clostridium septicum*. (Courtesy of Dr. John Huff.) (See also Figs. 20-6 and 36-3.)

virus in the brains of infected animals or feline leukemia virus in infected cells (see Figure 36-3).

Indirect Fluorescent Antibody Tests

Indirect fluorescent antibody tests are used to detect antibodies in serum or to identify antigens in tissues or cell cultures. When testing for antibodies, antigen is employed as a tissue smear, section, or cell culture on a slide or coverslip. This is incubated in a serum suspected of containing antibodies to that antigen. The serum is then washed off, leaving only specific antibodies bound to the antigen (Figure 16-4). These bound antibodies may be visualized after incubating the smear in FITC-labeled antiglobulin. When unbound antiglobulin is removed by washing and the slide examined, fluorescence indicates that antibody was present in the test serum. The quantity of antibody in the test serum may be estimated by examining increasing dilutions of serum on different antigen preparations.

The indirect fluorescent antibody test has two advantages over the direct technique. Since each antibody molecule binding to antigen will itself bind several labeled antiglobulin molecules, the fluorescence will be considerably brighter than in the direct test. Similarly, by using antiglobulins specific for each immunoglobulin class, the class of the specific antibody may also be determined.

Particle Concentration Fluorescence Immunoassays

Immunofluorescence assays can be automated and quantitated by means of particle immunoassays (Figure 16-5). For example, antigen-coated, submicrometer polystyrene particles can be mixed with test serum. After incubation,

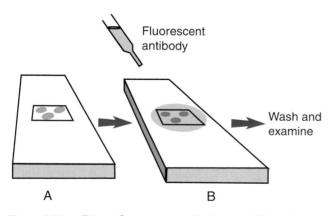

Fluorescent antibody

A   B

Wash and examine

Figure 16-2. Direct fluorescent antibody assay. This technique is used to detect antigen by means of FITC-labeled antibody.

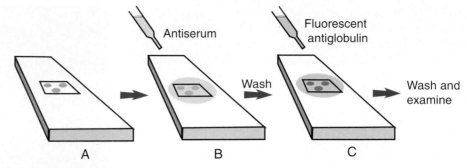

Figure 16-4. The indirect fluorescent antibody test may be used to detect either antigen or antibody. The antigen, in a section smear or culture, will bind antibody from serum. After washing, this antibody may be detected by binding to FITC-labeled antiglobulin.

the particles are recovered by vacuum filtration, washed to remove unbound antibody, and exposed to a fluorescent antiglobulin. After filtering the suspension again and washing to remove unbound antiglobulin, the particle suspension can be placed in a spectrofluorometer and the intensity of particle-bound fluorescence measured. This provides a measure of the level of antibodies in serum. A very useful variation on this is the competitive assay used as a rapid test for antibodies to *Brucella abortus* in cattle. In this case, *Brucella* antigen–coated polystyrene particles are mixed with a standard amount of fluorescent anti-*Brucella* serum and the serum under test. If positive, the unlabeled test serum inhibits the binding of fluorescent antibodies to the particles. The more antibody in the test serum, the greater will be the inhibition of fluorescent antibody binding.

Flow Cytometry

Flow cytometry, a fluorescent antibody technique used to identify cell surface antigens, is described in Chapter 9. It involves labeling a cell suspension with a fluorescent monoclonal antibody to a specific cell surface antigen.

The washed cell suspension is then passed across a laser beam and the characteristics of the labeled and unlabeled cells are determined. Flow cytometry provides a rapid quantitative technique for the analysis of complex cell mixtures and the identification of cell immunophenotypes.

IMMUNOENZYME ASSAYS

Among the most important immunoassays employed in veterinary medicine are the ELISAs. As with other primary binding tests, ELISAs may be used to detect and measure either antibody or antigen.

Microwell ELISA Tests

In the most common form of indirect ELISA for antibodies, microwells in polystyrene plates are first coated with an antigen solution (Figure 16-6). Proteins bind firmly to polystyrene, so that after unbound antigen is removed by vigorous washing the tubes remain coated with a layer of antigen. The coated tubes can be stored until required. The serum under test is added to the

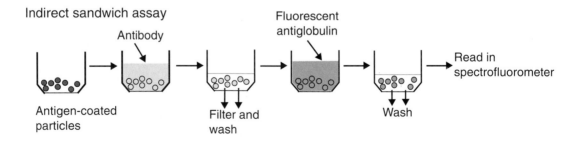

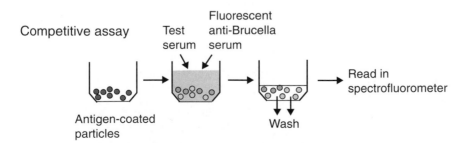

Figure 16-5. Principle of the particle concentration fluorescence immunoassay.

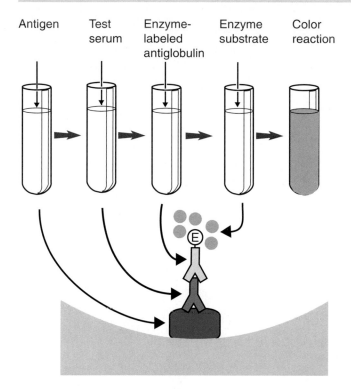

Figure 16-6. The indirect ELISA technique. Antigen is bound to the walls of a polystyrene tube. The presence of bound antibody is detected by means of an enzyme-labeled antiglobulin. Addition of the enzyme substrate leads to a color change proportional to the amount of bound antibody.

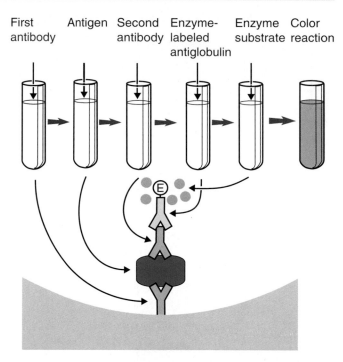

Figure 16-7. The antibody sandwich ELISA. Antigen is bound to the plate by means of an antibody. The presence of that bound antigen is detected by sequential addition of a second antibody and an enzyme-labeled antiglobulin. Addition of the enzyme substrate leads to a color change proportional to the amount of bound antigen.

tubes so that antibodies in the serum may bind to the antigen on the tube wall. After incubation and washing to remove unbound antibody, the presence of any bound antibodies is detected by addition of an antiglobulin chemically linked to an enzyme. This complex binds to the antibody and, following incubation and washing, may be detected and measured by addition of the enzyme substrate. The enzyme and substrate are selected so that a colored product develops in the tube. The intensity of the color that develops is therefore proportional to the amount of enzyme-linked antiglobulin that is bound, which in turn is proportional to the amount of antibody present in the serum under test. The color intensity may be estimated visually or, preferably, by spectrophotometry.

A modification of this technique, the antibody sandwich ELISA, is used to detect antigen (Figure 16-7). First polystyrene tubes are coated with specific antibody (capture antibody). The antigen solution is then added so that the capture antibody binds any antigen present. This is followed, after washing, by specific antibody, enzyme-labeled antiglobulin, and substrate, as described for the indirect technique. In this test, the intensity of the color reaction is related directly to the amount of bound antigen. Because these tests involve the formation of antibody-antigen-antibody layers, they are called sandwich ELISAs. Sandwich ELISAs are used to detect circulating virus in blood from cats with feline leukemia.

Another common modification is the labeled-antigen ELISA. This is favored in manufactured diagnostic kits. The antigen is bound to the plate before testing (Figure 16-8). The antibody to be tested is added, followed, after washing, by labeled antigen. The antibody binds the labeled antigen to the plate. This technique works well for testing whole blood because not all the unbound immunoglobulin has to be washed out.

A competitive ELISA can be used to measure hapten molecules or viral antigens (Figure 16-9). In this technique, antibody coats the inside wall of the microwell. In a single reaction, antigen from the test sample and enzyme-labeled antigen compete for the antibody-binding sites. The amount of labeled antigen bound to the solid phase (microwell) is inversely related to the concentration of antigen present in the test sample. This technique clearly has some speed advantages over other ELISA techniques. It can be made very sensitive if the sample antigen is permitted to react with the antibody before the labeled antigen conjugate is added.

Western Blotting

One solution to the problem of identifying protein antigens in a complex mixture is by use of a technique called Western blotting. This is a three-stage primary binding test (Figure 16-10). Stage 1 involves electrophoresis of

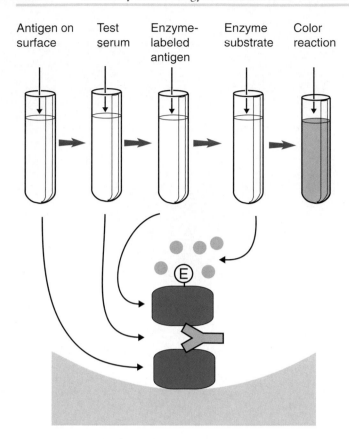

Figure 16-8. The labeled antigen ELISA. The serum under test is added to an antigen-coated plate. Bound antibodies are then detected by an enzyme-labeled antigen.

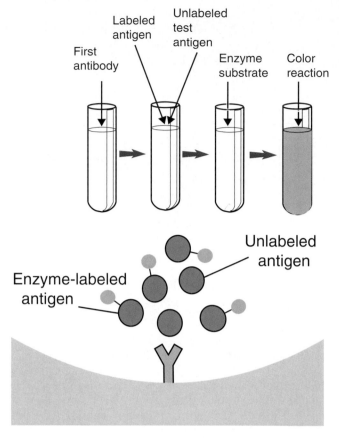

Figure 16-9. The competitive ELISA test. Labeled and unlabeled antigen compete for binding to antibody. Addition of the enzyme substrate leads to a color change inversely proportional to the amount of test antigen bound.

a protein mixture on gels so that each component is resolved into a single band. Stage 2 involves blotting or transfer of these protein bands to an immobilizing paper. This is accomplished by placing a nitrocellulose membrane on top of the gel to be transferred and sandwiching the two between sponges saturated with buffer. The sandwich is supported between rigid plastic sheets and placed in a buffer reservoir and an electrical current is passed between the sponges. The protein bands are rapidly transferred from the gel to the nitrocellulose membrane without loss of resolution.

The third stage involves visualization of transferred antigens by means of an enzyme immunoassay or radioimmunoassay. When an enzyme immunoassay is employed the membrane is first incubated in specific antiserum. After the membrane has been washed an enzyme-labeled antiglobulin solution is added. When this is removed by washing, substrate is added and a color develops in the bands where the antibody has bound to antigen. When isotope-labeled antiglobulin is used, an autoradiograph must be made and the labeled band identified by darkening of a photographic emulsion. Western blotting has proven very useful in identifying the important antigens in complex microorganisms or parasites (Figure 16-11). A variation of the Western blot is the dot blot. Antigen

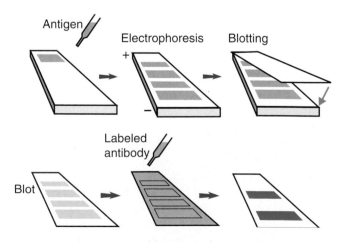

Figure 16-10. Western blotting technique. Serum is separated by electrophoresis and blotted onto nitrocellulose paper; the antigen bands are revealed by use of specific antibody and an enzyme- or isotope-labeled antiglobulin. The blotting stage may be a passive transfer or an electric potential may be used to accelerate the blotting process.

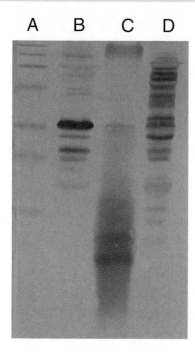

Figure 16-11. An allergic response to soy in dogs as detected by Western blotting. Soy extracts were first electrophoresed and blotted. The blot was then exposed to serum from a dog that was highly allergic to soy. The presence of bound IgE was detected by exposure to labeled anti-canine IgE. Each band represents an antigen from soy recognized by the dog's IgE. *A*, Prestained molecular weight markers. *B*, Globulin fraction of whole soy. *C*, Hydrolyzed soy globulin. *D*, Whey fraction of whole soy. (Courtesy of Dr. Robert Kennis.)

solution is drawn through a nitrocellulose filter so that any protein binds to the membrane. The presence of the antigen can be determined using specific antiserum and enzyme-labeled antiglobulin in sequence. After exposure to enzyme substrate, the presence of a stained dot is a positive reaction. (Use of nasal washings as a source of the antigen, such as when detecting respiratory viruses, is called a snot-blot!).

It is possible to put large numbers of different monoclonal antibodies as small dots on a single membrane or sheet. They may then be exposed to a complex labeled antigen mixture such as a cell protein extract, and after washing and developing, the relative concentrations of many different antigens can be visualized. This is known as an antibody microarray.

ELISAs can be used to test fluids other than blood. For example, saliva or tears can be tested for the presence of feline leukemia virus. In most cases these are simply modified versions of the serum ELISA tests. However, in one such test, a hard plastic swab with antibody to feline leukemia virus bound to the tip is rubbed throughout the cat's mouth. The antibodies on the swab are protected by a sugar coating that is removed by soaking before the test. The antibody on the swab will bind any viral antigen in the saliva. The swab is then incubated in a tube containing enzyme-labeled monoclonal antibodies against feline leukemia virus antigens. After washing, the swab is placed in a solution of the enzyme substrate and the color change noted. This technique is much less sensitive than testing blood directly but is very convenient.

Immunohistochemistry

Enzymes conjugated to immunoglobulins or antiglobulins can be used to locate specific antigens in tissue sections. Horseradish peroxidase is the most widely employed label. The tests are performed in a manner similar to the immunofluorescence tests. Thus in the direct immunoperoxidase test, the tissue section is treated with the enzyme-labeled antibody. After washing, the tissue is incubated in the appropriate enzyme substrate. Bound antibody is detected by the presence of a brown deposit at the site of antibody binding (Figure 16-12). In the indirect test, bound antibody is detected by means of a labeled antiglobulin. This technique has a very significant advantage over the immunofluorescence techniques in that the tissue can be examined by conventional light microscopy and can be stained so that structural relationships are easier to see.

DISPOSABLE IMMUNOASSAY DEVICES

Recent years have seen the development of simple immunoassays that can be employed in the clinic and will give useful information in a very short time. The most commonly used is the sandwich or excess reagent assay. These assays simply provide all necessary reagents in excess, and the sample to be tested becomes the limiting

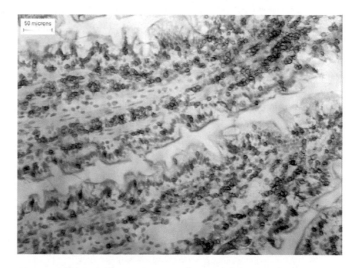

Figure 16-12. Immunoperoxidase technique showing α/β T cells in the lamina propria and epithelium of canine duodenum. Cells binding the monoclonal antibody are exposed to peroxidase-labeled specific antiglobulin. The presence of the peroxidase is revealed as a brown deposit. (From German AJ, Hall EJ, Moore PF, et al: *J Comp Pathol* 121:249-263, 1999.)

feature. Most disposable devices use this form of assay because the use of excess reagents makes the accurate metering of the sample unnecessary. Examples include immunofiltration and immunochromatography assays.

Immunofiltration

Membrane filter or flow-through devices are systems based on use of a capture antibody immobilized onto a membrane filter (Figure 16-13). One simple method uses a nylon membrane with a high immobilizing ability. The membrane, with antibody attached, is set on a support base connected to an absorbent bed. A test sample, such as blood containing antigen, flows through the membrane, followed sequentially at specific times by defined volumes of labeled antibody conjugate, wash solution, and enzyme substrate. A positive result, where antigen has bound, may be visualized as a colored dot or the creation of a plus sign. In this test, the negative sign area is formed by material that binds the enzyme conjugate (or by enzyme coupled to the matrix) and the other vertical bar that forms the plus sign is formed by capture antibody bound to the matrix. A modification, which allows the use of a whole-blood sample, includes either a blood-solubilizing dilution system or a prefilter to

remove cells. Because of the high surface area within these membranes, assay times can be significantly reduced. This form of test is commonly employed for the diagnosis of feline leukemia, feline immunodeficiency virus, and heartworm infections.

Immunochromatography

To make assays even faster and easier to read, immunochromatography assays are being increasingly employed. In their simplest form, these involve allowing an antigen solution (such as infected blood) to flow through a porous strip. As the solution passes through the strip it first passes through a zone where it meets and solubilizes dried labeled antibody conjugate and forms immune complexes. The antibody may be labeled with either colloidal gold (pink color) or colloidal selenium (blue color). The fluid then flows through a detection zone containing immobilized antibody against the antigen. This captures any immune complexes. As a result, a pink or blue line develops in the detection zone (Figure 16-14). Results are read by reading the line at a specific location. This simple procedure permits multiple samples to be analyzed in a simple one-step procedure. A positive control band can be developed as well and the use of an effective prefilter can permit the use of whole blood. This assay is used for the detection of heartworm or feline leukemia antigens.

The system can be manufactured in several different formats. For example, the sample containing the antigen of interest can be applied to a porous membrane at one end of the strip. Then capillary action can draw the solution through a conjugate pad, a solid-phase detection zone, and into an absorption pad. Buffer may be added to speed the flow of antigen solution. In another form of

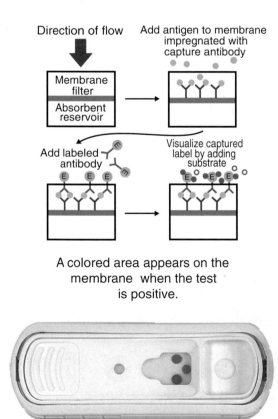

A colored area appears on the membrane when the test is positive.

Figure 16-13. Immunofiltration technique. Captured antibody is immobilized on a membrane and reagent samples are allowed to flow through sequentially. The final labeled product is seen as a colored bar or dot. In practice this method is used in the form of a plastic-mounted kit. (Courtesy of Idexx Inc.)

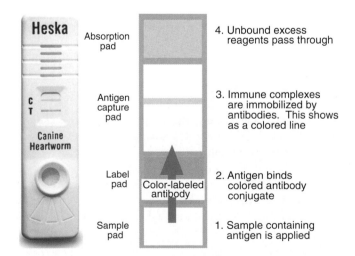

Figure 16-14. Immunochromatography. A sample containing antigen flows through a porous strip and positive reactions are shown by the appearance of a colored band. (Courtesy of Heska Inc.)

this assay, the antigen solution is dropped onto a pad containing antibody. This is followed by wash buffer that drives the immune complexes through the pad to an area containing the second antibody. The immune complexes are captured at this point. Then buffer can be applied at the other end of the pad and used to flush labeled antibody back to the detection zone where it forms a colored band.

ANTIBODY LABELS

Although radioisotopes and enzymes have been commonly used as labels for primary binding tests, both have disadvantages. For example, isotopes may have a short half-life, are potentially hazardous, and may require expensive detection devices. Enzymes, though stable and relatively cheap, are large molecules that may inhibit antibody activity or lose enzymatic activity in the process of being conjugated to antiglobulin. One alternative is to use the small molecule biotin and its specific binding protein, avidin. Biotin can bind to proteins without affecting their biological activity. Avidin binds very strongly and specifically to biotin and may be conjugated with enzymes.

The most popular enzymes used in ELISAs include alkaline phosphatase, horseradish peroxidase, and β-galactosidase. Enzyme assays involving the production of luminescent products, such as luciferase, may be many times more sensitive than conventional enzyme assays but require sophisticated instruments to measure the luminescence produced. Colored dyes linked to antibodies have been used in dipstick assays. Reagents linked to ferritin or colloidal gold may be used to identify the location of antigens on cell surfaces examined by electron microscopy because such labels are electron dense. As described above, colloidal gold and colloidal selenium are colored and so can be used as labels in simple immunochromatography tests.

SECONDARY BINDING TESTS

The reactions between antigens and antibodies are commonly followed by a secondary reaction. Thus if antibodies combine with soluble antigens in solution, the resulting complexes may precipitate. If antigens are particulate (e.g., bacteria or red blood cells), then antibodies may make them clump or agglutinate. If an antibody can activate the classical complement pathway and the antigen is on a cell surface, then cell lysis may result.

PRECIPITATION

If a solution of soluble antigen is mixed with a strong antiserum, the mixture becomes cloudy within a few minutes, and then flocculent; finally a precipitate settles to the bottom of the tube within an hour. The precipitate consists of antigen–antibody complexes. If increasing amounts of soluble antigen are mixed with a constant amount of antibody, the amount of precipitate that develops is determined by the relative proportions of the reactants. No obvious precipitate is formed at low antigen concentrations. As the amount of antigen increases, larger quantities of precipitate form until the amount is maximal. However, with the addition of yet more antigen, the amount of precipitate gradually diminishes, until none is observed in tubes containing a large excess of antigen (Figure 16-15). Horse antibodies behave in a somewhat different fashion, producing a distinct flocculation over a very narrow range of antigen concentrations (Figure 16-16). This is a particular property of the IgG3 subclass.

In the first stage of these reactions, only a little antigen is complexed to antibody and little precipitate is deposited. In the tubes where most precipitation occurs, both antigen and antibody are completely complexed and neither can be detected in the supernatant fluid. This is called the equivalence zone, and the ratio of antibody to antigen is optimal. When antigen is added to excess, little precipitate is formed, although soluble immune complexes are present and free antigen may be detected in the supernatant fluid.

This result is due to the fact that antibodies are usually bivalent and therefore can cross-link only two epitopes at a time, but complex antigens are generally multivalent, possessing many epitopes (Figure 16-17). Where there is excess antibody, each antigen molecule is covered with antibody, preventing cross-linkage and thus precipitation. When the reactants are in optimal proportions, the ratio of antigen to antibody is such that cross-linking and lattice formation are extensive. As this lattice grows it becomes insoluble and eventually precipitates. In mixtures where antigen is in excess, each antibody molecule is bound to two antigen molecules. Further cross-linkage is impossible, and since these complexes are small and soluble, no precipitation occurs. Mononuclear phagocytes are most efficient at binding and removing complexes formed at optimal proportions and in antibody excess. Small immune complexes formed in antigen excess are poorly removed by phagocytic cells but are deposited in vessel walls and in glomeruli, where they cause type III hypersensitivity reactions (Chapter 28).

Immunodiffusion

One simple method of demonstrating precipitation of antigen by antibody is immunodiffusion or gel diffusion. Round wells, about 5 mm in diameter and about 1 cm apart, are cut in a layer of clear agar. One well is then filled with soluble antigen and the other with antiserum; the reactants diffuse out radially. Where the reactants meet in optimal proportions an opaque white line of precipitate appears (Figure 16-18).

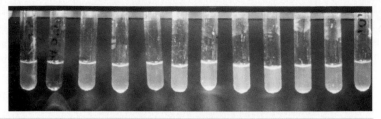

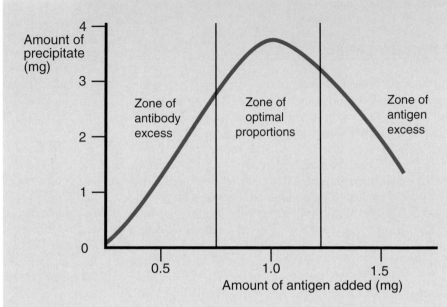

Figure 16-15. Effect of mixing increasing amounts of antigen (bovine serum) with a constant amount of antibody (rabbit antiserum). The tube with the greatest amount of precipitate is the one in which the ratio of antigen to antibody is optimal. A quantitative precipitation curve of this test shows this effect graphically.

If the solutions used contain several different antigens and antibodies, each component is unlikely to reach optimal proportions in exactly the same position. Consequently, a separate line of precipitate is produced for each interacting set of antigens and antibodies. This test can be used to determine the relationship between antigens. If two antigen wells and one antibody well are set up as in Figures 16-18 and 16-19, then lines will form between each antigen well and the antibody well. If these two lines join, the two antigens are probably identical. If the lines cross, then the two antigens are completely different. If the lines merge with spur formation, a partial identity exists, indicating that one antigen possesses epitopes not present in the other. The Coggins test is a gel diffusion method used to detect antibodies against equine infectious anemia virus in horse serum. In this test an extract of infected horse spleen or a cell culture antigen reacts with the serum of the horse under test in agar gel, and the development of a line of precipitate constitutes a positive reaction. A similar test is used to identify cattle infected with bovine leukemia virus.

Radial Immunodiffusion

If an antigen solution is placed in a well and allowed to diffuse into agar in which specific antiserum has been incorporated, then a ring of precipitate will form around the antigen well. The area of this ring is directly related to the amount of antigen added to the well. A standard curve may therefore be constructed using known amounts of antigen (Figure 16-20). Unknown solutions of antigen can then be accurately assayed by comparing the ring diameters from unknowns with the standard curve.

Immunoelectrophoresis and Related Techniques

Although conventional gel diffusion techniques give a separate precipitation line for each antigen–antibody system in a mixture, it is often difficult to resolve all the

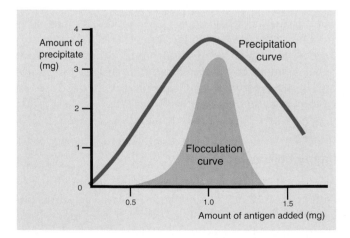

Figure 16-16. Quantitative precipitation curve of the type obtained when horse serum is used as a source of antibody. Flocculation occurs only over a narrow range of antigen–antibody mixtures.

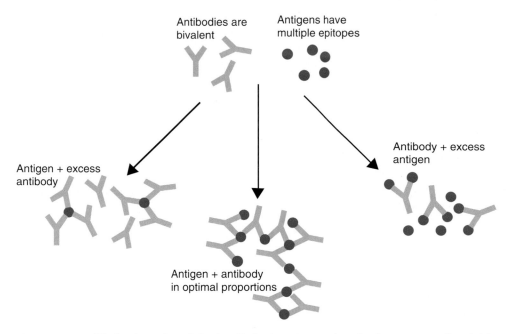

Figure 16-17. Mechanism of precipitation. In both antigen and antibody excess, small, soluble, immune complexes are produced. However, at optimal proportions, large insoluble complexes are generated.

components in a complex mixture. One way to improve the resolution of the system is by separating the antigen mixture by electrophoresis before undertaking immunodiffusion. This technique is called immunoelectrophoresis and is it used to identify proteins in body fluids (Figure 16-21).

Immunoelectrophoresis involves the electrophoresis of the antigen mixture in agar gel in one direction. A trough is then cut in the agar just to one side and parallel to this line of separated proteins. Antiserum is placed in this trough and allowed to diffuse laterally. When the diffusing

antibodies encounter antigen, curved lines of precipitate are formed. One arc of precipitation forms for each of the constituents in the antigen mixture. This technique can resolve the proteins of normal serum into 25 to 40 distinct precipitation bands (Figure 16-22). This

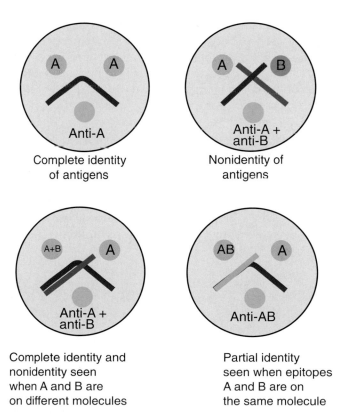

Complete identity
of antigens

Nonidentity of
antigens

Complete identity and
nonidentity seen
when A and B are
on different molecules

Partial identity
seen when epitopes
A and B are on
the same molecule

Figure 16-19. Gel diffusion technique to determine the relationship of two antigens.

Figure 16-18. Precipitation in agar gel. Antigen and antibody diffusing from their respective wells precipitate in a region where optimal proportions are achieved. In this example, the antigen is identical in both top wells. As a result, the precipitation lines fuse to show complete identity.

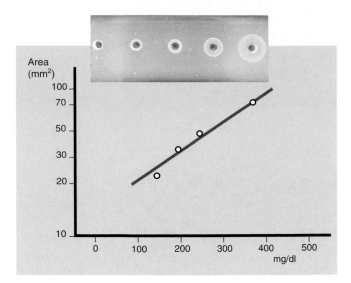

Figure 16-20. Radial immunodiffusion. The area of precipitation is proportional to the concentration of antigen. In this case antiserum to bovine IgA is incorporated in the agar and is used to measure bovine serum IgA levels.

technique is used to identify the absence of a normal serum protein as in animals with a congenital deficiency of some complement components. It is also used to detect the presence of excessive amounts of an individual component, as in animals with myeloma (Figure 11-23).

If, instead of being permitted to passively diffuse into agar-containing antiserum as in the radial immunodiffusion technique, the antigen is driven into the antiserum agar by electrophoresis, then the ring of precipitation around each well becomes deformed into a rocket shape. The length of the rocket is proportional to the amount of antigen placed in each well. This technique is called rocket electrophoresis.

TITRATION OF ANTIBODIES

Although the simple detection of antibodies or antigen is sufficient for many purposes, it is usually desirable to quantitate the reaction. One way of measuring specific antibody levels is by titration. The serum under test is diluted in a series of decreasing concentrations (Figure 16-23). Each dilution is then tested for activity. The reciprocal of the highest dilution giving a positive reaction, called the titer, provides an estimate of the amount of antibody in that serum.

AGGLUTINATION

Because antibodies are bivalent they can cross-link particulate antigens such as bacteria or foreign red cells, resulting in their clumping or agglutination. Antibodies differ in their ability to cause agglutination; for example, IgM antibodies are more efficient than IgG antibodies (Table 16-2). If excess antibody is added to a suspension of antigenic particles, then, just as in the precipitation reaction, each particle may be so coated by antibody that agglutination is inhibited. This lack of reactivity at high concentrations of antibody is termed a prozone. Another cause of prozone formation is the presence of antibodies that cannot cause agglutination. These nonagglutinating antibodies are also called incomplete antibodies. The reason for their lack of agglutinating activity is not completely understood; one possibility is that the epitopes with which they react lie deep within the surface coat of the particle, so deep that cross-linking cannot occur. An alternative suggestion is that they are capable of only restricted movement in their hinge region, causing them to be functionally monovalent.

Antiglobulin Tests

If it is necessary to test for the presence of nonagglutinating antibodies on the surface of particles such as bacteria or erythrocytes, then a direct antiglobulin test may be used. The washed particles are mixed with an antiglobulin, and if immunoglobulins are present on their surface, then agglutination will occur (Figure 16-24).

Passive Agglutination

Since agglutination is a much more sensitive technique than precipitation, it is sometimes useful to convert a precipitating system to an agglutinating one (Figure 16-25).

Figure 16-21. Technique of immunoelectrophoresis (see text for details).

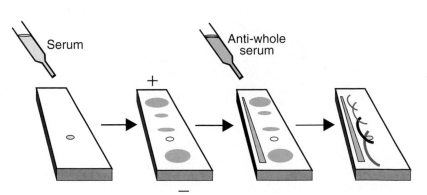

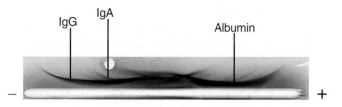

Figure 16-22. Immunoelectrophoresis of pig serum showing the lines of precipitation produced by some of the major serum proteins. (See also Figure 11-23.)

TABLE 16-2
Role of Specific Immunoglobulin Classes in Serological Assays

Property	IgG	IgM	IgA	IgG (T)
Agglutination	+	+++	+	−
Complement activation	+	+++	−	−
Precipitation	+++	+	±	±
Time of appearance (days)	3–7	2–5	3–7	3–7
Time to peak titer (days)	7–21	5–14	7–21	7–21

This may be done by chemically linking soluble antigen to inert particles such as erythrocytes, bacteria, or latex beads. Erythrocytes are among the best particles for this purpose, and tests that employ coated erythrocytes are called passive hemagglutination tests.

An interesting modern variant of hemagglutination tests is the use of bifunctional monoclonal antibodies. A bifunctional monoclonal antibody can be made by breaking the bonds between the two heavy chains so that two identical halves are formed. Two halves from different immunoglobulins are then joined to produce a molecule that can cross-link two different epitopes. For example, a bifunctional antibody can be made whereby one antigen-binding site is directed against canine red blood cells and the other against adult heartworm (*Dirofilaria immitis*) antigen (Figure 16-26). When this reagent is mixed with whole blood from a heartworm-infected dog, it cross-links the heartworm antigen to the red cells, resulting in visible hemagglutination within a few minutes.

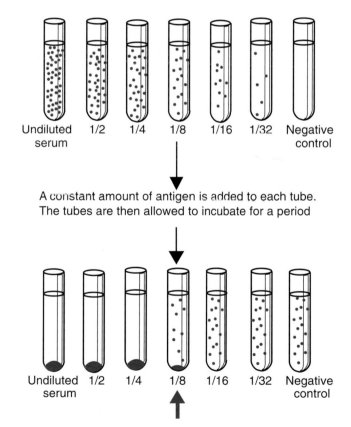

A constant amount of antigen is added to each tube. The tubes are then allowed to incubate for a period

Figure 16-23. Principle of antibody titration. Serum is first diluted in a series of tubes. A constant amount of antigen is then added to each tube and the tubes are incubated. At the end of the incubation period, the last tube in which a reaction has occurred is identified. In this example, agglutination has occurred in all tubes up to a serum dilution of 1:8. The agglutination titer of the serum is said to be 8.

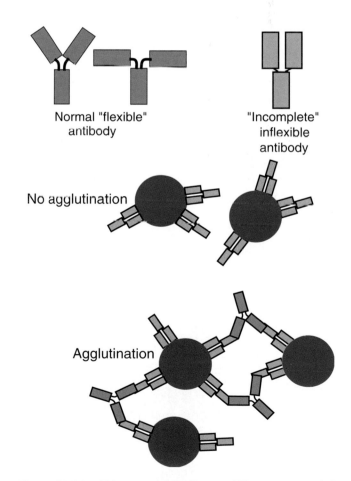

Figure 16-24. Direct antiglobulin test. The presence of the antiglobulin is required to agglutinate particles coated with nonagglutinating antibody.

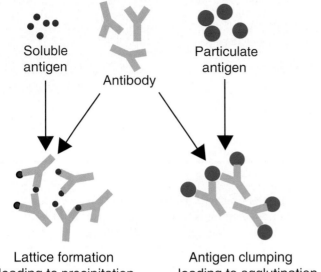

Figure 16-25.   Relationship between precipitation and agglutination. This is essentially a consequence of the size of the antigenic particle. Large particles agglutinate. Small particles and soluble molecules precipitate.

VIRAL HEMAGGLUTINATION AND ITS INHIBITION

Some viruses can bind and agglutinate mammalian and avian red cells. This virus-induced hemagglutination may assist in characterizing an unknown virus. Inhibition of viral hemagglutination by antibody can be used either as

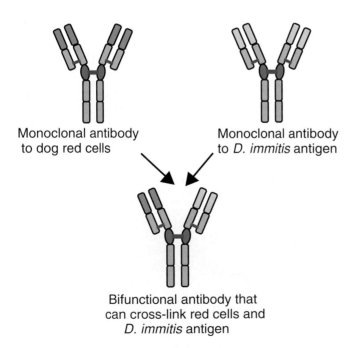

Figure 16-26.   Use of bifunctional antibodies to cross-link two different epitopes. In this example the antibody cross-links canine red cells with heartworm antigens. If the antibody is mixed with infected dog blood it will cause visible hemagglutination.

a method of identifying a specific virus or to measure antibody levels in serum. Hemagglutinating organisms include orthomyxoviruses and paramyxoviruses, alphaviruses, flaviviruses, and bunyaviruses as well as some adenoviruses, reoviruses, parvoviruses, and coronaviruses. They also include some mycoplasma such as *Mycoplasma gallisepticum*.

COMPLEMENT FIXATION

The activation of the classical complement pathway by antibody bound to antigen results in the generation of membrane attack complexes that can disrupt cell membranes. If the antibody is bound to red cells, these are ruptured and hemolysis occurs. This phenomenon can be used to measure serum antibody levels in a test called the complement fixation test.

The complement fixation test is performed in two parts. First, antigen and antibodies (the serum under test deprived of its complement by heating at 56° C) are incubated in the presence of normal guinea pig serum as a source of complement. (Guinea pig serum is most commonly used because its complement lyses sheep red cells well.) After the antigen–antibody–complement mixture reacts, the amount of free complement remaining in the mixture is measured by adding an indicator system consisting of antibody-coated sheep red cells. Lysis of these cells (seen as the development of a transparent red solution) is a negative result because it indicates that complement was not activated and that antibody was absent from the serum under test (Figure 16-27). Absence of lysis (seen as a cloudy red cell suspension), indicating that complement was consumed (or fixed), is a positive result. It is usual to titrate the serum being tested so that, if antibodies are present in that serum, as it is diluted the reaction in each tube will change from no lysis (positive) to lysis (negative). The titer is the highest dilution of serum in which no more than 50% of the red cells are lysed.

Cytotoxicity Tests

Complement may cause membrane damage, not only to erythrocytes but also to nucleated cells and to protozoa. Antibodies against cell surface antigens thus may be measured by reacting target cells with antibody and complement and estimating the resulting cell death. This form of assay is employed in the identification of major histocompatibility complex class I molecules.

ASSAYS IN LIVING SYSTEMS

If an organism or antigen possesses biological activity, antibodies can be measured by their ability to neutralize this activity. The activities that may be neutralized

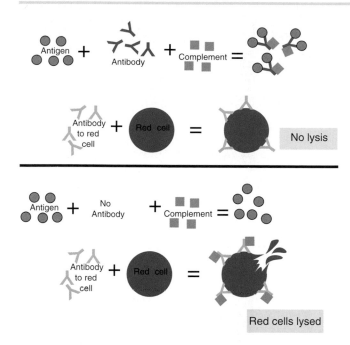

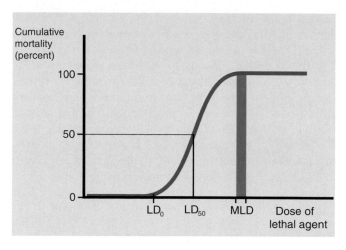

Figure 16-28. A cumulative mortality curve showing how the LD_{50} provides a more accurate estimate of the lethal effects of a toxin than either the LD_0 or the MLD.

Figure 16-27. Principle of the complement fixation test. Complement, if fixed by antigen and antibody, is unavailable to lyse the target cells in the indicator system. In the absence of antibody the complement remains unfixed and is available to lyse the indicator system.

include hemolysis of erythrocytes, lysis of nucleated cells, and disease or death in animals. Reactions such as these are subject to a high degree of variability because they tend to change gradually over a wide range of doses of organism or antigen. For this reason, results obtained from a single positive or negative neutralization test are usually of little use. For example, 0.003 mg of tetanus toxin may kill some mice in a test group, but about five times that dose is required to kill all mice in the same group. In addition, if an attempt is made to assess the lowest dose of tetanus toxin that will kill all the animals in a group (the minimal lethal dose), it is found to be highly variable. It is equally difficult to estimate with precision the highest dose of toxin that will just fail to kill all test animals. The most precise method of measuring the lethal effects of a toxin has therefore been to estimate the dose that will just kill 50% of a group of test animals (Figure 16-28). In practice, it is usually not possible to arrive at this 50% end point by direct experimentation, and it is necessary to calculate it by plotting the results against the dose of toxin given and arriving at the 50% end point by calculation.

In the example cited in the previous paragraph, the lethality of the toxin can be estimated by measuring the dose required to kill 50% of a group of experimental animals. This is called the LD_{50}. Similarly, the dose of complement that just lyses 50% of a red cell suspension is called the CH_{50}. The dose of organisms that infects

50% of animals is the ID_{50}, the dose that just infects 50% of tissue cultures is the $TCID_{50}$, and the dose of antiserum or vaccine that protects 50% of challenged animals is the PD_{50}.

Neutralization Tests

Neutralization tests estimate the ability of antibody to neutralize the biological activity of antigen when mixed with it in vitro. These tests may be used to identify bacterial toxins such as *Clostridium perfringens* α-toxin or staphylococcal α-toxin.

Viruses may be prevented from infecting cells after specific antibody has combined with and blocked their critical attachment sites. This reaction is the basis of the neutralization tests that are employed either for the identification of unknown viruses or for the measurement of specific antiviral antibody. Neutralization tests are highly specific and extremely sensitive. Thus, antiserum to coliphage T4 will neutralize phage-induced lysis of *Escherichia coli* because antibodies can block the receptor on the phage tail, thus preventing its attachment to a bacterium. A single antibody molecule is sufficient to cause this blockage, and a phage neutralization test may therefore detect as little as 0.00005 mg of antibody.

Protection Tests

A protection test is a form of neutralization test carried out entirely in vivo. The protective properties of a specific antiserum are measured by administering it in increasing dilutions to a group of test animals, which may then be challenged with a standard dose of pathogenic organisms or toxin. Although protection tests provide a direct measure of the therapeutic efficacy of an antiserum, they are also subject to great experimental variation because of differences among animals. Thus animals differ in their susceptibility to infection and in a number of other factors, such as the rate of absorption of antiserum, the level of activity of the mononuclear phagocyte system, and the half-life of the passively administered immunoglobulin. As in neutralization tests, meaningful results can be obtained only if large numbers of animals are employed and if the challenge does is carefully standardized. It is usual to use a dose of organisms or toxin containing a known number of LD_{50} or ID_{50}. Similarly, the protective effect of an antiserum may be expressed in PD_{50}, the dose required to protect 50% of a group of animals.

DIAGNOSTIC APPLICATIONS OF IMMUNOLOGICAL TESTS

Obviously, the presence of antibodies to a specific organism in an animal's serum indicates previous exposure to an epitope present on that organism. It does not, however, prove that infection exists or that any concurrent disease is actually caused by the organism in question. An immune response to an invading microorganism generates specific antibodies. These are a heterogeneous mixture. The specificity of the serum will reflect the dominant specificity of the antibody mixture. For example, the fact that the sera of most healthy horses contain antibodies to *Salmonella enterica var. typhimurium* does not prove that most horses have salmonellosis. Thus, the presence of antibodies to an organism in a single serum sample is rarely of diagnostic significance. Only if at least two samples are taken 1 to 3 weeks apart and at least a fourfold rise in titer is shown can a diagnosis be made. This should be done only in conjunction with careful analysis of clinical factors.

A second feature that must be considered in the interpretation of serological results is the possibility of errors. Technical errors are usually prevented by incorporation of appropriate controls into the test system. Other errors, however, are largely unavoidable. These may be of two types: false-positive results and false-negative results. A test in which a large proportion of the positive results is false is considered to be nonspecific, whereas one with a very high proportion of false-negative results is considered to be insensitive. In general, the level of such errors is set by the criteria used to differentiate positive from negative reactions (Figure 16-29). If these criteria are adjusted so that the number of false-positive results is reduced, then there will be an increasing proportion of false-negative results encountered, and vice versa. Thus, highly sensitive tests tend to be relatively nonspecific and highly specific tests are generally insensitive. The establishment of criteria in reading tests and, from this, the sensitivity and specificity of a test are determined both by the requirements of the test procedure and by the importance of false-positive and false-negative reactions. In ideal tests, it would be

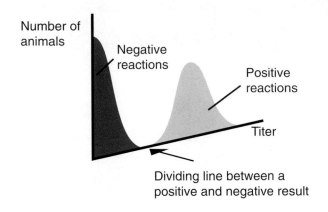

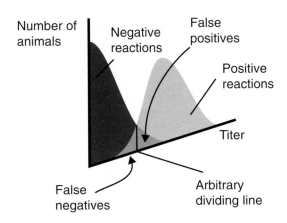

Figure 16-29. Schematic diagrams depicting the errors associated with immunological tests. The top diagram depicts an ideal test in which there is no ambiguity in interpreting test results. The bottom diagram depicts a more typical test in which an arbitrary line must be used to separate positive from negative results. By moving this dividing line the relative proportions of false-positive and false-negative results may be changed.

desirable for the criteria used in interpreting the test results to be so obvious and absolute that each test would be absolutely sensitive and specific. Unfortunately, such ideal tests are uncommon.

As has been evident from the discussions earlier in this chapter, the advantages and disadvantages of each immunodiagnostic test vary according to the specific requirements of the investigator, the nature of the antigen employed, and the complexity, sensitivity, and specificity of each method. In general, the selection of a diagnostic test represents a compromise among its sensitivity, its specificity, and its complexity, that is, the number of steps involved, the degree of technical expertise required, its cost, and the nature of the equipment needed to conduct the test. Although precise guidelines cannot be drawn, it is usually most appropriate to use the most sensitive and specific test that can be satisfactorily performed with the available technical assistance and equipment, at the lowest cost.

SOURCES OF ADDITIONAL INFORMATION

Bolton AE: Antisera for radioimmunoassay, *Irish Vet J* 35: 143-153, 1981.

Boto WMO, Powers KG, Levy DA: Antigens of *Dirofilaria immitis* which are immunogenic in the canine host: detection by immuno-staining of protein blots with the antibodies of occult dogs, *J Immunol* 133:975-980, 1984.

Bradley GA, Calderwood Mays MB: Immunoperoxidase staining for the detection of autoantibodies in canine autoimmune skin disease; comparison of immunofluorescence results, *Vet Immunol Immunopathol* 26:105-113, 1990.

Carter GR, Moojen V: A summary of serologic tests used to detect common infectious diseases of animals, *Vet Med/Small Anim Clin* 76:1725-1730, 1981.

Cripps AW, Husband AJ, Scicchitano R, Sheldrake RF: Quantitation of sheep IgG_1, IgA and IgM and albumin by radioimmunoassay, *Vet Immunol Immunopathol* 8:137-147, 1985.

Diamond BA, Yelton DE, Scharff MD: Monoclonal antibodies: a new technology for producing serologic reagents, *N Engl J Med* 304:1344-1349, 1981.

Friedman H, Linna TJ, Prier JE (eds): *Immunoserology in the diagnosis of infectious diseases*, University Park Press, 1979, Baltimore.

Gerstman BB, Cappucci DT: Evaluating the reliability of diagnostic test results, *J Am Vet Med Assoc* 188:248-251, 1986.

Golden CA: Overview of the state of the art of immunoassay screening tests, *J Am Vet Med Assoc* 198:827-830, 1991.

Gwozdz JM, Thompson KG, Murray A, et al: Comparison of three serological tests and an interferon-γ assay for the diagnosis of paratuberculosis in experimentally infected sheep, *Aust Vet J* 78:779-783, 2000.

McVicker JK, Rouse GC, Fowler MA, et al: Evaluation of a lateral-flow immunoassay for use in monitoring passive transfer of immunoglobulins in calves, *Am J Vet Res* 63: 247-250, 2002.

Rose NR, Friedman H (eds): *Manual of clinical immunology*, 2nd ed, American Society of Microbiology, 1980, Washington, DC.

Schultz RD, Adams LS: Immunologic methods for detection of humoral and cellular immunity, *Vet Clin North Am (Small Anim Prac)* 8:721-753, 1978.

Scott MA, Kaiser L, Davis JM, Schwartz KA: development of a sensitive immunoradiometric assay for detection of platelet-surface-associated immunoglobulins in thrombocytopenic dogs, *Am J Vet Res* 63:124-136, 2002.

Sutherland SS: Immunology of bovine brucellosis. *Vet Bull* 50:359-368, 1980.

Voller A, deSavigny D: Enzyme linked immunosorbent assay (ELISA), In: *Techniques in clinical immunology* (RA Thompson, ed). Blackwell Science, 1981, London.

Wilchek M, Bayer EA: The avidin–biotin complex in immunology, *Immunol Today* 5:39-43, 1984.

Williams JD, Heck FC, Davis DS, Adams LG: Comparison of results from five serologic methods used for detecting *Brucella abortus* antibody activity in coyote sera, *Vet Immunol Immunopathol* 29:79-88 1991.

Worthington RW: Serology as an aid to diagnosis: uses and abuses, *N Z Vet J* 30:93-97, 1982.

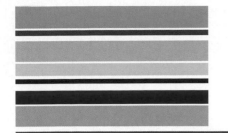

T-Cell Function and the Destruction of Cell-Associated Invaders

CHAPTER 17

Antibodies bind to invading organisms in the circulation or tissue fluids, hastening their elimination. However, not all foreign organisms are found outside cells. All viruses and some bacteria grow inside cells in sites inaccessible to antibody. Antibodies are therefore of limited usefulness in defending the body against these invaders. Viruses and other intracellular organisms are eliminated by other mechanisms. Either the infected cell is killed rapidly so that the invader has no time to grow or the infected cell develops the ability to destroy the intracellular organism. In general, organisms such as viruses that enter the cell cytoplasm or nucleus are killed through cytotoxicity, whereas organisms such as bacteria or parasites that reside within cytoplasmic vacuoles are destroyed through cell activation. T cells mediate both processes. The antigens that trigger these responses arise from intracellular locations and are therefore called endogenous antigens.

ENDOGENOUS ANTIGENS

As described in Chapter 6, every time a cell makes a protein, a sample is processed and small peptides are carried to the cell surface bound to the antigen-binding groove of MHC class I molecules (Figure 17-1). If these peptides are not recognized by T cells, then no response is triggered. If, however, the peptide–MHC complex binds to a T-cell receptor (TCR), then that T cell is triggered to respond. Thus when a cell is infected by a virus, T cells may recognize many of the peptides from viral proteins. The T cells that respond to these endogenous antigens are CD8$^+$. CD8 is the receptor that T cells use to bind MHC class I molecules.

PROGRAMMED CELL DEATH

All old, surplus, damaged, or abnormal cells that would otherwise interfere with normal tissue functions must be promptly removed from the body. These cells are killed by programmed cell death where the cell plays an active role in its own demise. Apoptosis is the best characterized form of programmed cell death. Apoptosis is characterized by membrane blebbing, flipping of phosphatidylserine in the plasma membrane, nuclear fragmentation, and activation of a family of cell suicide proteases called caspases. There are two major pathways of apoptosis. One pathway is triggered by cytokines such as tumor necrosis factor-α (TNF-α) acting through specific receptors. This is called the extrinsic or "death receptor" pathway. The other pathway is triggered by the release of cytochrome c from mitochondria and so is known as the intrinsic or mitochondria-dependent pathway (Figure 17-2). In cells dying through the extrinsic pathway, ligand binding to death receptors leads to the formation of a death-inducing signaling complex (DISC). This complex contains caspase 8 and caspase 10. In cells dying through the intrinsic pathway, cytochrome c triggers the formation of a complex polymer called an apoptosome. The apoptosome recruits and activates caspase 9. Irrespective of their origin, the caspases then initiate an enzyme cascade that degrades cytoplasmic and skeletal proteins and leads to endonuclease activation and cell death. Apoptotic cells characteristically fragment their DNA into many low-molecular-weight fragments. This fragmentation may be responsible for the characteristic chromatin condensation. In apoptotic cells dying by either pathway, the nuclear chromatin condenses against the nuclear membrane (Figure 17-3). Affected cells shrink

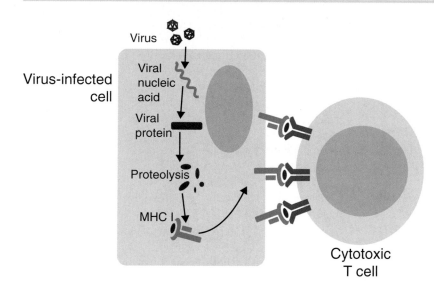

Figure 17-1. Processing of endogenous antigen. Endogenous antigen is first broken down into small peptides and inserted into the antigen-binding groove of MHC class I molecules. When presented on a cell surface, antigen bound to MHC class I antigens triggers a cytotoxic T-cell response.

and detach from the surrounding cells. Eventually nuclear fragmentation and cytoplasmic budding occur and form cell fragments called apoptotic bodies (Figure 17-4).

As cells die, the lipid phosphatidylserine is exposed on their surface. This lipid binds to receptors on macrophages and dendritic cells and triggers phagocytosis. It also triggers the release of anti-inflammatory cytokines such as transforming growth factor-β (TGF-β) while inhibiting the release of proinflammatory cytokines such as TNF-α.

When dendritic cells phagocytose apoptotic cells, they process the protein molecules from these cells and present them as antigen–MHC complexes on their surface. However, they do not express costimulatory molecules at this time. As a result, any T cells that recognize this antigen are not costimulated. They will be selectively

turned off and tolerance results. The anti-inflammatory cytokines will also tend to ensure that T cells remain unresponsive.

If cells are severely damaged as a result of trauma, toxicity, or microbial invasion, they will die and undergo necrosis. (Apoptosis is an active process; necrosis is a passive process). Cells killed by necrosis trigger inflammation. Thus HMG-1 (Box 4-2) from the cell nucleus is a potent inflammatory mediator. Likewise, when dendritic cells engulf necrotic cells, they not only process their proteins into MHC–antigen complexes, but they also express costimulatory molecules. T cells that recognize this antigen will therefore be turned on. Thus a cell killed by a virus will trigger significant inflammation and provoke a potent T-cell response to the viral antigens.

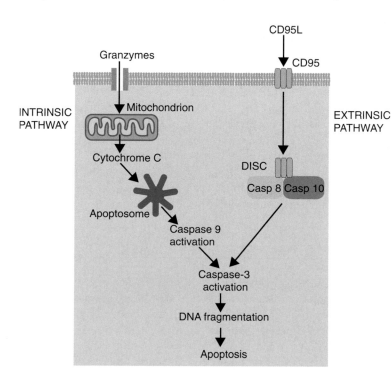

Figure 17-2. The two pathways by which apoptosis may be triggered. Both lead to caspase activation, DNA fragmentation, and cell death. The intrinsic pathway is activated by ligation of death receptors such as CD95 and formation of the death-inducing signaling complex (DISC). The intrinsic pathway is initiated by multiple damage signals, including injection of granzymes, and leads to the release of cytochrome C from mitochondria, the formation of an apoptosome, and activation of caspase 9.

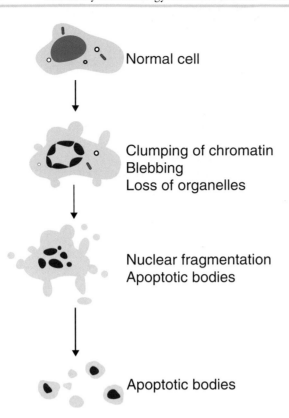

Normal cell

Clumping of chromatin
Blebbing
Loss of organelles

Nuclear fragmentation
Apoptotic bodies

Apoptotic bodies

Figure 17-3. Major morphological features of cell death by apoptosis.

CELL COOPERATION

During the generation of a primary immune response, CD8[+] cytotoxic T cells cannot respond to infected cells by themselves alone. There are about 10^{13} nucleated cells in a human-sized body and possibly several hundred native T cells with receptors for any individual viral

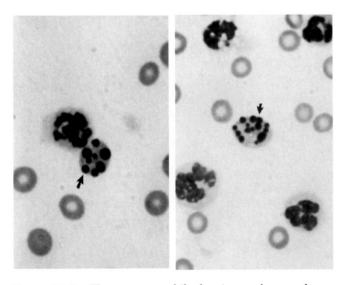

Figure 17-4. Two rat neutrophils showing nuclear condensation and fragmentation characteristic of apoptosis. (Courtesy of Ms. K Kennon.)

antigen. Clearly it would be almost impossible for these T cells to find individual virus-infected cells by themselves. The antigen must first be brought to them. Naive cytotoxic T cells in fact remain within lymphoid tissues and antigen is carried to them by dendritic cells. A subset of dendritic cells takes up endogenous antigen and attaches it to their MHC class I molecules. This is then carried to the lymphoid organs where it is presented to CD8[+] T cells. If they are to respond to this processed antigen these CD8[+] cells must also be costimulated by CD4[+] Th1 cells. Costimulation is only effective if both CD8[+] and CD4[+] T cells recognize antigen on the same antigen-presenting cell. Thus a T helper cell first interacts with the antigen-presenting dendritic cell in the normal way through CD40 and its ligand CD154. Immature dendritic cells express low levels of MHC and costimulatory molecules and are ineffective cell stimulators. T helper cells, however, activate the dendritic cells, up-regulating their expression of MHC and stimulating production of molecules such as interleukin-12 (IL-12) and the T-cell chemotactic chemokine CCL22. Only when it is fully activated can a dendritic cell successfully trigger a cytotoxic T-cell response.

The activated dendritic cells present peptides associated with MHC class I molecules to CD8[+] T cells. They can do this readily if the dendritic cells are themselves infected. However, they may also present peptides from nonreplicating organisms or dying infected cells. Thus by processing dying cells, dendritic cells activate T cells against endogenous antigens. These cytotoxic T-cell functions do not require CD40/CD154 interaction. The activated cytotoxic T cells receive three key signals. The first is IL-12 secreted by activated dendritic cells. The second signal comes from the endogenous antigen/MHC class I complex on an abnormal cell. The third signal comes from IL-2 and interferon-γ (IFN-γ) secreted by Th1 cells. Once all signals are received, the CD8 T cells will respond.

In CD8 T cells, different responses are triggered by different levels of stimulation. Thus T-cell cytotoxicity can be readily induced by a much lower threshold than cytokine synthesis. Likewise, although activated cytotoxic T cells can be readily stimulated by brief exposure to antigen, naive T cells have to be stimulated for several hours before responding. However, the required stimulation time can be shortened by increasing TCR occupancy or by providing more costimulation.

CYTOTOXIC T-CELL RESPONSES

Once fully activated, CD8[+] T cells leave the lymphoid organs and seek infected cells by themselves. When an activated CD8[+] T cell recognizes an MHC–antigen complex expressed on another cell and its TCR is occupied, then it kills the target cell. Although most cells can be triggered to undergo apoptosis by specific signals, the cytotoxic T cell is able to induce apoptosis in any cell it recognizes. Recognition of a single peptide–MHC class I complex on a target cell is sufficient to trigger this cytotoxicity. Cytotoxic T cells are larger than unstimulated lymphocytes and are pyroninophilic, reflecting the presence of many ribosomes and their ability to synthesize proteins (Figure 17-5).

Once activated, cytotoxic T cells kill their targets through one of two apoptotic pathways. One pathway involves the secretion of proteins called perforins and granzymes (the perforin pathway) (Figure 17-6). This kills cells through the intrinsic route. The other pathway kills cells through a death receptor called CD95 or fas (the CD95 pathway) (Figure 17-7). Both pathways require physical contact between the cytotoxic T cell and its target. These two pathways account for all the cytotoxic activity of T cells because if both are knocked out the T-cell cytotoxicity is completely abolished. The perforin pathway is used primarily to destroy virus-infected cells whereas the CD95 pathway is used to destroy unwanted T cells.

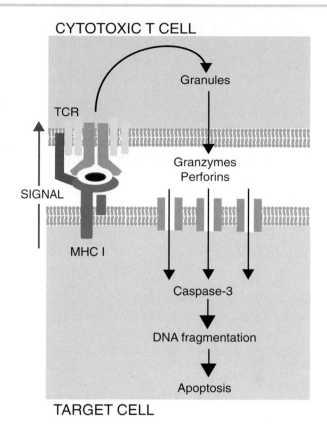

Figure 17-6.   The perforin pathway by which T cells kill targets.

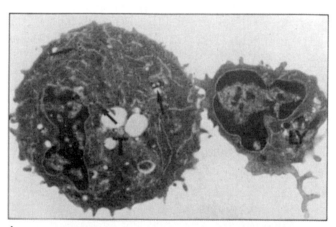

A

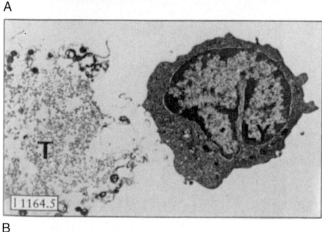

B

Figure 17-5.   Destruction of target cells by cytotoxic T cells. **A,** Conjugation between a peritoneal exudate lymphocyte (the small cell on the right) and a target cell. Note the lysosome-like bodies *(LY)* and the nuclear fragmentation of the target cell *(T)*. **B,** A lymphocyte with the remains of a lysed target cell. (From Zagury D et al: *Eur J Immunol* 5:881, 1975.)

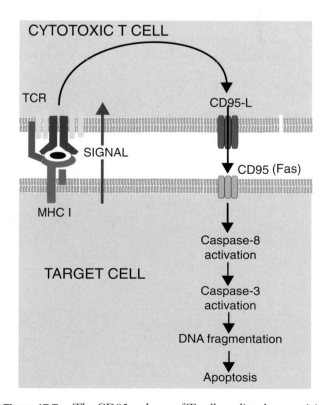

Figure 17-7.   The CD95 pathway of T-cell-mediated cytotoxicity.

Cytotoxic T cell killing is highly efficient. Movies show that the cytotoxic T lymphocyte can kill a target cell within 2 to 10 minutes. They are also serial killers that can move on to kill other cells within 5 to 6 minutes.

The Perforin Pathway

This pathway is used primarily to kill virus-infected cells. The killing process can be divided into three phases: adhesion, lethal hit, and cell death (Figure 17-6).

The Adhesion Phase

The CD8–TCR complex on a cytotoxic T cell binds to MHC I molecules on the target cell surface and an immunological synapse rapidly forms around the contact area. The TCRs and other signaling molecules cluster at the center of the complex while they are surrounded by rings of adhesion molecules (Figure 17-8). CD8-MHC type I binding is usually necessary for a successful cytotoxic T-cell response, and experimentally antibodies against CD8 can block cytotoxic target recognition. The blocking effect of this anti-CD8 can be overcome by increasing the concentration of either MHC or antigen on the surface of the target cell. Thus the CD8 molecules simply enhance the binding between a T cell and its target. If the TCR has a very high affinity for the target, then costimulation through CD8 molecules may not be necessary.

In addition to the signal from antigen–MHC–CD8 complexes located at the center of the synapse, cytotoxic T-cell responses require that costimulatory signals be transmitted between the T cell and its target. As with CD4 helper cells, CD8 cytotoxic cells are optimally activated only when their CD28 surface receptors bind to CD86 on the target cell at the center of the synapse. The additional signal generated by CD28-CD86 binding may permit cytotoxic T cells to kill target cells in the absence of IL-2 from Th1 cells. Tumors or virus-infected cells that express CD86 are much more sensitive to killing by cytotoxic T cells than target cells that fail to express this molecule. Additional adhesion between cytotoxic T cells and their target is mediated by binding between CD2 and CD58 (in nonrodents) or CD48 (in rodents) and between CD11a/CD18 (LFA-1) and CD54 (ICAM-1).

Contents of Cytotoxic T Cells

Cytotoxic T-cell granules contain two molecules needed for the cytotoxic process: perforins and granzymes. Cytotoxic T cells release the contents of these granules within the central area of the immunological synapse. It is thought that the close contact between the cell membranes in this central area stops the leakage of cytotoxic molecules and so reduces the risk of damage to nearby cells.

Perforins are glycoproteins produced by cytotoxic T cells and natural killer (NK) cells. Perforins penetrate the target cell membrane and aggregate to form tubular structures called membrane attack complexes (Figure 17-9). Two perforins have been identified: perforin P1 from T cells produces large (16 nm) lesions in target cell membranes, whereas perforin P2 is produced by NK cells and produces small (5 to 7 nm) lesions. The perforins are related to and act in a similar manner to C9, the molecule that forms the complement membrane attack complex.

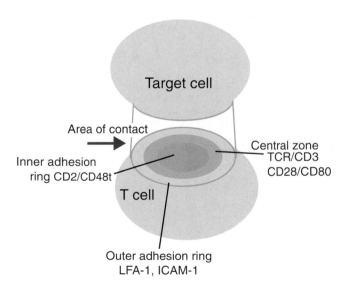

Figure 17-8. Structure of the immunological synapse that forms between a cytotoxic T cell and its target. The ring of adhesive proteins forms an effective "gasket" that prevents leakage of cytotoxic molecules into tissue fluidity.

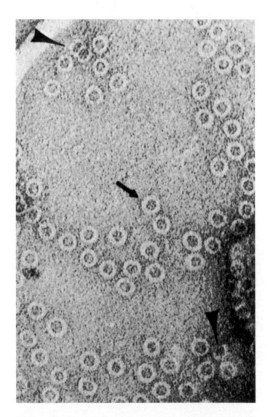

Figure 17-9. Perforins from human natural killer cells on the surface of a rabbit erythrocyte target. The arrowheads point to incomplete rings and double rings. (From Podack ER, Dennert G: *Nature* 301:44, 1983.)

Granzymes are a family of serine esterases found in lymphocyte granules where they account for about 90% of the total granule contents. Granzymes, especially granzyme B, can enter target cells in association with the perforins or via receptor-mediated endocytosis. Perforin activity in cytotoxic T cells is increased significantly by IL-2, IL-3, IL-4, and IL-6 and to a lesser degree by TNF-α and IFN-γ.

The Lethal Hit

The initiation of target cell apoptosis is called the lethal hit. The first step in the lethal hit process occurs within a few minutes of binding to the target as the T cells orient their microtubule organizing center, their Golgi complex, and their granules toward the target cell. The granules move toward the contact site. After the T cell comes into contact with its target, a synapse forms, and the T-cell granule contents are secreted into the intercellular space of the immunological synapse. Once the granules contact the target their perforins and granzymes are released. The perforins immediately aggregate to form polyperforins and insert themselves into the target membranes so that they form transmembrane channels. Between 12 and 18 monomers aggregate to form a membrane attack complex. Granzyme B then enters the target cell, either by injection through the central pore of the perforin complex or by endocytosis. Granzyme B in turn triggers the release of mitochondrial cytochrome *c* and the intrinsic apoptosis pathway. As described above, the cytochrome *c* activates an apoptosome that in turn activates caspase 9 and the caspase cascade. Once activated, the caspase cascade initiates a series of reactions leading to endonuclease activation, DNA fragmentation, and cell death.

Within seconds after contact between a T cell and its target, the organelles and the nucleus of the target cell show apoptotic changes. The T cell can then disengage itself and move on to find another target. It is not clear just how the cytotoxic T cell is itself not damaged during the lethal hit process, although it is likely that the structure of the synapse ensures that the perforin is correctly oriented to the target.

The CD95 (Fas) Pathway

The second mechanism of T-cell-mediated cytotoxicity involves its use of molecules called CD95L (or CD178 or fas-ligand) and their receptor CD95 (or fas). CD95L is a protein expressed on activated CD8+ T cells and on NK cells. It binds to death receptors on target cells called CD95 (or fas). When a T cell contacts its target, CD95L binds to CD95 and the CD95 trimerizes. This leads to the formation of a death-inducing signaling complex that contains caspase 8 and caspase 10 (Figure 17-2). These enzymes in turn activate caspase 3 and trigger the apoptosis cascade.

The CD95L-CD95 system regulates T-cell development. When activated T cells have completed their task of killing their targets, they themselves undergo CD95-mediated apoptosis to down-regulate the immune response.

In mice, *lpr* (lymphoproliferation) and *gld* (generalized lymphoproliferative disease) are loss-of-function mutations in the genes encoding CD95 and CD95L, respectively. Both mutations cause accumulation of activated T cells and accelerate autoimmune diseases. For example, *lpr* mice do not express CD95 on their thymocytes. As a result the thymocytes do not undergo apoptosis (negative selection) and are released into the secondary lymphoid organs. Here they proliferate excessively, resulting in a gross increase in the size of their lymphoid organs (lymphadenopathy). Because self-reactive cells are not destroyed, many of these cells react against self-antigens and *lpr* mice develop an autoimmune disease similar to systemic lupus erythematosus (Chapter 34).

Other Cytotoxic Pathways

TNF-β [also called lymphotoxin-α (LT-α)], a cytokine secreted by some cytotoxic T cells probably has a similar mode of action to CD95L. When produced by antigen-stimulated T cells, TNF-β acts in one of two ways. Either it binds to LT-β in the T-cell membrane to form a heterodimeric complex that kills target cells on contact or, alternatively, the secreted form binds to TNF-β death receptors on target cells and so triggers their apoptosis. Structural changes are seen by 2 to 3 hours, and by 16 hours more than 90% of target cells exposed to TNF-β are dead.

Granulysin is an antibacterial peptide found in the granules of both cytotoxic T cells and NK cells. It is secreted after T-cell activation and can kill target cells as well as a wide variety of extracellular pathogenic bacteria, fungi, and parasites. It shares homology with other proteins that attack lipid membranes called saposins. These are not pore-forming proteins but molecules that activate lipid-degrading enzymes such as sphingomyelinases. As a result, an increase in saposins increases ceramide content and ceramide can induce apoptosis. The importance of granulysin lies in ensuring that lysed cells do not release viable bacteria. For example, cytotoxic T cells can control *Listeria monocytogenes* and *Mycobacterium tuberculosis* infections simply by killing infected cells. One problem with this process is that viable bacteria released from the killed cells might infect healthy cells. In order to avoid this, the cytotoxic T cells release granulysin. This kills not only infected macrophages but also the intracellular bacteria.

CYTOTOXIC T-CELL SUBSETS

As pointed out in Chapter 10, there are two CD4+ T helper cell subsets, Th1 and Th2. Each subset is characterized by the mixture of cytokines it secretes. Subsets of

CD8+ T cells have also been identified in rodents, where they are called Tc1 and Tc2. Tc1 cells secrete IL-2 and IFN-γ but not IL-4, whereas Tc2 cells secrete IL-4 and IL-5 but not IFN-γ. Both Tc1 and Tc2 secrete granulocyte-macrophage colony-stimulating factor (GM-CSF) and IL-3. Within the Tc1 subset some but not all clones secrete IL-2. IL-6 and IL-10 are synthesized in high amounts by Tc2 cells and in low amounts by Tc1 cells. A third subset, Tc0, has an unrestricted cytokine profile. Unlike helper cells that can differentiate readily into Th1 or Th2 cells, CD8+ T cells show a strong preference for the Tc1 phenotype. Differentiation into Tc2 requires exposure to large amounts of IL-4. Tc1 cells exposed to IL-4 in this way permanently lose their ability to secrete IL-2. All three subsets are cytotoxic.

Another way of classifying cytotoxic T cells is on the basis of CD8 expression. Thus in mice there are CD8+ cytotoxic T cells that kill *M. tuberculosis*-infected macrophages using granulysin and so destroy the mycobacteria. Mice also have a population of double-negative cells (CD4−CD8−) that kill targets through the CD95 pathway but do not inhibit mycobacterial growth.

In humans and mice, a large proportion of γ/δ T cells can recognize mycobacteria. *Mycobacterium tuberculosis*-activated γ/δ T cells express IL-2 receptor, secrete IL-2, and can kill target cells infected with this organism.

OTHER MECHANISMS OF CELLULAR CYTOTOXICITY

T-cell-mediated cytotoxicity is not the only way by which the cells of the immune system can destroy abnormal cells (Table 17-1; Figure 17-10). For example, cells that possess the antibody receptors FcγRI or FcγRII may bind to foreign target cells or bacteria through specific antibodies and then become cytotoxic. These cytotoxic cells may include monocytes, eosinophils, neutrophils, B cells, and NK cells (Chapter 31). The mechanism of this antibody-dependent cell-mediated cytotoxicity (ADCC) is unclear. However, neutrophils and eosinophils probably act by releasing oxidants. ADCC is slower and less efficient than direct T-cell-mediated cytotoxicity, taking from 6 to 18 hours to occur.

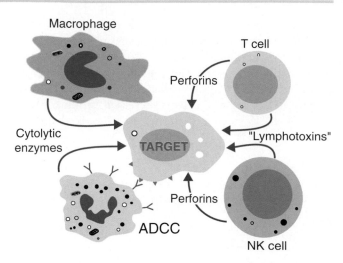

Figure 17-10. Major pathways by which the cells of the immune system can kill nucleated target cells. These targets would normally be tumor cells or virus-infected cells.

Whether or not a macrophage participates in ADCC depends on the level of expression of its FcR and on its degree of activation. Macrophage-activating cytokines such as IFN-γ or GM-CSF promote macrophage ADCC. Macrophages may also destroy target cells in a slow, antibody-independent process. For example, when they ingest bacteria or parasites, macrophages release nitric oxide, proteases, and TNF-α. The nitric oxide will kill nearby bacteria and cells. TNF-α is, of course, cytotoxic for some tumor cells.

MACROPHAGE ACTIVATION

Although killing of infected cells by triggering apoptosis is an important defense mechanism, there are occasions where such an extreme measure is not needed. It may be sufficient simply to activate macrophages so that these cells can effectively destroy invaders. For example, bacteria such as *L. monocytogenes*, *M. tuberculosis*, and *Brucella abortus*, and protozoa such as *Toxoplasma gondii* survive and multiply inside normal macrophages. Antibodies are therefore ineffective against these organisms. Protection against this type of infection develops as a result of macrophage activation (Figure 17-11).

TABLE **17-1**
A Comparison of the Three Major Mechanisms of Cell-Mediated Cytotoxicity

Cytotoxic Cells	Time (hr)	Mechanism	MHC Restricted	Antigen Specific
NK cells	24	NK-mediated cytotoxicity	No	No
Normal lymphocytes or macrophages with FcγR with specific antibody	6	ADCC activity	No	Yes
Primed T cells	1	T-cell mediated cytotoxicity	Yes	Yes

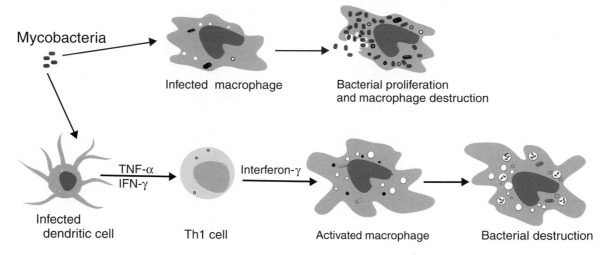

Figure 17-11.   Normal macrophages are killed by growing intracellular bacteria. IFN-γ released by Th1 cells can activate macrophages and so enable them to kill otherwise resistant intracellular bacteria.

Macrophages are activated by exposure to two signals. One signal is the cytokine IFN-γ. IFN-γ primes macrophages for activation but does not do so by itself. The second signal comes from TNF-α or, indirectly, from inducers of TNF-α production such as bacterial lipopolysaccharides. In practice, therefore, macrophages can be activated by innate mechanisms or by T-cell-mediated mechanisms (Figure 17-12). Thus the innate pathway is triggered when macrophages encounter microbial PAMPS such as mycobacterial glycolipids or lipoproteins through their toll-like receptors. These receptors signal to the cell and up-regulate the production of TNF-α. The TNF-α then stimulates NK cells to secrete IFN-γ. IFN-γ binds to its receptor on macrophages, signals through a JAK-STAT pathway, and initiates activation.

In the T-cell-mediated pathway, processed antigen triggers Th1 cells to secrete IFN-γ. The IFN-γ primes macrophages as described above. The necessary TNF-α comes from microbial invasion. The second signal for complete macrophage activation may also be generated by interaction between CD40 on the macrophage and CD154 on a T cell. It is likely that the innate pathway works in the early stages of an infection, whereas the T-cell dependent mechanisms come into operation later.

Macrophages activated by IFN-γ and TNF-α (M1 cells) secrete increased amounts of many proteins. These include the cytokines TNF-α, IL-1α, IL-6, CXCL8, and IL-12. As a result they induce a strong Th1 response. Macrophage-derived nitric oxide also has an effect on T cells (Figure 17-13). By activating guanyl cyclase it causes a rise in cyclic guanosine monophosphate, which in turn causes increased expression of the IL-12 receptor but has no effect on the IL-4 receptor. This also results in enhanced Th1 activity. Activated macrophages secrete proteases, which activate complement components. They secrete interferons, as well as thromboplastin, prostaglandins, fibronectins, plasminogen activator, and the complement components C2 and B. They express increased

quantities of MHC class II molecules on their surface and so have an enhanced ability to process antigen.

M1 macrophages are enlarged and show increased membrane activity (especially ruffling), increased formation of pseudopodia, and increased pinocytosis (uptake of fluid droplets) (Figure 17-14). They move more rapidly

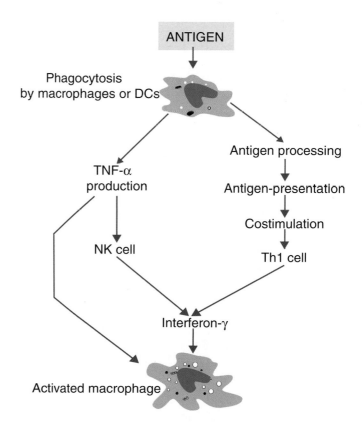

Figure 17-12.   The two pathways by which macrophages can be activated. One involves IFN-γ production by natural killer cells and is thus an innate pathway. The other is mediated by IFN-γ from Th1 cells and so is an acquired response.

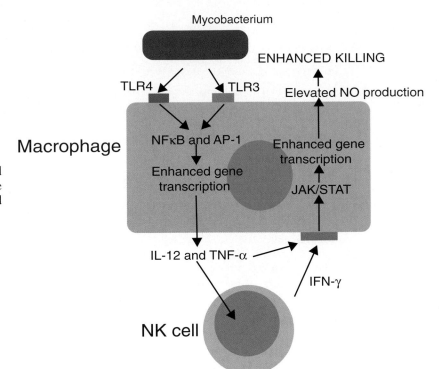

Figure 17-13. Macrophages may be activated through two linked pathways. Thus they may be activated by bacteria acting through TLR3 and TLR4 or by NK cells acting through IFN-γ.

in response to chemotactic stimuli. They contain increased amounts of lysosomal enzymes and respiratory burst metabolites, and they are more avidly phagocytic than normal cells. They produce greatly increased amounts of nitric oxide synthase 2 (NOS2). As a result, they can kill intracellular organisms or tumor cells by generating high levels of nitric oxide. The nitric oxide can destroy nearby tumor cells and intracellular bacteria such as *L. monocytogenes* (Figure 17-15). IFN-γ-activated macrophages can also inhibit the growth of intracellular bacteria such as *Legionella pneumophila* by limiting the availability of iron. They do this by down-regulating their transferrin receptors (CD71) so that less transferrin

is endocytosed and by reducing the concentration of intracellular ferritin, the major iron storage protein in macrophages. All these changes reduce the ability of the cells to support microbial growth.

On occasion, macrophage activation may result in a different type of polarized response whereby the cells differ in receptor expression, cytotoxic function, and cytokine production (Figure 17-16). For example, macrophages activated through their FcγR or under the influence of Th2 cytokines such as IL-4, IL-10, and IL-13 may become M2 cells. These M2 cells are functionally immunosuppressive and anti-inflammatory. Instead of producing nitric oxide, they use arginase to produce

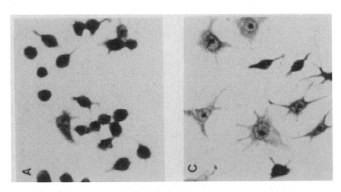

Figure 17-14. Stained cultures of mouse macrophages grown under identical conditions: *Left,* Normal unstimulated macrophages. *Right,* Macrophages activated by exposure to IFN-γ and acemannan. Note the cytoplasmic spreading of the activated cells. These cells secrete large quantities of cytokines and nitric oxide. Original magnification ×400. (Courtesy of Dr. Linna Zhang.)

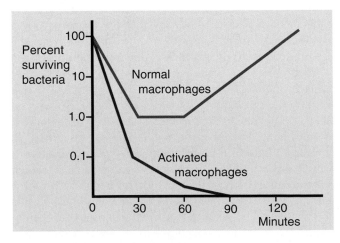

Figure 17-15. The destruction of *Listeria monocytogenes* when mixed in vitro with cultures of normal macrophages and "activated" macrophages from *Listeria*-infected mice.

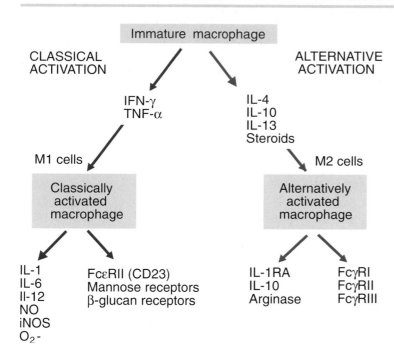

Figure 17-16. Depending on their cytokine exposure, macrophages may be activated in the classical sense (M1 cells) or become alternatively activated (M2 cells). M2 cells likely have a major regulatory role.

ornithine. This important regulatory process is discussed in Chapter 18.

The importance of these activation pathways can be seen in tuberculosis. Thus mycobacteria that enter the lungs are readily phagocytosed by alveolar macrophages that mount a respiratory burst and secrete proinflammatory cytokines. These cytokines act on NK cells triggering IFN-γ production and limited macrophage activation. This rapid innate response can slow mycobacterial growth significantly. Nevertheless these macrophages cannot destroy the bacteria by these mechanisms alone. However, after several days, recruitment of T cells occurs. The T cells are stimulated by mycobacteria-infected dendritic cells secreting IL-12, TNF-α, and IFN-α. As a result, responding Th1 cells are stimulated to secrete IFN-γ and fully activate the macrophages about 10 days after onset of infection (Table 17-2). In most individuals, this level of activation is sufficient to control the infection.

Cytotoxic T cells can interact with infected macrophages. For example, cytotoxic T cells generated in cattle infected with *M. bovis* will specifically kill infected macrophages . This cytotoxicity is mediated by both WC1⁺ γδ and CD8⁺ T cells. Presumably any *Mycobacteria* released are killed by granulysin.

Delayed Hypersensitivity Reactions

When certain antigens are injected into the skin of a sensitized animal, a slowly developing inflammatory response, taking many hours to develop, may occur at the injection site. This is a T-cell-mediated response called delayed hypersensitivity. Delayed hypersensitivity reactions are classified as type IV hypersensitivity reactions (Chapter 29). An important example of a delayed hypersensitivity reaction is the tuberculin response (the skin reaction that occurs following an intradermal injection of tuberculin).

T-CELL MEMORY

In contrast to the prolonged antibody response, the effector phase of T-cell responses is relatively brief. Indeed, cytotoxicity is seen only in the presence of antigen. This is logical. Sustained cytotoxic activities or overproduction of cytokines can cause tissue damage.

Naive T cells are long-lived resting cells that continuously recirculate between the bloodstream and lymphoid organs. Once they encounter antigen these cells respond rapidly and multiply fast in an effort to keep pace with the growth of invading pathogens. The number of responding cells may increase more than 1000-fold within a few days. They reach a peak 5 to 7 days after infection,

TABLE 17-2		
Effects of Cytokines on Macrophage Function		
Cytokine	Major Source	Effect
IL-2	Th1 cell	Activates
IFN-γ	Th1 cell, NK cell	Activates
IFN-α/β	Macrophages, T cells	Activates
TNF-α	Macrophages, Th1 cells	Activates
TNF-β	Th1 cells	Activates
GM-CSF	Many cell types	Activates
IL-4	Th2 cells	Suppresses
IL-10	Th2 cells, macrophages	Suppresses
IL-13	Th2 cells	Suppresses
TGF-β	T cells	Suppresses

when pathogen-specific, cytotoxic T cells can comprise 50% to 70% of total CD8+ T cells. Once the infection has cleared most of these cells are superfluous. Therefore the vast majority are destroyed by apoptosis 1 to 2 weeks after infection. Elimination of excess cytotoxic T cells is a tightly controlled process involving the CD95L-CD95 system. (In the absence of either CD95 or CD95L, you will recall, mice develop lymphoid hyperplasia and autoimmunity.) The survivors of this stage become long-lived memory cells. In acute viral infections, memory T cells probably develop only when antigen is eliminated. In chronic or persistent infections, cytotoxic T cells probably persist.

The number of surviving memory cells is directly related to the intensity of the primary response. Thus in general only 5% to 10% of the peak number of cytotoxic T cells produced survive to become memory T cells. Survival may be a function of duration of exposure to antigen. Cells exposed to antigen for prolonged periods may die whereas cells exposed only briefly may live. The observation that overwhelming viral infections can exhaust the T-cell pool and impair memory is consistent with this idea.

Memory T cells can be distinguished from naive T cells by their immunophenotype, by secreting a different mixture of cytokines, and by their behavior. For example, memory T cells are CD44+ and express high levels of IL-2Rβ, a receptor that binds both IL-2 and IL-15. They express increased amounts of adhesion molecules so they can bind more efficiently to antigen-presenting cells. They produce more IL-4 and IFN-γ and respond more strongly to stimulation of their TCR. Their enhanced responses may also be due to possession of higher affinity IL-2 receptors. They continue to divide, very slowly, in the absence of antigen. This division requires IL-15 and is inhibited by IL-2. Thus the persistence of memory T cells is regulated by the balance between IL-15 and IL-2.

SOURCES OF ADDITIONAL INFORMATION

Anderson CF, Mosser DM: A novel phenotype for an activated macrophage: the type 2 activated macrophage, *J Leukocyte Biol* 72:101-106, 2002.

Bevan MJ: Remembrance of things past, *Nature* 420:748-749, 2002.

Carter LL, Dutton RW: Relative perforin- and Fas-mediated lysis in T1 and T2 CD8 effector populations, *J Immunol* 155:1028-1031, 1995.

Cohen JJ: Apoptosis, *Immunol Today* 14:126-130, 1993.

Dooms H, Abbas AK: Life and death in effector T cells, *Nat Immunol* 9:797-798, 2002.

Green DR, Beere HM: Gone but not forgotten, *Nature* 405: 28-29, 2000.

Krammer PH: CD95's deadly mission in the immune system, *Nature* 407:789-795, 2000.

Liu CC, Young LHY, Young JD: Lymphocyte-mediated cytolysis and disease, *N Engl J Med* 335: 1651-1659 1996.

Lowin B, Hahne M, Mattmann C, Tschopp J: Cytolytic T-cell cytotoxicity is mediated through perforin and Fas lytic pathways, *Nature* 370:650-652, 1994.

MacDonald HR: T before NK, *Science* 296:481-482, 2002.

Nagata S: Fas ligand and immune evasion, *Nat Med* 2:1306-1307, 1996.

O'Rourke AM, Mescher MF: The roles of CD8 in cytotoxic T lymphocyte function, *Immunol Today* 14:183-187, 1993.

Pinkoski MJ, Waterhouse NJ, Heibein JA, et al: Granzyme B-mediated apoptosis proceeds predominantly through Bcl-2-inhibitable mitochondrial pathway, *J Biol Chem* 276: 12060-12067, 2001.

Rouvier E, Luciani MF, Golstein P: Fas involvement in Ca(2+)-independent T cell-mediated cytotoxicity, *J Exp Med* 177: 195-200, 1993.

Smyth MJ, Ortaldo JR: Mechanisms of cytotoxicity used by human peripheral blood CD4+ and CD8+ T cell subsets, *J Immunol* 151:740-747, 1993.

Sprent J, Tough DF: Lymphocyte life-span and memory, *Science* 265:1395-1400, 1994.

Squier MKT, Sehnert AJ, Cohen JJ: Apoptosis in leukocytes, *J Leukocyte Biol* 57:2-10, 1995.

Stenger S, Hanson DA, Teitelbaum R, et al: An antimicrobial activity of cytolytic T cells mediated by granulysin, *Science* 282:121-125, 1998.

Stinchcombe JC, Bossi G, Booth S, Griffiths GM: The immunological synapse of CTL contains a secretory domain and membrane bridges, *Immunity* 15:751-761, 2001.

Suda T, Takahashi T, Golstein P, Nagata S: Molecular cloning and expression of the fas ligand, a novel member of the tumor necrosis factor family, *Cell* 75:1169-1178, 1993.

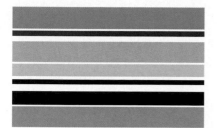

Regulation of the Acquired Immune Response

CHAPTER 18

The acquired immune system is a superbly sophisticated defense system. Thus it can recognize and respond to foreign invaders and can learn from the experience so that the body responds faster and more effectively when exposed to the invader a second time. However, there is a risk associated with this—the risk of damaging normal body components. One of the main reasons that the acquired immune system is so complex is that considerable effort must be put into ensuring that it will only attack foreign or abnormal tissues and will ignore normal healthy tissues. As might be anticipated, many different mechanisms ensure that the chances of autoimmune responses are minimized. In addition, the immune responses must be carefully regulated to ensure that they are appropriate with respect to both quality and quantity (Figure 18-1).

Since both T and B lymphocytes generate their repertoire of antigen-binding receptors at random, it is clear that the initial production of self-reactive cells cannot be prevented. An animal cannot control the amino acid sequences and hence the antigen specificity of these receptors. Tolerance induction therefore requires that lymphocytes with receptors that can bind self-antigens are destroyed or, at a minimum, irreversibly switched off.

TOLERANCE

Tolerance is the name given to the specific immunological unresponsiveness of an individual to an antigen. Physiologically this tolerance is directed against self-antigens from normal tissues. In 1948 Burnet and Fenner first suggested that the development of tolerance was determined by the maturity of antigen-sensitive cells when they first encounter antigens. They suggested that lymphocytes would not respond to an antigen if they first met that antigen early in fetal life.

Support for this suggestion came from observations on chimeric calves. In 1945 Ray Owen noted that when cows are carrying twin calves, blood vessels in the two placentas might fuse. As a result, the blood of the twins intermingles freely, and bone marrow stem cells from one animal colonize the other. Each calf is born with a mixture of blood cells, some of its own and some originating from its twin. In dizygotic (nonidentical) twins this is called a chimera. The foreign blood cells persist indefinitely in spite of being genetically dissimilar. Each chimeric calf is fully tolerant to the presence of its twin's blood cells (Figure 18-2). Burnet and Fenner suggested that this could only happen because each calf was exposed to the foreign cells early in fetal life during a period when

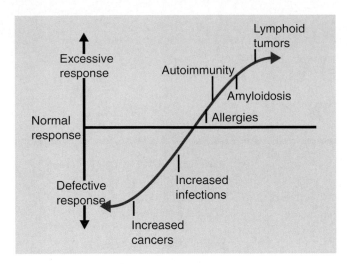

Figure 18-1.   Some of the bad things that can happen if the immune system is not carefully regulated.

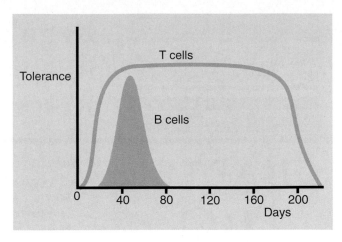

Figure 18-3.   The duration of tolerance in T cells and B cells. T cells are much more easily rendered tolerant than B cells. Once tolerant, they remain that way for much longer.

antigen-sensitive lymphocytes become tolerant upon encountering antigens. Cells from an unrelated calf would be rejected normally if administered after birth. Medawar and his colleagues conducted a variation of this "natural" experiment by inoculating the spleen cells from mice of one inbred strain (A) into the newborns of a second inbred strain (CBA). When the CBA mice grew to maturity, they

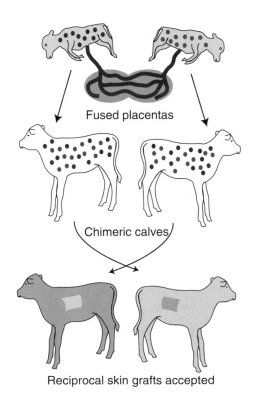

Figure 18-2.   Fusion of the placentas of dizygotic twin calves results in the development of calf chimeras. Hematopoietic stem cells from each animal colonize the bone marrow of the other. Each chimera is tolerant to its twin's cells and so will accept a skin graft from its twin despite the genetic differences.

would accept skin grafts from strain A mice but not from unrelated strains. This tolerance was very clearly demonstrated when Medawar's group succeeded in having a skin graft from a black mouse grow on a white one.

By reconstituting lethally irradiated mice with T and B cells derived from normal or tolerant donors, tolerance can be shown to occur in both lymphocyte populations. However, their susceptibility to tolerance induction differs considerably. Thus T cells can be made tolerant rapidly and easily, and remain in that state for more than 100 days (Figure 18-3). In contrast, B cells develop tolerance much more slowly (about 10 days as compared with 24 hours for T cells) and return to normal within 50 days. Since T helper cells are required for both cell- and antibody-mediated immune responses, an animal may be functionally tolerant even though its B cells are not.

T-CELL TOLERANCE

Selection of the T-Cell Receptor

The ability of a T cell to respond to an antigen depends on having receptors that can bind that antigen. In the absence of such T cells tolerance will result (Figure 18-4). Although theoretically the body may use any of the many possible combinations of α/β or γ/δ T-cell receptors (TCRs) generated by the processes outlined in Chapter 14, far fewer receptors are actually used by mature T cells than might be anticipated. Several processes limit receptor diversity. First, the mechanisms used to generate TCR diversity inevitably result in the production of nonfunctional receptors. For example, two thirds of possible gene arrangements will be out of frame. Presumably cells bearing these nonfunctional TCRs undergo apoptosis. Second, there is positive selection of T cells carrying receptors that can bind the animal's own major

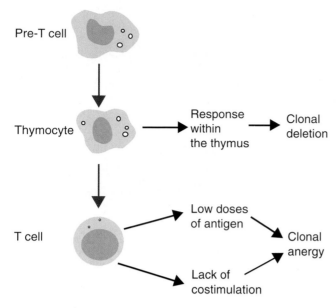

Figure 18-4. The two principal ways by which T cells can be made tolerant.

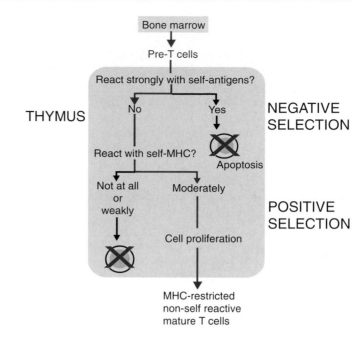

Figure 18-5. How the thymus regulates the production of T cells by positive and negative selection. Surviving T cells are unreactive to autoantigens yet can still recognize foreign antigenic peptides in association with MHC molecules.

histocompatibility complex (MHC) molecules. After all, the T cell must be able to respond to antigen fragments in association with the MHC of the antigen-presenting cell. T cells that cannot recognize their own MHC must also be eliminated. Third, T cells with receptors for self-antigens that may be able to mount damaging autoimmune responses are killed. This killing is called negative selection or clonal deletion, and is a major mechanism of self-tolerance.

Negative Selection

As T cells mature within the thymus, antigen receptors appear on their surface. Positive selection ensures that the cells that recognize self-MHC molecules survive. At this point, however, the cells whose receptors bind too strongly to self-antigens are killed (Figure 18-5). The timing and extent of this killing depend on the affinity of the TCR for a self-antigen. T cells that bind self-antigens strongly are killed earlier and more completely than weakly binding cells. Thus the T-cell population that eventually leaves the thymus has been purged of danger-ous, self-reactive cells.

One problem regarding the concept of negative selec-tion is the presence of self-antigens in the thymus. We normally think of each tissue or cell type possessing its own tissue-specific antigens. Thus "skin antigens" are restricted to the skin whereas "liver antigens" are restricted to the liver. However, studies have shown that the epithelial cells in the thymic medulla are unique in that they show "promiscuous" gene expression. These thymic epithelial cells contain a transcription regulator (called the autoimmune regulator, or aire) that promotes the expression of many different proteins once thought to be restricted to other tissues. Examples include

insulin, thyroglobulin, and myelin basic protein. In this way, the thymic epithelial cells ensure that self-reactive T cells encounter many normal tissue antigens within the thymus and are therefore eliminated. Defects in the *aire* gene lead to the development of multiple autoimmune diseases. In addition, some antigens are taken up by macrophages and B cells and carried to the thymus. T cells are also exposed to these antigens and those self-reactive cells eliminated. However, this raises another question: What about self-antigens that are not expressed in, or do not enter, the thymus? For example, antigens in the eye, testis, or brain are not processed in this way, and as a result tolerance to these antigens may not fully develop.

Additional evidence for the importance of negative selection is seen in *lpr* mice. These mice experience severe autoimmunity and excessive T cell proliferation as a result of mutations in the gene coding for CD95 (fas). CD95, you may remember, is a key component of the death receptor apoptotic pathway (Chapter 17). Because of the *lpr* mutation, the death receptor pathway is blocked. As a result, negative selection of T cells cannot occur, self-reactive thymocytes survive, and autoimmu-nity develops.

It is not entirely clear how both positive and negative selection can occur within the thymus and not cause removal of all T cells. Thus in one case self-reactive T cells are selected, and in the other they are destroyed. One favored hypothesis suggests that although all cells that can bind self-MHC molecules are positively selected, only those that bind MHC molecules with very low or very high affinity are subsequently deleted. Thus the moderate-affinity clones survive and are able to recognize foreign antigens. An additional factor that probably determines whether a cell will live or die is the amount of antigen presented to cells within the thymus. Thus if the concentration of a specific antigen is high (as one might anticipate for a self-antigen), multiple TCRs will be occupied on each thymocyte. This level of binding may trigger apoptosis and thus negative selection. In contrast, if only low concentrations of an antigen are available, these will occupy only a few TCRs on each thymocyte. This level of signal may cause positive selection and thymocyte proliferation.

Receptor Editing

When the antigen receptors of a developing B or T lymphocyte bind to self-antigens, the cell is killed by apoptosis. However, cell death is not instantaneous. Cell maturation stops and since the RAG genes are still active, the "antiself" cell is given a brief reprieve during which time it has a second chance to translocate its antigen receptor genes. This may result in production of new receptors that do not bind self-antigens. This process is called receptor editing. If a cell successfully edits its receptors then its maturation can proceed. Failure to do so will result in cell death.

Clonal Anergy

Negative selection is an imperfect process. Some low-affinity antiself T cells may escape from the thymus, and these must be suppressed by other mechanisms. This form of suppression is called clonal anergy. Clonal anergy, the prolonged, antigen-specific suppression of T-cell function, depends on the costimulatory signals delivered to a T cell.

As pointed out in Chapter 10, binding of an antigen to a TCR is by itself insufficient to trigger T-cell responses. Indeed, occupation of the TCR by an antigen in the absence of additional costimulation turns off a T cell. For example, protein solutions normally contain some aggregated molecules. These aggregated molecules are readily taken up and processed by dendritic cells and thus are highly immunogenic. If a solution of such a protein, such as bovine gamma globulin, is ultracentrifuged so that all the aggregates are removed, then the aggregate-free solution will induce tolerance when injected into adult rabbits. This tolerance is antigen specific because it is directed only against the bovine gamma globulin. It occurs because the T helper cells were exposed to free soluble antigens while they failed to receive the costimulatory signals normally provided by an antigen-presenting cell and so are turned off (Figure 18-6).

Binding to the TCR by an antigen activates the tyrosine kinases and phospholipase C of the T cell and raises its intracellular Ca^{2+}. However, this is not sufficient

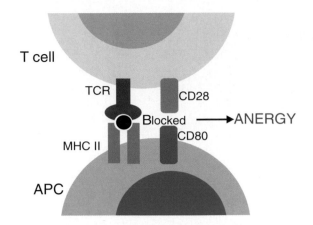

Figure 18-6. Clonal anergy will develop if a T-cell receptor is stimulated by antigen in the absence of simultaneous costimulation through the CD28/CD80 or CD28/CD86 pathway.

to fully activate the cell. In fact it triggers a repressor gene that makes the cell turn off. Only if interleukin-12 (IL-12) binds to its receptor *and* CD28 binds to CD80 will the induction of the repressor be blocked and the cell activated. Anergic Th1 cells produce about 1% to 3% of normal IL-2 levels and much less IL-3 and interferon-γ (IFN-γ). Once induced, this anergy can last for several weeks.

Very high doses of an antigen can also induce a form of clonal anergy called immune paralysis (Figure 18-7). The high doses of the antigen probably bypass antigen-presenting cells, reach the T helper cell receptors directly, and make the cells anergic.

B-CELL TOLERANCE

Unlike the TCR repertoire, antibody diversity is generated in B cells in two phases. The first phase occurs by gene segment rearrangement or gene conversion in the

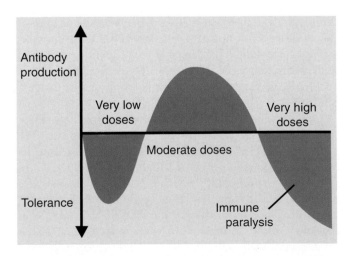

Figure 18-7. Capacity of different doses of antigen to induce tolerance. Both very low and very high doses can induce tolerance. Moderate doses, in contrast, induce an immune response.

primary lymphoid organs; the second phase involves random somatic mutation in germinal centers in secondary lymphoid organs. B cells therefore have several opportunities to become reactive to self-antigens, and it has been determined that 55% to 75% of early immature B cells are self-reactive! Selection against self-reactive B cells begins at an early stage in the cell's development. Nevertheless, self-reactive B cells can be readily found in lymphoid organs. These cells do not necessarily make autoantibodies. If not all the components necessary for a B-cell response are present (i.e., antigen-presenting cells and T helper cells) or if regulatory T cells are active, the B cell may become anergic (Figure 18-8). Since their response depends on costimulation by T helper cells, the failure of B cells to produce autoantibodies may simply result from a lack of appropriate T helper cells rather than any change in the B cells themselves. However, this is not a foolproof method of preventing self-reactivity. When T cells are tolerant but B cells are not, autoantibody production may be stimulated by the use of either cross-reacting epitopes or a foreign carrier molecule to stimulate nontolerant T helper cells (Figure 32-2). Thus, other mechanisms must also ensure B-cell tolerance. These mechanisms include clonal abortion, clonal anergy, clonal exhaustion, and blockage of B-cell receptors.

Clonal Abortion

Immature B cells can be made tolerant once they have successfully arranged their V-region genes and are committed to express complete IgM molecules on their surface provided they encounter antigens before they fully mature. When they bind self-antigen strongly, the B-cell receptor (BCR) transmits a signal that arrests cell development and triggers apoptosis. An immature B-cell

population can be rendered tolerant by one millionth of the dose of an antigen required to make mature B cells tolerant. B cells of young animals may also be unable to regenerate cell surface immunoglobulins after synapse formation. Clonal abortion occurs only if B cells encounter an antigen early in their development within the bone marrow. Other mechanisms of deleting self-reactive peripheral B cells are needed to suppress cells that become self-reactive as a result of somatic mutation. This involves the development of clonal anergy.

Clonal Anergy

As with T cells, B-cell clonal anergy results if the B cells encounter antigens in the absence of appropriate costimulation. B cells are difficult to maintain in a tolerant state, however, and will recover activity fairly rapidly unless steps are taken to maintain tolerance. Self-reactive B cells must also bind to a critical threshold of self-antigen to be made tolerant. This results in selective silencing of the high-affinity B cells. Presumably the failure of low-affinity antiself B cells to become tolerant poses little threat of autoimmune disease because the low-affinity antibodies produced do not cause tissue destruction.

Other Tolerance Mechanisms

B cells subjected to repeated exhaustive antigenic stimulation might be stimulated to differentiate into short-lived plasma cells. If all B cells develop into plasma cells, then no memory B cells will remain to respond to subsequent doses of antigen and tolerance will result. Some polymeric antigens such as pneumococcal polysaccharide can bind irreversibly to B-cell receptors. These antigens thus effectively freeze the B-cell membrane and block

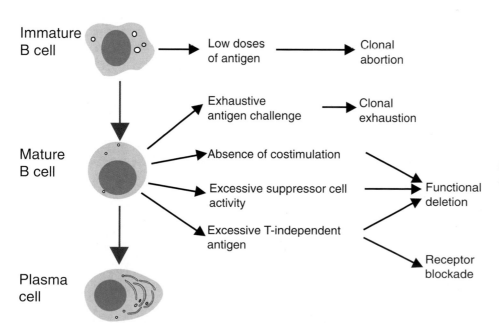

Figure 18-8. The ways in which B cells can be made tolerant.

any further responses by these cells. The B cells will recover when the antigen is removed.

Orally administered proteins may induce tolerance. The mechanism underlying this oral tolerance depends on the amount of an antigen fed. Thus high doses induce clonal deletion and anergy whereas lower doses induce the development of regulatory cells. Orally administered antigens have been used to suppress experimental autoimmune diseases.

B cells, like T cells, can undergo receptor editing. Thus if a B cell responds to self-antigens the cell may have an opportunity to generate a second set of light chains. If the second set of BCRs does not bind to self-antigens, the B cell may continue its development. If the second set is self-responsive, then the cell can try to generate yet another receptor. B cells have four opportunities to produce a functional, nonself-binding receptor. If all attempts fail, the cell will die.

INCOMPLETE TOLERANCE

Tolerance need not be total, and it can be generated in selected segments of the immune system. For example, tolerance in the response involving a single immunoglobulin class can be produced, and IgE-producing B cells are much more readily suppressed than those producing IgG or IgM. As a result it is possible to decrease susceptibility to allergies by desensitizing injections of an antigen (Chapter 26).

DURATION OF TOLERANCE

The duration of tolerance depends on the persistence of an antigen and on the ability of the bone marrow to generate fresh antigen-sensitive cells. When an antigen is completely metabolized, tolerance fades. If, however, an antigen is persistent (such as occurs in calf chimeras or with an animal's own tissue antigens), then tolerance also persists. This is because, in the continued presence of an antigen, newly formed antigen-sensitive cells will be killed as soon as their receptors bind self-antigen. Treatment that promotes bone marrow activity, such as low-dose irradiation, hastens the fading of tolerance, whereas immunosuppressive drug treatment has the opposite effect. It is possible to break tolerance to some self-antigens, such as thyroglobulin or myelin basic protein (Chapter 32), by administering the antigen with a potent immunostimulating adjuvant such as Freund's complete adjuvant.

CONTROL OF IMMUNE RESPONSES

Tolerance is not the only mechanism of immune regulation employed by the body. The magnitude of immune responses must also be regulated. An inadequate immune response may lead to immunodeficiency and increased susceptibility to infection. An excessive immune response may result in the development of allergies or autoimmunity (Chapter 26). Failure to control the burst of lymphocyte proliferation that occurs during immune responses may lead to the development of lymphoid cell tumors. Failure to control the immune response to the fetus may lead to abortion (Chapter 30). The immune responses must therefore be carefully regulated to ensure that they are appropriate in both quality and quantity. As might be anticipated, many different control mechanisms exist.

ANTIGEN REGULATION OF IMMUNE RESPONSES

Acquired immune responses are antigen driven. They commence only on exposure to an antigen, and once its concentration drops below a critical threshold, the responses stop. If an antigen persists, then the stimulus persists and, as a result, the immune response is prolonged. Thus a prolonged response occurs after immunization with poorly metabolized antigens such as the bacterial polysaccharides, or with antigens incorporated in oil or insoluble adjuvants so that the antigen cannot be rapidly eliminated. Persistence of low levels of an antigen maintains protective immunity. Persistence of high levels of an antigen can cause hypersensitivity

T and B cells tend to respond optimally to antigens presented for 3 to 5 days. T cells respond poorly, if at all, to antigens (e.g., self-antigens) that are continuously present in lymphoid organs. This is because persistence of antigens eventually activates and deletes all T cells responding to that antigen. Antigens that do not reach organized lymphoid tissues, irrespective of their origin, fail to induce either an immune response or tolerance. Thus self-antigens restricted to sites such as the brain, or infectious agents such as papilloma viruses that never enter lymphoid organs, are ignored by the immune system.

Antibody responses are also regulated by antigen. Thus, rigid polymeric antigens such as those on a bacterial surface or antigens linked to polyclonal activators such as lipopolysaccharide can induce B-cell responses in the absence of T-cell help. On the other hand, nonpolymeric, flexible antigens such as soluble proteins induce B-cell responses only in the presence of CD4+ T cells. Antigen concentration also affects this because the lower the antigen concentration, the greater the need for T-cell help.

Antigen Processing and Immune Regulation

The nature of the immune response may vary in different parts of the body as a result of processing by different dendritic cell populations. Langerhans cells seem especially suited for promoting T-cell responses (delayed hypersensitivity) whereas follicular dendritic cells prime

B cells. DC1 cells are optimized to present antigens to Th1 cells whereas DC2 cells present antigens to Th2 cells. Adjuvants also influence the type of immune response through their effects on antigen-presenting cells. Thus, lipids conjugated to protein antigens commonly induce delayed hypersensitivity rather than antibody production and localize in T- rather than B-cell areas of lymphoid tissues. T-independent antigens do not require T-cell help since they possess multiple epitopes and strongly stimulate B cells. However, they may stimulate B cells excessively and so cause tolerance.

ANTIBODY REGULATION OF IMMUNE RESPONSES

Antibodies or immune complexes generally suppress immune responses. In general, IgG antibodies suppress the production of both IgM and IgG antibodies whereas IgM antibodies tend to suppress only the further synthesis of IgM. Specific antibodies tend to suppress a specific immune response better than nonspecific immunoglobulins. An excellent example of this is seen in the method employed to prevent hemolytic disease of the newborn in humans (Chapter 27). In this disease a mother who lacks the Rhesus factor (Rh) antigen makes antibodies against Rh antigens on the red blood cells of her fetus. If the mother is given antibodies against this antigen at the time of her exposure to fetal red blood cells at birth, she will be completely blocked from making anti-Rh.

This negative feedback of antibodies on B cells can be explained in molecular terms. Thus B cells express the immunoglobulin receptor CD32 (FcγRII). If antibodies are present, they will occupy these receptors. If these receptor-bound antibodies bind to an antigen that is also bound to a BCR, the two receptors will become cross-linked. The cross-linking will therefore draw a BCR and CD32 close together (Figure 18-9). As a result, their signal transduction molecules interact and a critical tyrosine residue is phosphorylated. This in turn activates a phosphatase that inhibits BCR signal transduction and blocks B-cell activation. This pathway serves as a feedback mechanism whereby B-cell activation is suppressed by antibody and so prevents uncontrolled B-cell responses.

In diseases in which serum immunoglobulin levels are abnormally high, as in patients with myelomas (Chapter 11), these feedback mechanisms depress normal antibody synthesis and patients become very susceptible to infections. A similar phenomenon occurs in newborn animals that acquire antibodies from their mother. The presence of this maternal antibody, while conferring protection, effectively inhibits immunoglobulin synthesis and prevents the successful vaccination of newborn animals (Figure 18-10).

The regulation of serum IgG levels is also mediated through the MHC class Id immunoglobulin receptor, FcRn. In addition to transferring immunoglobulins

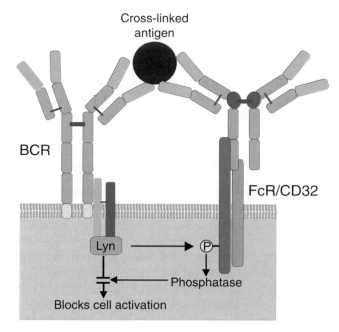

Figure 18-9. Cross-linkage of a B-cell receptor with antibody with CD32, an Fc receptor, by antibody and antigen can turn off a B cell by activating a phosphatase that in turn blocks signaling by tyrosine kinase.

across the newborn intestinal wall, FcRn is widely distributed on endothelial cells in muscle, vasculature, and hepatic sinusoids. Mice that lack FcRn have IgG with an unusually brief serum half-life. It is suggested that immunoglobulins binding to FcRn are protected from degradation. If FcRn expression remains constant, IgG levels remain stable. If IgG levels rise, then the surplus will fail to bind FcRn and so be degraded. Conversely, if IgG levels drop, then a greater proportion will bind to FcRn and be protected.

The class, as well as the quantity, of immunoglobulins produced during an immune response is also regulated. Most unstimulated B cells have both IgM and IgD surface immunoglobulins. During the course of an immune

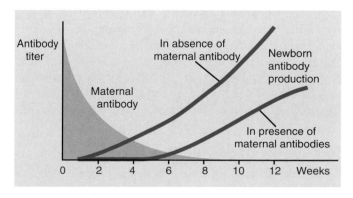

Figure 18-10. The presence of maternal antibody in a newborn animal effectively delays the onset of immunoglobulin synthesis through a negative feedback process.

response, these cells switch to the production of IgM, IgG, IgA, or IgE, and this class switch is controlled by T helper cells. In animals given T-independent antigens, there is no switch from IgM to IgG production, and a persistent low-level IgM response ensues (Figure 11-12). Neonatal bursectomy in birds may also result in a failure of the IgM-to-IgG switch.

INHIBITORY RECEPTORS

A key feature of the acquired immune system is that, while poised to launch a potent array of destructive mechanisms against invaders, the body can maintain control of the process. It is critically important to limit and eventually terminate a response by inactivating or eliminating pathways that are no longer required. This regulation involves the extensive use of inhibitory receptors. They are especially important in diminishing the activity of lymphocytes once they have completed their task. They provide a crucial safeguard against inappropriate immune responses. Thus activation and inhibition must be paired in order to initiate and terminate immune responses. In some cases activating and inhibitory receptors recognize similar ligands, so that the net outcome is a product of the relative strength of these signals. Loss of inhibitory signals is often associated with autoimmunity or hypersensitivity.

B-Cell Inhibitory Receptors

An excellent example of an inhibitory receptor is CD32-B1 (FcγRII). This immunoglobulin receptor is found on B cells as well as on macrophages, neutrophils, and mast cells. When it cross-links to the BCR through antigen and antibody it prevents signaling by the BCR and blocks B-cell activation and proliferation. It is through this mechanism that negative feedback by antibodies is achieved. This receptor when aggregated by antibody binding sends a signal to the B cell that triggers apoptosis. Animals deficient in this receptor produce large amounts of autoantibodies. Given that another receptor, FcγRIII, stimulates B cells, modulation of B-cell responses can be achieved by regulating the ratio of FcγRII to FcγRIII. Macrophage activation is regulated in a similar manner, and activated macrophages have a high FcγRIII-to-II ratio. Other B-cell inhibitory receptors include CD5, CD22, CD66a, and CD72. A deficiency of any of these results in uncontrolled B-cell proliferation.

T-Cell Inhibitory Receptors

CD28 and CTLA4 on T cells both bind the same ligand (CD80) but deliver antagonistic signals. CD28 is an activator whereas CTLA4 is an inhibitor. A deficiency of CTLA4 leads to uncontrolled T-cell proliferation and autoimmunity.

REGULATORY CELLS

Although much immune regulation is "passive" in that self-reactive lymphocytes are eliminated, it is clear that "active" regulation involving the activities of regulatory cells is also important. Many of the cells engaged in immune responses are known to have a regulatory function. These include T cells, macrophages, dendritic cells, and natural suppressor cells.

Regulatory T Cells

Some T-cell populations can suppress immune responses and have been called regulatory T cells (T$_R$ cells). They are CD4$^+$, they express the activation marker CD25, and they secrete IL-10 and/or transforming growth factor-β (TGF-β) to suppress other T-cell responses. T$_R$ cells can suppress the proliferation of T helper cells in response to an antigen and prevent experimental autoimmune disease. In the absence of an antigen, these T$_R$ cells prevent inappropriate T-cell activation. When an animal is infected, activated dendritic cells secreted IL-6, which overrides the suppressive effects of T$_R$ cells and permits an effector T-cell response to occur.

Oral administration of an antigen may induce the appearance of T$_R$ cells. Thus CD4$^+$ T-cell clones from the mesenteric lymph nodes of these tolerant animals secrete TGF-β, with various amounts of IL-4 and IL-10. These T$_R$ cells can suppress a variety of immune responses, including experimental autoimmunity.

Many of the regulatory activities of T cells reflect the antagonistic functions of Th1 and Th2 cells. For example, IFN-γ from Th1 cells can suppress IgE production whereas IL-10 from Th2 cells is suppressive for dendritic cell IL-12 production and thus for the production of cytokines by Th1 cells. Likewise IL-4 may suppress IL-2-mediated B-cell proliferation.

CD8$^+$ T cells can also secrete cytokine mixtures typical of Th1 or Th2 cells, so that a CD8$^+$ cell secreting IL-10 could be an effective suppressor cell. Another possible suppressive mechanism could involve the stimulation of cytotoxic T cells by antigen presented on B cells. Since some cytotoxic T cells are MHC class II restricted, they could potentially kill B cells presenting antigens in the conventional manner.

Interleukin-10

IL-10 was first described as an inhibitor of cytokine synthesis produced by Th2 cells. However, it is now clear that IL-10 can also be produced by Th1 cells, T$_R$ cells, CD8$^+$ T cells, dendritic cells, monocytes, B cells, mast cells, eosinophils, and keratinocytes. Thus IL-10 can inhibit the production of many cytokines, including IL-1α, IL-1β, IL-5, IL-6, CXCL8, IL-12, tumor necrosis factor-α (TNF-α), granulocyte-macrophage colony-stimulating factor (GM-CSF), and granulocyte colony-stimulating factor (G-CSF). It down-regulates

MHC class II and costimulatory molecule expression on dendritic cells and macrophages. In addition, IL-10 enhances the production of IL-1RA, an anti-inflammatory cytokine. IL-10 inhibits not only Th1 but also many Th2 responses. IL-10 or IL-10-treated dendritic cells can induce a long-lasting, antigen-specific, anergic state in both CD4$^+$ and CD8$^+$ T cells. It is interesting to note that pigs that become tolerant to a foreign kidney graft appear to possess T cells producing unusually large amounts of IL-10.

Regulatory Macrophages

Although activation of macrophages by IFN-γ is well recognized, it is only recently that an alternative macrophage activation pathway mediated by Th2 cytokines has been recognized. Thus, under some circumstances, macrophages may be activated in such a way that they suppress rather than enhance immune responses. These are called M2 cells, and their production is called "alternative activation." This type of activation enables M2 cells to participate in tolerance induction, regulate inflammation, and participate in tissue repair processes. Alternative activation is induced by the Th2 cytokines IL-4 and IL-13. As a result M2 cells show increased expression of the macrophage mannose receptor, the β-glucan receptor, and CD163; enhanced endocytosis and antigen processing; and increased MHC II expression. M2 macrophages produce anti-inflammatory cytokines such as IL-10, TGF-β, and IL-1RA. They do not show enhanced killing functions because IL-4 and IL-13 promote the production of arginase, which generates ornithine rather than nitric oxide (see Figure 17-16).

In healthy animals, M2 macrophages are normally found in the placenta and lung where they inhibit unwanted inflammatory reactions. They can also be found in healing tissues, where they are associated with angiogenesis.

Regulatory macrophages may be immunosuppressive. Thus placental and alveolar macrophages inhibit dendritic cell antigen presentation and can inhibit mitogen responses in lymphocytes. These regulatory macrophages are responsible for control of granuloma formation as well as for skin tolerance induced by UVB radiation.

Dendritic cells may also be activated in this way and so be immunosuppressive. Thus treatment of dendritic cells with IL-10 can block their ability to activate Th1 cells while preserving their ability to promote Th2 responses. A subpopulation of human dendritic cells has been shown to produce indoleamine 2,3-dioxygenase (IDO). This enzyme removes tryptophan and increases the production of metabolites that promote apoptosis. IDO is therefore a potent inhibitor of T cell proliferation and survival. It is known to play a key role in preventing immunological rejection of the fetus (Chapter 30).

Natural Suppressor Cells

Natural suppressor (NS) cells are large granular lymphocytes that secrete proteins that have suppressor cell–inducing activity. They suppress B- and T-cell proliferation as well as immunoglobulin production. NS cells occur normally in the adult bone marrow and neonatal spleen and possibly regulate innate immune responses. Potent NS activity develops in animals undergoing a graft-versus-host disease (Chapter 30).

When Do Regulatory Cells Work?

Regulatory cell activities have been described as regulating almost all aspects of immune reactivity. Regulatory T cells are claimed to be responsible for antigenic competition; lack of immune responses in the newborn; immunosuppression following trauma, burns, or surgery; prevention of autoimmunity; some cases of hypogammaglobulinemia; and blocking of responses to mitogens. These regulatory cells are found in some tumor-bearing animals where they block tumor rejection and in pregnant animals where they block rejection of the fetus. They also occur in individuals unresponsive (anergic) to tuberculosis infection.

Suppressor T cells induced by oral administration of an antigen (oral tolerance) may be selectively neutralized by a population of γ/δ T cells found in intestinal epithelium called contrasuppressor (Tcs) cells. As a result of the activities of Tcs cells an immune response may proceed in the intestinal wall in the presence of active suppression throughout the rest of the body.

REGULATION OF APOPTOSIS

The thymus of the mouse releases about a million new T cells into the circulation every day. Presumably a cow would produce many more. In order to keep the number of lymphocytes in the mouse body relatively constant, a million must also die. Likewise, the mouse bone marrow releases about 10^7 B cells daily and an equivalent number must die. In addition, lymphocytes divide in response to antigens. To keep the number of lymphocytes constant, all this proliferation must be balanced by the removal of cells by apoptosis. Apoptosis also removes autoreactive lymphocytes and limits the clonal expansion of lymphocytes during an immune response. This homeostatic system is carefully tuned because if it fails excess lymphocytes can cause lymphoid tumors or autoimmunity. The regulation depends on providing cell populations with survival signals. If these are inadequate, then cells will die. These regulatory signals probably differ among subpopulations since the loss of some cells, such as naive T cells, is not compensated for by an increase in memory T cells. These signals are likely provided by a cytokine mixture since we know that many cytokines, such as

IL-2, IL-4, IL-9, and IL-21, regulate lymphocyte survival by inhibiting apoptosis.

Apoptosis in lymphocytes is mediated by intracellular proteases. The best characterized of these are cysteine proteases belonging to the caspase family. These proteases are constitutively expressed as inactive precursors in lymphocytes. Their activity is modulated by proteins of the bcl-2 family. Thus, in a quiescent cell, survival depends on the ongoing presence of bcl-2. Animals lacking bcl-2 progressively lose lymphocytes and become immunodeficient. Cell receptors also regulate apoptosis. Thus survival is signaled through IL-2, IL-4, IL-7, and IL-15 receptors whereas cell death is signaled through Fas (CD95) and TGF-β. Adherence receptors such as integrins also regulate the survival of quiescent B and T cells. Thus if a lymphocyte does not traffic to the lymphoid organs it may be destroyed by apoptosis. These sites contain adhesion receptor ligands that allow long-term lymphocyte survival. Thus, together cytokine and adhesion receptors ensure the survival of quiescent lymphocytes.

Once a lymphocyte has been activated, it becomes less likely to undergo apoptosis unless it gets inappropriate or conflicting signals. The stronger the antigenic signals, the greater is the resistance to apoptosis. However, activated lymphocytes also become more susceptible to induction of cell death through the TNF receptors and CD95. Thus, activation of T cells by antigen causes expression of CD95L. As a result, they become sensitive to CD95-mediated killing. However, the CD95 pathway is normally blocked by costimulatory signals such as those transmitted through CD28 on T cells and CD40 on B cells. The production of cytokines by T cells also promotes their survival. If an antigen or costimulatory signal is lost, then the activated cell becomes sensitive to CD95-induced apoptosis. This is why lymphocytes are eliminated at the end of the immune response. Lymphocyte activation, while temporarily protecting lymphocytes against apoptosis, will also ensure that these cells can eventually be removed. Thus, CD40 up-regulates CD95 on B cells and IL-2 primes T cells for subsequent killing by CD95L.

NEURAL REGULATION OF IMMUNITY

The central nervous and immune systems regulate each other. Thus, the central nervous system signals the immune system through hormonal and neuronal pathways. The immune system signals the central nervous system through cytokines.

For example, it has been known for many years that mental attitudes, especially stress, significantly influence resistance to infectious diseases (Figure 18-11). One obvious example is shipping fever. This is a complex pneumonia of cattle primarily caused by several viral respiratory pathogens with secondary infection by

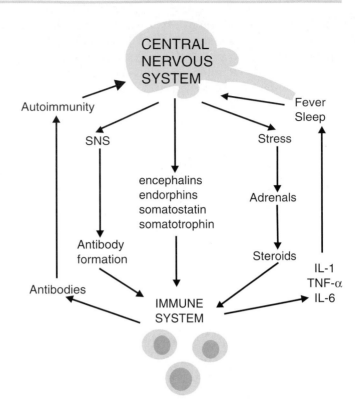

Figure 18-11.   Some of the ways in which the central nervous system and the immune system interact.

Mannheimia hemolytica. It develops in cattle that have been transported in confined spaces for long distances (and hence, many hours) with minimal feed and water and usually after rapid weaning and castration. The stress involved in the shipping process is sufficient to make these cattle highly susceptible to pneumonia. Stress can depress T-cell responses to mitogens, natural killer (NK) activity, IL-2 production, and expression of IL-2R on lymphocytes. Reduction in stress can have a reverse effect.

Stress can be due to something as simple as early weaning, which reduces IL-2 production in piglets. Stress in pregnant sows results in immunosuppression of their offspring. Thus confinement stress late in pregnancy results in the birth of piglets whose T and B cells have a reduced ability to respond to mitogens. Both morbidity and mortality are increased in piglets from stressed sows. A different form of stress may be a key factor in mammalian social structures. Thus, the social structure of animal populations is regulated by social dominance established in many cases by fighting. Once a hierarchy is established, fighting is reduced because each individual animal knows its social status. If new individuals are introduced into a group, or a dominant animal loses its position, stresses occur as a result of new tensions. It has been shown that there is a relationship between social status and disease susceptibility. Thus morbidity and mortality among pigs challenged with pseudorabies virus were highest among subordinate animals. Dominant pigs had lymphocytes that were more responsive to virus antigens. This of course makes sense from an evolutionary point of view in that the least reproductively fit animals were more likely to die of disease, but it is difficult to separate cause and effect in this phenomenon. Were subordinate animals immunosuppressed because they were under stress as a result of their lowly status? Alternatively, could it be that those animals with a highly effective immune system were healthier and thus better able to reach high social status within the population? Were dominant animals better fed than subordinates? Certainly high levels of social stress are found in confined, crowded animal populations.

When the behavior of pigs is examined, they can be divided into two groups: aggressive animals that tend to fight other animals and then may flee rapidly, and passive animals that tend to cope with stress by withdrawing gradually from stressful situations. These differences are associated with different behavioral, physiological, and endocrine responses to stress. When the immune reactivity of each type of pig was examined, significant differences were also found. Thus aggressive pigs had higher in vitro and in vivo cell-mediated immune responses but lower humoral responses than passive animals. This suggests that there were differences in the relative Th1 and Th2 responses of these animals. However, when these animals were stressed, the aggressive ones showed a much greater drop in these responses than the passive animals. It was also of interest to note that certain MHC class I haplotypes were not evenly distributed between the groups. Thus differences in the way animals cope with stress are reflected in differences in immune reactivity. It should also be noted that immune responses differ in their susceptibility to stress, and some are relatively resistant to stressors.

In looking for the mechanisms of this stress effect, it is clear that key roles are played by the products of the hypothalamic-pituitary-adrenal cortical axis and by the sympathetic-adrenal medullary axis. For example, the adrenal cortex is stimulated by adrenocorticotrophic hormone from the pituitary under the influence of corticotrophin-releasing hormone from the hypothalamus. As a result, glucocorticoids are secreted and are profoundly suppressive for T-cell function through the NF-κB pathway. Other mechanisms may involve noradrenaline signaling leading to nuclear factor-κB (NF-κB) activation in mononuclear cells. It may also involve direct signaling from nerves in lymphoid organs. Cells of the immune system have receptors for the opioid peptides. Neuropeptides such as enkephalins and endorphins are released during stress. These can bind to receptors on lymphocytes and influence their activity. Thus the generation of cytotoxic T cells is enhanced by metenkephalin and β-endorphin. α-Endorphin suppresses antibody formation and β-endorphin reverses this suppressive effect. Other neuropeptides that can influence the immune system include adrenocorticotropic hormone, oxytocin,

vasoactive intestinal peptide, somatostatin, prolactin, and substance P. Certain sites in the brain influence immune function by controlling neurotransmitter function or the autonomic nervous system. The pituitary influences the activity of the thymus, so that, for example, growth hormone injections augment the level of thymulin in dogs.

Many parts of the immune system are well supplied by nerves. For example nerves are linked to Langerhans cells in the skin. By releasing neuropeptides, these nerves can depress the antigen presenting ability of these Langerhans cells. This might explain why "hot spots" in dogs worsen with anxiety. Noradrenergic nerves innervate the thymus, the splenic white pulp, and the lymph nodes. They influence blood flow, vascular permeability, and lymphocyte migration and differentiation. Surgical or chemical sympathectomy of the spleen enhances antibody production and can induce changes in the distribution of lymphocyte subpopulations. Thus NK cell activity appears to be modulated directly by the preoptic nucleus of the hypothalamus through the splenic nerve. Denervated skin shows reduced inflammation following tissue damage and heals more slowly.

Immune responses are also modulated by environmental factors. Thus changes in day length (photoperiod) influence immune responses. These effects can be complex, but in general reduced day length appears to promote immune reactivity. The effect appears to be mediated through the hormone melatonin.

Finally, the innate immune system can influence nervous function. For example, cytokines such as IL-1, IL-6, and TNF-α induce "sickness behavior" including fever, fatigue, depressed activity, and excessive sleep. All these are closely associated with the immune response to infectious agents and chronic inflammation.

SOURCES OF ADDITIONAL INFORMATION

Anderson MS, Venanzi ES, Klein L, et al: Projection of an immunological self shadow within the thymus by the aire protein, *Science* 298:1395-1401, 2002.

Cohen JJ: Programmed cell death in the immune system, *Adv Immunol* 50:55-85, 1992.

Downing JEG, Miyan JA: Neural immunoregulation: emerging roles for nerves in immune homeostasis and disease, *Immunol Today* 21:281-289, 2000.

El-Lethey H, Huber-Eicher B, Jungi TW: Exploration of stress-induced immunosuppression in chickens reveals both stress-resistant and stress-susceptible antigen responses, *Vet Immunol Immunopathol* 95:91-101, 2003.

Fuchs EJ, Matziger P: B cells turn off virgin but not memory T cells, *Science* 258:1156-1158, 1992.

Gimmi CD, Freeman GJ, Gribben JG, et al: Human T-cell clonal anergy is induced by antigen presentation in the absence of B7 costimulation, *Proc Natl Acad Sci U S A* 90:6586-6590, 1993.

Gordon S: Alternative activation of macrophages, *Nat Rev Immunol* 3:23-34, 2003.

Green DR, Cotter TG: Apoptosis in the immune system, *Semin Immunol* 4:355-362, 1992.

Grohmann U, Fallarino F, Puccetti I: Tolerance, dendritic cells, and tryptophan: much ado about IDO, *Trends Immunol* 24:242-249, 2003.

Hartley SB, Cooke MP, Fulcher DA, et al: Elimination of self-reactive B lymphocytes proceeds in two stages: arrested development and cell death, *Cell* 72:325-335, 1993.

Hessing MJC, Coenen GJ, Vaiman M, Renard C: Individual differences in cell-mediated and humoral immunity in pigs, *Vet Immunol Immunopathol* 45:97-113, 1995.

Hessing MJC, Scheepens CJM, Schouten WGP, et al: Social rank and disease susceptibility in pigs, *Vet Immunol Immunopathol* 43:373-387, 1994.

Jekins MK, Miller RA: Memory and anergy: challenges to traditional models of T lymphocyte differentiation, *FASEB J* 6:2428-2433, 1992.

Kahled AR, Durum SK: Lymphocide: cytokines and the control of lymphoid homeostasis, *Nat Rev Immunol* 2:817-830, 2002.

Koide J, Engleman EG: Differences in surface phenotype and mechanism of action between alloantigen-specific CD8+ cytotoxic and suppressor T cell clones, *J Immunol* 144:32-40, 1990.

Marrack P, Kappler JW: How the immune system recognizes the body, *Sci Am* 269:81-89, 1993.

Mills CD, Kinkaid K, Alt JM, et al: M1/M2 macrophages and the Th1/Th2 paradigm, *J Immunol* 164:6166-6173, 2000.

Moldofsky II, Lue FA, Davidson JR, Gorczynski R: Effects of sleep deprivation on human immune functions, *FASEB J* 3:1972-1977, 1989.

Munn DH, Sharma MD, Lee JR, et al: Potential regulatory function of human dendritic cells expressing indoleamine 2,3-dioxygenase, *Science* 297:1867-1870, 2002.

Padgett DA, Glaser R: How stress influences the immune response, *Trends Immunol* 24:444-448, 2003.

Pasare C, Medzhitov R: Toll pathway-dependent blockade of CD4+CD25+ T cell-mediated suppression of dendritic cells, *Science* 300:1033-1036, 2003.

Posselt AM, Barker CF, Tomaszewski JE, et al: Induction of donor-specific unresponsiveness by intrathymic islet transplantation, *Science* 249:1293-1295, 1990.

Ramsdell F, Fowlkes BJ: Maintenance of in vivo tolerance by persistence of antigen, *Science* 257:1130-1138, 1992.

Reichlin S: Neuroendocrine–immune interactions, *N Engl J Med* 329:1246-1253, 1993.

Tuchscherer M, Kanitz E, Otten W, Tuchscherer A: Effects of prenatal stress on cellular and humoral immune responses in neonatal pigs, *Vet Immunol Immunopathol* 86:195-203, 2002.

Webster JI, Tonelli L, Sternberg EM: Neuroendocrine regulation of immunity, *Annu Rev Immunol* 20:125-163, 2002.

Yellon SM, Tran LT: Photoperiod, reproduction and immunity in select strains of inbred mice, *J Biol Rhythms* 17:65-75, 2002.

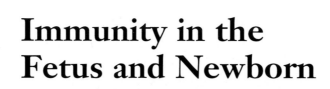

Immunity in the Fetus and Newborn

CHAPTER 19

When a mammal is born, it emerges from the sterile uterus into an environment where it is immediately exposed to a host of microorganisms from its mother and from the surrounding environment. Its surfaces, such as the gastrointestinal tract, eventually develop a dense, complex microbial population. If it is to survive, the newborn animal must be able to control microbial invasion within a very short time. In practice, the acquired immune system takes some time to become fully functional, and innate mechanisms are probably responsible for the initial resistance to infection. In some species with a short gestation period, such as mice, the acquired immune system may not even be fully developed. In animals with a long gestation period, such as the domestic mammals, the acquired immune system is fully developed at the time of birth but cannot function at full adult levels for several weeks. The complete development of acquired immunity depends on antigenic stimulation. The proper development of B cells and BCR diversity requires clonal selection and antigen-driven cell multiplication (Chapter 11). Thus, newborn mammals are vulnerable to infection for the first few weeks of life. They need assistance in defending themselves at this time. This temporary help is provided by the mother in the form of antibodies and possibly T cells. The passive transfer of immunity from mother to newborn is essential for survival.

DEVELOPMENT OF THE IMMUNE SYSTEM

The development of the immune system in the mammalian fetus follows a consistent pattern. The thymus is the first lymphoid organ to develop, followed closely by the secondary lymphoid organs. B cells appear soon after the development of the spleen and lymph nodes, but antibodies are not usually found until late in fetal life, if at all (Box 19-1). The ability of the fetus to respond to antigens develops very rapidly after the lymphoid organs appear, but all antigens are not equally capable of stimulating fetal lymphoid tissue. The immune system develops in a series of steps, each step permitting the fetus to respond to more antigens. These steps are driven by a gradual increase in the use of gene conversion or somatic mutation to increase antibody diversity. The ability to mount cell-mediated immune responses develops at the same time as antibody production. Data from humans suggest that T-cell receptor diversity is limited in the fetus and neonate and that cytokine production may be low. This may simply be due to the absence of memory cells in the fetus and neonate, reflecting their lack of exposure to foreign antigens.

Calf. The immune system of the calf develops early in fetal life. Although the gestation period of the cow is 280 days, the fetal thymus is recognizable by 40 days postconception. The bone marrow and spleen appear at

BOX 19–1

Although the immune responses of marsupials are usually slower to develop than those of placental mammals, their immune system may develop remarkably early. Thus the opossum, *Didelphis marsupialis*, is born after only 12 or 13 days gestation and can make antibodies to *Salmonella typhi* and bacteriophage f2 after 5 days in the pouch (17 or 18 days after conception).

55 days. Lymph nodes are found at 60 days, but Peyer's patches do not appear until 175 days (Figure 19-1). Peripheral blood lymphocytes are seen in fetal calves by day 45, IgM$^+$ B cells by day 59, and IgG$^+$ B cells by day 135. The time of appearance of serum antibodies depends on the sensitivity of the techniques used. It is therefore no accident that the earliest detectable immune responses are those directed against viruses, using highly sensitive virus neutralization tests. Calves have been reported to respond to rotavirus at 73 days, to parvovirus at 93 days, and to parainfluenza 3 virus at 120 days. Calf blood lymphocytes can respond to mitogens between 75 and 80 days, but this ability is temporarily lost around the time of birth as a result of high serum steroid levels.

Lamb. The gestation period of the ewe is about 145 days. MHC class I positive cells can be detected by day 19, and MHC class II positive cells can be found by day 25. The thymus and lymph nodes are recognizable by 35 and 50 days postconception, respectively, but the Peyer's patches appear only at 60 days. Blood lymphocytes are seen in fetal lambs by day 32, and CD4$^+$ and CD8$^+$ cells

appear in the thymus by 35 to 38 days. B cells are detectable at 48 days in the spleen and by that time have already rearranged their Vλ genes. C3 receptors appear by day 120 but Fc receptors do not appear until the animal is born. Fetal liver lymphocytes can respond to phytohemagglutinin by 38 days. Lambs can produce antibodies to phage φx 174 at day 41 and reject skin allografts by day 77. Some fetal lambs can produce antibodies to Akabane virus by as early as 50 days postconception. Antibodies to Cache Valley virus can be provoked by day 76, to SV40 virus by day 90, to T4 phage by day 105, to bluetongue virus by day 122, and to lymphocytic choriomeningitis virus by day 140. The proportions of α/β and γ/δ T cells change as lambs mature. Thus, one month before birth 18% of blood T cells are γ/δ$^+$. By one month after birth they constitute 60% of blood T cells.

Piglet. The gestation period of the sow is about 115 days. The first SWC3$^+$ leukocytes can be found in the yolk sac and liver on day 17. The thymus develops by 40 days postconception and is colonized by two waves of T-cell progenitors beginning on day 38. γ/δ T cells appear first in the thymus and then peripheral blood. α/β T cells develop later but their numbers grow rapidly so that they predominate late in gestation. The intestinal lymphoid tissues are devoid of T cells at birth. CD4$^+$ T cells appear in the intestine at two weeks of age and CD8$^+$ T cells appear at 4 weeks. Their proliferation appears to be driven by the intestinal microflora. IgM$^+$ B cells can be found in blood by day 50. Fetal piglets can produce antibodies to parvoviruses at 58 days and can reject allografts at approximately the same time. Blood lymphocytes can respond to mitogens between 48 and 54 days. Natural killer (NK) cell activity does not develop until several weeks after birth, although cells with an NK phenotype can be identified in the fetal pig. B cells are the first lymphocytes to appear in peripheral blood. The number of circulating B cells rises significantly between 70 and 80 days. The response to antigens in the fetus is essentially of the IgM type, but newborn and fetal piglets also produce a small immunoglobulin that may not have light chains. It is interesting to note also that B cells can be found in the thymus of newborn pigs.

The molecular development of the antibody repertoire has been followed in the developing pig. Thus, VDJ rearrangement is first seen in the fetal liver at day 30. However, the fetal piglet does not use all its *IGHV* or *IGHD* genes initially. Likewise, N-region addition does not occur before day 40, suggesting that the onset of terminal deoxynucleotidyltransferase activity occurs after that time. IgM, IgA, and IgG transcripts were present from 50 days in all major lymphoid organs. Piglets are thus born with relatively limited B cell diversity. B cell numbers increase for the first 4 weeks after birth, but their antigen-binding repertoire does not begin to expand until 4 to 6 weeks of age. Similar studies on rabbits have shown that the fetal immunoglobulin

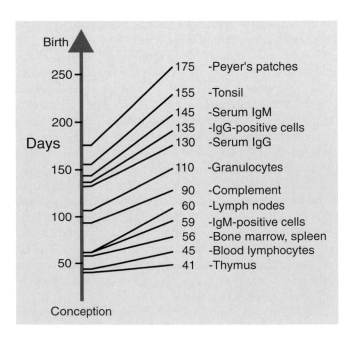

Figure 19-1. Progressive development of the immune system in the fetal calf.

repertoire does not diversify until after birth and this appears to be stimulated by bacterial colonization of the gastrointestinal tract. CD4+ CD8+ T cells and CD2+ B cells do not appear in gnotobiotic animals and are absolutely dependent on contact of the immune system with live microorganisms.

Foal. The gestation period of the mare is about 340 days. Lymphocytes are seen first in the thymus around 60 to 80 days postconception. They are found in the mesenteric lymph node and intestinal lamina propria at 90 days and in the spleen at 175 days. Blood lymphocytes appear at around 120 days. A few plasma cells may be seen at 240 days. Graft-versus-host disease, a cell-mediated response, has developed in immunodeficient foals transplanted with tissues from a 79-day-old fetus. The equine fetus can respond to coliphage T2 at 200 days postconception and to Venezuelan equine encephalitis virus at 230 days. Newborn foals have detectable quantities of IgM and IgG and occasionally IgG3 in their serum. Like other large herbivores, the foal has a well-developed ileal Peyer's patch that eventually involutes.

Puppy. The gestation period of the bitch is about 60 days. The thymus differentiates between days 23 and 33, and fetal puppies can respond to phage φX174 on day 40. Blood lymphocytes will respond to phytohemagglutinin by 45 days postconception, and these cells can be detected in lymph nodes by 45 days and in the spleen by 55 days. The ability to reject allografts also develops around day 45, although rejection is slow at this stage, and puppies may be made tolerant by intrauterine injection of an antigen before day 42. Thymic seeding of T cells to the secondary lymphoid organs and the development of humoral immune responses are therefore relatively late phenomena in the dog compared with these phenomena in the other domestic animals.

Kitten. Data on the ontogeny of the kitten are limited. B cells are seen in the fetal liver at 42 days postconception. Fetal kittens do make some IgG that can be detected in their serum before suckling, although this may be due to antibodies crossing the placenta.

Chick. Stem cells arise in the yolk sac membrane and migrate to the thymus and bursa at 5 to 7 days incubation. These cells differentiate within the bursa, and follicles develop by day 12. Lymphocytes with surface IgM may be detected in the bursa by day 14, and antibodies to keyhole limpet hemocyanin and to sheep erythrocytes may be produced by 16 and 18 days incubation, respectively. Lymphocytes with surface IgY develop on day 21 around the time of hatching, whereas IgA-positive cells first appear in the intestine 3 to 7 days after hatching. Vaccination of 18-day embryonated eggs is commonly employed in the modern poultry industry. The major vaccine employed is against the Marek's disease herpesvirus but extension of the technology to other antigens is in progress.

Development of Phagocytic Capability

In the fetal pig, neutrophils at 90 days postconception are fully capable of phagocytosing bacteria such as *Staphylococcus aureus*. However, they are deficient in bactericidal activity, which only reaches adult levels 10 days later. Near birth, the phagocytic and bactericidal capacity of these neutrophils declines as a result of an increase in fetal steroid levels. After birth, macrophages have depressed chemotactic responsiveness, and they are also able to support the growth of some viruses that macrophages from adult animals do not. Virucidal activity is gradually acquired, although this process appears to be under thymic influence. The macrophages from neonatally thymectomized mice do not acquire this resistance, perhaps as a result of a deficiency of interferon-γ (IFN-γ). The serum of newborn animals is also deficient in some complement components, resulting in a poor opsonic activity that is reflected in an increased susceptibility to infection. The neutrophils of newborn foals have altered locomotion as compared to their dams. However, phagocytosis and bactericidal activity were no different in fetal foal cells than in mare cells. Serum C3 increases rapidly after birth in newborn piglets and reaches adult levels by 14 days of age.

Interesting changes occur in the distribution of macrophages in the newborn pig. Thus, in newborn piglets there are very few pulmonary intravascular macrophages. However, during the first few days after birth, blood monocytes adhere to the pulmonary capillary endothelium and differentiate into macrophages. Thus, in the newborn piglet 75% of particles are cleared from the blood in the liver and spleen. By 2 months of age 75% are cleared in the lungs. The alveolar macrophages of newborn pigs have poor phagocytic activity, but this is effectively acquired by seven days of age.

The Immune System and Intrauterine Infection

Although the fetus is not totally defenseless, it is less capable than the adult of combating infection. Its acquired immune system is not fully functional; as a result, some infections may be mild or unapparent in the mother but severe or lethal in the fetus. Examples include bluetongue, infectious bovine rhinotracheitis [bovine herpesvirus 1 (BHV-1)], bovine virus diarrhea (BVD), rubella in humans, and the protozoan infection toxoplasmosis. Fetal infections commonly trigger an immune response as shown by lymphoid hyperplasia and elevated immunoglobulin levels. For this reason the presence of any immunoglobulins in the serum of a newborn, unsuckled animal suggests infection in utero.

In general, the response to these viruses is determined by the state of immunological development of the fetus. For example, if bluetongue virus vaccine, which is nonpathogenic for normal adult sheep, is given to pregnant ewes at 50 days postconception, it causes severe lesions in the nervous system of fetal lambs, including hydranencephaly and retinal dysplasia, whereas if it is given at 100 days postconception or to newborn lambs, only a mild inflammatory response is seen. Bluetongue virus vaccine given to fetal lambs between 50 and 70 days postconception may be isolated from lamb tissues for several weeks, but if given after 100 days, reisolation is not usually possible. Akabane virus acts in a similar fashion in lambs. If given before 30 to 36 days postconception it causes congenital deformities. If given to older fetuses it provokes antibody formation and is much less likely to cause malformations.

Piglets that receive parvovirus before 55 days postconception will usually be aborted or stillborn. After 72 days, however, piglets will normally develop high levels of antibodies to the parvovirus and survive.

Prenatal infection of calves with BHV-1 results in a fatal disease, in contrast to postnatal infections, which are relatively mild. The transition between these two types of infection occurs during the last month of pregnancy.

The effects of the timing of viral infection are well seen with bovine viral diarrhea virus (BVDV). Thus, if a newly pregnant cow is infected early in pregnancy (up to 50 days), she may abort. On the other hand, infections occurring between 50 and 120 days, before the fetus develops immune competence, lead to asymptomatic persistent infection because the calves develop tolerance to the virus (Figure 19-2). These calves are viremic yet, because of their tolerance, fail to make antibodies or T cells against the virus. Some of these calves may show minor neurologic problems and failure to thrive, but many are clinically normal. If the cow is infected with BVDV between 100 and 180 days postconception, calves may be born with severe malformations involving the central nervous system and eye, as well as have jaw defects, atrophy, and growth retardation. Vaccines containing modified live BVDV may have a similar effect if administered at the same time. Calves infected after 150 to 180 days gestation are usually clinically normal.

Since they are specifically tolerant to BVD, persistently infected calves shed large quantities of virus in their body secretions and excretions and so act as the major source of BVDV for other animals in a herd. The persistently infected calves may also produce neutralizing antibodies if immunized with a live BVD vaccine of a serotype different from that of the persistent virus. Despite this, the original virus will persist in these animals. These persistently infected calves grow slowly and often die of opportunistic infections such as pneumonia before reaching adulthood. (BVD has a tropism for lymphocytes and is immunosuppressive.) They also have depressed neutrophil phagocytic and bactericidal functions.

BVD viruses occur in two distinct biotypes: cytopathic and noncytopathic. (The name derives from their behavior in cell culture, not their pathogenicity in animals.) Noncytopathic strains do not trigger type I interferon production and therefore can survive in calves and cause persistent infections. Cytopathic strains induce interferon production and cannot cause persistent infection. These cytopathic strains do, however, cause mucosal disease (MD), a severe enteric disease leading to profuse diarrhea and death (Figure 19-3). Mucosal disease develops as a result of a mutation in a nonstructural viral gene that changes the BVDV biotype from noncytopathic to cytopathic while the animal fails to produce neutralizing antibodies or T cells. The cytopathic strain can spread between tolerant animals and lead to a severe mucosal disease outbreak. Both cytopathic and noncytopathic viruses can be isolated from these animals. Recombination may also occur between persistent noncytopathic strains and cytopathic strains administered in vaccines and lead to MD outbreaks. Although some of the lesions in MD are attributable to the direct pathogenic effects of the BVD virus, glomerulonephritis and other immune-complex-mediated lesions also develop. The reasons for this are unclear but may reflect superinfection or the production of non-neutralizing antibodies. Because persistently infected calves can reach adulthood and breed, it is possible for BVD infection to persist indefinitely within carrier animals and their progeny. Epidemiological studies suggest that between 0.4% and 1.7% of cattle in the United States are persistently infected in this way.

Figure 19-2. The effects of bovine viral diarrhea virus infection on development of the fetal calf depend on the timing of infection. As with adult animals, there is considerable individual variation in resistance to infection. Persistently infected calves may show minor neurological problems or failure to thrive.

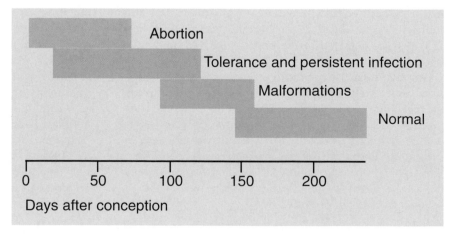

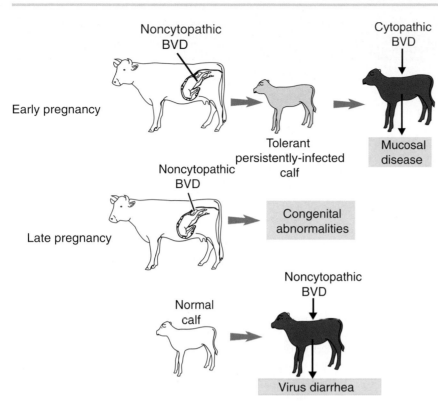

Figure 19-3. The relationship of mucosal disease to persistent infection with bovine viral diarrhea (BVD) virus in tolerant cattle. Calves persistently infected with noncytopathic BVDV and then superinfected with cytopathic BVD virus develop mucosal disease.

IMMUNE RESPONSE OF NEWBORN ANIMALS

After developing in the sterile environment of the uterus, mammals are born into an environment rich in microorganisms. The young of domestic animals are capable of mounting both innate and acquired immune responses at birth. However, any acquired immune response mounted by a newborn must be a primary response with a prolonged lag period and low concentrations of antibodies. The newborn animal also tends to produce immune responses skewed toward a Th2 rather than Th1 cytokine pattern. Some Th1 cytokines, such as IFN-γ, appear to cause placental damage; therefore, this skewing is probably not accidental and may be a result of hormonal influences during pregnancy. Over the first months of life, the immune responses usually revert to the balanced adult pattern.

Unless immunological assistance is provided, newborn animals may be killed by organisms that present little threat to an adult. This immunological assistance is provided by antibodies transferred from the mother to her offspring through colostrum. Maternal lymphocytes may also be transferred to the fetus through the placenta or to newborn animals through colostrum and transintestinal migration, but the biological significance of this is unclear.

TRANSFER OF IMMUNITY FROM MOTHER TO OFFSPRING

The route by which maternal antibodies reach the fetus is determined by the structure of the placenta. In humans

and other primates, the placenta is hemochorial; that is, the maternal blood is in direct contact with the trophoblast. This type of placenta allows maternal IgG but not IgM, IgA, or IgE to transfer to the fetus. Maternal IgG enters the fetal bloodstream; therefore, the newborn human infant has circulating IgG levels comparable to those of its mother.

Dogs and cats have an endotheliochorial placenta in which the chorionic epithelium is in contact with the endothelium of the maternal capillaries. In these species 5% to 10% of IgG may transfer from the mother to the puppy or kitten, but most is obtained through colostrum.

The placenta of ruminants is syndesmochorial; that is, the chorionic epithelium is in direct contact with uterine tissues, whereas the placenta of horses and pigs is epitheliochorial and the fetal chorionic epithelium is in contact with intact uterine epithelium. In animals with these types of placenta, the transplacental passage of immunoglobulin molecules is totally prevented, and their newborn are entirely dependent on antibodies received through the colostrum.

Secretion and Composition of Colostrum and Milk

Colostrum contains the accumulated secretions of the mammary gland over the last few weeks of pregnancy together with proteins actively transferred from the bloodstream under the influence of estrogens and progesterone. Therefore, it is rich in IgG and IgA but also contains some IgM and IgE (Table 19-1). The predominant immunoglobulin in the colostrum of most of the major domestic animals is IgG, which may account for 65% to 90% of its total antibody content; IgA and the

TABLE   19-1
Colostral and Milk Immunoglobulin Levels in Domestic Animals

Species	Fluid	Immunoglobulin (mg/dL)				
		IgA	IgM	IgG	IgG3	IgGb
Horse	Colostrum	500–1500	100–350	1500–5000	500–2500	50–150
	Milk	50–100	5–10	20–50	5–20	0
Cow	Colostrum	100–700	300–1300	2400–8000		
	Milk	10–50	10–20	50–750		
Ewe	Colostrum	100–700	400–1200	4000–6000		
	Milk	5–12	0–7	60–100		
Sow	Colostrum	950–1050	250–320	3000–7000		
Bitch	Colostrum	500–2200	14–57	120–300		
	Milk	110–620	10–54	1–3		
Queen	Colostrum	150–340	47–58	4400–3250		
	Milk	240–620	0	100–440		

other immunoglobulins are usually minor but significant components. As lactation progresses and colostrum changes to milk, differences among species emerge. In primates and humans, IgA predominates in both colostrum and milk. In pigs and horses, IgG predominates in colostrum but its concentration drops rapidly as lactation proceeds, so that IgA comes to predominate in milk. In ruminants, IgG1 is the predominant immunoglobulin class in both milk and colostrum (Figure 19-4).

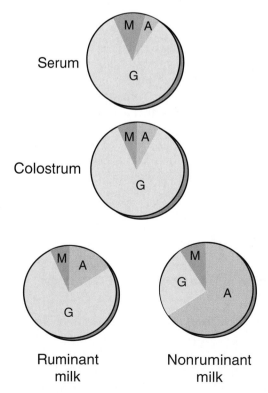

Figure 19-4. Relative concentrations of the major immunoglobulin classes in serum, colostrum, and the milk of ruminants and nonruminants.

All of the IgG, most of the IgM, and about half of the IgA in bovine colostrum are derived from serum. In milk, in contrast, only 30% of the IgG and 10% of the IgA are so derived; the rest are produced locally in the udder. Colostrum also contains secretory component both in the free form and bound to IgA. Colostrum is also rich in cytokines. For example, bovine colostrum contains IL-1β, IL-6,TNF-α, and IFN-γ. It has been suggested that these cytokines promote the development of the immune system in the young animal.

Absorption of Colostrum

Young animals that suckle soon after birth take colostrum into their gastrointestinal tract. Thus naturally suckled calves ingest an average of 2 L of colostrum although individual calves can ingest as much as 6 L. In these young animals, the level of protease activity in the digestive tract is low and is further reduced by trypsin inhibitors in colostrum. Therefore, colostral proteins are not degraded and used as food but instead reach the small intestine intact. Colostral immunoglobulins bind to special Fc receptors on the intestinal epithelial cells of newborns called FcRn. These are also expressed on mammary gland ductal and acinar cells, and are probably involved in the active secretion of IgG into colostrum. FcRn is an MHC class Id molecule with a large α chain and β2-microglobulin. It is probably found in all mammals and is very similar to the Fc receptor found on the yolk sac of the chicken. Once bound to cell surface FcRn, immunoglobulins are endocytosed by intestinal epithelial cells and passed into the lacteals and possibly the intestinal capillaries. Eventually the absorbed immunoglobulin reaches the systemic circulation, and newborn animals thus obtain a massive transfusion of maternal immunoglobulins.

Domestic mammals differ in the selectivity and duration of intestinal permeability. In the horse and pig, protein absorption is selective, IgG and IgM are preferentially absorbed, whereas IgA mainly remains in the intestine. In ruminants, absorption is unselective and all immunoglobulin classes are absorbed, although IgA is gradually excreted. Young pigs and probably other young animals have large amounts of free secretory component in their intestine. Colostral IgA and, to a lesser extent, IgM can bind this secretory component, which may then inhibit immunoglobulin absorption.

The duration of intestinal permeability varies between species and among immunoglobulin classes. In general, permeability is highest immediately after birth and declines after about 6 hours, perhaps because of the replacement of FcRn⁺ intestinal epithelial cells by a cell population that does not express the receptor. As a rule, absorption of all immunoglobulin classes will have dropped to a very low level after approximately 24 hours. Feeding colostrum tends to hasten this closure while a delay in feeding results in a slight delay in closure (up to 33 hours). The presence of the mother may be associated with increased immunoglobulin absorption. Thus calves fed measured amounts of colostrum in the presence of the mother will absorb more immunoglobulins than calves fed the same amount in her absence. In laboratory studies where measured amounts of colostrum are fed, there is a great variation (25% to 35%) in the quantity of immunoglobulins absorbed. Management should ensure that foals or calves ingest at least 1 L of colostrum within 6 hours of birth. In piglets, the ability to absorb immunoglobulins may be retained for up to 4 days if milk products are withheld.

Unsuckled animals normally have very low levels of immunoglobulins in their serum. The successful absorption of colostral immunoglobulins immediately supplies them with serum IgG at a level approaching that found in adults (Figure 19-5). Peak serum immunoglobulin levels are normally reached between 12 and 24 hours after birth. After absorption ceases, these passively acquired antibodies decline through normal metabolic processes. The rate of decline differs among immunoglobulin classes, and the time taken to decline to unprotective levels depends on their initial concentration.

As intestinal absorption is taking place, a simultaneous proteinuria may occur. This is due to intestinal absorption of proteins such as β-lactoglobulin that are sufficiently small to be excreted in the urine. In addition, the glomeruli of newborn animals are permeable to macromolecules. Thus, the urine of neonatal ruminants contains intact immunoglobulin molecules. This proteinuria ceases spontaneously with the termination of intestinal absorption.

The secretions of the mammary gland gradually change from colostrum to milk. Ruminant milk is rich in IgG1 and IgA. Nonruminant milk is rich in IgA. For the first few weeks in life, while protease activity is low, these immunoglobulins can be found throughout the intestine and in the feces of young animals. As the digestive ability of the intestine increases, eventually only secretory IgA molecules remain intact. The amount of IgA in the intestine can be large; for instance, a 3-week-old piglet may receive 1.6 g daily from sow's milk.

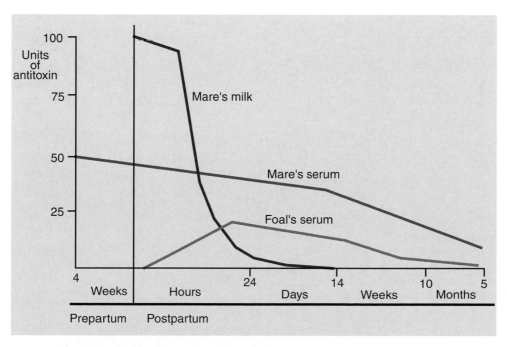

Figure 19-5. *Clostridium perfringens* antitoxin levels in serum, colostrum, and milk of six pony mares and in the serum of their foals from birth to 5 months. (After Jeffcott LB: *J Comp Pathol* 84:96, 1974.)

FAILURE OF PASSIVE TRANSFER

The absorption of IgG from colostrum is required for the protection of a young animal against septicemic disease. The continuous intake of IgA or IgG1 from milk is required for protection against enteric disease. Failure of these processes predisposes a young animal to infection.

There are three major reasons for failure of passive transfer through colostrum. First, the mother may produce insufficient or poor-quality colostrum (production failure). Second, there may be sufficient colostrum produced but inadequate intake by the newborn animal (ingestion failure). Third, there may be a failure of absorption from the intestine despite an adequate intake of colostrum (absorption failure).

Production Failure

Since colostrum represents the accumulated secretions of the udder in late pregnancy, premature births may mean that insufficient colostrum has accumulated. Valuable colostrum may also be lost from animals as a result of premature lactation or excessive dripping before birth. Colostral IgG levels also vary between individuals with up to 28% of mares producing low-quality colostrum. It is not possible to assess colostral quality simply by looking at it. Its IgG content should be assessed using a colostrometer (a modified hydrometer) to measure its specific gravity. This is normally in the range of 1.060 to 1.085, equivalent to an IgG concentration of 3000 to 8500 mg/dL. Colostrum with an IgG level of less than 3000 mg/dL may be inadequate to protect a foal and supplemental, high-quality colostrum may be required.

Ingestion Failure

In sheep or pigs, an inadequate intake may result from multiple births because the amount of colostrum produced does not rise in proportion to the number of newborns. It may be due to poor mothering, an important problem among young, inexperienced mothers. It also may be due to weakness in the newborn, to a poor suckling drive, or to physical problems such as damaged teats or jaw defects.

Absorption Failure

Failure of intestinal absorption is a major cause for concern in any species. It is especially important in horses not only because of the value of many foals but also because even with good husbandry, about 25% of newborn foals fail to absorb sufficient quantities of immunoglobulins. Alpacas also appear to experience a disproportionate number of cases of failure of passive transfer. Foals require serum IgG concentrations of at least 800 mg/dL after receiving colostrum to ensure protection. Foals that have less IgG than this are at increased risk of infection. If their IgG level fails to reach 400 mg/dL severe infections are assured (Figure 19-6).

Diagnosis of Failure of Passive Transfer

The success of passive transfer cannot be evaluated in a foal until about 18 hours after birth, when antibody absorption is essentially complete. Several assays for serum immunoglobulins are available. The most rapid and economic procedure is the zinc sulfate turbidity test, which involves mixing a zinc sulfate solution with foal serum. Zinc sulfate makes globulins insoluble. In total failure of transfer, the reaction mixture remains clear. In sera with an IgG level of more than 400 mg/dL the mixture becomes cloudy. As an alternative to visual inspection, the optical density of the mixtures can be read in a spectrophotometer and the IgG concentration read off a standard curve. Other similar techniques include precipitation by glutaraldehyde or by sodium sulfite.

Single radial immunodiffusion is a more accurate method in that it is both quantitative and specific for IgG. As described in Chapter 16, known standards are

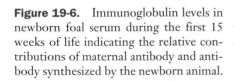

Figure 19-6. Immunoglobulin levels in newborn foal serum during the first 15 weeks of life indicating the relative contributions of maternal antibody and antibody synthesized by the newborn animal.

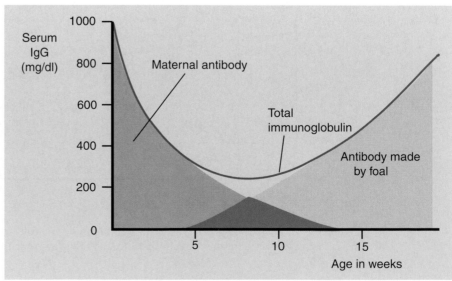

compared with the test serum by measuring the diameter of precipitation produced in agar gel containing an antiserum to equine IgG. A diagnosis of failure of passive transfer is made in foals if IgG levels are less than 400 mg/dL and partial failure of passive transfer if IgG levels are between 400 and 800 mg/dL. Unfortunately radial immunodiffusion is expensive and takes 18 to 24 hours to give a result.

A third method of measuring IgG levels is by use of a latex agglutination test. The latex particles are coated with antiequine IgG. In the presence of IgG they agglutinate. This test can be performed in about 10 minutes using either whole foal blood or serum. It appears to be reliable and rapid.

It is also possible to use a semiquantitative membrane-filter enzyme-linked immunosorbent assay (ELISA) test to measure IgG in a foal's serum. The color intensity of the reaction on the test filter is compared to color calibration spots. A variant technique uses a dipstick ELISA. Less satisfactory techniques include serum protein electrophoresis and refractometry.

Management of Failure of Passive Transfer

An IgG concentration higher than 800 mg/dL is preferred, but foals with immunoglobulin levels higher than 400 mg/dL will generally remain healthy and do not require treatment. About 75% of foals with IgG levels between 200 and 400 mg/dL will also remain healthy. However, they should be carefully watched and treated with antibiotics at the first signs of bacterial infection. Any foals with total failure of passive transfer or foals younger than 3 weeks with partial failure of passive transfer should be treated. Foals with plasma IgG concentrations less than 200 mg/dL, foals that have not nursed within 6 hours of birth, and foals that have received colostrum with IgG of less than 1000 mg/dL (specific gravity less than 1.050) should receive additional colostrum. Two to three liters of good-quality colostrum (IgG of more than 7000 mg/dL) should be given by bottle or nasogastric tube in three or four doses at hourly intervals. The colostrum must be free of antibodies to the foal's erythrocytes (Chapter 27). Colostrum can be obtained from mares that have more than is needed for their own young. It can be stored frozen at $-15°$ C to $-20°$ C for up to one year. If stored colostrum is unavailable, fresh colostrum from primiparous mares can be used. If colostrum is not available, serum or plasma may be administered orally. A large volume (up to 9 L) may be required, since serum IgG is not well absorbed and its concentration is much less than that found in colostrum.

In foals that are older than 15 hours, oral absorption ceases and an intravenous plasma infusion must be given. Ideally the dose to be used can be calculated in order to attain an IgG level of at least 400 mg/dL. Frozen horse plasma is available commercially although this may not contain antibodies against local pathogens. Alternatively the plasma may be obtained from local donors. Blood should be collected aseptically with heparin or sodium citrate. The plasma is collected after the erythrocytes settle and is stored frozen until used. The plasma must be prechecked for antierythrocyte antibody and must be free of bacterial contamination. The transfusion should be given slowly while the foal is monitored for untoward reactions. All foals receiving supplemental colostrum or plasma should have their IgG levels rechecked 12 to 24 hours later.

Considerations similar to those described above apply to failure of passive transfer in the calf. Calves with serum IgG less than 1000 mg/dL at 24 to 48 hours of age have mortality rates more than twice than that of calves with higher IgG levels. Commercially available colostrum may be enriched in specific antibodies to protect the calf against potential pathogens such as K99 *Escherichia coli*, rotaviruses, and coronaviruses, the major causes of calf diarrhea.

Colostral transfer of immunity is essential for the survival of young animals, but it may also cause problems. If a mother becomes immunized against the red cells of her fetus, colostral antibodies may cause massive erythrocyte destruction in the newborn animal, a condition called hemolytic disease of the newborn (discussed at length in Chapter 27).

CELL-MEDIATED IMMUNITY IN MILK

Colostrum is full of lymphocytes. For example, sow colostrum contains between 1×10^5 and 1×10^6 lymphocytes/mL. Of these lymphocytes, 70% to 80% are T cells. The CD4/CD8 ratio is approximately 0.57, which is lower than the ratio in blood (1.4). Bovine colostrum also contains up to 1×10^6 lymphocytes/mL, about half of which are T cells. There are usually very few lymphocytes in milk. These colostral lymphocytes may survive up to 36 hours in the intestine of newborn calves, and some penetrate the intestinal wall through the epithelium of Peyer's patches and reach the lacteal ducts or the mesenteric lymph nodes. Within 2 hours after receiving colostrum that contained labeled cells, piglets had maternal lymphocytes in their bloodstream. It is possible that cell-mediated immunity is transferred to newborn animals in this way. Piglets that had received these colostral cells showed enhanced responses to mitogens compared to control animals. Cell-containing and cell-free colostrum have been compared for their ability to protect calves against enteropathic *E. coli*. The calves receiving colostral cells excreted significantly fewer bacteria than the animals receiving cell-free colostrum. The concentration of IgA- and IgM-specific antibodies against *E. coli* in the serum of neonatal calves was higher in those that received colostral cells than in those that did not. The calves that received colostral cells had better responses to the mitogen concanavalin A and to foreign antigens such as sheep erythrocytes. The mechanisms of this protective effect are unclear.

DEVELOPMENT OF ACQUIRED IMMUNITY IN NEONATAL ANIMALS

Local Immunity

The intestinal lymphoid tissues of neonatal animals respond rapidly to an ingested antigen. For example, calves orally vaccinated with coronavirus vaccines at birth are resistant to virulent coronavirus within 3 to 9 days. Likewise, piglets vaccinated orally 3 days after birth with transmissible gastroenteritis virus (TGE) vaccines develop neutralizing antibodies in the intestine 5 to 14 days later. Much of this early resistance is attributable to innate production of interferon α/β, but there is an early intestinal IgM response that switches to IgA by 2 weeks. In the young animal, the IgA response appears earlier and reaches adult levels well before the other immunoglobulins. This rapid response of the unprimed intestinal tract is also seen in germ-free pigs. In these animals, antibody synthesis in the intestine can be detected by 4 days after infection with *E. coli*.

Systemic Immunity

The antibodies acquired by a young animal as a result of ingesting its mother's colostrum, maternal antibodies, will inhibit the ability of the newborn to mount its own immune response. As a result, very young animals are unable to respond to active immunization using vaccines. This inhibition is B cell–specific and T cell responses are largely unaffected. It depends on the relative concentrations of maternal antibody and the dose of vaccine administered.

Several different mechanisms have been suggested as mediating this suppression. One of the simplest is the rapid neutralization of live viral vaccines by the maternal antibody. This would prevent viral replication and provide insufficient antigen to prime B cells. However, data from human infants and domestic mammals indicate that sufficient antigen is present to prime T cells. Likewise, this mechanism could not account for inhibition of the immune response to nonliving vaccines.

A second proposed mechanism suggests that the inhibition results from antibodies binding to B-cell Fc receptors and blocking BCR signaling. However, recent studies on mice whose Fc receptors have been deleted (FcR knockout mice) have shown that the ability of maternal antibodies to inhibit antibody responses is unaffected. This clearly cannot be the mechanism involved. Likewise, the suggestion that maternal antibodies bind antigen, which is then removed by Fc-dependent phagocytosis, cannot be correct.

A third suggested mechanism is that maternal antibodies simply mask the epitopes on vaccine antigens and so prevent their recognition by the animal's B cells. This suggestion is compatible with the selective inhibition of B cell responses, the lack of inhibition of T cell

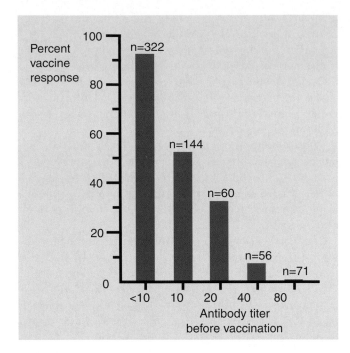

Figure 19-7. Effect of the presence of maternal antibodies to canine parvovirus in 653 puppies on their response to a modified live parvovirus vaccine. The prevaccination antibody titer profoundly inhibits the response of the puppies to the vaccine. (From Carmichael LE: *Compend Contin Educ Prac Vet* 5:1043-1054, 1983.)

responses, and with the evidence that, at least in humans and mice, high doses of antigen can overcome maternal immunity. Thus for a given vaccine dose, an immune response can be elicited only when maternal antibody titers fall below a critical threshold (Figure 19-7).

In the absence of maternal antibodies, the newborn animal is able to make antibodies soon after birth. For example, if calves fail to suckle and are therefore hypogammaglobulinemic, they will begin to make their own antibodies by about 1 week of age. In calves that have suckled and thus possess maternal antibodies, antibody synthesis does not commence until about 4 weeks of age. Likewise, colostrum-deprived piglets respond well to pseudorabies virus by 2 days after birth, but if they have suckled antibody production does not begin until 5 to 6 weeks after birth. Colostrum-deprived lambs synthesize IgG1 at 1 week and IgG2 by 3 to 4 weeks. In colostrum-fed lambs, however, IgG2 synthesis does not occur until 5 to 6 weeks old.

Vaccination of Young Animals

Because maternal antibodies inhibit neonatal immunoglobulin synthesis, they prevent the successful vaccination of young animals. This inhibition may persist for many months, its length depending on the amount of antibodies transferred and the half-life of the immunoglobulins involved. This problem can be illustrated using the example of vaccination of puppies against canine distemper.

Maternal antibodies, absorbed from the puppy's intestine, reach maximal levels in serum by 12 to 24 hours after birth. From then on their levels decline slowly through normal protein catabolism. The catabolic rate of proteins is exponential and is expressed as a half-life. Thus, the half-life of antibodies to distemper and canine infectious hepatitis is 8.4 days, and the half-life of antibodies to feline panleukopenia is 9.5 days. Experience has shown that, *on average*, the level of maternal antibodies to distemper in puppies declines to insignificant levels by about 10 to 12 weeks, although in some animals antibodies may disappear by 6 weeks whereas in others they can persist for up to 16 weeks. In a population of puppies, the proportion of nonimmune animals therefore increases gradually from a very few or none at birth, to almost all at 10 to 12 weeks. Consequently very few newborn puppies can be successfully vaccinated; most can be protected by 10 to 12 weeks. Rarely, a puppy may be 15 or 16 weeks old before it can be successfully vaccinated. If canine distemper were not so common, it would be sufficient to delay vaccination until all puppies were about 12 weeks old, when success could be almost guaranteed. In practice, a delay of this type means that an increasing proportion of puppies, fully susceptible to disease, would be without immune protection—an unacceptable situation. Nor is it feasible to vaccinate all puppies repeatedly at short intervals from birth to 12 weeks, a procedure that would ensure almost complete protection; therefore, a compromise must be reached.

The earliest age to vaccinate a puppy or kitten with a reasonable expectation of success is between 6 and 9 weeks (Box 19-2). If the young animal is at unusually high risk of disease, then it may be appropriate to begin vaccination somewhat earlier. Colostrum-deprived orphan pups may be vaccinated at 2 weeks of age. Normal puppies should be given distemper, two adenovirus, parvovirus, leptospirosis, and parainfluenza vaccines. In puppies a second dose should be given at 9 to 12 weeks and a third at 13 to 16 weeks. Rabies vaccine may also be given at 16 weeks. In kittens an appropriate protocol would be to vaccinate against viral rhinotracheitis, calicivirus, and panleukopenia at 6 to 9 weeks, 9 to 12 weeks, and 12 to 14 weeks; feline leukemia vaccine can be given twice at 9 to 12 and 12 to 14 weeks; with rabies vaccine being given at 12 weeks. There are many similar alternative vaccination protocols, all aimed at conferring early protection while leaving as few puppies as possible unprotected (Figure 19-8).

Similar considerations apply when vaccinating large farm animals. The prime factor influencing the duration of maternal immunity is the level of antibodies in the mother's colostrum. Thus in foals maternal antibodies to tetanus toxin can last for 6 months and antibodies to equine arteritis virus for as long as 8 months. Antibodies to bovine virus diarrhea may persist for up to 9 months in calves. The half-lives of maternal antibodies against equine influenza and equine arteritis virus antigens in the

---

BOX 19–2

Measles Vaccine

An alternative approach to overcoming the problems caused by maternal immunity to canine distemper has been the use of measles vaccine. Measles virus shares a major antigen, the F antigen, with canine distemper virus. The two viruses also possess distinctly different hemagglutinins (HA antigens). Generally, the presence of antibodies directed against both F and HA antigens are required for effective virus neutralization and complete protection, but antibodies to the individual antigens give partial protection. Thus maternal anti-distemper HA antibodies cannot prevent measles infection of puppy cells. The measles virus F antigen may then prime the puppy's immune system. As a result, measles vaccine given to puppies at 6 weeks of age may induce a protective response in spite of the presence of a high level of anti-distemper HA antibody.

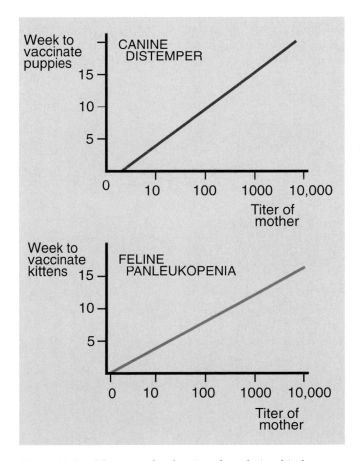

Figure 19-8. Nomographs showing the relationship between the antibody titer of the mother and the age at which to vaccinate her offspring with modified live virus vaccine. (Data from Scott FW, Csiza CK, Gillespie JH: *J Am Vet Med Assoc* 156: 439-453, 1970 [FPL]; and Baker JA, Robson DS, Gillespie JH, et al: *Cornell Vet* 49:158-167, 1959 [CD].)

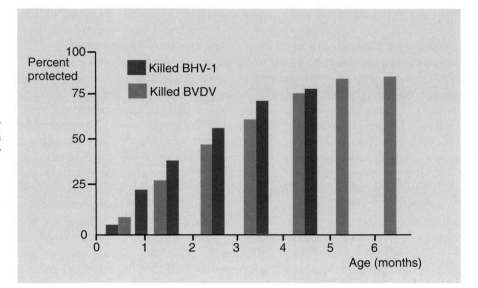

Figure 19-9. Effectiveness to two inactivated viral vaccines in calves between birth and 6 months of age. (Data courtesy of Dr. RJ Schultz.)

foal are 32 to 39 days. As in puppies, a young foal may have unprotective levels of maternal antibodies long before it can be vaccinated. Maternal antibodies, even at low levels, effectively block immune responses in young foals and calves, so that premature vaccination may be ineffective. The effectiveness of vaccines increases progressively after the first 6 months of life (Figure 19-9). A safe rule is that calves and foals should be vaccinated no

earlier than 3 to 4 months of age followed by one or two revaccinations at 4-week intervals. The precise schedule will depend on the vaccine used and the species to be vaccinated. Animals vaccinated before 6 months of age should always be revaccinated at 6 months or after weaning to ensure protection.

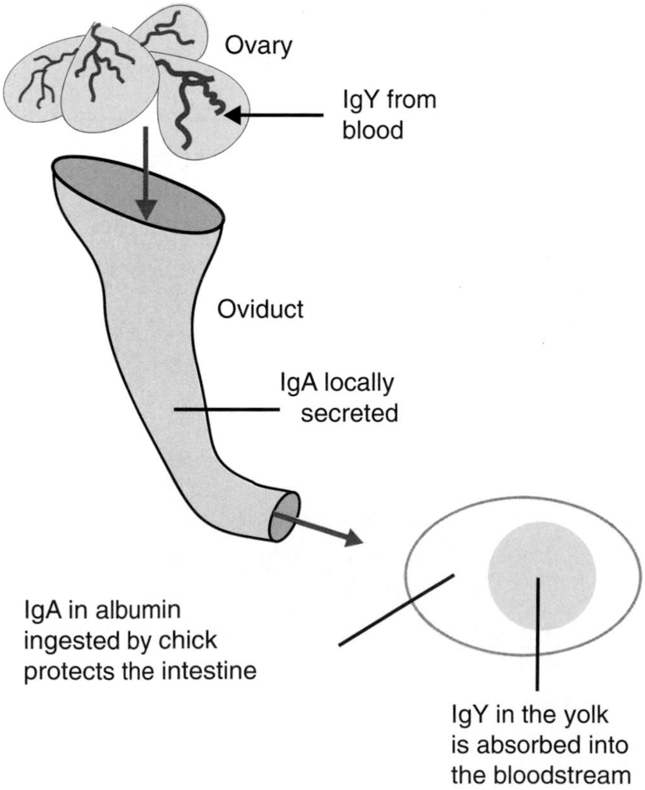

PASSIVE IMMUNITY IN THE CHICK

Newly hatched birds emerge from the sterile environment of the egg and, like mammals, require temporary immunological assistance. Serum immunoglobulins are actively transported from the hen's serum to the yolk while the egg is still in the ovary. (The immunoglobulin binds to an Fc receptor similar to mammalian FcRn.) In the fluid phase of egg yolk, IgY is therefore found at levels equal to or greater than those in hen serum. In addition, as the fertilized ovum passes down the oviduct, IgM and IgA from oviduct secretions are acquired with the albumin (Figure 19-10). As the chick embryo develops in ovo it absorbs the yolk IgY, which then appears in its circulation. At the same time, the IgM and IgA from the albumin diffuse into the amniotic fluid and are swallowed by the embryo. Thus when a chick hatches it possesses IgY in its serum and IgM and IgA in its intestine. The newly hatched chick does not absorb all its yolk sac antibodies until about 24 hours after hatching. These maternal antibodies effectively prevent successful vaccination until they disappear between 10 and 20 days after hatching.

Figure 19-10. Passive transfer of immunity from the hen to the chick.

SOURCES OF ADDITIONAL INFORMATION

Aldridge B, Garry F, Adams R: Role of colostral transfer in neonatal calf management: failure of acquisition of passive immunity, *Compend Contin Educ Prac Vet* 14:265-270, 1992.

Bernadina WE, van Leeuwen MAW, Hendrikx WML, et al: Serum opsonic activity and neutrophil phagocytic capacity of newborn lambs before and 24–36 h after colostrum uptake, *Vet Immunol Immunopathol* 29:127-138, 1991.

Butler JE, Weber P, Sinkora M, et al: Antibody repertoire development in fetal and neonatal piglets. VIII. Colonization is required for newborn piglets to make serum antibodies to T-dependent and type 2, T-independent antigens, *J Immunol* 169:6822-6830, 2002.

Crawford TB, Perryman LE: Diagnosis and treatment of failure of passive transfer in the foal, *Equine Prac* 2:17-23, 1980.

Hope JC, Sopp P, Howard CJ: NK-like CD8+ cells in immunologically naive neonatal calves that respond to dendritic cells infected with *Mycobacterium bovis* BCG, *J Leukoc Biol* 71:184-194, 2002.

Kruse-Elliott K, Wagner PC: Failure of passive antibody transfer in the foal, *Compend Contin Educ Prac Vet* 6:702-706, 1984.

Lejan C: A study by flow cytometry of lymphocytes in sow colostrum, *Res Vet Sci* 57:300-304, 1994.

Levy JK, Crawford PC, Collante WR, Papich MG: Use of adult cat serum to correct failure of passive transfer in kittens, *J Am Vet Med Assoc* 219:1401-1405, 2001.

Lunn DP: Pediatric immunology and vaccination, *AAEP Proc* 43:49-56, 1997.

Mackay CR, Maddox JF, Brandon MR: Thymocyte subpopulations during early fetal development in sheep, *J Immunol* 136:1592-1599, 1986.

Pollock JM, Rowan TG, Dixon JB, et al: Estimation of immunity in the developing calf: cellular and humoral responses to keyhole limpet hemocyanin, *Vet Immunol Immunopathol* 29:105-114, 1991.

Reynolds JD, Morris B: The evolution and involution of Peyer's patches in fetal and postnatal sheep, *Eur J Immunol* 13:627-635, 1983.

Ricks CA, Avakian A, Bryan T, et al: In ovo vaccination technology, *Adv Vet Med* 41:495-515, 1999.

Riedel-Caspari G: The influence of colostral leukocytes on the course of experimental *Escherichia coli* infection and serum antibodies in neonatal calves, *Vet Immunol Immunopathol* 35:275-288, 1993.

Schnulle PM, Hurley WL: Sequence and expression of the FcRn in the porcine mammary gland, *Vet Immunol Immunopathol* 91:227-231, 2003.

Sun J, Hayward C, Shinde R, et al: Antibody repertoire development in fetal and neonatal piglets. I. Four VH genes account for 80 percent of VH usage during 84 days of fetal life, *J Immunol* 161:5070-5078, 1998.

Tlaskalova-Hogenova H, Mandel L, Trebichavsky I, et al: Development of immune responses in early pig ontogeny, *Vet Immunol Immunopathol* 43:135-142, 1994.

Van Maanen C, Bruin G, deBoer-Luijtze E, et al: Interference of maternal antibodies with the immune response of foals after vaccination against equine influenza, *Vet Q* 14:13-17, 1992.

Vivrette S: Colostrum and oral immunoglobulin therapy in newborn foals, *Compend Contin Educ Prac Vet* 23:286-291, 2001.

Washington EA, Kimpton WG, Cahill RNP: Changes in the distribution of $\alpha\beta$ and $\gamma\delta$ T cells in blood and lymph nodes from fetal and postnatal lambs, *Dev Comp Immunol* 16:493-501, 1992.

Williams PP: Immunomodulating effects of intestinal absorbed maternal colostral leukocytes by neonatal pigs, *Can J Vet Res* 57:1-8, 1993.

Wilson CB, Penix L, Weaver WM, et al: Ontogeny of T lymphocyte function in the neonate, *Am J Reprod Immunol* 28:132-135, 1992.

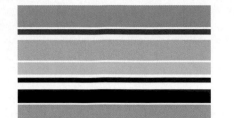

Immunity at Body Surfaces

Although mammals possess an extensive array of innate and acquired defense mechanisms within tissues, it is at their surfaces that invading microorganisms are first encountered and largely repelled or destroyed (Figure 20-1). Although the skin is the most obvious of these surfaces, it in fact represents only a small fraction of the area of the body exposed to the exterior. The areas of the mucous membranes of the intestine and respiratory tracts are at least 200 times larger. These surfaces are defended by both innate and acquired protective mechanisms.

INNATE PROTECTIVE MECHANISMS

One of the most important functions of the skin is to present a barrier to invading microorganisms. It presents a strong physical barrier supplemented by continuous desquamation, desiccation, and a low pH because of fatty acids in sebum. In addition, the skin carries a resident bacterial flora that excludes other bacteria and fungi. If this skin flora is disturbed, its protective properties are reduced, and microbial invasion may result. Thus skin infections tend to occur in areas such as the axilla or groin, where both pH and humidity are relatively high. Similarly, animals forced to stand in water or mud show an increased frequency of foot infections as the skin becomes sodden, its structure breaks down, and its resident flora changes in response to alterations in the local environment. The importance of the resident flora

is well seen in the intestine, where it is essential not only for the control of potential pathogens but also for the digestion of foods such as cellulose in the diet of herbivores. In addition, the natural development of the immune system in species such as the rabbit depends on the simulation provided by intestinal microflora.

Because they have no bacterial flora, gnotobiotic (germ-free) pigs or mice have hypoplastic secondary lymphoid organs that do not develop germinal centers, and their immunoglobulin levels are only about 2% of normal. If the natural flora of the intestine is eliminated or its composition drastically altered (by aggressive antibiotic treatment, for example), an overgrowth of potential pathogens may occur, leading to severe colitis. The flora of the digestive tract normally acts competitively against potential invaders through mechanisms that supplement the other physical defenses of this system (Figure 20-2). Thus in the mouth, the flushing activity of saliva is complemented by the generation of peroxidases from streptococci. In single stomached animals the gastric pH may be sufficiently low to have a bactericidal or virucidal effect, although this varies greatly among species and among meals. The dog, for instance, has a relatively low gastric pH relative to that of the pig. Similarly, the pH in the center of a mass of ingested food may not necessarily drop to low levels, and some foods such as milk are potent buffers.

Farther down the intestine, the resident bacterial flora keeps the pH and oxygen tension low. The intestinal flora is also influenced by the diet; for instance, the

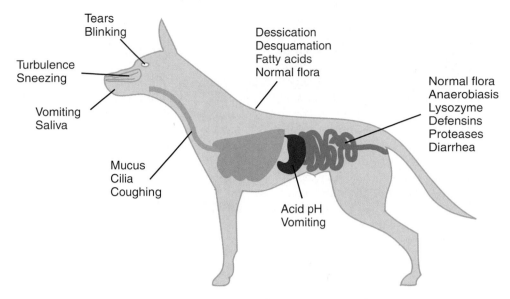

Figure 20-1. Some innate surface protection mechanisms.

intestine of milk-fed animals is colonized largely by lactobacilli, which produce large quantities of bacteriostatic lactic and butyric acids. These acids inhibit colonization by potential pathogens such as *Escherichia coli*, so that young animals suckled naturally tend to have fewer digestive disturbances than animals weaned early in life. In the large intestine the bacterial flora mainly consists of strict anaerobes.

Alpha defensins are secreted by specialized intestinal epithelial cells called Paneth cells. These enteric defensins, known as cryptdins, accumulate within intestinal crypts and can achieve very high concentrations locally. They prevent bacteria from entering the crypts and so protect enterocytes from invasion. In cattle, expression of cryptdin genes has been detected, throughout the small intestine and colon. These bovine cryptdins are secreted as active molecules as opposed to the human and mouse molecules that are secreted as inactive precursors and activated by trypsin within the intestine.

Lysozyme, the antibacterial and antiviral enzyme, is synthesized in the gastric mucosa and in macrophages within the intestinal mucosa. As a result, it is found in large quantities in intestinal fluid. Paneth cells secrete both lysozyme and cryptdins.

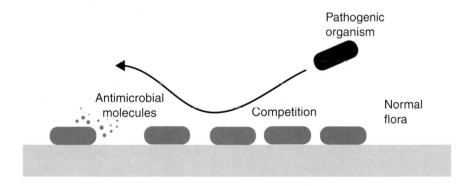

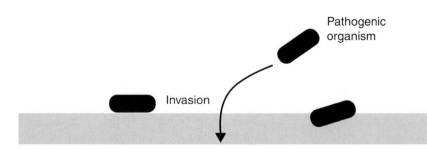

Figure 20-2. The role of the normal bacterial flora in excluding pathogens from body surfaces by competition. In the absence of a normal flora, the invading organisms face no competition and can readily colonize and invade surfaces.

In the urinary system, the flushing action and low pH of urine generally provide adequate protection; however, when urinary stasis occurs, urethritis resulting from the unhindered ascent of pathogenic bacteria is not uncommon. In adult animals, the vagina is lined by a squamous epithelium composed of cells rich in glycogen. When these cells desquamate, they provide a substrate for lactobacilli that, in turn, generate large quantities of lactic acid, which protects the vagina against invasion. Glycogen storage in the vaginal epithelial cells is stimulated by estrogens and thus occurs only in sexually mature individuals.

The mammary gland uses several different defense mechanisms. In a non-lactating animal, a keratin plug blocks the teat orifice and so excludes bacteria. In a lactating animal, the flushing action of the milk helps to prevent invasion by some potential pathogens, whereas milk itself contains many innate antibacterial substances (called lactenins). These antibacterial agents include complement, lysozyme, lactoferrin, and lactoperoxidase. Lactoferrin competes with bacteria for iron and makes it unavailable for their growth. It also enhances the neutrophil respiratory burst. Milk contains high concentrations of lactoperoxidase and thiocyanate (SCN^-) ions. In the presence of exogenous hydrogen peroxide, lactoperoxidase can oxidize the SCN^- to bacteriostatic products such as $OSCN^-$.

$$H_2O_2 + SCN^- \rightarrow OSCN^- + H_2O$$

The hydrogen peroxide may be produced by bacteria, such as streptococci or by the oxidation of ascorbic acid. Some strains of streptococci are resistant to this bacteriostatic pathway, since they have an enzyme that reduces the SCN^-. The phagocytic cells released into the mammary gland in response to irritation also contribute to antimicrobial resistance not only through their phagocytic efforts but also by providing additional lactoferrin, hydrogen peroxide, and lysosomal peroxidases. The binding of bovine lactoferrin to unencapsulated *Streptococcus agalactiae* can activate the classical complement pathway. The lactoferrin is apparently able to substitute for antibodies and activate C1q.

The respiratory tract differs from other body surfaces in that it is in intimate connection with the interior of the body yet it is required by its very nature to allow unhindered access of air to the alveoli. The system obviously requires a filter. Particles suspended in the air entering the respiratory tract are largely removed by turbulence that directs them onto its mucus-covered walls, where they adhere. The turbulence is caused by the conformation of the turbinate bones, the trachea, and the bronchi. This turbulence filter serves to remove particles as small as 5 μm before they reach the alveoli (Figure 20-3).

A blanket of sticky mucus produced by goblet cells covers the walls of the upper respiratory tract. The mucus gel traps soluble host defense molecules such as defensins, lysozyme, and IgA and thus has antimicrobial activity. This mucus layer is in continuous flow, being carried from the bronchioles up the bronchi and trachea by ciliary action or backward through the nasal cavity to the pharynx. Here the dirty mucus is swallowed and presumably digested in the intestinal tract. Particles smaller than 5 μm that can bypass this mucociliary escalator and reach the alveoli are phagocytosed by alveolar macrophages. Once these cells have successfully ingested particles, they migrate to the mucus escalator and are also carried to the pharynx and eliminated.

LYMPHOID TISSUES

Because of the importance of preventing infection through mucosal surfaces, these surfaces contain large amounts of lymphoid tissue. These mucosal lymphoid tissues fall into two groups: sites where antigens are processed and immune responses are initiated (inductive sites) and sites where antibodies and cell-mediated responses are mounted (effector sites).

Inductive Sites

Some mucosal lymphoid tissues possess all the components required to initiate an immune response: T cells, B cells, and dendritic cells. These include the tonsils in the pharynx, Peyer's patches, solitary lymphoid nodules, and the appendix in the intestine, and numerous lymphoid nodules in the lung. These lymphoid tissues are known by their acronyms. Thus GALT (gut-associated lymphoid tissue) is the collective term for all the lymphoid nodules, Peyer's patches, and individual lymphocytes found in the intestinal walls. Similarly, BALT is the acronym used for the bronchus-associated lymphoid tissue in the lungs. These organized lymphoid tissues, unlike lymph nodes, do not encounter foreign antigens delivered through afferent lymph but sample it directly from the lumen.

The surface of the intestine is covered by a layer of intestinal epithelial cells (enterocytes) that form intercellular tight junctions and which thus form an effective barrier to both microbes and macromolecules. (Molecules larger than about 2 kDa are excluded.) Obviously, some aggressive invasive bacteria can damage and penetrate enterocytes directly and so trigger local inflammatory and immune responses. However, it is also clear that there is an interplay between the antigen-processing cells in the intestinal wall and antigens in the lumen. Thus there are two other important routes by which organisms and macromolecules can penetrate the intact intestinal wall and be directed toward the intestinal lymphoid tissues. One route involves specialized cells (M cells) located directly over aggregates of lymphoid tissue or Peyer's patches; the other involves dendritic cells that reside in the submucosa but extend their cytoplasmic processes between the epithelial cells into the intestinal lumen. The tight junctions remain intact but antigen

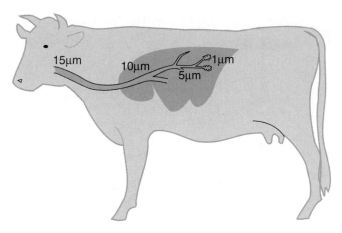

Figure 20-3. The influence of particle size on the site of deposition of particles within the respiratory tract. Only the smallest particles can penetrate deeply and gain access to the alveoli.

samples can be transported within the dendritic cell cytoplasm. This latter route provides a mechanism whereby noninvasive bacteria and macromolecules can be sampled and presented to nearby T cells.

Peyer's patches are the largest of the mucosal lymphoid tissues. A newborn calf normally has about 100 Peyer's patches, and these may cover as much as half of the ileal surface. Collectively, therefore, the intestine contains more lymphocytes than the spleen. In ruminants and pigs there are two types of Peyer's patch that differ in location, structure, and functions. The ileocecal Peyer's patches are primary lymphoid organs, whereas the jejunal Peyer's patches are secondary lymphoid organs. In lambs, these ileocecal patches increase in size from birth to 6 months of age and then regress, leaving only a small

scar in adults. In contrast, the jejunal patches persist throughout adult life and play a major role in intestinal defense. Both types of Peyer's patch consist of masses of lymphocytes arranged in follicles and covered with an epithelium that contains specialized cells called M cells (They have microfolds rather than microvilli on their surface.) (Figure 20-4). M cells take up antigens from the intestinal lumen and present them directly to nearby lymphocytes. M cells may transport soluble macromolecules such as IgA, small particles, and even whole organisms. (Some pathogens such as salmonellae, *Yersinia*, *Listeria*, *M. tuberculosis*, and the reoviruses may take advantage of the M cells and use them to gain access to the body.) The proportion of M cells in the follicle-associated epithelium varies from 10% in humans and mice, to 50% in rabbits, and to 100% in the terminal ileum of pigs and calves.

Effector Sites

Although Peyer's patches contain large numbers of lymphocytes, most IgA is produced in diffuse lymphoid nodules and in isolated plasma cells located in the walls of the intestine, in bronchi, in salivary glands, and in the gallbladder. These cells constitute at least 80% of all plasma cells in the body. As a result, more IgA is produced every day than all other immunoglobulin classes combined.

B Cells

The intestinal wall contains B cells that respond to antigen by differentiating into plasma cells. Some of these responding B cells migrate to regional lymph nodes and into intestinal lymphatics, from which they reach the thoracic duct and enter the bloodstream. These circulating

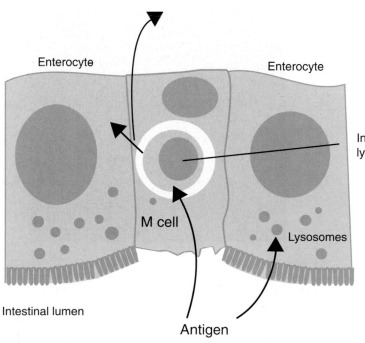

Figure 20-4. The role of M cells as antigen-processing cells in the intestinal wall. Antigen that enters enterocytes is usually rapidly degraded in lysosomes. Antigen that enters M cells is not degraded. It may be presented directly to intraepithelial lymphocytes within the M cell or, alternatively, permitted to pass along the intercellular space to the tissue fluid. From here, it will be carried to the draining lymph nodes.

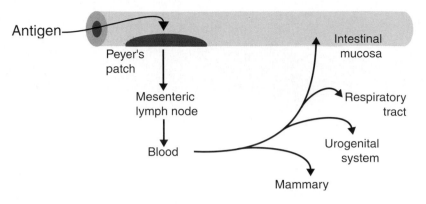

Figure 20-5. When stimulated by antigen, IgA-producing B cells are produced in inductive sites, such as the Peyer's patches. They then leave the intestine and circulate in the bloodstream. They all eventually settle on other surfaces, such as the lung, the mammary gland, and other regions of the gastrointestinal tract—effector sites. It is this transfer of antibody-producing cells in the mammary gland that ensures that milk contains IgA antibodies directed against intestinal pathogens.

IgA-positive B cells have an affinity for all body surfaces. As a result, they end up not only in the intestinal tract but also in the respiratory tract, urogenital tract, and mammary gland. Thus antigen priming at one location will permit antibodies to be synthesized and secondary responses to occur at locations remote from the priming site (Figure 20-5). The movement of IgA-positive B cells from the intestine to the mammary gland is especially important, since it provides a route by which intestinal immunity can be transferred to the newborn through milk. Oral administration of antigen to a pregnant animal will thus result in the appearance of IgA antibodies in its milk. In this way, the intestine of the newborn animal will be flooded by antibodies directed against intestinal pathogens. T cells originating within the Peyer's patches also home specifically to the intestinal mucosa. This results from the use of specialized vascular addressins that determine lymphocyte migration patterns. For example, the mucosal vascular addressin cell adhesin molecule (MadCAM-1) is expressed only on the high endothelial venules of Peyer's patches and on venules in intestinal lamina propria and the mammary gland. Its ligand is the lymphocyte integrin α4/β7. As a result, B and T cells that express this integrin home preferentially to the intestine and the mammary gland.

T Cells

Both α/β and γ/δ T cells are found on body surfaces, but in different locations. Thus in the intestine, α/β T cells are found in the lamina propria, whereas γ/δ T cells are found beneath and between enterocytes, where they are known as intraepithelial lymphocytes (IELs) (Figure 20-6). The number and location of these IELs suggest that they play a key role in the defense of the gastrointestinal tract, although there are species differences. Thus 5% of IEL in humans, 50% in mice, and up to 90% in ruminants carry γ/δ TCR. A high proportion of intestinal T cells are CD8+ (85% in humans, 77% in pigs, 24% in sheep). The CD8 molecules on these IELs consist of α/α homodimers in contrast to the CD8 α/β heterodimers found on conventional α/β T cells. Instead of binding to MHC class II as in conventional responses, CD8 on IELs binds to a MHC class Ib molecule called TL (thymus-leukemia) antigen. TL antigen is expressed exclusively on enterocytes. The binding of T cells to TL molecules appears to suppress

T cell function and thus prevents the killing of enterocytes by the T cells. Conversely, enterocytes secrete stem cell factor and IL-7, so they may promote γ/δ T cell survival.

IELs tend to use unusual Vγ and Vδ genes to form the TCR antigen-binding site. These genes are not expressed in other lymphoid organs, suggesting that the IEL T cells are specialized for epithelial surveillance.

The suggestion that γ/δ IEL may be a novel cell lineage is confirmed by the observation that they are found in neonatally thymectomized mice. They originate within the

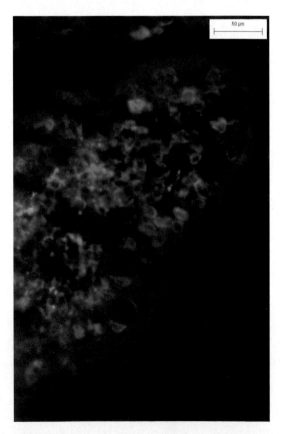

Figure 20-6. Double-color immunofluorescence showing a canine duodenal villous tip stained with monoclonal antibodies to αβ TCR and γδ TCR. The αβ T cells are stained green and are located in the interior of the villus. The γδ T cells are stained red and are clearly located within the intestinal epithelium. (From German AJ, Hall EJ, Moore PF, et al: *J Comp Pathol* 121:249-263, 1999.)

bone marrow and mature within cryptopatches, clusters of cells located just under the enterocytes. Cryptopatches each contain several hundred immature T cells with the surface markers c-kit (CD117, the receptor for SCF) and IL-7R (CD 127). IELs are MHC class II–positive, and they may act as antigen-presenting cells on their own. IELs do not proliferate in response to conventional antigens. It is possible that their lack of proliferative response may be due to an absence of CD5 and CD28. Some γ/δ T cells have contrasuppressor activity and can prevent the development of oral tolerance within the intestinal lymphoid tissues (Chapter 18). They may also regulate B cell IgA responses. Some have NK activity, whereas others are cytotoxic T cells that may attack parasites within the intestinal lumen. One unique property of γ/δ T cells is that they can recognize antigens directly without prior processing. They secrete cytokines such as IFN-γ in response. The interferon can in turn stimulate macrophages and nearby enterocytes to secrete nitric oxide. This nitric oxide may serve a protective role in the intestinal mucosa.

Globule leukocytes, once thought to be degranulated mast cells, have been demonstrated to be a subset of γ/δ T cells in the cat and goat. They contain large eosinophilic cytoplasmic granules, but their nucleus resembles that in lymphocytes. Their function is unknown.

Ruminant γ/δ T cells recirculate continuously between epithelial surfaces such as the skin or intestinal epithelium and the bloodstream. In sheep, they are primarily located in skin near the basal layer of the epidermis and in the dermis close to hair follicles and sebaceous glands. They are uncommon in wool-covered skin but are present in large numbers in skin that is not covered by wool. In addition, they are found in the epithelium of the tongue, esophagus, trachea, and bladder.

ACQUIRED PROTECTIVE MECHANISMS

Body surfaces are protected by both antibody- and cell-mediated immune processes. The antibodies produced on mucosal surfaces include IgA, IgM, IgE, and IgG. Some of these, most notably IgA and possibly IgM, act by immune exclusion (Figure 20-7). The others, especially IgE and IgG, destroy antigen within the surface tissues by immune elimination.

Immune Exclusion

Immunoglobulin A
Immunoglobulin A predominates in surface secretions; it is found in significant amounts in saliva, intestinal fluid, nasal and tracheal secretions, tears, milk, colostrum, urine, and the secretions of the urogenital tract (Figure 20-8). IgA appears to have evolved specifically to protect body surfaces (Table 20-1). Thus in swine 90% of immunoglobulin-containing cells in the intestinal lamina propria contain IgA.

Th2 cells are the predominant helper cells found in surface tissues. When appropriately stimulated, these

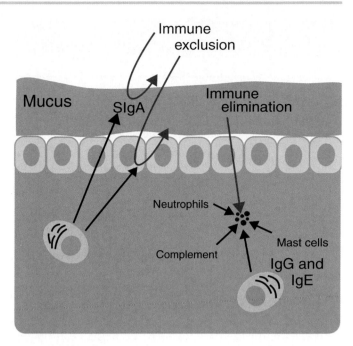

Figure 20-7. Two key defensive mechanisms are employed on mucosal surfaces. The most important is immune exclusion, an effect primarily mediated by IgA. If antigens gain access to the mucosa, they are then destroyed by IgG- and IgE-mediated processes by immune elimination.

Th2 cells secrete a mixture of cytokines that result in the preferential production of IgA and IgE. Transforming growth factor-α (TGF-α) is the key cytokine that triggers this switch to IgA production (Figure 20-9), whereas IL-6 is essential for the terminal differentiation of IgA-producing plasma cells. Other Th2 cytokines, such as IL-4, IL-5, and IL-10, promote these processes.

The IgA monomer has a molecular weight of about 160 kDa and is a typical four-chain, Y-shaped molecule

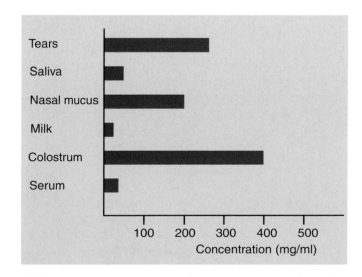

Figure 20-8. Typical immunoglobulin A levels in bovine body fluids. In other species, milk and colostral IgA concentrations may be considerably higher.

TABLE   20-1
Approximate IgA Levels in the Serum and Various Secretions of the Domestic Animals

Animal	Secretion (mg/dl)					
	Serum	Colostrum	Milk	Nasal Mucus	Saliva	Tears
Horse	170	1000	130	160	140	150
Cow	30	400	10	200	56	260
Sheep	30	400	10	50	90	160
Pig	200	1000	500	—	—	—
Dog	100	250	400	—	—	—
Cat	200	100	24	—	54	—
Chicken	50	—	—	—	20	15

(Figure 13-6). It is usually secreted as a dimer or larger polymer bound together by a J chain. IgA has several extra cysteine residues in its heavy chains. As a result, the short interchain disulfide bonds compact the chains and shield vulnerable bonds from proteases.

IgA is synthesized and secreted by plasma cells in the intestinal submucosa, especially in the crypt region. This dimeric IgA binds to a glycoprotein receptor for polymeric immunoglobulin (pIgR) on the basal surface of enterocytes (Figure 20-10). Once bound, the receptor forms disulfide bonds with the Ca2 domain of one of the IgA monomers. The complex of IgA and pIgR is then endocytosed and actively transported across the enterocyte. When it reaches the exterior surface, the endocytic vesicle fuses with the plasma membrane and exposes the IgA to the intestinal lumen. The extracellular domains of the pIgR are then cleaved by proteases so that the IgA, with the receptor peptide still attached (secretory IgA), is released into the lumen. The receptor peptide is called secretory component. The production, transport, and secretion of secretory component occurs even in the absence of IgA so that free secretory component is found in high concentrations in intestinal secretions.

IgA is not bactericidal and activates complement only by the alternate and lectin pathways. It can neutralize viruses, as well as some viral and bacterial enzymes, and it can act as an opsonin and function in some antibody-dependent cellular cytotoxicity (ADCC) systems. Its most important function however, is to prevent the adherence of bacteria and viruses to epithelial surfaces—immune exclusion. If bacteria or viruses cannot adhere to enterocytes, they simply pass along with the intestinal contents and are expelled without doing any harm.

Because IgA is transported through enterocytes, it can also act inside these cells (Figure 20-11). Thus IgA can bind to newly synthesized viral proteins inside epithelial cells and interrupt viral replication. In this way, the IgA can prevent viral growth before the integrity of the epithelium is damaged. This is a unique example of an antibody acting in an intracellular location. The second unique function of intracellular IgA is to excrete foreign antigens. Thus IgA can bind to antigens that have penetrated to the submucosa. Once bound, the IgA-antigen complexes will bind to pIgR and be actively transported across the enterocytes into the intestinal lumen. IgA can therefore act at three different levels to exclude foreign antigens: within the submucosa, within enterocytes, and within the intestinal lumen.

In some species, such as rats, rabbits, and chickens, up to 75% of the IgA produced within the intestinal wall may diffuse into the portal blood circulation and be carried to the liver (Figure 20-12). In these species, hepatocytes have pIgR on their surface. The bloodborne IgA thus binds to hepatocytes and is carried across the hepatocyte cytoplasm to be released into the bile canaliculi. Bile is therefore the major route by which IgA reaches the intestine in these species. It is also a route by which antigens bound to circulating IgA can be removed from the body. The reader should note, however, that in the major domestic mammals (dogs, ruminants, and swine), less than 5% of IgA enters the bile.

IgA binds to the pIgR on enterocytes and hepatocytes before being transported to the intestinal lumen or bile.

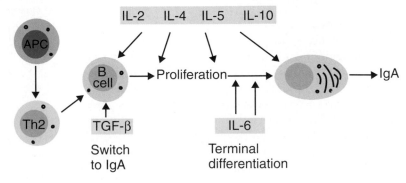

Figure 20-9. The control of IgA production. TGF-β is primarily responsible for the IgM-to-IgA switch. Terminal differentiation of IgA-producing plasma cells is mainly mediated by IL-6. Other cytokines are also important in the process.

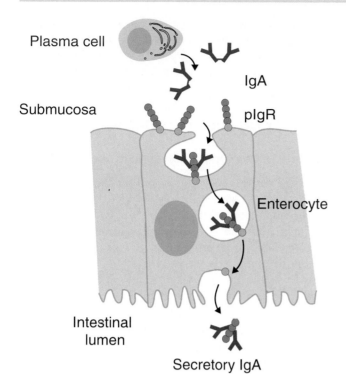

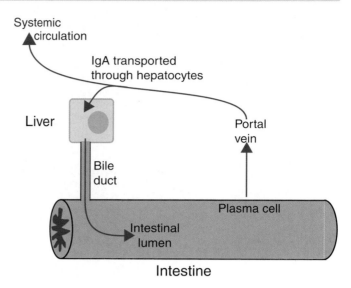

Figure 20-10. IgA is secreted by mucosal plasma cells and binds to receptors (pIgR) on the interior surface of intestinal enterocytes. The bound IgA is taken into the enterocytes and passed in vesicles to the cell surface. Once in the intestinal lumen, the pIgR is cleaved from the cell and remains bound to the IgA. In this state it is called secretory component and serves to protect the IgA from degradation.

Figure 20-12. Some IgA, instead of being secreted directly into the intestine, as shown in Figure 20-10, may be carried to the liver, where it is passed through the hepatocytes into the bile duct. In some species, such as the rat, this is a very important pathway. In others it is much less significant. For example, only about 5% of IgA reaches the intestine by this route in humans.

In addition, IgA-antigen complexes can bind to monocytes and macrophages, neutrophils, and eosinophils through the low-affinity receptor FcαR1 (CD89). When IgA-opsonized particles bind to the FcαR on phagocytic cells, they can trigger superoxide production, opsonization, ADCC, and the release of inflammatory mediators. IgA also adheres selectively to Peyer's patch M cells, which appear to possess an IgA receptor that is not FcαR1. This mediates the transport of IgA from the lumen to the underlying lymphoid tissues and explains how an animal may be able to mount a secondary immune response to an antigen in the intestine, even in the presence of IgA.

Immunoglobulin M
The earliest immunoglobulins found in the intestine of the newborn are of the IgM class. IgM will also bind to pIgR and is carried through the enterocyte to the lumen. Because of its structure, however, SIgM is much more susceptible than SIgA to proteases.

Immune Elimination

Immunoglobulin E
Because IgA does not activate complement, it functions by immune exclusion. There is a second line of defense, however, which destroys antigen that penetrates the mucosal barrier, (immune elimination). This process is mediated by IgE. Cells producing IgE are mainly found on body surfaces rather than in the lymph nodes or spleen. IgE attaches to mast cells within the walls of the intestine, respiratory tract, and in the skin. Thus, if invading organisms evade the IgA and gain access to the tissues, IgE-mediated responses will be triggered (Figure 20-13).

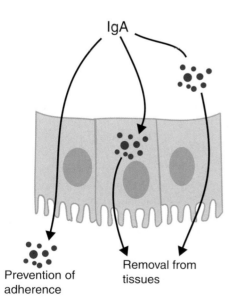

Figure 20-11. IgA is unique in that it can act in three locations. It can bind antigen in tissue fluid or in enterocytes as well as in the intestinal lumen. The bound antigen in tissues or enterocytes is carried to the intestinal lumen.

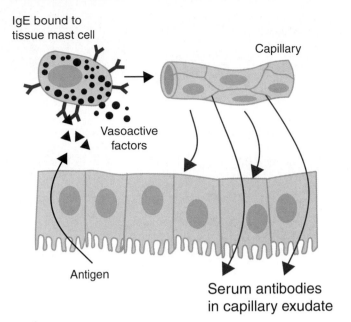

Figure 20-13. The IgE response in the intestinal wall. Antigen reaches IgE-sensitized mast cells to cause their degranulation. As a result of this, vasoactive factors are released. These cause increased vascular permeability and exudation of serum IgG antibodies.

These responses involve rapid degranulation of mast cells and the release of their vasoactive molecules into the surrounding tissues. As described in Chapter 2, these molecules cause acute inflammation, increase the permeability of small blood vessels, and promote fluid leakage between enterocytes, leading to the outflow of fluid containing large quantities of IgG into the intestinal lumen.

This process occurs, for example, when parasitic worms invade the intestinal mucosa. IgA has little effect on these invaders, so they have no difficulty in burrowing into the superficial layers of the mucosa. When parasite antigens encounter sensitized mast cells, however, the release of vasoactive molecules together with the local inflammation, changes in blood flow, and intestinal motility may be sufficient to force the parasite to disengage—a phenomenon called "self-cure" (Chapter 25).

Thus IgA and IgE work in concert. IgA normally is the first line of defense, and IgE serves as a back-up system. If IgA production is defective, the IgE response may be triggered to excess. As a result, low levels of IgA result in increased IgE production and the development of allergic responses to food and inhaled antigens.

Immunoglobulin G

In ruminants (especially cattle), IgG1, not IgA, is the major secretory immunoglobulin in colostrum and milk. This is due to selective transfer from the bloodstream into the mammary gland. On other body surfaces in ruminants, however, IgA remains the predominant immunoglobulin, although IgG1 is also present at high concentrations. IgG2 is also transferred into the intestine and saliva in ruminants. IgG may be of greater protective significance in the respiratory tract than in the intestine since there it is less likely to be degraded by proteases.

IMMUNITY ON SPECIFIC SURFACES

Immunity in the Gastrointestinal Tract

One of the central questions in immunology is how the immune system reacts relatively weakly to food antigens and normal flora but still has the ability to respond to intestinal pathogens. The intestinal immune system cannot selectively ignore antigens. A T cell cannot "know" that one antigen comes from food whereas another comes from an intestinal virus. Thus we now recognize that the intestinal immune system is responsive to food antigens and the normal flora. It is likely that in normal animals, there is more immune activity in the intestine than in all other lymphoid tissues combined. It has been estimated, for example, that more than 80% of the body's activated B cells are found in the intestine.

The intestine is the most important route of entry for foreign antigens and contains a major portion of the lymphoid tissue of the body. The antigens that may enter the body from the intestine include food proteins, commensal gut flora, and invading pathogens. The gut epithelium must serve as the major barrier to invading pathogens, while at the same time permitting the absorption of nutrients. It has been argued that the body must ensure that the intestinal immune system excludes food antigens to prevent the systemic immune system from being overwhelmed by vast amounts of foreign antigen.

It has been estimated that about 2% of ingested protein is absorbed as peptide fragments large enough to be recognized by the immune system, although a very much smaller fraction (<0.002%) is absorbed intact. This protein readily reaches the portal circulation, but little passes the liver and enters the systemic circulation. Presumably the Kupffer cells of the liver effectively capture food antigens. Antibodies produced locally may bind to adsorbed antigen and generate immune-complexes that are removed as the blood passes through the liver. Thus if a calf is fed a defined dietary antigen such as soy protein, although it is initially well absorbed, the animal soon begins to make IgA antibodies against it. Once these antibodies are produced and immune exclusion develops, the amount of protein absorbed drops significantly. If a new novel protein is introduced into the feed, it too will be initially absorbed until IgA is produced against it. Thus a prime role for IgA may be to exclude food antigens from the circulation.

If a small amount of dietary antigen gains access to the general circulation in adults, a systemic immune response may be prevented by the activities of regulatory T cells and oral tolerance develops to the antigen. Oral tolerance may involve either cellular suppression or clonal anergy and is generally directed against Th1 cells. The determining factor in deciding which mechanism is involved in this tolerance is probably the dose of antigen. Low doses invoke active suppression. High doses provoke clonal anergy. To ensure that immune exclusion continues to operate, the intestinal mucosa is rich in contra-suppressor cells (Chapter 18).

Vast numbers of bacteria live within the gastrointestinal tract. These commensal bacteria invade the gastrointestinal tract soon after birth and drive the normal development of the immune system in species such as pigs and rabbits. Germ-free animals fail to fully develop their intestinal lymphoid tissues. It is probable that the host mounts persistent but ineffective immune responses against these organisms. This is probably due to their location. Commensal bacteria largely reside in the intestinal lumen behind a glycocalyx barrier that keeps them from direct contact with enterocytes. Persistent IgA responses will have a similar effect. On the other hand, pathogens such as *E. coli* or *S. enterica* can cross the glycocalyx and either attach to enterocytes or release damaging toxins. These will trigger the host defenses.

The gastrointestinal mucus barrier is also critical to the defense of body surfaces. Not only does it serve as a physical barrier keeping pathogens and chemicals away from the enterocytes, but it also traps and expels pathogens. Rich in defensins and lysozyme, it is an insuperable barrier to many potentially pathogenic bacteria and viruses.

If pathogenic bacteria penetrate the intestinal mucosa and gain access to the lacteals and portal vessels, they are subsequently trapped in the mesenteric lymph nodes and liver. Other organisms may enter the body through surface lymphoid tissues. For instance, the epithelium at the bottom of the tonsillar crypts is very thin (Figure 20-14). Viruses may enter the body by this route and multiply locally in the tonsil before spreading elsewhere.

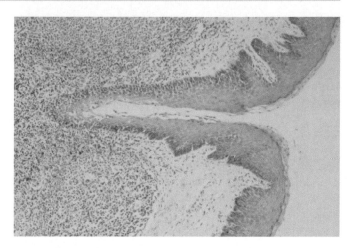

Figure 20-14. A section of pig tonsil showing a tonsillar crypt. Note how thin the epithelium is at the base of the crypt. An easy invasion route for many organisms. Original magnification ×150. (Courtesy of Dr S Yamashiro.)

Microbial antigens presented in the intestine tend to stimulate a more intense immune response than do dietary antigens. This may be due to differences in penetration of the mucosa and the development of immune elimination rather than immune exclusion. Oral vaccination may help to protect against those diseases to which an animal is susceptible for only a short period. Giving a diet containing killed *E. coli* to calves and pigs has resulted in a reduced incidence of diarrhea, a better feed conversion, and an improved overall health of the animals. Live oral transmissible gastroenteritis vaccine may also be given to pregnant sows to stimulate an intestinal IgA response and seed antibody-producing cells to the udder. This results in the appearance of specific antibodies in colostrum, and in the protection of suckling piglets.

Immunity in the Mammary Gland

The protective mechanisms of the udder are presumably not at their most effective in that biological anomaly, the modern dairy cow. The flushing action of the milk helps to prevent invasion by some potential pathogens while milk itself contains bacterial inhibitors (lactenins) and phagocytic cells. In addition, milk contains IgA, secretory component, and IgG1. The IgA and secretory component are closely associated with the milk fat globules. In simple-stomached animals, IgA predominates, whereas in ruminants, IgG1 does.

IgA is locally synthesized in the mammary tissue, although many of the IgA-producing cells in the gland are derived from precursors originating in the intestine. These cells are a source of antibodies against intestinal pathogens. IgG1, in contrast, is selectively transferred by active transport from serum using the FcRn receptor on mammary gland epithelial cells.

BOX 20–1

How to Suppress Intestinal Inflammation

Bacteria that seek to invade the intestinal wall normally must survive in the face of a potent inflammatory response. Some organisms do this by suppressing inflammation. *Salmonella enterica pullorum,* the cause of fowl typhoid, is such an organism. It effectively suppresses inflammation by preventing activation of the transcription factor NF-κB. NF-κB is normally bound to its inhibitor IκB so that it cannot move to the nucleus and activate genes. If IκB is phosphorylated, ubiquitinated, and degraded, NF-κB is released. The NF-κB then moves to the nucleus and switches on the genes for various cytokines and chemokines that serve as inflammatory mediators. *S. enterica pullorum* prevents the ubiquitination and degradation of IκB. As a result NF-κB remains inhibited, and tissues invaded by *S. enterica pullorum* do not become inflamed.

If antigen is infused into a lactating mammary gland, it tends to be promptly flushed out again in the milk. If it is infused into a nonlactating gland, then a local immune response develops in which IgA and IgG1 predominate. Unfortunately, because of the continuous removal of milk, antibody concentrations in this fluid remain low (<100 mg/dl) even though, over a period of time, the amount of immunoglobulin produced by the udder may be considerable. In acute mastitis, the inflammatory response leads to the influx of actively phagocytic cells, especially neutrophils, and to the exudation of serum proteins. As a result immunoglobulin levels in mastitic milk may rise to levels at which they can exert a protective influence (~8000 mg/dl).

Because the local immune response in the udder is relatively ineffective in preventing infection, attempts to vaccinate against mastitis-causing organisms have been generally unsuccessful. Nevertheless, recent advances have produced encouraging results. Thus an *S. aureus* vaccine that stimulates the production of antibodies against the pseudocapsule appears to be effective. This pseudocapsule interferes with the ability of milk leukocytes to phagocytose *S. aureus*. Antibodies induced by the vaccine promote opsonization and destruction of the bacteria. A vaccine designed to stimulate antibody production against staphylococcal α toxin, as well as the pseudocapsule, has reduced the incidence of mastitis following a challenge infection by 50%. Encouraging results have also been obtained by the use of a J5 mutant vaccine against coliform bacteria (Chapter 23). The vaccine, given to cattle at drying off, 30 days later, and at calving, appears to be highly effective.

Colostrum is rich in macrophages and lymphocytes. These macrophages can process antigen, and when cultured, their supernatant fluids can enhance IgA production from blood lymphocytes. Milk lymphocytes may survive for some time in the intestine and may transfer some immunity to the newborn animal (Chapter 19).

Immunity in the Urogenital Tract

The predominant immunoglobulin in cervico-vaginal mucus is IgA, whereas within the uterus it is IgG. If bacteria such as *Campylobacter fetus* infect the genital tract, vaginal IgA antibodies immobilize and agglutinate the organisms. If the mucus membrane becomes inflamed, IgG antibodies from serum will also assist in protection. *C. fetus* infections are associated with the presence of many mononuclear cells, as well with delayed skin reactions (type IV hypersensitivity), and it is possible that cell-mediated immunity is also involved in resistance to this local infection. Similar local immune responses may also be directed against other organisms that cause infections of the cervix and vagina, and the presence of agglutinating antibodies in vaginal mucus may be used as a diagnostic test for brucellosis, campylobacteriosis, and trichomoniasis. (The local immune response to trichomoniasis is largely mediated by IgE; see Chapter 25.) Preputial washings of bulls infected with *C. fetus* may contain agglutinins. These are largely IgG1 with some IgM and IgA. IgA is present in small amounts in normal urine, produced presumably by lymphoid tissues in the walls of the urinary tract. In nephritis cases however, IgG may also be found in large amounts in urine because of the breakdown in the glomerular barrier.

Immunity in the Respiratory Tract

Unlike the intestine, which is exposed to large quantities of foreign material on a daily basis, the respiratory tract is exposed to very small amounts of foreign material, usually in the form of inhaled particles or aerosols. Large particles are usually trapped in the upper respiratory tract, and only the smallest actually penetrate to the lung. Indeed, the lungs are normally sterile. The respiratory tract contains lymphoid nodules in the walls of the bronchi, as well as lymphocytes distributed diffusely throughout the lung and the walls of the airways (Figure 20-15). M cells may be associated with these lymphoid nodules, as well as with nasal mucosal lymphoid tissues. The immunoglobulin synthesized in these tissues is mainly secretory IgA, especially in the upper regions of the respiratory tract. This IgA is bound to the mucus layer through secretory component and so enhances the clearance of adherent bacteria. pIgR is expressed at low levels on bronchial epithelial cells. In the bronchioles and alveoli, however, the secretions contain a large proportion of IgG, the concentration of which is intermediate between the levels in the trachea and in serum. IgE is also synthesized in significant amounts in the lymphoid tissues of the upper respiratory tract. As on other body surfaces, IgA in the

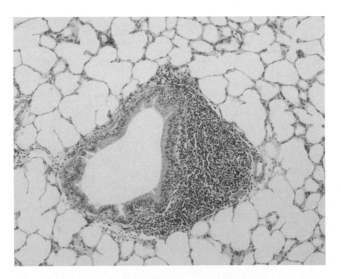

Figure 20-15. Lymphoid follicle found in the bifurcation of an airway in a section of calf lung. This type of bronchus-associated lymphoid tissue is a key component of the defenses of the respiratory tract. (From a specimen kindly provided by Drs. NH McArthur and LC Abbott.)

respiratory tract probably protects by immune exclusion, whereas IgG and IgE act by immune elimination (see Figure 20-13).

Many cells may be washed out of the airways of the lung by lavage with saline. In dogs, about 80% of bronchoalveolar cells are macrophages and 13% are lymphocytes, of which about half are T cells (Table 20-2). In healthy horses, 54% of the cells in bronchoalveolar washes are macrophages, 41% are lymphocytes, and 2% are neutrophils. In sheep, B cells are less than 10% of the lung lymphocyte population. These lung T cells can produce cytokines, and alveolar macrophages are activated following infection with *Listeria monocytogenes*. Cell-mediated immune reactions are therefore readily provoked among the cells within the lower respiratory tract.

The lungs of the majority of domestic species (pigs, horses, sheep, goats, cattle, cats) differ from rodent, human, or dog lungs in that they contain large numbers of intravascular macrophages (Chapter 4). It has been estimated that these macrophages cover 16% of the lung capillary surface in young pigs. As a result of the presence of these cells, the lungs of these species can clear more bacteria from the blood than can the liver and spleen. In pigs, pulmonary intravascular macrophages are damaged by porcine reproductive and respiratory syndrome virus. As a result, infected animals are more likely to develop *Streptococcus suis* pneumonia. There is debate as to whether lung macrophages are effective antigen-presenting cells. There is, however, a dense network of dendritic cells within airway epithelium and alveoli.

Immunity on the Skin

The skin is the first line of defense against many microbial invaders. It carries out this function effectively; few bacteria can penetrate intact skin unaided. The skin has a multitude of innate defenses ranging from its own microbial flora to the production of potent antimicrobial peptides. It also participates in the acquired immune system through the use of the Langerhans cell network. These Langerhans cells can bind exogenous antigen and may present it to nearby helper T cells. In the domestic species most of the epidermal T cells have γ/δ TCRs. In cattle for example, 44% of dermal T cells are γ/δ-positive.

Keratinocytes have MHC class II molecules on their surface and can synthesize and secrete IL-1, IL-6, and CXCL8. There is evidence to suggest that a T cell subpopulation selectively homes to the skin. Thus if an antigen is injected intradermally, such as occurs when a tick bites an animal, the antigen is trapped by Langerhans cells and presented to skin T cells, thus stimulating a rapid and effective immune response. A similar reaction occurs when reactive chemicals are painted on the skin. If skin is subjected to severe ultraviolet irradiation, the Langerhans cells are destroyed and the protective mechanisms in the skin are effectively suppressed. Skin washings contain immunoglobulins. For example, in cattle, serum IgM, IgG1, and IgG2 cross the skin by transudation, but the IgA appears to be locally synthesized.

VACCINATION ON BODY SURFACES

When animals are vaccinated against organisms that cause local infections of body surfaces, such as the intestinal or respiratory tracts, it makes sense to stimulate an IgA response. In order to do this, the vaccine antigen must be applied locally. Unfortunately, this is not always easy. Inactivated antigens are usually ineffective in triggering an IgA response since they are immediately washed or sneezed off when applied to mucous membranes. (A notable exception occurs when high levels of vaccine antigens are incorporated in feed.) The only way a significant IgA response can be triggered is to use live vaccines, by which the vaccine organism can temporarily invade mucous membranes. The vaccine must persist for a sufficient time to trigger an immune response yet not cause significant damage. Good examples of such vaccines are the respiratory tract vaccines against bovine or feline rhinotracheitis. Even some of these vaccines may cause a transient conjunctivitis or tracheitis. Other examples of effective live oral vaccines include polio vaccine in humans and transmissible gastroenteritis vaccine in piglets.

Systemic vaccination against these surface infections will provide limited immunity, since small quantities of IgG may be transferred from serum to the mucosal surface. Indeed, many currently available vaccines simply work by stimulating high levels of IgG antibodies in blood. These are effective, because once an invading organism causes tissue damage and triggers an inflammatory response, the site of invasion is flooded by IgG.

TABLE 20-2 Composition of Cells in Canine Bronchoalveolar Lavage Fluid	
Cell	**Percentage (Range)**
Macrophages	79.4 (71-87)
Lymphocytes	13.5 (7-20)
Eosinophils	3.6 (0-14)
Mast cells	2.1 (0-5)
Epithelial cells	0.8 (0-6)
Neutrophils	0.6 (0-2)
LYMPHOCYTE PERCENTAGES	
T cells	52.0 (34-69)
CD4+	21.9 (10-32)
CD8+	17.8 (6-25)
CD4/CD8 ratio	1.3 (0.8-2.4)

From Vail, DM, Mahler PA, Soergel SA: *Am J Vet Res* 56:282-285, 1995.

Nevertheless, this is clearly not an efficient way of providing immunity.

Once a protective IgA response has been stimulated, other difficulties may arise. For example, secondary immune responses are sometimes difficult to induce on surfaces, and multiple doses of vaccine may not increase the intensity or duration of the local immune response. This is not caused by any intrinsic defect but occurs because high levels of IgA can block antigen absorption and prevent it from reaching antigen-presenting cells.

SOURCES OF ADDITIONAL INFORMATION

Autenrieth LB, Schmidt MA: Bacterial interplay at intestinal mucosal surfaces: implications for vaccine development, *Trends Microbiol* 8:457-463, 2000.

Barratt MEJ, Twohig BMA, Hall H, Porter P: Hypersensitivity to dietary components in young farm animals: immunization of calves for IgE antibody responses, *Res Vet Sci* 39:62-65, 1985.

Bonneville M, Janeway CA, Ito K, et al: Intestinal intraepithelial lymphocytes are a distinct set of γδ T cells, *Nature* 336: 479-481, 1988.

Brandtzaeg P: Molecular and cellular aspects of the secretory immunoglobulin system, *APMIS* 103:1-19, 1995.

Craven N, Williams MR: Defense of the bovine mammary gland against infection and prospects for their enhancement, *Vet Immunol Immunopath* 10:71-127, 1985.

Hogenesch H, Felsburg PJ: Development and functional characterisation of T cell lines from canine Peyer's patches, *Vet Immunol Immunopathol* 23:29-39, 1989.

Jepson MA, Clark MA: Studying M cells and their role in infection, *Trends Microbiol*, 6:359-365, 1998.

Lambolez F, Rocha B: A molecular gut reaction, *Science* 294:1848-1849, 2001.

Liebler EM, Pohlenz JF, Woode GN: Gut-associated lymphoid tissue in the large intestine of calves. I. Distribution and histology, *Vet Pathol* 25:503-508, 1988.

Mantis NJ, Cheung MC, Chintalacharuvu KR, et al: Selective adherence of IgA to murine Peyer's patch M cells: evidence for a novel IgA receptor, *J Immunol* 169:1844-1851, 2002.

Mazanec MB, Kaetzel CS, Lamm ME et al: Intracellular neutralization of virus by immunoglobulin A antibodies, *Proc Natl Acad Sci USA* 89:6901-6905, 1992.

Neish AS, Gewirtz AT, Zeng H, et al: Prokaryotic regulation of epithelial responses by inhibition of IκB-α ubiquitination, *Science* 289:1560-1563, 2000.

Nickerson SC: Bovine mammary gland: structure and function; relationship to milk production and immunity to mastitis, *Agri-Practice* 15:8-18, 1994.

Pabst R, Binns RM: The immune system of the respiratory tract in pigs, *Vet Immunol Immunopathol* 43:151-156, 1994.

Phalipon A, Cardona A, Kraehenbuhl J, et al: Secretory component: a new role in secretory IgA-mediated immune exclusion in vivo, *Immunity* 17:107-115, 2002.

Pickles K, Pirie RS, Rhind S, et al: Cytological analysis of equine bronchoalveolar fluid. Part 2: comparison of smear and cytocentrifuged preparations, *Equine Vet J* 34: 292-296, 2002.

Ridyard AE, Nuttall TJ, Else RW, et al: Evaluation of Th1, Th2, and immunosuppressive cytokine mRNA expression within the colonic mucosa of dogs with idiopathic lymphocytic-plasmacytic colitis, *Vet Immunol Immunopathol* 86: 205-214, 2002.

Solari R, Kraehenbuhl JP: The biosynthesis of secretory component and its role in the transepithelial transport of IgA dimers, *Immunol Today* 6:17-20. 1985.

Stokes CR, Bailey M, Wilson AD: Immunology of the porcine gastrointestinal tract, *Vet Immunol Immunopathol* 43: 143-150, 1994.

Van Egmond M, Damen CA, van Spriel AB, et al: IgA and the IgA Fc receptor, *Trends Immunol* 22:205-211, 2001.

Weiner HL: Oral tolerance, *Proc Natl Acad Sci USA* 91: 10762-10765, 1994.

Wold AE, Dahlgren UIH, Hanson LA, et al: Differences between bacterial and food antigens in mucosal immunogenicity, *Infect Immun* 57:2666-2673, 1989.

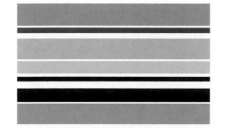

Vaccines and
Their Production

CHAPTER
21

Vaccination has proved to be by far the most efficient and cost-effective method of controlling infectious diseases in humans and animals. The eradication of smallpox from the globe, the elimination of hog cholera and brucellosis from many countries, as well as the control of diseases such as foot-and-mouth disease, canine distemper, pseudorabies, and rinderpest, would not have been possible without the use of effective vaccines. Vaccine technology continues to advance rapidly, especially through the use of modern molecular techniques and with our increased understanding of immune mechanisms and ways to optimize immune responses to achieve maximal protection.

TYPES OF IMMUNIZATION PROCEDURES

There are two basic methods by which any animal may be made immune to an infectious disease (Figure 21-1): passive and active immunization. Passive immunization produces temporary immunity by transferring antibodies from a resistant to a susceptible animal. These passively transferred antibodies give immediate protection, but since they are gradually catabolized, this protection wanes and the recipient eventually becomes susceptible to reinfection.

Active immunization, in contrast, involves administering antigen to an animal so that it responds by mounting an immune response. Reimmunization or exposure to infection in the same animal will result in a secondary immune response and greatly enhanced immunity. The

disadvantage of active immunization is that, as with all acquired immune responses, protection is not conferred immediately. However, once established, immunity is long-lasting and capable of restimulation (Figure 21-2).

PASSIVE IMMUNIZATION

Passive immunization requires that antibodies be produced in a donor animal by active immunization and that these antibodies be given to susceptible animals in order to confer immediate protection. Serum containing these antibodies (antisera) may be produced against a wide variety of pathogens. For instance, they can be produced in cattle against anthrax, in dogs against distemper, in cats against panleukopenia, and in humans against measles. They are most effective protecting animals against toxigenic organisms such as *Clostridium tetani* or *C. perfringens*, using antisera raised in horses. Antisera made in this way are called immune globulins and are commonly produced in young horses by a series of immunizing injections. The toxins of the clostridia are proteins that can be denatured and so made nontoxic by treatment with formaldehyde. Formaldehyde-treated toxins are called toxoids. Donor horses are first injected with toxoids, but once antibodies are produced, subsequent injections may contain purified toxin. The responses of the horses are monitored, and once their antibody levels are sufficiently high, they are bled. Bleeding is undertaken at intervals until the antibody level drops, when the animals are again boosted with antigen. Plasma is

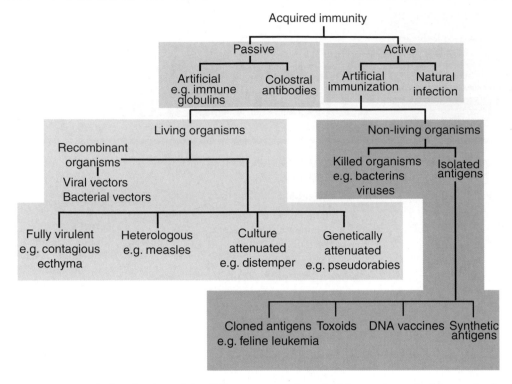

Figure 21-1.   A classification of the different types of acquired immunity and of the methods employed to induce protection.

separated from the horse blood, and the globulin fraction that contains the antibodies is concentrated, titrated, and dispensed.

To standardize the potency of different immune globulins, comparison must be made with an international biological standard. In the case of tetanus immune globulin, this is done by comparing the dose necessary to protect guinea pigs against a fixed amount of tetanus toxin with the dose of the standard preparation of immune globulin required to do the same. The international standard immune globulin for tetanus toxin is a quantity held at the State Serum Institute in Copenhagen.

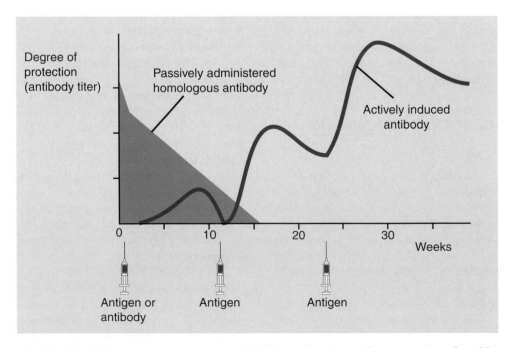

Figure 21-2.   The levels of serum antibody (and hence the degree of protection) conferred by active and passive methods of immunization.

An international unit (IU) of tetanus immune globulin is the specific neutralizing activity contained in 0.03384 mg of the international standard. The U.S. standard unit (AU) is twice the international unit.

Tetanus immune globulin is given to animals to confer immediate protection against tetanus. At least 1500 IU of immune globulin should be given to horses and cattle; at least 500 IU to calves, sheep, goats, and swine; and at least 250 IU to dogs. The exact amount should vary with the amount of tissue damage, the degree of wound contamination, and the time elapsed since injury. Tetanus immune globulin is of little use once the toxin has bound to its target receptor and clinical signs appear.

Although immune globulins give immediate protection, some problems are associated with their use. For instance, when horse tetanus immune globulin is given to horses, it will persist for a relatively long time, being removed only by catabolism. If, however, it is given to a cow or dog, it will be perceived as foreign material, elicit an immune response, and be rapidly eliminated (Figure 21-3). To reduce antigenicity, immune globulins are usually treated with pepsin to destroy their Fc region and leave intact only the portion of the immunoglobulin molecule required for toxin neutralization—the F(ab)'$_2$ fragment.

If circulating horse antibody is still present by the time the recipient animal mounts an immune response, the immune-complexes formed may cause a type III hypersensitivity reaction called serum sickness (Chapter 28). If repeated doses of horse immune globulin are given to an animal of another species, this may provoke IgE production and anaphylaxis (Chapter 26). Finally, the presence of high levels of circulating horse antibody may interfere with active immunization against the same antigen. This is a phenomenon similar to that seen in newborn animals passively protected by maternal antibodies (Box 21-1).

Monoclonal antibodies are another source of passive protection for animals. These are, however, mainly made

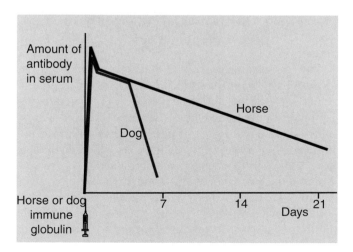

Figure 21-3. The fate of passively administered immune globulin when given to a homologous species (horse) or to a heterologous species (dog).

BOX 21-1

Serum Hepatitis of Horses

On rare occasions, horses may develop hepatitis 30 to 70 days after administration of a product such as tetanus immune globulin. Certain serum mixtures or a single vaccine batch may be associated with a high incidence of the disease. Its etiology, mechanism of transmission, and pathogenesis are unknown. Occasional cases have been described in untreated horses living with affected animals, suggesting that a virus may transmit the disease. Nevertheless, experimental transmission and serological testing have failed to reveal a causal agent. The disease is severe, with 53% to 88% mortality. Clinical signs include icterus, excessive sweating, and neurological abnormalities. Clinical chemistry indicates severe liver damage with high liver enzyme levels, ammonia, and bilirubin.

---

by mouse-mouse hybridomas and thus are mouse immunoglobulins. They will therefore stimulate an immune response when given to animals of other species. Nevertheless, mouse monoclonal antibodies against the K99 pilus antigens of *Escherichia coli* can be given orally to calves to protect them against diarrhea caused by this organism. A mouse monoclonal antibody to lymphoma cells has been successfully used in the treatment of dogs with this tumor. Now that methods have been developed to produce monoclonal antibodies from domestic animal cells (xenohybridomas; see Chapter 11), it is likely that they too will have a place in infectious disease control.

ACTIVE IMMUNIZATION

Active immunization has several advantages compared with passive immunization. These include the prolonged period of protection and the recall and boosting of this protective response by repeated injections of antigen or by exposure to infection. An ideal vaccine for active immunization should therefore give prolonged strong immunity. This immunity should be conferred on both the animal immunized and any fetus carried by it. In obtaining this strong immunity, the vaccine should be free of adverse side effects. The ideal vaccine should be cheap, stable, and adaptable to mass vaccination; ideally, it should stimulate an immune response distinguishable from that due to natural infection so that immunization and eradication may proceed simultaneously.

In addition to the requirements listed above, effective vaccines must have other critical properties. First, antigen must be delivered efficiently so that antigen-presenting cells can process antigen and release appropriate cytokines. Second, both T and B cells must be stimulated so that they generate large numbers of memory cells. Third, helper and effector T cells must be generated to several epitopes in the vaccine so that individual variations in

MHC class II polymorphism and epitope properties are minimized. Finally, the antigen must be able to stimulate memory cells in such a way that protection will last as long as possible.

Living and Killed Vaccines

Unfortunately, two of the prerequisites of an ideal vaccine—high antigenicity and absence of adverse side effects—are often incompatible. Modified live vaccines infect host cells and undergo viral replication. The infected cells then process endogenous antigen. In this way live viruses trigger a response dominated by CD8+ cytotoxic T cells, a Th1 response. This may be hazardous because the vaccine viruses may themselves cause disease or persistent infection (called residual virulence). Killed organisms, in contrast, act as exogenous antigens. They commonly stimulate responses dominated by CD4+ Th2 cells. This may not be the most appropriate response to some organisms, but it may be safer.

The practical advantages and disadvantages of vaccines containing living or killed organisms are well demonstrated in the vaccines available against *Brucella abortus* in cattle. *B. abortus* is a cause of abortion in cattle, and vaccination has been used historically to control the disease. Brucella infections are best controlled by a T cell–mediated immune response, and a vaccine containing a living avirulent strain of *B. abortus* is required for the control of this infection. Older *Brucella* vaccines, especially strain 19, caused a life-long immunity in cows and successfully prevented abortion. Unfortunately, strain 19 vaccine also caused systemic reactions: swelling at the injection site, high fever, anorexia, listlessness, and a drop in milk yield. Strain 19 could cause abortion in pregnant cows, orchitis in bulls, and undulant fever in humans. To eradicate brucellosis, serological tests are used to identify infected animals, and strain 19 caused an antibody response that was difficult to distinguish from a natural infection.

Because of the disadvantages associated with the use of strain 19, considerable efforts were made to find a better alternative. Unfortunately, killed vaccines (strain 45/20) protected cattle for less than 1 year. More recently, a live attenuated strain of *B. abortus* called RB-51 has been used in cattle in the United States. This is a rough mutant that fails to produce the lipopolysaccharide O antigen. As a result, it produces a strong Th1 response, but unlike strain 19 does not induce false-positive results in the standard diagnostic tests such as card agglutination, complement fixation, or tube agglutination. It is therefore possible to distinguish between vaccinated and infected cattle. RB-51 is less pathogenic for cattle than strain 19, and it is not shed in nasal secretions, saliva, or urine. RB-51 will not cause abortion in pregnant cattle. It will, however, cause disease in accidentally exposed humans, and because of its failure to stimulate antibody production, this may be difficult to diagnose.

TABLE 21-1 **The Relative Merits of Living and Dead Vaccines**	
Living Vaccines	**Inactivated Vaccines**
Few inoculating doses required	Stable on storage
Adjuvants unnecessary	Unlikely to cause disease through residual virulence
Less chance of hypersensitivity	
Induction of interferon	Unlikely to contain live contaminating organisms
Relatively cheap	

The advantages of vaccines such as 45/20 that contain killed organisms are that they are safe with respect to residual virulence and are relatively easy to store, since the organisms are already dead (Table 21-1). These advantages of killed vaccines correspond to the disadvantages of live vaccines, such as strain 19 or RB-51. That is, some live vaccines may possess residual virulence, not only for the animal for which the vaccine is made but also for other animals. They may revert to a fully virulent type or spread to unvaccinated animals. Thus some vaccine strains of porcine reproductive and respiratory syndrome virus (PRRSV) vaccine may be transmitted to unvaccinated pigs causing persistent infection and disease. Live vaccines always run the risk of contamination with unwanted organisms; for instance, outbreaks of reticuloendotheliosis in chickens in Japan and Australia have been traced to contaminated Marek's disease vaccines. A major outbreak of bovine leukosis in Australia resulted from contamination of a batch of babesiosis vaccine containing whole calf blood. Abortion and death have occurred in pregnant bitches that received a vaccine contaminated with bluetongue virus. Contaminating mycoplasma may also be present in some vaccines. Scrapie has been spread in mycoplasma vaccines. Finally, vaccines containing living attenuated organisms require care in their preparation, storage, and handling to avoid killing the organisms. Thus maintaining the cold chain can account for 20% to 80% of the cost of a vaccine in the tropics.

The disadvantages of killed vaccines parallel the advantages of living vaccines. Thus, the use of adjuvants to increase effective antigenicity can cause severe inflammation or systemic toxicity, whereas multiple doses or high individual doses of antigen increase the risk for producing hypersensitivity reactions, as well as increasing costs. In general, vaccines containing living organisms tend to induce a stronger Th1-dominated immunity than vaccines containing killed organisms. One reason for this is that the living vaccine virus may invade host cells and induce interferon production, thus conferring early protection on susceptible animals. Killed vaccines are more likely to stimulate a Th2 response. For many organisms, especially viruses, a Th1 response may well be more appropriate.

Inactivation

Organisms killed for use in vaccines must remain as antigenically similar to the living organisms as possible. Therefore crude methods of killing that cause extensive changes in antigen structure as a result of protein denaturation are usually unsatisfactory. If chemicals are used, they must not alter the antigens responsible for stimulating protective immunity. One such chemical is formaldehyde, which cross-links proteins and nucleic acids and confers structural rigidity. Proteins can also be mildly denatured by acetone or alcohol treatment. Alkylating agents that cross-link nucleic acid chains are also suitable for killing organisms, since by leaving the surface proteins of organisms unchanged, they do not interfere with antigenicity. Examples of alkylating agents include ethylene oxide, ethyleneimine, acetylethyleneimine and β-propiolactone, all of which have been used in veterinary vaccines. Many successful vaccines containing killed bacteria (bacterins) or inactivated toxins (toxoids) can be made relatively simply by the use of these agents. Some vaccines may contain mixtures of these components. For example, some vaccines against *Mannheimia hemolytica* contain both killed bacteria and inactivated bacterial leukotoxin.

Attenuation

Virulent living organisms cannot normally be used in vaccines. Their virulence must be reduced so that, although still living, they can no longer cause disease. This process of reduction of virulence is called attenuation. The level of attenuation is critical to vaccine success. Under-attenuation will result in residual virulence and disease; overattenuation will result in an ineffective vaccine. The traditional methods of attenuation were empirical, and there was little understanding of the changes induced by the attenuation process. They usually involved adapting organisms to growth in unusual conditions so that they lost their adaptation to their usual host. For example, the Bacille Calmette-Guérin (BCG) strain of *Mycobacterium bovis* was rendered avirulent by being grown for 13 years on bile-saturated medium. The strain of anthrax currently used in vaccines was rendered avirulent by growth in 50% serum agar under an atmosphere rich in CO_2 so that it lost its ability to form a capsule. *Brucella abortus* strain 19 vaccine was grown under conditions in which there was a shortage of nutrients. Unfortunately, genetic stability cannot always be guaranteed in these attenuated strains. Back-mutation may occur, and vaccine organisms may redevelop virulence.

A more reliable method of making bacteria avirulent is by genetic manipulation. For example, a modified live vaccine is available that contains streptomycin-dependent *Mannheimia hemolytica* and *P. multocida*. These mutants depend on the presence of streptomycin for growth. When they are administered to an animal, the absence of streptomycin will eventually result in the death of the bacteria, but not before they have stimulated a protective immune response.

Viruses have traditionally been attenuated by growth in cells or species to which they are not naturally adapted. For example, rinderpest virus, which is normally a pathogen of cattle, was first attenuated by growth in rabbits. Eventually, a successful tissue culture-adapted rinderpest vaccine devoid of residual virulence was developed. Similar examples include the adaptation of African horse sickness virus to mice and of canine distemper virus to ferrets. Alternatively, mammalian viruses may be attenuated by growth in eggs. For example, the Flury strain of rabies was attenuated by prolonged passage in eggs and lost its virulence for normal dogs and cats.

The most commonly used method of virus attenuation has been prolonged tissue culture. It is usual to culture cells from the species to be vaccinated in order to reduce the side effects resulting from the administration of foreign tissues. In these cases virus attenuation is accomplished by culturing the organism in cells to which they are not adapted. For example, virulent canine distemper virus preferentially attacks lymphoid cells. For vaccine purposes, therefore, this virus was cultured repeatedly in canine kidney cells, as a result of which its virulence was lost.

Some vaccines use, instead of artificially attenuated organisms, antigenically related organisms normally adapted to another species. For example, measles virus has been used to protect dogs against distemper, and bovine virus diarrhea virus can protect swine against hog cholera.

Under some circumstances it is possible to use fully virulent organisms for immunization just as the Chinese once did with smallpox. Vaccination against contagious ecthyma of sheep is of this type. Contagious ecthyma (orf) is a viral disease of lambs that causes massive scab formation around the mouth, prevents feeding, and results in a failure to thrive. The disease has little systemic effect. Lambs recover completely within a few weeks and are immune from then on. It is usual to vaccinate lambs by rubbing dried, infected scab material into scratches made in the inner aspect of the thigh. The local infection at this site has no untoward effect on the lambs, and they become solidly immune. Because the vaccinated animals may spread the disease however, they must be separated from unvaccinated animals for a few weeks.

MODERN VACCINE TECHNOLOGY

Although both killed and modified live vaccines have been successful in controlling many infectious diseases, there is always a need to make them more effective, cheaper, and safer (Figure 21-4). The use of modern molecular techniques can produce new and improved vaccines. The U.S. Department of Agriculture (USDA) classifies these vaccines into three categories (Table 21-2).

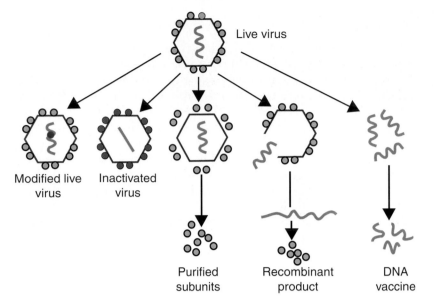

Figure 21-4.   A schematic diagram showing some of the different ways in which a virus and its antigens may be treated in order to produce a vaccine.

Antigens Generated by Gene Cloning (Category I)

Gene cloning can be used to produce large quantities of purified antigen. In this process, DNA coding for an antigen of interest is first isolated. This DNA is then inserted into a bacterium, yeast, or other cell, and the recombinant antigen is expressed. The first successful use of gene cloning to prepare an antigen in this way involved foot-and-mouth disease virus (Figure 21-5). This virus is extremely simple. The protective antigen (VP1) is well recognized, and the genes that code for this protein have been mapped. The RNA genome of the foot-and-mouth disease virus was isolated and transcribed into DNA by the enzyme reverse transcriptase. The DNA was then carefully cut by restriction endonucleases so that it only contained the gene for VP1. This DNA was then inserted into an *E. coli* plasmid, the plasmid inserted into *E. coli*, and the bacteria grown. The recombinant bacteria synthesized large quantities of VP1 that was harvested, purified, and incorporated into a vaccine. The process is highly efficient since 4×10^7 doses

of foot-and-mouth vaccine can be obtained from 10 L of *E. coli* grown to 10^{12} organisms per ml. Unfortunately, the immunity produced is inferior to that produced by killed virus and requires a 1000-fold higher dose to induce comparable protection.

The first commercially available category I recombinant veterinary vaccine was made against feline leukemia virus. The major envelope protein of FeLV, gp70, is the antigen largely responsible for inducing a protective

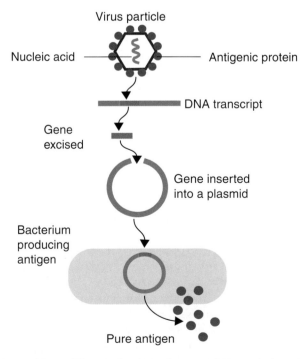

Figure 21-5.   The production of a recombinant viral protein for use in a vaccine. The gene coding for the viral antigen of interest is cloned into another organism, in this case a bacterium, and produced in very large quantities.

TABLE 21-2	
The USDA Classification of Genetically Engineered Veterinary Biologics	
Category	**Description**
I	Vaccines that contain inactivated recombinant organisms or purified antigens derived from recombinant organisms
II	Vaccines containing live organisms that contain gene deletions or heterologous marker genes
III	Vaccines that contain live expression vectors expressing heterologous genes for immunizing antigens or other stimulants

immune response in cats. Thus the gene for gp70 (a glycoprotein of 70 kDa) plus a small portion of a linked protein called p15e (a protein of 15 kDa from the envelope) was isolated and inserted into *E. coli* that then synthesized large amounts of p70. This recombinant p70 is not glycosylated and has a molecular weight of just over 50 kDa. Once cloned, the recombinant protein is harvested, purified, mixed with a saponin adjuvant, and used as a vaccine.

Another example of a recombinant vaccine is one directed against the Lyme disease agent, *Borrelia burgdorferi*. Thus the gene for OspA, the immunodominant outer surface lipoprotein of *B. burgdorferi*, was cloned into *E. coli*. The recombinant protein expressed by the *E. coli* is purified and used as a vaccine when combined with adjuvant. This vaccine is unique since ticks feeding on immunized animals ingest the antibody. The antibodies then kill the bacteria within the tick midgut and prevent their dissemination to the salivary glands. They thus prevent transmission by the vector.

Gene cloning techniques are useful in any situation in which pure protein antigens need to be synthesized in large quantities. Unfortunately, pure proteins are often poor antigens because they are not effectively delivered to antigen-sensitive cells and they may not be correctly folded. In addition, they may be inefficient antigens because of MHC restriction. An alternative method of delivering a recombinant antigen is to clone the gene of interest into an attenuated living carrier organism.

Genetically Attenuated Organisms (Category II)

Attenuation by prolonged tissue culture can be considered as a primitive form of genetic engineering. The desired result is the development of a strain of organism that cannot cause disease. This may be difficult to achieve and reversion to virulence is an ever-present risk. Molecular genetic techniques, however, make it possible to modify the genes of an organism so that it becomes irreversibly attenuated. The USDA classifies these as category II vaccines. They are now available against the herpesvirus that causes pseudorabies in swine. The enzyme thymidine kinase (TK) is required by herpesviruses to replicate in nondividing cells such as neurons. Viruses from which the TK gene has been removed can infect nerve cells but cannot replicate and cannot therefore cause disease (Figure 21-6). As a result, these vaccines not only confer effective protection but also block cell invasion by virulent pseudorabies viruses and so prevent the development of a persistent carrier state.

Genetic manipulation can also be used to make "marker vaccines." Thus for example, pseudorabies virus synthesizes two glycoprotein antigens called gX and gI. These are potent antigens yet neither is essential for viral growth or virulence. They are expressed by all field isolates of this virus. Animals infected with the field virus will make antibodies to gX and gI. It has proved possible

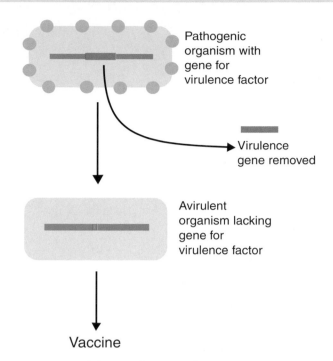

Figure 21-6. The production of an attenuated virus by removal of a gene required for virulence. Genes coding for major antigens detected by serological techniques can also be removed, ensuring that vaccinated animals can be distinguished from naturally infected ones.

to construct an attenuated pseudorabies virus that lacks either gX or gI and can be used as a vaccine. Vaccinated pigs will not make antibodies to gX or gI, but naturally infected pigs will. The vaccine will not cause positive serological reactions in ELISA tests for gX or gI, and the presence of antibodies to gX and gI in a pig is evidence that the animal has been exposed to field strains of pseudorabies virus. This type of vaccine, called a DIVA vaccine (*d*ifferentiate *i*nfected from *v*accinated *a*nimals), should be of great assistance in eradicating specific infectious diseases much more economically and rapidly than conventional methods.

Live Recombinant Organisms (Category III)

Genes coding for protein antigens can be cloned directly into a variety of organisms. Instead of being purified, the recombinant organism itself may then be used as a vaccine. The USDA classifies these as category III vaccines (Figure 21-7). Experimental recombinant vaccines have used adenoviruses, herpesviruses, and bacteria such as BCG or *Salmonella*, but the organisms that have been most widely employed for this purpose are poxviruses such as vaccinia, fowlpox, or canarypox. These viruses are easy to administer by dermal scratching or by ingestion. They have a large genome that makes it relatively easy to insert a new gene (up to 10% of its genome can be replaced by foreign DNA), and they can express high levels of the new antigen. Moreover, these recombinant

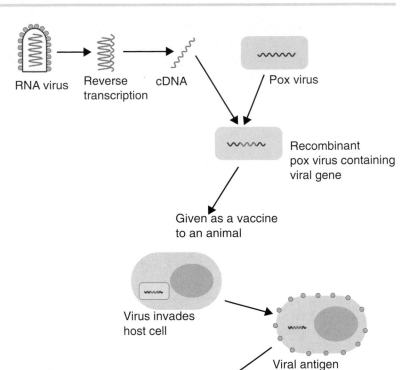

Figure 21-7.   The production of a vaccinia recombinant vaccine. Vaccinia is selected because it has room to spare in its genome, and it is easy to administer to an animal. Thus rabies-vaccinia recombinants can be given orally.

proteins undergo appropriate processing steps including glycosylation and membrane transport within the pox virus. A good example of such a vaccine is the vaccinia virus recombinant, which contains the gene for the rabies envelope glycoprotein or G protein. The G glycoprotein forms the characteristic spikes on the surface of rabies virus. This glycoprotein is the only rabies antigen capable of inducing virus-neutralizing antibody and conferring protection against rabies. Infection with this rabies-vaccinia recombinant results in the production of antibodies to the G protein and the development of immunity. This vaccine has been successfully used as an oral vaccine administered to wild carnivores in a bait. This form of the vaccine can be distributed by dropping from aircraft. Thus in Belgium, oral rabies vaccine dropped from the air effectively terminated fox rabies, spreading through the Ardennes (Figure 21-8). It has been used in Ontario to prevent the spread of fox rabies, in New Jersey to prevent the spread of raccoon rabies, and in Texas to block the spread of coyote rabies. For example, since 1995, 17.5 million doses of recombinant rabies vaccine have been spread over 255,500 square miles (661,745 sq km) over Texas with great success.

Effective category III vaccines have also been developed for rinderpest; these consist of a vaccinia or capripox vector containing the hemagglutinin (H) or fusion (F) genes of rinderpest virus. The recombinant capripox vaccine has the benefit of protecting cattle against both rinderpest and lumpy skin disease. The vaccinia virus can be further attenuated by inactivation of its thymidine kinase and hemagglutinin genes. This has the advantage that it does not cause pock lesions in vaccinated animals. Swinepox has been tested as a potential vector for pseudorabies in pigs.

The first category III vaccine approved by the USDA was against the Newcastle disease virus. The carrier organism is a fowlpox virus, into which Newcastle disease HA and F genes have been incorporated. It has the benefit of conferring immunity against fowlpox as well.

Polynucleotide Vaccines

Another method of vaccination involves injection, not of a protein antigen but of DNA that encodes foreign antigens. For example, the DNA coding for a vaccine antigen can be inserted into a bacterial plasmid, a piece of circular DNA that acts as a vector (Figure 21-9). The vaccine gene is placed under the control of a strong mammalian promoter sequence. When the genetically engineered plasmid is injected intramuscularly into an animal, it may be taken up by host cells. The DNA is then transcribed into mRNA and translated into endogenous vaccine protein (Figure 21-10). The plasmid, unlike viral vectors, cannot replicate in mammalian cells. Transfected host cells express the vaccine protein and express it, as other endogenous antigens, in association with MHC class I molecules. This can lead to the development not only neutralizing antibodies but also, since the antigen is endogenous, of cytotoxic T cells. Expressed antigens will

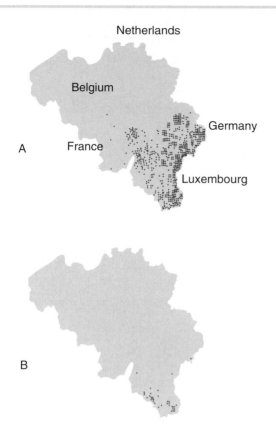

Figure 21-8. The geographical distribution of cases of wild animal rabies in Belgium. **A,** In 1989. **B,** In 1992 and 1993, following the introduction of an oral rabies-vaccinia recombinant vaccine. A remarkable example of the effectiveness of a recombinant vaccine. (From Brochier B, Boulanger D, Costy F, Pastoret PP: *Vaccine* 12:1368-1371, 1994.)

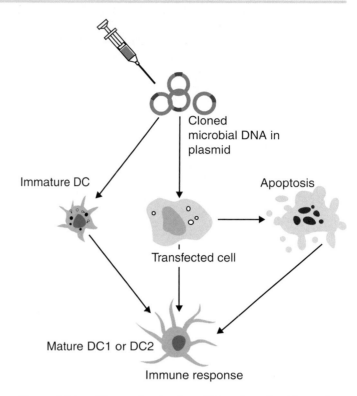

Figure 21-9. The mechanism by which polynucleotide vaccines can work. The DNA that enters a cell is functional and can code for endogenous antigens.

have authentic tertiary structure and posttranslational modifications such as glycosylation. The immune response is also enhanced since the bacterial DNA contains unmethylated CpG motifs that are recognized by TLR-9 and stimulate the activation of dendritic cells. These in turn promote a strong Th1 response with resulting strong immunity to viruses or intracellular bacteria. This approach has been applied experimentally to produce vaccines against bovine herpes, avian influenza, lymphocytic choriomeningitis, canine and feline rabies, canine parvovirus, bovine viral diarrhea, feline immunodeficiency virus, feline leukemia virus, pseudorabies, influenza, foot-and-mouth disease virus, bovine herpesvirus-1, and Newcastle disease. Although theoretically producing a response similar to that induced by attenuated live vaccines, these nucleic acid vaccines are ideally suited to prepare vaccines against organisms that are difficult or dangerous to grow in the laboratory.

DNA vaccines appear to be able to induce immunity in the presence of very high titers of maternal antibody. Although the maternal antibodies block serological

responses, the development of strong memory responses is not impaired.

Polynucleotide vaccines must be delivered inside target cells. This can be done by intramuscular injection or by "shooting" the DNA plasmids directly through the skin adsorbed onto microscopic gold beads fired by a "gene gun." Although intramuscular injection is very inefficient because the transfection rate is low (about 1% to 5% of myofibrils in the vicinity of an intramuscular injection site), the expression can persist for at least 2 months. The gene products are either treated as endogenous antigens and displayed on the cell surface or secreted and presented to antigen-processing cells.

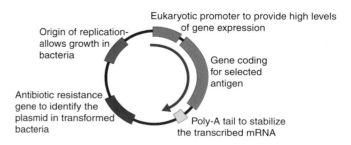

Figure 21-10. The structure of a typical DNA plasmid used for vaccination purposes. In addition to coding for the antigen in question, the plasmid carries an antibiotic resistance marker so that its fate may be traced.

This processed antigen thus preferentially stimulates a Th1 response associated with IFN-γ production. The use of a gene gun is a more efficient procedure since some of this DNA is taken up by the animal's dendritic cells directly and it minimizes degradation. By bypassing TLR-9, this material appears to preferentially stimulate a Th2 response. This is, of course, of major practical significance. Viral DNA in eye drops can induce an IgA response in the tears and bile of recipients.

Immunization with purified DNA in this way allows presentation of viral antigens in their native form, which are synthesized in the same way as antigens during a viral infection. This is a great improvement over the use of recombinant proteins, in which case it has proved difficult to create the proteins in the correct conformation. Another advantage is that it is possible to select only the genes for the antigen of interest rather than using a complex carrier organism with its own large gene pool and antigenic mass.

As far as safety is concerned, one theoretical disadvantage is the potential for the vaccine DNA to integrate into the host genome and possibly activate oncogenes or inhibit tumor suppressor genes. Experience suggests that this is a low risk. The presence of an antibiotic-resistant gene in these plasmids also runs the risk of transferring this resistance to bacteria. This can be avoided by the use of other markers.

Synthetic Peptides

If the structure of a protective epitope is known, it may be chemically synthesized and used alone in a vaccine. The procedures involved include a complete sequencing of the antigen of interest, followed by identification of its important epitopes. The epitopes may be predicted by the use of computer models of the protein or by the use of monoclonal antibodies to identify the critical protective components. Experimental synthetic vaccines have been developed against hepatitis B, diphtheria toxin, foot-and-mouth-disease virus, canine parvovirus, and influenza A, and they provoke some protective immunity (Box 21-2).

BOX 21-2

Reverse Vaccinology

Now that complete bacterial genomes are available, it is possible to identify potential vaccine antigens by computer analysis. This analysis can rapidly identify novel potential vaccine candidates. These antigens can then be rapidly screened and tested. Thus, for example, the genome of the recently emerged coronavirus disease, SARS, was sequenced within a month of its discovery. Vaccine targets have been identified, and vaccines are now being tested.

ADJUVANTS

To maximize the effectiveness of vaccines, especially those containing killed organisms, it has been common practice to add substances called adjuvants together with the antigen. Adjuvants can greatly enhance the body's response to vaccines and are essential if long-term memory is to be established to soluble antigens. The mechanisms of adjuvant action are only poorly understood, a problem that has hampered rational adjuvant development and that has made adjuvant selection somewhat empirical. In general, however, adjuvants work through one of three mechanisms (Figure 21-11). Depot adjuvants simply serve to protect antigens from rapid degradation and so prolong immune responses. A second group consist of particles that effectively deliver antigen to antigen-presenting cells. A third group—immunostimulatory adjuvants—consists of molecules that enhance cytokine production.

Depot Adjuvants

Some adjuvants simply delay the elimination of antigens and thus permit an immune response to last longer. The immune system, being antigen driven, responds to the presence of antigen and terminates that response once antigen is eliminated. The rate of antigen elimination can be slowed by mixing it with an insoluble, slowly degraded adjuvant. Examples of depot-forming adjuvants include aluminum salts, such as aluminum hydroxide, aluminum phosphate, and aluminum potassium sulfate (alum) (Table 21-3). When antigen is mixed with one of these salts and injected into an animal, a macrophage-rich granuloma forms in the tissues. The antigen within this granuloma slowly leaks into the body and so provides a prolonged antigenic stimulus. Antigens that normally persist for only a few days may be retained in the body for several weeks by this technique. These depot adjuvants influence only the primary immune response and have little effect on secondary immune responses. Aluminum based adjuvants also have the disadvantage that while promoting antibody responses, they have little stimulatory effect on cell-mediated responses.

An alternative method of forming a depot is to incorporate the antigen in a water-in-oil emulsion (called Freund's incomplete adjuvant). The light mineral oil stimulates a local, chronic inflammatory response, and as a result, a granuloma or abscess forms around the site of the inoculum. The antigen is slowly leached from the aqueous phase of the emulsion. Newer oil-based adjuvants hold promise of allowing us to select whether we wish to stimulate Th1 or Th2 responses, depending on the animal's specific needs.

These depot adjuvants will cause significant tissue irritation and destruction. Mineral oils are especially irritating. Nonmineral oils, although less irritating, are also less effective. Tissue damage induced by adjuvants may also promote immune responses since the products

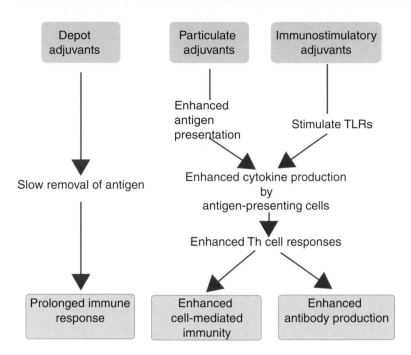

Figure 21-11. The three major groups of adjuvants and the ways in which these may act to enhance immune responses triggered by vaccine antigens.

of inflammation and cell death can stimulate the activities of dendritic cells and macrophages.

Particulate Adjuvants

The immune system can generally trap and process particulate antigens such as bacteria or other microorganisms much more efficiently than soluble antigens. As a result, many attempts have been made to incorporate antigens into readily phagocytosable particles. These adjuvants include emulsions, microparticles, ISCOMs, and liposomes and all are designed to deliver antigen efficiently to antigen presenting cells. They commonly are of similar size to bacteria and are readily endocytosed by antigen-presenting cells. Biodegradable microparticles incorporating antigens are usually designed to be readily phagocytosed. Liposomes are lipid-based microparticles containing antigens that are readily trapped and processed. ISCOMS are complex lipid-based microparticles described below. All of these particulate adjuvants may be made

TABLE 21-3
Some Common Adjuvants

Type	Adjuvant	Mode of Action
Depot adjuvants	Aluminum phosphate	Slow-release antigen depot
	Aluminum hydroxide	Slow-release antigen depot
	Alum	
	Freund's incomplete adjuvant	
Immunostimulatory adjuvants	Anaerobic corynebacteria	Macrophage stimulator
	BCG	Macrophage stimulator
	Muramyl dipeptide	Macrophage stimulator
	Bordetella pertussis	Lymphocyte stimulators
	Lipopolysaccharide	Macrophage stimulator
	Saponin	Stimulates antigen processing
	Lysolecithin	Stimulates antigen processing
	Pluronic detergents	Stimulates antigen processing
	Acemannan	Macrophage stimulator
	Glucans	Macrophage stimulator
	Dextran sulfate	Macrophage stimulator
Particulate adjuvants	Liposomes	Stimulates antigen processing
	ISCOMS	Stimulates antigen processing
	Microparticles	Stimulates antigen processing
Mixed adjuvants	Freund's complete adjuvant	Water-in-oil emulsion plus *Mycobacterium*

more potent by incorporating microbial immunostimulants. They are not yet widely employed in veterinary vaccines.

Immunostimulatory Adjuvants

These adjuvants exert their effects by promoting cytokine production. Many of them are complex microbial products that often represent pathogen-associated molecular patterns (PAMPS). These molecules activate dendritic cells and macrophages through toll-like receptors and stimulate the secretion of key cytokines such as IL-12. These cytokines in turn promote helper T cell responses and drive and focus the acquired immune responses. Depending on the specific microbial product, they may enhance either Th1 or Th2 responses.

Commonly employed microbial immunostimulants include lipopolysaccharides (or their derivatives). These enhance antibody formation if given at about the same time as the antigen. They have no effect on cell-mediated responses, but they can break tolerance, and they have a general immunostimulatory activity, which is reflected in a nonspecific resistance to bacterial infections. Killed anaerobic corynebacteria, especially *Propionibacterium acnes*, have a similar effect. When used as adjuvants, these bacteria enhance antibacterial and antitumor activity. *Bordetella pertussis*, the cause of whooping cough, also prolongs and enhances immunological memory and stimulates macrophage activity. *B. pertussis* may selectively enhance Th2 responses and IgE production. Microbial CpG DNA also appears to be a potent immunostimulatory adjuvant for Th1 responses.

Another group of immunostimulatory adjuvants are the saponins (triterpene glycosides), derived from the bark of a South American tree called *Quillaja saponaria*. Saponins have both toxic and adjuvant activities. However, fractionation can isolate those that have potent adjuvant activity yet are relatively nontoxic. Saponin-based adjuvants may selectively stimulate Th1 activity, since they direct antigens into endogenous processing pathways and enhance costimulatory activity. A purified saponin is used as an adjuvant in a recombinant feline leukemia vaccine. Toxic saponin mixtures are used in anthrax vaccines, where they destroy tissue at the site of injection so that the anthrax spores may germinate. Saponin is also employed as an adjuvant for foot-and-mouth disease vaccines. DEAE dextran may be an effective substitute for saponins in some vaccines.

Mixed Adjuvants

Very powerful adjuvants can be constructed by combining a particulate or depot adjuvant with an immunostimulatory agent. For example, an oil-based depot adjuvant can be mixed with killed *Mycobacterium tuberculosis* incorporated into the water-in-oil emulsion. The mixture is called Freund's complete adjuvant (FCA). Not only does FCA form a depot, but the tubercle bacilli contain muramyl dipeptide (*n*-acetylmuramyl-L-alanyl-D-isoglutamine), a molecule that activates macrophages and dendritic cells through toll-like receptors. FCA works best when given subcutaneously or intradermally and when the antigen dose is relatively low. It acts specifically to stimulate T cell function. FCA promotes IgG production over IgM. It inhibits tolerance induction, favors delayed hypersensitivity reactions, accelerates graft rejection, and promotes resistance to tumors. FCA can be used to induce some experimental autoimmune diseases, such as experimental allergic encephalitis and thyroiditis (Chapter 32). It also stimulates macrophages, promoting their phagocytic and cytotoxic activities.

Use of oil-based adjuvants in animals intended for human consumption is problematic, since the oil may spoil the meat. Use of FCA is unacceptable in food animals, not only because of the mineral oil but also because the mycobacteria in the adjuvant may induce a positive skin reaction to tuberculin, a critical drawback in any area in which tuberculosis is controlled by skin testing.

ISCOMS are stable complexes containing cholesterol, phospholipid, saponin, and antigen. Micelles may be constructed using protein antigens and a matrix of a saponin mixture called Quil A. These immune-stimulating complexes (ISCOMs) are effective adjuvants with few adverse side effects. They are highly effective in targeting antigens to the professional antigen-processing cells, while the saponin activates these cells and so promotes cytokine production and the expression of costimulatory molecules. Depending on the antigen employed, ISCOMs can stimulate either Th1 or Th2 responses.

Given that many adjuvants act by stimulating cytokine production, it is logical that many cytokines can serve as effective adjuvants. Most cytokines tested in this way have unacceptable toxicity, although IL-12 appears to be especially effective in this regard, since as a Th1 cell stimulator, it enhances IFN-γ production.

By far the most widely employed adjuvants in commercial veterinary vaccines are the depot adjuvants such as aluminum hydroxide, aluminum phosphate, or aluminum potassium sulfate (alum). These adjuvants are produced in the form of a colloidal suspension to which the antigenic material is adsorbed. They are stable on storage, and although they produce a small local granuloma on inoculation, they do not track or make large parts of the carcass unsuitable for consumption. These adjuvants are therefore considered the most suitable type for animals at present.

SOURCES OF ADDITIONAL INFORMATION

Aucouturier J, Dupuis L, Ganne V: Adjuvants designed for veterinary and human vaccines, *Vaccine* 19:2666-2672, 2001.
Ada G: Vaccines and vaccination, *N Engl J Med* 345:1042-1051, 2001.

Babiuk LA: Vaccination: a management tool in veterinary medicine, *Vet J* 164:188-201, 2002.

Babiuk LA, Pontarollo R, Babiuk S, et al: Induction of immune responses by DNA vaccines in large animals, *Vaccine* 21:649-658, 2003.

Brochier B, Boulanger D, Costy F, Pastoret PP: Towards rabies elimination in Belgium by fox vaccination using a vaccinia-rabies recombinant virus, *Vaccine* 12:1368-1371, 1994.

Cardenas L, Clements JD: Oral immunization using live attenuated *Salmonella* spp. as carriers for foreign antigens, *Clin Microbiol Rev* 5:328-342, 1992.

Chattergoon M, Boyer J, Weiner MB: Genetic immunization: a new era in vaccines and immune therapeutics, *FASEB J* 11:753-763, 1997.

Dalsgaard K, Hilgers L, Trouve G: Classical and new approaches to adjuvant use in domestic food animals, *Adv Vet Sci Comp Med* 35; 121-160, 1990.

Dunham SP: The application of nucleic acid vaccines in veterinary medicine, *Res Vet Sci* 73:9-16, 2002.

Fischer L, Barzu S, Andreoni C, et al: DNA vaccination of neonatal piglets in the face of maternal immunity induces humoral memory and protection against a virulent pseudorabies virus challenge, *Vaccine* 21:1732-1741, 2003.

Guglick MA, MacAllister CG, Ely RW, Edwards WC: Hepatic disease associated with administration of tetanus antitoxin in eight horses, *J Am Vet Med Assoc* 206:1737-1740, 1995.

Jiang W, Baker HJ, Swango LJ, et al: Nucleic acid immunization protects dogs against challenge with virulent parvovirus, *Vaccine* 10:601-607, 1998.

Krishnan S, Haensler J, Meulien P: Paving the way towards DNA vaccines, *Nature Med* 1:521-522, 1995.

Langeveld JPM, Kamstrup S, Uttenthal A: Full protection against mink enteritis virus with new generation canine parvovirus vaccines based on synthetic peptide or recombinant protein. *Vaccine* 13:1033-1037, 1995.

Mengeling WL, Vorwald AC, Lager KM, et al: Identification and clinical assessment of suspected vaccine-related field strains of porcine reproductive and respiratory syndrome virus, *Am J Vet Res* 60:334-340, 1999.

Modlin RL: A toll for DNA vaccines, *Nature* 408:659-660, 2000.

O'Hagan DT, MacKichan ML, Singh M: Recent developments in adjuvants for vaccines against infectious diseases, *Biomol Eng* 18:69-85, 2001.

Romero CH, Barrett T, Kitching RP, et al: Protection of cattle against rinderpest and lumpy skin disease with a recombinant capripox virus expressing the fusion protein gene of rinderpest virus, *Vet Rec* 135:152-154, 1994.

Russell PH, Mackie A: Eye-drop DNA can induce IgA in the tears and bile of chickens, *Vet Immunol Immunopathol* 10:327-332, 2001.

Singh M, O'Hagan D: Advances in vaccine adjuvants, *Nature Biotechnology* 17:1075-1081, 1999.

Yamanouchi K, Barrett T, Kai C: New approaches to the development of virus vaccines for veterinary use, *Rev Sci Tech* 17:641-653, 1998.

Yamanouchi K, Inui K, Sugimoto M, et al: Immunization of cattle with a recombinant vaccinia vector expressing the haemagglutinin gene of rinderpest virus, *Vet Rec* 132:152-156, 1993.

Yancey RJ: Recent advances in bovine vaccine technology, *J Dairy Sci* 76:2418-2436, 1993.

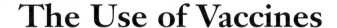

The Use of Vaccines

Vaccination has proved to be by far the most efficient and cost-effective method of controlling major infectious diseases in domestic animals. When first developed, many vaccines were of limited efficacy and induced severe adverse effects, although these effects were considered acceptable when measured against the risks of acquiring disease. The vaccination protocols developed at that time reflected the short duration of immunity induced by these vaccines. Ongoing developments in vaccine design and production have resulted in great improvements in both vaccine safety and effectiveness. These improvements have led to a reassessment of the relative risks and benefits of vaccination and have resulted in changes in vaccination protocols. Thus vaccination is not always an innocuous procedure and may occasionally cause sickness or death. For this reason, the use of any vaccine should be accompanied by a risk:benefit analysis on the need for administration of a vaccine conducted by the veterinarian in consultation with an animal's owner. Vaccination protocols should be customized to each animal, giving due consideration to the seriousness and zoonotic potential of the agent, the animal's exposure risk, and any legal requirements relating to vaccination.

The two major factors that determine vaccine usage are safety and efficacy. We must always be sure that the risks of vaccination do not exceed those associated with the chance of contracting the disease itself. Thus it may be inappropriate to use a vaccine against a disease that is rare, is readily treated by other means, or is of little clinical significance. In addition, because the detection of antibodies is a common diagnostic procedure, unnecessary use of vaccines may complicate diagnosis based on serology and perhaps make eradication of a disease impossible. Because of this, the decision to use vaccines for the control of any disease must be based on considerations not only of the degree of risk associated with the disease but also of the availability of superior control or treatment procedures.

The second major consideration is vaccine efficacy. Vaccines are not always effective. Thus in some diseases, such as equine infectious anemia, Aleutian disease in mink, and African swine fever, poor or no protective immunity can be induced even with the best vaccines. In other diseases, such as foot-and-mouth disease in pigs, the immune response is transient and relatively ineffective, so that successful vaccination is very difficult to achieve.

As a result of these considerations, some investigators have recommended that animal vaccines be divided into categories based on their importance. The first category consists of essential (or core) vaccines—those vaccines that are required in that they protect against common, dangerous diseases and that a failure to use them would place an animal at significant risk of disease or death. The second category consists of optional (or non-core) vaccines. These are directed against diseases for which the risks associated with not vaccinating may be low. In many cases, risks from these diseases are determined by the location or lifestyle of an animal. The use of these optional vaccines would be determined by a veterinarian on the basis of exposure risk. A third category consists of those vaccines that may have no application in routine vaccination but might be used under very special circumstances. These are vaccines that would be directed against diseases of little clinical significance or vaccines whose risks do not significantly outweigh their benefits. Of course, all vaccine usage should be conducted on the basis of informed consent. An animal's owner should be made aware of the risks and benefits involved before seeking approval to vaccinate.

When vaccines are used to control disease in a population of animals rather than in individuals, the concept of herd immunity should also be considered. This herd immunity is the resistance of an entire group of animals to a disease as a result of the presence, in that group, of a proportion of immune animals. Herd immunity reduces the probability of a susceptible animal meeting an infected one so that the spread of disease is slowed or terminated. If it is acceptable to lose individual animals from disease while preventing epizootics, it may be possible to do this by vaccinating only a proportion of the population.

ADMINISTRATION OF VACCINES

Most vaccines are administered by injection. All such vaccines should be injected carefully and with due regard to the anatomy of the animal. Thus care must be taken not to injure or introduce infection into any animal. All needles used must be clean and sharp. Dirty or dull needles can cause tissue damage and infection at the injection site. The skin at the injection site must be clean and dry, although excessive use of alcohol should be avoided. Vaccines are provided in a standard dose, and this dose should not be divided to account for an animal's size. Doses are not formulated to account for body weight or age. (There must be a sufficient amount of an antigen to trigger the cells of the immune system and provoke an immune response. This amount is not related to body size.) Vaccination by subcutaneous or intramuscular injection is the simplest and most common method of vaccine administration. This approach is obviously excellent for small numbers of animals and for diseases in which systemic immunity is important. In some diseases, however, systemic immunity is not as important as local immunity, and it is perhaps more appropriate to administer the vaccine at the site of

potential invasions. Therefore intranasal vaccines are available for infectious bovine rhinotracheitis of cattle; for *Streptococcus equi* infections in horses; for feline rhinotracheitis, *Bordetella bronchiseptica*, coronavirus, and calicivirus infections; for canine parainfluenza and *Bordetella*; and for infectious bronchitis and Newcastle disease in poultry. Unfortunately, these methods of administration require that each animal be dealt with on an individual basis. When animal numbers are large, other methods must be employed. For example, aerosolization of vaccines enables them to be inhaled by all the animals in a group. This technique is employed in vaccinating against canine distemper and mink enteritis on mink ranches and against Newcastle disease in poultry. Alternatively, the vaccine may be put in the feed or drinking water, as is done with *Erysipelothrix rhusiopathiae* vaccines in pigs and against Newcastle disease, infectious laryngotracheitis, and avian encephalomyelitis in poultry.

Vaccination is now the most important method of preventing infectious diseases in farmed fish, in which it may significantly reduce mortality. Most commercial vaccines consist of inactivated products that are administered, either by intraperitoneal injection or, preferably, by immersing the fish in a dilute antigen solution. Immersion results in the antigen being deposited on mucosal surfaces such as the gills or oral cavity, and some may be swallowed.

Multiple-Antigen Vaccines

For convenience, it has become common to employ mixtures of organisms within single vaccines. For respiratory diseases of cattle, for example, vaccines are available that contain infectious bovine rhinotracheitis (BHV-1), bovine virus diarrhea (BVD), parainfluenza 3 (P13), and even *M. hemolytica*. Dogs may be given vaccines containing all of the following organisms: canine distemper virus, canine adenovirus-1, canine adenovirus-2, canine parvovirus-2, canine parainfluenza virus, leptospira bacterin, and rabies vaccine. These mixtures may be used when exact diagnosis is not possible and may protect animals against several infectious agents with economy of effort. However, it can also be wasteful to use vaccines against organisms that may not be causing problems. When different antigens in a mixture are inoculated simultaneously, competition occurs between antigens. Manufacturers of multiple-antigen vaccines take this into account and modify their mixtures accordingly. Vaccines should never be mixed indiscriminately, since one component may dominate the mixture and interfere with the response to the other components.

Some veterinarians have questioned whether the use of complex vaccine mixtures leads to less than satisfactory protection or increases the risk for adverse side effects. The suggestion that these multiple-antigen vaccines can overload the immune system is unfounded, nor is there any evidence to support the contention that the risk for adverse effects increases disproportionately when more components are added to vaccines. Certainly such vaccines should be tested to ensure that all components induce a satisfactory response. Licensed vaccines provided by a reputable manufacturer will generally provide satisfactory protection against all components.

Recent studies on mink receiving repeated multiple antigen vaccines have suggested that vaccinated animals may have significantly more immunoglobulins deposited in their glomeruli than animals receiving monovalent vaccine. This may be due to immune complex deposition or perhaps to individual components within the multivalent product. There was no evidence of alterations in renal function, so the significance of this finding is unclear.

Vaccination Schedules

Although it is not possible to give exact schedules for each of the veterinary vaccines available, certain principles are common to all methods of active immunization. Thus most vaccines require an initial series in which protective immunity is initiated, followed by revaccination (booster shots) at intervals to ensure that this protective immunity remains at an adequate level.

Initial Series

Because maternal antibodies passively protect newborn animals, it is not usually possible to successfully vaccinate animals very early in life. If stimulation of immunity is deemed necessary at this stage, the mother may be vaccinated during the later stages of pregnancy, the vaccinations being timed so that peak antibody levels are achieved at the time of colostrum formation. Once an animal is born, successful active immunization is effective only after passive immunity has waned. Since it is impossible to predict the exact time of loss of maternal immunity, the initial vaccination series will generally require administration of at least two and possibly more doses. Administration of vaccines to young animals is discussed in Chapter 19.

Revaccination

As pointed out in Chapter 10, the phenomenon of immunological memory is not well understood; yet it is the persistence of memory cells after vaccination that provides an animal with long-term protection. This may also be associated with persistent antibody production so that a vaccinated animal may have antibodies present in its bloodstream for many years after exposure to a vaccine. The reasons for this are unclear. It was originally believed that this persistence reflected the continuing presence of live antigens in an animal and was thus associated with the use of modified live vaccines. However, antibodies to some killed viral vaccines may be equally persistent. More recent evidence suggests that long-lived antibody-producing cells are stimulated to survive by nonspecific microbial molecules.

Duration of Immunity

Revaccination schedules depend on duration of immunity (Table 22-1) This in turn depends on antigen content, whether the vaccine consists of living or dead organisms, and its route of administration. In the past, relatively poor vaccines may have required frequent administration, perhaps as often as every 6 months, in order to maintain an acceptable level of immunity. Newer, modern vaccines usually produce a long-lasting immunity, especially in companion animals, and some may require revaccination only once every 2 or 3 years. Even killed viral vaccines may protect individual animals against disease for many years. Unfortunately, the minimal duration of immunity has, until recently, rarely been measured, and reliable figures are not available for many vaccines. Likewise, although serum antibodies can be monitored in vaccinated animals, tests have not been standardized and there is no consensus regarding the interpretation of these antibody titers. Nor is there much information available regarding long-term immunity on mucosal surfaces. In general, immunity against feline panleukopenia, canine distemper, canine parvovirus, and canine adenovirus is considered to be relatively long-lived (>2 years). On the other hand, immunity to feline rhinotracheitis, feline calicivirus, and chlamydophila, is

TABLE 22-1

Estimated Minimum Duration of Immunity (DOI) of Select Commercially Available Canine Vaccine Antigens

Vaccine	Estimated Minimum DOI	Estimated Relative Efficacy (%)
ESSENTIAL		
Canine distemper (MLV)	≥7 years	>90
Canine distemper (R)	≥1 year	>90
Canine parvovirus-2 (MLV)	≥7 years	>90
Canine adenovirus-2 (MLV)	≥7 years	>90
Rabies virus (K)	≥3 years	>85
OPTIONAL		
Canine coronavirus (K or MLV)	N/A	N/A
Canine parainfluenza (MLV)	≥3 years	>80
Bordetella bronchiseptica (ML)	≤1 year	≤70
Leptospira canicola (K)	≤1 year	≤50
L. grippotyphosa (K)	≤1 year	N/A
L. icterohaemorrhagiae (K)	≤1 year	≤75
L. pomona (K)	≤1 year	N/A
Borrelia burgdorferi (K)	1 year	≤75
B. burgdorferi OspA (R)	1 year	≤75
Giardia lamblia (K)	≤1 year	N/A

From Paul MA, Appel M, Barrett R, et al: *J Am Anim Hosp Assoc* 39: 119-131, 2003.
MLV, Modified live virus; *K,* killed, *R,* recombinant.

believed to be relatively short. One problem in making these statements is variability among individual animals and among different types of vaccine. Thus recombinant canine distemper vaccines may induce immunity of much shorter duration than conventional, modified live vaccines. There may be a great difference between the shortest and longest duration within a group of animals. Duration of immunity studies are confounded by the fact that in many cases older animals already show increased innate resistance. Different vaccines within a category may differ significantly in their composition, and although all vaccines may induce immunity in the short term, it cannot be assumed that all confer long-term immunity. Manufacturers use different master seeds and different methods of antigen preparation. The level of immunity required for most of these diseases is unknown. Likewise, a significant difference exists between the minimal level of immunity required to protect most animals and the level of immunity required to ensure protection of all animals.

Annual revaccination has been the rule for most animal vaccines since this approach is administratively simple and has the advantage of ensuring that an animal is regularly seen by a veterinarian. Recent information, however, indicates that some animal vaccines such as those against canine distemper or feline herpesvirus may induce protective immunity that can last for many years and that annual revaccination using these vaccines may be unnecessary. Unfortunately, there is insufficient information available on many vaccines to determine minimum vaccination intervals. A veterinarian should always assess the relative risks and benefits to an animal in determining the use of any vaccine and its frequency of administration. It may therefore be good practice to use serum antibody assays such as ELISAs, if available, to provide guidance on revaccination intervals. Persistent antibody titers may indicate protection, but this is not guaranteed, especially if cell-mediated immune mechanisms are important for protection. Likewise, animals with low or undetectable serum antibody levels may still be protected either because of cell-mediated immunity, or simply because of the persistence of memory B cells capable of responding rapidly to reinfection.

Notwithstanding the discussion above, animal owners should be made aware that protection against an infectious disease can only be maintained reliably when vaccines are used in accordance with the protocol approved by the vaccine licensing authorities. The duration of immunity claimed by a vaccine manufacturer is the minimum duration of immunity that is supported by the data available at the time the vaccine license is approved. This must always be taken into account when discussing revaccination protocols with an owner.

The timing of initial vaccinations may also be determined by the disease. Some diseases are seasonal, and vaccines may be given before disease outbreaks are expected. Examples of these include the vaccine against the lungworm *Dictyocaulus viviparus* given in early summer just before the anticipated lungworm season, the vaccine against anthrax given in spring, and the vaccine against *Clostridium chauvoei* given to sheep before turning them out to pasture. Bluetongue of lambs is spread by midges (*Culicoides varipennis*) and is thus a disease of midsummer and early fall. Vaccination in spring will therefore protect lambs during the susceptible period.

VACCINATION STRATEGIES

Although vaccination is a powerful tool for the control of infectious disease, its potential to prevent the spread of a disease or to eliminate a disease depends on selecting correct control strategies. If an infectious disease outbreak, such as one caused by foot-and-mouth virus, is to be rapidly controlled, it is vitally important to select the correct population for vaccination. The success of any mass vaccination program depends both on the proportion of animals vaccinated and the efficacy of the vaccine. Neither of these factors will reach 100%, so it is essential to target the vaccine effectively. It is also the case that vaccines do not confer immediate protection, so the strategy employed will depend on the rate of spread of an infection. Vaccines may thus be given either prophylactically, in advance of an outbreak, or reactively, in response to an existing outbreak. Both strategies have advantages and disadvantages. In general, prophylactic vaccination greatly reduces the potential for a major epidemic of a disease such as foot-and-mouth disease by reducing the size of a susceptible population. The effectiveness of this approach can be greatly enhanced by identifying high risk individuals and ensuring that they are protected in advance of an outbreak.

It is generally not feasible to vaccinate an entire population of animals once a disease outbreak has occurred. However, two effective reactive vaccination strategies include "ring-vaccination," which seeks to contain an outbreak by establishing a barrier of immune animals around an infected area, and "predictive-vaccination," which seeks to vaccinate the animals on farms likely to contribute most to the future spread of disease. Reactive vaccination in this way can ensure that an epidemic is not unduly prolonged. A prolonged "tail" to an epidemic commonly results from the disease "jumping" to a new area. Well-considered, predictive vaccination may well prevent these jumps. Thus in an ideal situation a combination of prophylactic and reactive vaccination will likely yield the most effective results.

VACCINE ASSESSMENT

To assess the efficacy of a vaccine, animals must first be vaccinated and then challenged. The percentage of vaccinated animals that survive this challenge can then be measured. It is important, however, to determine the percentage of nonvaccinated control animals that also survive the challenge. The true efficacy of a vaccine, called the preventable fraction (PF), is calculated as follows:

$$PF = \frac{(\% \text{ of controls dying} - \% \text{ of vaccinates dying})}{\% \text{ of controls dying}}$$

For example, a challenge that kills 80% of controls and 40% of vaccinates shows that the PF of the vaccine is as follows:

$$PF = \frac{80 - 40}{80} = 50\%$$

Good, effective vaccines should have a PF of at least 80%. Obviously, less effective vaccines are acceptable if safe and if nothing better is available.

FAILURES IN VACCINATION

There are many reasons why a vaccine may fail to confer protective immunity on an animal (Figure 22-1).

Incorrect Administration

In many cases vaccine failure is due to unsatisfactory administration. For example, a live vaccine may have died as a result of poor storage, the use of antibiotics in conjunction with live bacterial vaccines, the use of chemicals to sterilize syringe, or the excessive use of alcohol when swabbing the skin. Sometimes, animals given vaccines by nonconventional routes may not be protected. When large flocks of poultry or mink are to be vaccinated, it is common to administer the vaccine either as an aerosol or in drinking water. If the aerosol is not evenly distributed throughout a building, or if some animals do not drink, they may receive insufficient vaccine. Animals that subsequently develop disease may be interpreted as cases of vaccine failure.

Correct Administration but Failure to Respond

Occasionally, a vaccine may actually be ineffective. The method of production may have destroyed the protective epitopes, or there may simply be insufficient antigen in the vaccine. Problems of this type are uncommon and can generally be avoided by using only vaccines from reputable manufacturers.

More commonly, an animal may simply fail to mount an immune response. The immune response, being a

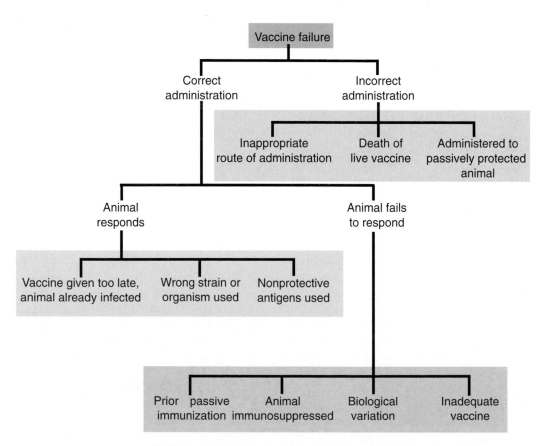

Figure 22-1.   A classification of the causes of vaccine failure.

biological process, never confers absolute protection and is never equal in all members of a vaccinated population. Since the immune response is influenced by a large number of genetic and environmental factors, the range of immune responses in a large random population of animals tends to follow a normal distribution. This means that most animals respond to antigens by mounting an average immune response, whereas a few will mount an excellent response and a small proportion will mount a poor immune response (Figure 22-2). This group of poor responders may not be protected against infection in spite of having received an effective vaccine. Therefore, it is essentially impossible to protect 100% of a random population of animals by vaccination. The size of this unreactive portion of the population will vary between vaccines, and its significance will depend on the nature of the disease. Thus, for highly infectious diseases against which herd immunity is poor and in which infection is rapidly and efficiently transmitted, such as foot-and-mouth disease, the presence of unprotected animals could permit the spread of disease and would thus disrupt control programs. Likewise, problems can arise if the unprotected animals are individually important; for example, companion animals. In contrast, for diseases that are inefficiently spread, such as rabies, 70% protection may be sufficient to effectively block disease transmission within a population and may therefore be quite satisfactory from a community health viewpoint.

Another type of vaccine failure occurs when the normal immune response is suppressed. For example, heavily parasitized or malnourished animals may be immuno-suppressed and should not be vaccinated. Some virus infections induce profound immunosuppression. Animals with a major illness or high fever should not normally be vaccinated unless for a compelling reason. Stress may reduce a normal immune response, probably because of increased steroid production; examples of such stress

include pregnancy, fatigue, malnutrition, and extremes of cold and heat. This type of immunosuppression is discussed in detail in Chapter 36. The most important cause of vaccine failure of this type is passively derived maternal immunity in young animals, as described in Chapter 19.

Correct Administration and Response

Even animals given an adequate dose of an effective vaccine may fail to be protected. If the vaccinated animal was incubating the disease before inoculation, the vaccine may be given too late to affect the course of the disease. Alternatively, the vaccine may contain the wrong strain of organisms or the wrong (nonprotective) antigens.

ADVERSE CONSEQUENCES OF VACCINATION

Vaccination continues to be the only safe, reliable, and effective way of protecting animals against the major infectious diseases. Nevertheless, the use of vaccines is not free of risk. Residual virulence and toxicity, allergic responses, disease in immunodeficient hosts, neurological complications and harmful effects on the fetus are the most significant risks associated with the use of vaccines (Figure 22-3). Veterinarians should use only licensed vaccines, and the manufacturer's recommendations should be carefully followed. Before using a vaccine, the veterinarian should consider both the likelihood that an adverse event will happen, as well as the possible consequences or severity of this event. These factors must be weighed against the benefits to the animal. Thus a common but mild complication may require a different consideration than a rare, severe complication.

The issue of the risk associated with vaccination remains, in large part a philosophical one, since the advantages of vaccination are well documented and extensive whereas the risk for adverse effects is poorly documented and, in many cases, largely theoretical (Box 22-1).

"Normal" Toxicity

By far the most common reactions to vaccines are local ones. For example, an immediate form of toxicity is the sting produced by some inactivating agents such as formaldehyde. This can present problems not only to the animal being vaccinated but also, if the animal reacts violently, to the vaccinator. More commonly, local swellings may develop at the reaction site. These may be firm or edematous and may be warm to the touch. They appear about one day after vaccination and can last for about a week. Unless an injection-site abscess develops, these swellings leave little trace. Vaccines containing killed gram-negative organisms may be intrinsically toxic owing to the presence of endotoxins that can cause cytokine release, leading to shock, fever, and leukopenia.

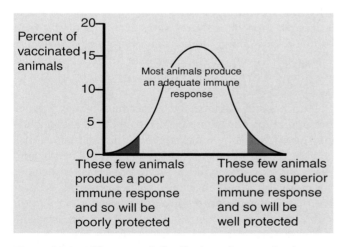

Figure 22-2.   The normal distribution of protective immune responses in a population of vaccinated animals. No vaccine can be expected to protect 100% of a population.

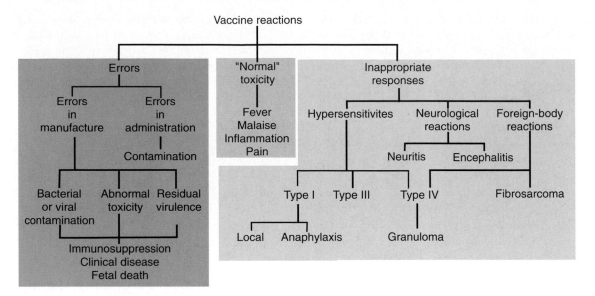

Figure 22-3.   A simple classification of the major adverse effects of vaccination.

Although such a reaction is usually only a temporary inconvenience to male animals, it may be sufficient to provoke abortion in pregnant females. Thus it may be prudent to avoid vaccinating pregnant animals unless the risks of not giving the vaccine are considered to be too great.

Inappropriate Responses

Vaccines may cause allergic reactions. For example, type I hypersensitivity can occur in response not only to the immunizing antigen but also to other antigens found in vaccines, such as egg antigens or antigens from tissue culture cells. All forms of hypersensitivity are more commonly associated with multiple injections of antigens and therefore tend to be associated with the use of killed vaccines. It is important to emphasize that a type I hypersensitivity is an immediate response to an antigen and

occurs within a few minutes or hours after exposure to an antigen. Reactions occurring more than 2 or 3 hours after administration of a vaccine are likely not type I hypersensitivity reactions.

Type III hypersensitivity reactions are also potential hazards. These may cause intense local inflammation, or they may present as a generalized vascular disturbance such as purpura. A type III reaction can occur in the eyes of dogs vaccinated against infectious canine hepatitis (Chapter 28). Some rabies vaccines may induce a local complement-mediated vasculitis leading to ischemic dermatitis and local alopecia. This type of reaction is most often seen in small dogs such as dachshunds, miniature poodles, Bichon Frises, and terriers.

Type IV hypersensitivity reactions may occur in response to vaccination, but a more common reaction is granuloma formation at the site of inoculation. This may be a response to depot adjuvants containing alum or oil. Vaccines containing a water-in-oil adjuvant produce larger and more persistent lesions at injection sites than vaccines containing alum and aluminum hydroxide. These lesions can be granulomas or sterile abscesses. If the skin is dirty at the injection site, these abscesses may become infected.

Under some circumstances vaccination may trigger autoimmunity. For example, an autoimmune encephalitis may be provoked by rabies vaccines that contain central nervous tissue. A polyneuritis (Gullain-Barré syndrome) has been associated with the use of certain virus vaccines (most notably swine influenza) in humans, and at least one case has been reported in a dog following vaccination with a polyvalent distemper-hepatitis-parvovirus vaccine (Chapter 33). The pathogenesis of this syndrome is unclear.

Postvaccinal canine distemper virus encephalitis is a rare complication that may develop after administration

---

BOX 22–1

Precise Figures?

Although figures for the prevalence of adverse reactions are difficult to obtain, data from the British National Suspected Adverse Reaction Surveillance Scheme suggest that in cats the incidence of adverse effects was 0.30 to 0.82 (mean 0.61) per 10,000 vaccine doses sold. In dogs the figure is lower (0.13 to 0.26; mean 0.21). Pedigree cats appeared to have a higher prevalence of adverse effects than nonpedigree cats. Adverse reactions appear to occur more often in male animals. In Australia, an adverse reaction rate of 0.2% to 0.4% has been reported (Table 22-2).

The United States Pharmacopeia Veterinary practitioners Reporting Program received 460 reports regarding adverse reactions to vaccines in the 1-year period 1997 to 1998.

TABLE 22-2
Reported Adverse Reactions From the British Suspected Adverse Reaction Surveillance Scheme 1995-1999

Disease Signs	Cats		Dogs	
	Incidence/1000 Doses	Number	Incidence/1000 Doses	Number
Anaphylaxis	0.026	33	0.018	53
Hypersensitivity	0.022	28	0.028	81
Urticaria	0	0	0.007	19
Local reactions	0.099	127	0.012	37
Sarcoma	0.021	26	0	0
Immune-mediated hemolytic anemia	0	0	0.001	4
Immune-mediated thrombocytopenia	0	0	0.002	5
Corneal edema	0	0	0.002	6
Polyarthritis	0.044	57	0.001	2
Upper respiratory tract lesions	0.028	36	0	0
Urticaria + lameness	0.006	8	0	0
Lameness/lethargy	0.071	91	0	0
Suspected no efficacy	0.027	35	0.016	46

From *Vet Rec* 150:126-134, 2002.

of a modified live canine distemper vaccine. The affected animal may show aggression, incoordination, and seizures or other neurological signs. The pathogenesis of this condition is unknown, but it may be due to residual virulence, increased susceptibility, or triggering of a latent paramyxovirus by the vaccine.

Errors in Manufacture or Administration

Some problems associated with vaccine use may be due to poor production or administration. Thus some modified live vaccines may retain the ability to cause disease. For example, some modified live herpes vaccines or calicivirus vaccines given intranasally may spread to the oropharynx and result in persistent infection. Indeed, such a virus vaccine may infect (and protect) other animals in contact. Even if these vaccines do not cause overt disease, they may reduce the rate of growth of an animal with significant economic consequences.

Another response to some vaccines is a mild immunosuppression. For example, some modified live parvovirus vaccines may cause a transient decrease in lymphocyte blastogenesis responses or even a lymphopenia in some puppies. Not all strains of canine parvovirus-2 are immunosuppressive, so it is difficult to determine the overall significance of this. Many polyvalent canine viral vaccines can cause a transient drop in absolute lymphocyte numbers and their responses to mitogens (Figure 36-2). This occurs although the individual components of these vaccines may not have this effect. Several vaccine combinations cause immunosuppression between 5 and 11 days after vaccination. Thus, for example, a combination of canine adenovirus type 1 or type 2 with canine distemper virus is especially suppressive of canine lymphocyte responses to mitogens. The mechanisms involved are unknown. The short duration

of the immunodeficiency state probably ensures that it rarely becomes clinically significant.

Vaccines such as bluetongue vaccine have been reported to cause congenital anomalies in the offspring of ewes vaccinated while pregnant. The stress from this type of toxic reaction may also be sufficient to reactivate latent infections; for example, activation of equine herpesvirus has been demonstrated following vaccination against African horse sickness. Mucosal disease may develop in calves vaccinated against bovine virus diarrhea.

Injection Site–Associated Sarcomas

Most vaccine site reactions in cats resolve rapidly. In some cats, however, tumors have developed at these injection sites many months after injection. They have typically been found in the cervical/interscapular and femoral regions (Figure 22-4). The appearance of these tumors has coincided with the introduction of new, potent, inactivated, adjuvanted vaccines such as those directed against rabies and feline leukemia. Most of these tumors are fibrosarcomas, but other types of malignant sarcomas have been observed. Epidemiological studies have linked the development of these tumors to vaccination. There appears to be a direct correlation with the irritancy of a substance and its ability to induce fibrosarcomas. Cats with fibrosarcomas occurring at sites where vaccines are currently administered were compared with cats that developed fibrosarcomas at nonvaccine injection sites. Cats receiving FeLV vaccine were 5.5 times more likely to develop a sarcoma at the injection site than cats that had not received a vaccine. There was a lesser association with rabies vaccination (twofold increase in risk). However, the risk was not enormously high In early studies it was calculated that 1 to 3.6 sarcomas developed per 10,000 FeLV and rabies vaccines

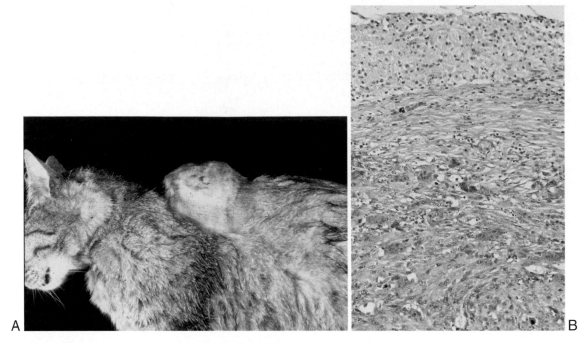

Figure 22-4. **A,** A postvaccinal sarcoma in a cat. Note its characteristic position over the scapulae, where the vaccine has been administered subcutaneously. **B,** A histological section of a postvaccinal sarcoma. This is a fibrosarcoma showing long interwoven bundles of spindle cells (H&E stain). (Courtesy of Dr. MJ Hendrick.)

administered. The risk did increase with the number of doses of vaccine administered—a 50% increase following one dose, a 127% increase following two doses, and a 175% increase following three or four vaccines given simultaneously. Vaccine-associated sarcomas tend to occur in younger animals and tend to be larger and more aggressive than sarcomas arising at other sites. In one study, injection site sarcomas developed on average 26 months after the last rabies vaccination given and 11 months after FeLV vaccination. Global, Web-based surveys suggest a somewhat lower prevalence of sarcomas (0.63 sarcomas/10,000 cats or 0.32 sarcomas/10,000 doses of all vaccines or one sarcoma from 31,000 doses administered). It must be pointed out, therefore, that the risks for developing a sarcoma are considerably smaller than the disease risks incurred by unvaccinated cats. Similar vaccination-related injection site sarcomas have been reported in ferrets.

The pathogenesis of these fibrosarcomas is unclear. The potent adjuvants found in modern vaccines will result in protection lasting for several years. In addition, these products are administered by the convenient subcutaneous route. As a result, an irritating adjuvant may persist at the injection site for a long time. Nevertheless, tumor development has also been associated with the use of nonadjuvanted vaccines and even with injection of substances other than vaccines, as well as the presence of persistent sutures.

Fibroblasts are stimulated to proliferate at sites of chronic inflammation and wound healing. Evidence suggests that in some of these fibroblasts the *sis* oncogene is activated. whereas in others, there appear to be defects in the tumor protective gene p53. The *sis* oncogene codes for the platelet-derived growth factor (PDGF) receptor, and vaccine-associated sarcomas have been found to express both PDGF and its receptor. Lymphocytes within these tumors are also PDGF-positive. In contrast, nonvaccine-associated tumors and normal cat lymphocytes are PDGF-negative. It has been suggested, therefore, that lymphocytes within the vaccine-associated sarcomas secrete PDGF, which then serves as a growth factor for the fibroblasts. This combination of abnormalities could result in the loss of growth control in the fibroblasts engaged in the chronic inflammatory process. There is no evidence that feline sarcoma virus, feline immunodeficiency virus, or feline leukemia virus causes these tumors.

To minimize the possibility of tumors developing at vaccination sites, it is recommended that when multiple vaccines are given, they be administered at standardized sites on the animal and away from sites where tumor management is difficult. For example, current recommendations are to inject rabies vaccine on the caudal half of the right side and FeLV vaccine on the caudal half of the left side of the cat's body ("rabies, right; leukemia, left"). If possible, the site of vaccine administration and the product used should be recorded for each vaccine to help in assessing risk factors. Nonadjuvanted vaccines appear to induce much less severe irritation and present a correspondingly lower risk for tumor formation. Successful treatment requires a combination of aggressive surgery and radiation.

Vaccine-Associated Autoimmune Disease

Although vaccination has been widely suspected of triggering autoimmune disease in animals, objective evidence of such an association is limited. The only data to suggest such a link were derived from a retrospective analysis of the history of dogs presenting with idiopathic autoimmune hemolytic anemia (AIHA) (Chapter 33). Thus 15 of 70 dogs with AIHA had been vaccinated within the previous month as compared with a randomly selected control group in which none had been vaccinated. Dogs with AIHA that developed within a month of vaccination differed in some clinical features from dogs with AIHA unassociated with prior vaccination. The disease was not associated with any specific type of vaccine. Although not conclusive, this association clearly requires confirmation.

PRODUCTION, PRESENTATION, AND CONTROL OF VACCINES

The production of veterinary vaccines is controlled by the Animal and Plant Health Inspection Service of the USDA in the United States, by the Health of Animals Branch of the Canada Department of Agriculture in Canada, and by the Veterinary Medicines Directorate in the United Kingdom. In general, regulatory authorities have the right to license establishments where vaccines are produced and to inspect these premises to ensure that the facilities are appropriate and that the methods employed are satisfactory. All vaccines must be checked for safety and potency. Safety tests include confirmation of the identity of the organism used and of the freedom of the vaccine from extraneous organisms (i.e., purity), as well as tests for toxicity and sterility. Because the living organisms or antigens found in vaccines normally die or degrade over a period of time, it is necessary to ensure that they will be effective even after storage. It is usual, therefore, to use an antigen in generous excess of the dose required to protect animals under laboratory conditions, and potency is tested both before and after accelerated aging. Vaccines that contain killed organisms, although much more stable than living ones, also contain an excess of antigens for the same reason. Vaccines approved for licensing on the basis of challenge exposure studies must usually show evidence of protection in 80% of vaccinated animals, whereas at the same time, at least 80% of the unvaccinated controls must develop evidence of disease after challenge exposure (the 80:80 efficacy guideline). The route and dose of administration indicated on the vaccine label should be scrupulously heeded since these were probably the only route and dose tested for safety and efficacy during the licensing process. Vaccines usually have a designated shelf life, and although properly stored vaccines may still be potent after the expiration of this shelf life, this should never be assumed. Correct storage and handling are essential.

All expired vaccines should be discarded. Adverse reactions should always be reported to the appropriate licensing authorities as well as to the vaccine manufacturer.

Because modified live vaccines carry with them the risks for residual virulence and for contamination with other agents, certain countries will not approve their use.

Inactivated vaccines are commonly available in liquid form and usually contain suspended adjuvant. These should not be frozen, and they should be shaken well before use. The presence of preservatives such as phenol or merthiolate will not control massive bacterial contamination, and multidose containers should be discarded after partial use. Many vaccines containing modified live viruses are susceptible to heat inactivation but are much more resistant if lyophilized. Remember, however, that intense sunlight and heat can destroy even lyophilized vaccines. They store well but should be kept cool and away from light and should only be reconstituted with the fluid provided by the manufacturer.

SOME ANTIBACTERIAL VACCINES

Toxoids

The immunoprophylaxis of tetanus is restricted to toxin neutralization. Tetanus toxoid in an aluminum hydroxide suspension is given for routine prophylaxis, and a single injection will induce protective immunity in 10 to 14 days. Conventional immunological wisdom would suggest that the previous use of immune globulin should interfere with the immune response to toxoid and must therefore be avoided. This is not a problem in practice, however, and both may be successfully administered simultaneously (at different sites) without problems. This may be because of the relatively small amount of immune globulin usually needed to protect animals.

Some veterinary vaccines combine both toxoid and killed bacteria in a single dose by the simple expedient of formolizing a whole culture. These products, sometimes called anacultures, are used to vaccinate against *Clostridium haemolyticum* and *C. perfringens*. Trypsinization of the anaculture may make it more immunogenic. Toxoids, usually incorporated with an alum adjuvant, are available for most clostridial diseases and for infections caused by toxigenic staphylococci.

Bacterins

Bacterin is the term used to describe vaccines containing killed bacteria. It is usual to kill the bacteria with formaldehyde and to incorporate them with alum or aluminum hydroxide adjuvants. As with other dead vaccines, the immunity produced by bacterins is relatively short-lived, usually lasting for not longer than 1 year and sometimes for a considerably shorter period. For instance, formolized swine erysipelas (*E. rhusiopathiae*) vaccine protects for only 4 to 5 months, and *S. equi* bacterins give immunity for less than 1 year, even though recovery from a natural case of strangles may confer a lifelong immunity in horses.

Bacterins may be improved by adding purified immunogenic antigens to the killed bacteria. Thus *E. coli* bacterins against enteric colibacillosis may be enriched and made much more effective by the addition of K88 or K99 pilus antigens. Antibodies to these antigens block binding of *E. coli* to the intestinal wall and thus contribute significantly to the protective immune response. Similarly, *Mannheimia* bacterins enriched in the leukotoxoid show improved efficacy over conventional bacterins. Purified bacterial components such as the surface antigens of *M. hemolytica* may also be effective vaccine components.

One problem encountered, especially when using coliform and *Campylobacter* vaccines, is strain specificity. Several different antigenic types of each organism commonly occur, and successful vaccination requires immunization with appropriate bacterial strains. This is sometimes not possible if a commercial vaccine must be employed. One method of overcoming this difficulty is to use autogenous vaccines. These are vaccines that contain organisms obtained either from infected animals on the farm where the disease problem is occurring or from the infected animal itself. These can be very successful if carefully prepared, since the vaccine will contain all the antigens required for protection in that particular location. As an alternative to the use of autogenous vaccines, some manufacturers produce polyvalent vaccines containing a mixture of antigenic types. For example, leptospirosis vaccines commonly contain up to five different serovars. This practice, although effective, is inefficient, since only a few of the antigenic types employed may be appropriate in any given situation.

A major advance in the development of vaccines against gram-negative bacteria is the use of common core antigens. As pointed out in Chapter 2, the outer layer of the gram-negative bacterial cell wall consists of lipopolysaccharide. This lipopolysaccharide consists of a variable oligosaccharide (O antigen) bound to a highly conserved core polysaccharide and lipid A. The O antigen varies greatly among gram-negative bacteria so that an immune response against one O antigen confers no immunity against bacteria bearing other O antigens. In contrast, the underlying core polysaccharide is similar among gram-negative bacteria of different species and genera. Thus an immune response directed against this common core structure has the potential to protect against a wide variety of different gram-negative bacteria.

Mutant strains of *E. coli* (J5) and *Salmonella enterica minnesota* or *S. enterica typhimurium* (Re) have been used as sources of core antigen. J5 is a rough mutant that is deficient in uridine diphosphate galactose 4-epimerase. As a result the organism makes an incomplete oligosaccharide side chain, having lost most of the outer lipopolysaccharide structure (Figure 2-2). Immunization with J5 thus provides protection against *E. coli*, *Klebsiella pneumoniae*, *A. pleuropneumoniae*, *Haemophilus influenzae* (type B), and *S. enterica typhimurium*. J5 has been reported to protect calves against organisms such as *S. enterica typhimurium* and *E. coli* and pigs against *A. pleuropneumoniae*. The most encouraging results have been obtained in protection against coliform mastitis.

Living Bacterial Vaccines

Successful living bacterial vaccines include strains 19 and RB51 of *B. abortus*. Another successful living vaccine is that employed for the prevention of anthrax. Older anthrax vaccines used Pasteur's technique of culturing the bacteria at a relatively high temperature (42° to 43° C) so that their virulence is reduced. The anthrax vaccines currently available for animals contain capsule-less mutants that remain capable of forming spores. The vaccine is prepared as a spore suspension and is administered with saponin.

A rough strain of *S. enterica dublin* (strain 51) is used in Europe to give good protection to calves when administered at 2 to 4 weeks of age. As discussed earlier, immunity to salmonellosis involves macrophage activation and is thus relatively nonspecific. For this reason, strain 51 may also give good protection against *S. enterica typhimurium*.

SOME ANTIVIRAL VACCINES

Because of the lack of antiviral drugs, vaccination is the only effective method for the control of most virus diseases in domestic animals. As a result, the development of viral vaccines is, in many ways, more advanced than the development of their bacterial counterparts. It has, for example, proved relatively easy to attenuate many viruses so that effective vaccines containing modified live viruses (MLV) derived from tissue culture are readily available.

As discussed in Chapter 21, MLV vaccines are usually good immunogens, but their use may involve certain risks. The most important problem encountered is residual virulence. One serious example of this was the development of clinical rabies in some dogs and cats following administration of older strains of MLV rabies vaccine. Some strains of infectious bovine rhinotracheitis and equine herpesvirus-1 vaccines may cause abortion when given to pregnant cows or mares, respectively, and MLV bluetongue vaccines may cause disease in fetal lambs if given to pregnant ewes (Chapter 19). More commonly, the residual virulence in these vaccines causes a mild disease. Thus intraocular or intranasal rhinotracheitis or calicivirus vaccines may cause a transient conjunctivitis or rhinitis in cats. MLV infectious bursal disease vaccines, some canine parvovirus-2 vaccines, and some bovine viral diarrhea vaccines can cause a mild immunosuppression.

Transient side effects such as these, which may otherwise be regarded as inconsequential, can be of major significance in the broiler chicken industry, where even a minor slowing in growth can have major economic results. Thus two strains of infectious bronchitis vaccine are available. The Massachusetts strain is mildly pathogenic but a good immunogen, whereas the Connecticut strain is nonpathogenic but a poor immunogen. It is common, therefore, in order to minimize complications, to use the Connecticut strain for primary vaccination and, if boosters are required, to use the Massachusetts strain subsequently. Similarly, of the two major vaccine strains of Newcastle disease, the LaSota strain is a good immunogen but may provoke mild adverse reactions. In contrast, the B1 strain is considerably milder but is less immunogenic, especially if given in drinking water.

Because of problems of this nature, persistent attempts have been made to minimize residual virulence in vaccines. One method involves the use of temperature-sensitive (ts) mutants. Ts strains of bovine herpesvirus-1, for example, will grow only at temperatures a few degrees lower than normal body temperature. When this organism is administered intranasally, it is able to colonize the relatively cool nasal mucosa but is unable to invade the rest of the body. Thus the vaccine can stimulate local immunity without incurring the risk for a systemic invasion. (It also has the advantage that its activity is not blocked by maternal immunity.) Some vaccine viruses may persist in vaccinated animals and cause a prolonged carrier state. Although this is a problem largely associated with herpesviruses, concerns have been expressed that the widespread use of MLV vaccines may serve to seed viruses into animal populations and that untoward consequences may develop in the future. This is a threat not to be taken lightly.

An alternative approach to overcoming the problems caused by modified live vaccines involves the increasing use of inactivated and subunit vaccines. Excellent inactivated vaccines are available against diseases such as foot-and-mouth disease, equine herpesvirus-4 (rhinopneumonitis), pseudorabies, feline panleukopenia, feline herpes (rhinotracheitis), and rabies. A genetically engineered subunit vaccine directed against the gp70 envelope antigen of feline leukemia virus is also available. At their best, these vaccines confer immunity comparable in strength and duration to that induced by MLV vaccines, with the assurance that they are free of residual virulence.

SOURCES OF ADDITIONAL INFORMATION

Buracco P, Martano M, Morello E, Ratto A: Vaccine-associated-like fibrosarcoma at the site of a deep non-absorbable suture in a cat, *Vet J* 163:105-107, 2002.

Coyne MJ, Burr JHH, Yule TD, et al: Duration of immunity in dogs after vaccination or naturally acquired infection, *Vet Rec* 149:509-515, 2001.

Coyne MJ, Burr JHH, Yule TD, et al: Duration of immunity in cats after vaccination or naturally acquired infection, *Vet Rec* 149:545-548, 2001.

Duval D, Giger U: Vaccine-associated immune-mediated hemolytic anemia in the dog, *J Vet Intern Med* 10:290-295, 1996.

Frank LA: Rabies vaccine-induced ischemic dermatitis in a dog, *Vet Allergy Clin Immunol* 6:9-12, 1998.

Gaskell RM, Gettinby G, Graham SJ, Skilton D: Veterinary products committee working group report on feline and canine vaccination, *Vet Rec* 150:126-134, 2002.

Gray A, Knivett S: Suspected adverse reactions, 1999, *Vet Rec* Sept:283-284, 2000.

Guglick MA, MacAllister CG, Ely RW, Edwards WC: Hepatic disease associated with administration of tetanus antitoxin in eight horses, *J Am Vet Med Assn* 206:1737-1740, 1995.

Hendrick MJ, Kass PH, McGill LD, Tizard IR: Post vaccinal sarcomas in cats, *J Nat Cancer Inst* 86:341-343, 1994.

HogenEsch H, Dunham AD, Scott-Moncrieff C, et al: Effect of vaccination on serum concentrations of total and antigen-specific immunoglobulin E in dogs, *Am J Vet Res* 63:611-616, 2002.

Keeling MJ, Woolhouse MEJ, May RM, et al: Modeling vaccination strategies against foot-and-mouth disease, *Nature* 421:136-142, 2003.

Langeveld JPM, Kamstrup S, Uttenthal A: Full protection against mink enteritis virus with new generation canine parvovirus vaccines based on synthetic peptide or recombinant protein, *Vaccine* 13:1033-1037, 1995.

McEntee MC, Page RL: Feline vaccine-associated sarcomas, *J Vet Intern Med* 15:176-182, 2001.

Mengeling WL, Vorwald AC, Lager KM, et al: Identification and clinical assessment of suspected vaccine-related field strains of porcine reproductive and respiratory syndrome virus, *Am J Vet Res* 60:334-340, 1999.

Meyer EK: Vaccine-associated adverse events, *Vet Clin North Am* 31:493-515, 2001.

Nalin DR: Evidence-based vaccinology, *Vaccine* 20:1624-1630, 2002.

Newman SJ, Johnson R, Sears W, Wilcock B: Investigation of repeated vaccination as a possible cause of glomerular disease in mink, *Can J Vet Res* 66:158-164, 2002.

Schrauwen E, Van Ham L: Postvaccinal acute polyradiculoneuritis in a young dog, *Progr Vet Neurol* 6:68-70, 1995.

Smith H: Reactions to strangles vaccination, *Aust Vet J* 71:257-258, 1994.

Twark L, Dodds WJ: Clinical use of serum parvovirus and distemper virus antibody titers for determining revaccination strategies in healthy dogs, *J Am Vet Med Assoc* 217:1021-1024, 2000.

Wilbur LA, Evermann JF, Levings RL, et al: Abortion and death in pregnant bitches associated with a canine vaccine contaminated with bluetongue virus, *J Am Vet Med Assoc* 204:1762-1765, 1994.

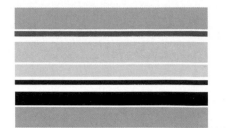

Acquired Immunity to Bacteria and Related Organisms

CHAPTER 23

Although animals live in an environment densely populated with bacteria, the vast majority of these organisms neither invade animal tissues nor cause disease. This is unsurprising for several reasons. First, the combined efforts of the innate and acquired immune systems are sufficient to prevent invasion. Second, even organisms that successfully invade the animal body gain very little by harming their host. On the contrary, illness or death of the host animal may well reduce the survival of the bacteria and is therefore normally avoided. Indeed, many bacteria are essential for the animal's well-being, since they maintain an environment on body surfaces that is hostile to other potential invaders. They also assist in the digestion of foods such as celluloses. Nevertheless, many commensal bacteria are also potential pathogens. For example, *Clostridium tetani* and *C. perfringens* are commonly found among the intestinal flora of horses, and *Bordetella bronchiseptica* is found in the nasopharynx of healthy swine. Bacterial disease is not, therefore, an inevitable consequence of the presence of pathogenic organisms on body surfaces. The development of disease is related to many other factors, including the response of the host, the presence of damaged tissues, the location of the bacteria within the body, and the disease-producing power (or virulence) of the bacteria. Only when the balance between host immunity and bacterial virulence is upset will disease or death result.

Antimicrobial immunity consists of an early innate response followed by a more sustained adaptive response. Recognition of invading bacteria through TLRs and other receptors induces inflammation, cytokine release, and complement activation. If this is insufficient to eliminate the invaders, acquired immune mechanisms take over. Thus dendritic cells and macrophages ingest invading bacteria and initiate acquired immunity by secreting cytokines and triggering both T and B cell responses. The importance of these innate defenses is emphasized by the observation that the resistance of chickens to *Salmonella enterica typhimurium* appears to be linked to allelic variations in TLR4.

ACQUIRED IMMUNITY

There are five basic mechanisms by which the acquired-immune responses combat bacterial infections (Figure 23-1). These are (1) the neutralization of toxins or enzymes by antibody, (2) the killing of bacteria by antibodies and complement, (3) the opsonization of bacteria by antibodies and complement, resulting in their phagocytosis and destruction, (4) the intracellular destruction of bacteria by activated macrophages, and (5) direct killing of bacteria by cytotoxic T cells and NK cells. The relative importance of each of these processes depends on the species of bacteria involved and on the mechanisms by which they cause disease.

Immunity to Toxigenic Bacteria

In disease caused by toxigenic bacteria such as the clostridia or *B. anthracis*, the immune response must not only eliminate the invading bacteria but also neutralize their toxins. Destruction of the bacteria may, however, be difficult if they are embedded in a mass of necrotic tissue, and toxin neutralization is a priority. Neutralization occurs when the antibody prevents the toxin from

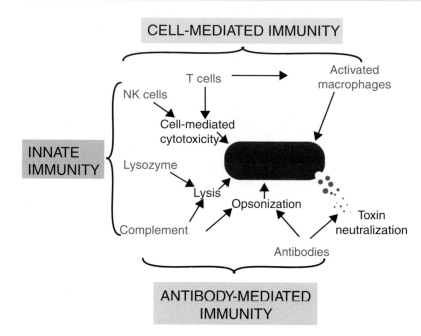

Figure 23-1. The mechanisms by which the immune responses can protect the body against bacterial invasion.

binding to its receptors on a target cell. The neutralization process therefore involves competition between receptors and antibodies for the toxin molecule. Once the toxin has combined with its receptors, antibodies are relatively ineffective in reversing this combination.

Immunity to Invasive Bacteria

Protection against invasive bacteria is usually mediated by antibodies directed against the surface antigens of the bacteria. Efficient phagocytosis requires that the surface of bacteria be coated with a layer of opsonin that will be recognized by neutrophils or macrophages. These opsonins are mainly antibodies or C3b (in addition to the innate opsonins such as MBL). Activation of complement by bacteria through the alternative and lectin pathways leads to the binding of C3b to their surface. Antibodies not only act as effective opsonins in their own right but also increase the binding of C3b by activating the classical complement pathway. Antibody directed against capsular (K) antigens may neutralize the antiphagocytic properties of the capsule, thus opsonizing the bacteria and permitting destruction by phagocytic cells to take place. In bacteria lacking capsules, antibodies directed against O antigens act as opsonins. A more subtle protective effect occurs when antibodies are produced against strains of *E. coli* carrying the pilus antigens K88 (F4) or K99 (F5). In this case, the antibodies interfere with the expression of the pilus antigens, and it has been claimed that they are eventually able to cause deletion of the genetic material (plasmid) that codes for these antigens. Once the adherence pili are deleted, these strains of *E. coli* cannot bind to the intestinal wall and thus are no longer pathogenic.

The importance of bacterial capsules in immunity is seen in anthrax. *B. anthracis* possesses both a capsule and an exotoxin. Antitoxic immunity is protective but slow to develop. In addition, toxin production tends to be prolonged, since the organism is encapsulated and phagocytic cells have difficulty eliminating it. As a result, death is usually inevitable in unvaccinated animals. The vaccine commonly employed against animal anthrax contains an unencapsulated but toxigenic strain of *B. anthracis*. Given in the form of spores that can germinate, the unencapsulated bacteria are eliminated by phagocytic cells before dangerous amounts of toxin are synthesized but not before antitoxic immunity is simulated.

Whereas some bacteria are phagocytosed and destroyed by neutrophils or macrophages or both, others are killed when free in the circulation. Bacteria may be destroyed by antibody and complement activated by the classical pathway. In unsensitized animals, the bacteria are destroyed by complement acting through the alternate or lectin pathways—innate defense mechanisms. Bacterial cell walls, lacking sialic acid, inactivate factor H and thus permit the production of the alternate C3 convertase (C3bBbP). As a result, the bacteria are either opsonized or lysed. The importance of this pathway is seen in bovine mycoplasma infections, in which pathogenic and nonpathogenic organisms may be differentiated on the basis of their ability to activate the alternate pathway. Nonpathogenic mycoplasmas activate the pathway; pathogenic ones do not.

Activation of the terminal complement components leads to the development of membrane attack complexes (MAC). These MACs may be unable to insert themselves into the complex carbohydrates of the microbial cell wall. However, lysozyme in the blood may digest the cell wall and enable the MACs to gain access to the lipid bilayer of the inner bacterial membrane.

Molecule for molecule, IgM is about 500 to 1000 times more efficient than IgG in opsonization and about 100 times more potent than IgG in sensitizing bacteria for complement-mediated lysis. During a primary immune response, therefore, the quantitative deficiency of the IgM response is compensated for by its quality, thus ensuring early and efficient protection.

The Heat-Shock Protein Response

Many new proteins are induced in cells by stresses that include a raised temperature, starvation, and exposure to oxygen radicals, toxins such as heavy metals, protein synthesis inhibitors, or viral infections. The heat-shock proteins (HSPs) are the best understood of these new proteins. HSPs are present in all organisms at very low levels at normal temperatures. Mild stress such as a low-grade fever will induce HSP production and increase their levels significantly. For example, HSP levels climb from 1.5% to 15% of the total protein in stressed *E. coli.* They increase thermotolerance so that the cells or organisms can function at a higher temperature by protecting their transcription and translation processes. There are three major bacterial heat-shock proteins: HSP 90, HSP 70, and HSP 60. (The number refers to their molecular weight.) When a bacterium is phagocytosed and exposed to the respiratory burst within a neutrophil, the stress results in the production of bacterial HSP. Thus HSP 60 is the dominant antigen induced by mycobacteria, *Coxiella burnetii*, *Legionella*, *Treponema*, and *Borrelia* infections. These HSPs are highly antigenic for several reasons. First, they are produced in abundance in the infected host; second, they are readily processed by antigen-presenting cells; third, the immune system may possess unusually large numbers of cells capable of responding to HSPs, and γ/δ^+ T cells may preferentially recognize bacterial HSPs. An anti-HSP response may therefore be a major defense against bacterial pathogens.

Immunity to Intracellular Bacteria

As discussed in Chapter 17, some bacteria such as *B. abortus*, *M. tuberculosis*, *Campylobacter jejuni*, *Rhodococcus equi*, *L. monocytogenes*, *Corynebacterium pseudotuberculosis*, *C. burnetii*, and some serovars of *S. enterica*, can readily grow inside macrophages. In addition, *L. monocytogenes* can travel from cell to cell without exposure to the extracellular fluid. Bacteria employ many different strategies to ensure their survival within macrophages (Figure 23-2). Some bacteria employ a resistant coat to protect themselves against lysosomal enzymes (Table 23-1). For example, the cell wall waxes of *C. pseudotuberculosis* make that organism resistant to lysosomal enzymes. Other bacteria ensure that they are never exposed to these enzymes by interfering with phagosomal maturation. *S. enterica typhimurium* prevents assembly of the

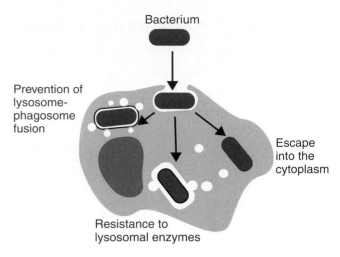

Figure 23-2. The mechanisms by which intracellular bacteria can evade intracellular destruction.

NOX complex. Mycobacteria, *Aspergillus flavus*, *B. abortus*, and *Chlamydophyla psittaci* can establish themselves within vacuoles that exclude proteases and oxidants by blocking lysosome-phagosome fusion. In the case of *M. tuberculosis*, the bacterium enters the macrophage via cholesterol-enriched membrane microdomains that are coated on the cytoplasmic side with a protein (tryptophan-aspartate–containing coat protein, or TACO) that prevents phagosome maturation. Thus lysosomes cannot fuse with the phagosome. They remain distributed within the cytoplasm, and the bacteria continue to survive and grow. Mycobacteria can also prevent acidification of phagosome by preventing fusion of the proton pump ATPase from the vacuolar membrane so that lysosomal cathepsins remain inactive. A third mechanism used to

TABLE   23-1
Facultative Intracellular Bacteria and Their Mechanisms of Survival

Organism	Method of Intracellular Survival
Brucella abortus	Resistant cell wall
	Prevents phagosome maturation
Corynebacterium pseudotuberculosis	Resistant cell wall
Listeria monocytogenes	Neutralizes respiratory burst
	Escapes into the cytosol
Mycobacterium tuberculosis	Lipid cell wall
	Prevents phagosome maturation
	Suppresses antigen presentation
	Detoxifies oxidants
Salmonella enterica	Prevents phagosome maturation
	Modifies endosomal trafficking
	Detoxifies oxidants
	Downregulates NOS2 and NOX
Rhodococcus equi	Survives in phagosomes

avoid destruction is simply to escape from the phagosome and persist free within the cytoplasm surrounded by a coat of polymerized actin. This method is employed by some mycobacteria and by *L. monocytogenes.*

Many bacteria manipulate the host's cytokine responses to their own advantage. The cytokines IFN-γ and TNF-α produced by primed T cells can activate macrophages, acidify the phagosomes, and kill the mycobacteria. To avoid this fate, mycobacteria may suppress the T cell responses by inducing synthesis of the regulatory cytokines IL-6, IL-10, and TGF-β by their host cells and so prolonging their own survival. IL-10 is especially effective in inhibiting macrophage activation, suppressing oxidant production, and downregulating antigen processing by reducing MHC class II expression.

Protection against intracellular bacteria is mediated by macrophage activation. Although macrophages from unimmunized animals are normally incapable of destroying these bacteria, this ability is acquired about 10 days after onset of infection when the macrophages are activated. This activation is mediated by IFN-γ released from sensitized Th1 cells. The response of these activated macrophages tends to be nonspecific, particularly in *Listeria* infections, and activated macrophages are able to destroy many normally resistant bacteria. IFN-γ, especially in association with TNF-α, greatly enhances the production of NO and NO_2^-. Thus an animal recovering from an infection with *L. monocytogenes* develops increased resistance to infection by *M. tuberculosis.* The development of these activated macrophages often coincides with the appearance of delayed (type IV) hypersensitivity responses to intradermally administered antigen (Chapter 29).

Both CD4+ and CD8+ cells are also involved in immunity to *Listeria.* CD8+ cytotoxic T cells lyse *Listeria-* or mycobacteria-infected cells and so complement the Th1 cells that secrete IFN-γ and activate macrophages.

It has been observed that protective immunity against intracellular bacteria cannot be induced by vaccines containing killed bacteria. Only vaccines containing living bacteria are protective. This difference is probably due to the differential stimulation of helper T cell populations by live and dead bacteria (Figure 23-3). Thus infection of mice with live *B. abortus* stimulates Th1 cells to secrete IFN-γ. Immunization of these mice with *Brucella* protein extracts induces Th2 cells to secrete IL-4. Live but not dead *L. monocytogenes* or *B. abortus* organisms induce macrophage secretion of TNF-α. Conversely, killed *Brucella* organisms stimulate IL-1 production to a greater extent than live bacteria. Resistance to these intracellular bacteria is generally short-lived, persisting for only as long as viable bacteria remain in the body. (An exception to this occurs in tuberculosis, in which case memory is prolonged.)

If, in a bacterial disease, it is observed that dead vaccines do not give good protection, that serum cannot confer protection, that antibody levels do not relate to resistance, and that delayed hypersensitivity reactions can be elicited to the bacterial antigens, then the possibility that cell-mediated immunity may play an important role in resistance to the causative organism should be considered and the use of vaccines containing living bacteria should be contemplated.

Modification of Bacterial Disease by Immune Responses

An animal's immune response will clearly influence the course and severity of an infection. At best, it will result in a cure. In the absence of a cure, however, the infection may be profoundly modified. This also depends on whether a cell-mediated or antibody response is generated. Thus the type of helper T cells used to control an infection may affect the course of disease. As described in

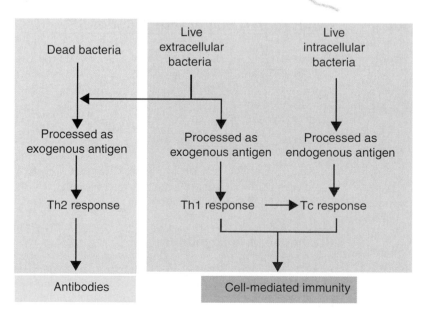

Figure 23-3. The type of immune response stimulated by bacteria depends on whether the bacteria are live or dead and whether they grow inside or outside cells.

Chapter 17, cell-mediated responses are usually required to control diseases caused by intracellular bacteria. Only activated macrophages can prevent the growth of these bacteria. Macrophage activation requires that Th1 cells produce IFN-γ. When the macrophages are activated, they can localize or cure these infections. If, in contrast, the immune response against these bacteria inappropriately stimulates Th2 responses, cell-mediated immunity fails to develop, macrophages are not activated, and chronic progressive disease results. This is readily seen in mycobacterial diseases. For example, in humans, leprosy occurs in two distinct forms called tuberculoid and lepromatous leprosy. Tuberculoid leprosy is characterized by an intense cell-mediated immune response with macrophage activation and minimal antibody responses to the leprosy bacillus. Lesions of this form of the disease contain very few organisms. In contrast, lepromatous leprosy is characterized by very high antibody levels and poor cell-mediated responses. The lesions of this disease contain enormous numbers of bacteria. The prognosis of lepromatous leprosy is much poorer than for tuberculoid leprosy.

A similar diversity of lesions is seen in Johne's disease of sheep. Some animals develop a lepromatous form of the disease, in which their intestinal lesions contain enormous numbers of bacteria (Figure 23-4) and little histological evidence of a cell-mediated response is present. In contrast, other sheep may develop a tuberculoid form of the disease, in which the lesions contain very few bacteria but large numbers of lymphocytes.

Humans with lepromatous leprosy mount an immune response, preferentially using Th2 cells that secrete IL-4 and IL-10. The IL-10 reduces the production of IL-12, which in turn decreases IFN-γ secretion by Th1 cells. Since IFN-γ is necessary for macrophage activation, this will reduce the patient's ability to control *M. leprae*. In contrast, patients who develop tuberculoid leprosy mount a response dominated by Th1 cells. Their lesions contain macrophages activated by IFN-γ. A similar dichotomy probably occurs in Johne's disease in sheep. Animals with the tuberculoid disease have T cells that are more responsive to antigen and produce more IL-2 and IFN-γ than sheep with the lepromatous disease (Figure 23-5). In contrast, sheep with the lepromatous disease have slightly higher antibody levels. It is likely, therefore, that sheep with tuberculoid Johne's disease mount an immune response in which Th1 cells predominate, whereas those with lepromatous disease mount primarily a Th2 response.

It must not be assumed from the above discussion that the specific Th subset involved in an immune response does not change once the response is established. Time-based studies have shown that immune responses to an organism can swing between Th1 and Th2 responses, perhaps several times, before a final response is established. This final response may well be a Th1 or Th2 response, or even some intermediate point in the Th1-Th2

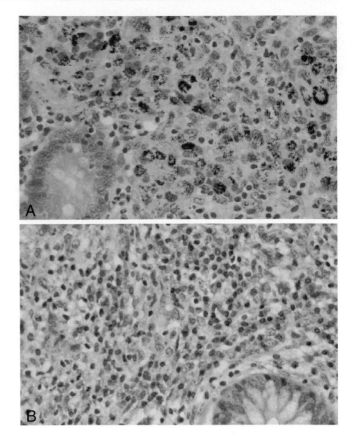

Figure 23-4. The two forms of Johne's disease in sheep. **A,** Section of terminal ileum from a case of lepromatous Johne's disease, showing abundant acid-fast organisms within large infiltrating macrophages. **B,** Section of terminal ileum from a case of tuberculoid Johne's disease, showing very few acid-fast bacteria and a significant lymphocyte infiltration. Ziehl-Nielsen stain. (Courtesy of Dr. CJ Clarke.)

spectrum. This variation appears to be a common feature of chronic infections such as tuberculosis.

EVASION OF THE IMMUNE RESPONSE

As pointed out previously, an invading microorganism becomes a pathogen because it can evade the immune defenses of its host. On the other hand, bacteria, like all organisms, seek to avoid their own destruction. They have therefore evolved an incredibly diverse array of mechanisms by which they overcome host innate and acquired immune responses and evade elimination. These mechanisms are of two general types: they may avoid recognition by the immune system or, alternatively, they may seek to resist immune effector mechanisms.

Prevention of Recognition

Campylobacter fetus ssp. *venerialis*, an organism that normally colonizes the male and female genital tracts in cattle, prevents immune recognition by changing its

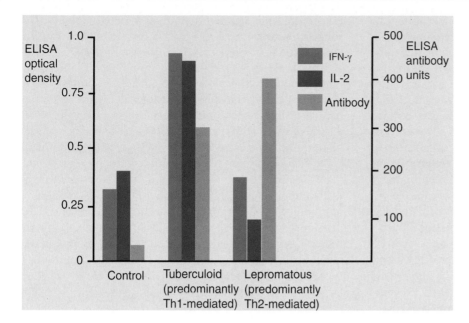

Figure 23-5. The differences in peripheral blood lymphocyte IL-2, IFN-γ and antibody production between sheep with the tuberculoid form and sheep with the lepromatous form of Johne's disease. Note that there is a marked tendency for the T cells from animals with the tuberculoid form of the disease to produce more Th1 cytokines than those with the lepromatous form. Despite this fact, animals with the latter form appear to produce more antibodies. (From data kindly provided by Dr. Chris Clarke and Mr. Charles Burrells.)

surface coat repeatedly. The destruction of most of this bacterial population by a local immune response leaves a small residue of bacteria that possesses new and different antigens. This residual population multiplies and is largely eliminated in turn by a second immune response, leaving organisms of a third antigenic type. This process of cyclical antigenic variation may be repeated for a prolonged period, resulting in a persistent infection. *Anaplasma marginale*, a bacterium that lives within bovine red cells, also shows sequential antigenic variation. As a result, the number of *Anaplasma* in blood cycles at 6- to 8-wcck intervals. The number of bacteria gradually increases and then declines rapidly as a result of an immune response. This is followed by a new antigenic variant that repeats the cycle. *A. marginale* is transmitted by ticks, so successful spread depends on maintenance of a high bacteremia.

Resistance to Effector Mechanisms

Bacteria can effectively block phagocytosis, Fc receptor function, cytotoxic T cell function, or complement activity. Many bacteria can survive within phagocytic cells. Some prevent recognition by phagocytic receptors. Thus the M protein of *Streptococcus equi* can reduce opsonization by interfering with the deposition of complement on the bacterial surface. *Streptococcus pyogenes* M protein can bind fibrinogen, which then masks C3b binding sites. It can also bind factor H, thus activating factor I and inactivating bound C3b. *S. aureus* also inhibits phagocytosis by means of protein A on its surface. Protein A attaches to the Fc region of IgG molecules. It prevents the immunoglobulin from binding to FcR on phagocytic cells and so inhibits opsonization. *Taylorella equigenitalis* can bind equine IgG and IgM in a similar manner.

Many bacteria interfere with complement activation. For example, *S. pyogenes* and *Streptococcus pneumoniae* can bind factor H, so promoting factor I activation and destruction of C3b. Other bacteria produce proteases that destroy many complement components. *S. enterica typhimurium* has a gene called *Rck* that confers resistance to complement-mediated lysis by preventing insertion of the membrane attack complex into the bacterial outer membrane. Other bacteria have surface structures that interfere with C3 convertase.

Bacteria such as enteropathogenic *E. coli*, *Yersinia pestis*, *M. tuberculosis*, and *Pseudomonas aeruginosa* secrete molecules that depress phagocytosis by neutrophils. In the case of *Pseudomonas*, for example, the bacterium uses a type III secretion system to inject toxins into the phagocytic cell. These toxins activate GTPases and disrupt intracellular signaling pathways. *S. aureus* can inhibit chemotaxis and phagocytosis by producing toxins such as streptolysin O that lyse neutrophil cell membranes. Several gram-negative bacteria of veterinary importance, such as *Mannheimia hemolytica*, *S. aureus*, and *Fusobacterium necrophorum*, secrete leukotoxins. Leukotoxins are primarily killers of leukocytes, especially granulocytes. They include several different molecules, but the most important are the RTX ("repeats in toxin") proteins. For instance, *Mannheimia haemolytica* secretes an RTX toxin that kills ruminant neutrophils, alveolar macrophages, and lymphocytes. This leukotoxin binds to the β2-integrin subunit, CD18, on ruminant leukocytes and induces activation with subsequent apoptosis of these cells. At high concentrations it produces transmembrane pores and necrosis. (This leukotoxin has been successfully incorporated in a vaccine against bovine respiratory disease). *Moraxella bovis* also secretes a leukotoxin for bovine neutrophils. *Actinobacillus pleuropneumoniae* secretes a toxin that kills porcine macrophages. *Mycoplasma mycoides*, and possibly other mycoplasmas, can kill bovine T cells. The fungal toxin aflatoxin is also immunosuppressive, reducing the resistance of poultry to *P. multocida* and to salmonellosis.

Other bacteria have mechanisms that reduce the killing ability of phagocytes. For example, the carotenoid pigments responsible for the color of *S. aureus* can quench singlet oxygen and permit the organism to survive the respiratory burst. *S. enterica typhimurium* can prevent assembly of the NOX complex and downregulate host NOS2 activity. *P. multocida* and *Histophilus somni* are also able to inhibit the respiratory burst. Brucella species secrete an inhibitor of TNF-α expression. Other protective devices employed by pathogenic bacteria include the production of proteases specific for IgA such as those produced by *Neisseria gonorrhoeae*, *H. influenzae*, and *S. pneumoniae*. These organisms can thus prevent opsonization and Fc receptor-mediated phagocytosis. *M. hemolytica* secretes a protease specific for bovine IgG1. *Pseudomonas aeruginosa* secretes a protease that caused cleavage and destruction of interleukin-2.

ADVERSE CONSEQUENCES OF THE IMMUNE RESPONSES

Although immune responses are beneficial in that they eliminate invading bacteria, this is not always the case. The immune responses can influence the course of a bacterial disease without producing a cure and in some situations may increase its severity. The adverse consequences of the immune responses correspond in their mechanisms to the hypersensitivity types described in Chapters 26 to 29. For example, a local type I hypersensitivity reaction is sometimes seen in sheep vaccinated against foot rot by means of *Fusobacterium necrophorum* vaccine, but in this case it is believed that the hypersensitivity may assist in preventing reinfection.

Type II (cytotoxic) reactions may account for the anemia seen in animals with salmonellosis. In these infections, bacterial lipopolysaccharides from disrupted bacteria are adsorbed onto erythrocytes. The subsequent immune response against the bacterium and its products therefore results in red cell destruction. Although a similar anemia is observed in leptospirosis, its mechanism is unknown, since antibodies produced by infected animals may agglutinate normal red cells taken from the same animal before infection.

Type III (immune complex) reactions may contribute to the development of arthritis in *Erysipelothrix rhusiopathiae* infections in pigs or to the development of intestinal lesions in Johne's disease due to *Mycobacterium paratuberculosis*. In the former case, bacterial antigen tends to localize in joints, where local immune-complex formation then results in inflammation and arthritis. Passively administered antiserum may therefore exacerbate the arthritis in these infected animals. In Johne's disease, type I or type III reactions occurring in the intestinal mucosa may increase the outflow of fluid and diarrhea. It is probable, however, that the intestinal lesions in this disease are etiologically complex, since diarrhea can be transferred to normal calves by either plasma or leukocytes, and antihistamines may reduce the diarrhea. Type III hypersensitivity reactions are involved in purpura hemorrhagica of horses, in which immune-complex lesions result from the animal's response to *S. equi*.

Although cell-mediated immune responses are manifestly beneficial, they do contribute to the development of granulomatous lesions in some chronic infections. The development of large granulomas, although serving to wall off invading bacteria and so prevent their spread, may also involve uninfected tissues. If these granulomas invade essential structures such as airways in the lungs or large blood vessels, damage may be severe.

SEROLOGY OF BACTERIAL INFECTIONS

Bacterial infections are often diagnosed by detecting the presence of specific serum antibodies. Thus the agglutination test is widely employed in the diagnosis of bacterial infections, particularly those involving gram-negative bacteria such as *Brucella* and *Salmonella*. The usual procedure in bacterial agglutination tests is to titrate serum (antibody) against a standard suspension of antigen. Bacteria are not, of course, antigenically homogeneous but are covered by a mosaic of many different antigens. Thus, motile bacteria will have flagellar (H) antigens, and agglutination by antiflagellar antibodies will produce fluffy cotton-like floccules as the flagella stick together, leaving the bacterial bodies only loosely agglutinated. Agglutination of the somatic (O) antigens results in tight clumping of the bacterial bodies so that the agglutination is finely granular in character. Many bacteria possess several O and H antigens, as well as capsular (K) and pilus (F) antigens. By using a set of specific antisera, it is therefore possible to characterize the antigenic structure of an organism and consequently to classify it. It is on this basis, for instance, that the 2400 or so different serovars of *S. enterica* are classified.

Flagella (H) antigens are destroyed by heating, whereas O antigens are heat-resistant and therefore remain intact on heat-killed bacteria. K antigens vary in their heat stability: the L antigen of *E. coli*, which is a capsular antigen, is heat-labile, whereas another K antigen, antigen A, is heat stable. *Salmonella typhi* possesses an antigen called Vi that, although heat stable, is removed from the bacterial cells by heating. The presence of K or Vi antigens on an organism may render them O-inagglutinable and thus complicate agglutination tests. It should also be pointed out that rough forms of bacteria do not form stable suspensions and therefore cannot be typed by means of agglutination tests.

Bacterial agglutination tests may be performed by mixing drops of reagents on glass slides or by titrating the reagents in tubes or wells in plastic plates. Tube agglutination tests are commonly used for such diseases as salmonellosis, brucellosis, tularemia, and campylobacteriosis. Slide agglutination tests are commonly used as screening tests. These include the *Brucella*-buffered antigen tests, in which killed, stained *Brucella* organisms are suspended in an acid buffer (pH 3.6). The dye used, either the red dye rose-bengal or a mixture of crystal violet and brilliant green, enables the test to be easily read. At this low pH, nonspecific agglutination by IgM antibodies is eliminated. The *Brucella*-buffered plate agglutination test has a specificity of as high as 99% and a sensitivity of 95%. The efficient and widespread use of these tests has eliminated bovine brucellosis from so many countries.

S. enterica pullorum infection in poultry can be diagnosed by a slide agglutination test, in which killed bacteria stained with gentian violet are mixed with whole chicken blood. Agglutination is readily seen if antibodies are present. Leptospirosis is diagnosed by a microscopic agglutination test, in which mixtures of living organisms and test serum are examined under the microscope for agglutination. This technique preferentially detects IgM antibodies and is thus an excellent test for detecting recent outbreaks, as well as for distinguishing between infected and vaccinated animals.

It is not mandatory that serum be used as the source of antibody for diagnostic tests. The presence of antibodies in body fluids other than serum, such as milk whey, vaginal mucus, or nasal washings, may be of more significance, especially if the infection is of a local or superficial nature. One such example is the milk ring test used to direct the presence of antibodies to *B. abortus* in milk (Figure 23-6). Fresh milk is shaken with bacteria stained with hematoxylin or triphenyl tetrazolium and is allowed to stand. If antibodies, especially those of the IgM or IgA classes, are present, the bacteria will clump and adhere to the fat globules of the milk and rise to the surface with the cream. If antibodies are absent, the stained bacteria will remain dispersed in the milk, and the cream, on rising, will remain white.

IMMUNITY TO FUNGAL INFECTIONS

Innate immune mechanisms against invasive fungi such as *Candida* or *Aspergillus* include activation of the alternate pathway of the complement system resulting in attraction of neutrophils and attempts by these neutrophils to ingest the invading hyphae or pseudohyphae. Because of their size, neutrophils cannot totally ingest the invading fungi. Nevertheless, by releasing their enzymes into the tissue fluid, neutrophils may severely damage fungal hyphae. Very small fungal fragments or spores may be ingested and destroyed by macrophages or by NK cells.

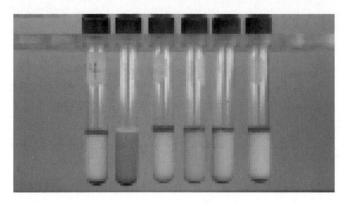

Figure 23-6.   The milk ring test. Stained *Brucella* remains suspended in the milk in a negative test but rises with the cream in a positive reaction. (Courtesy of Dr John Huff.)

Once established, fungal infections can be destroyed only by T cell–mediated mechanisms. Thus some species of *Aspergillus* are facultative intracellular parasites, and chronic or progressive fungal diseases are commonly associated with defects in the T cell system. T cells primarily function in fungal infections by activating macrophages and by promoting epidermal growth and keratinization. Some T and NK cells can exert a direct cytotoxic effect on yeasts such as *C. neoformans* and *C. albicans*. It is not uncommon for recovered animals to develop a type IV hypersensitivity to fungal antigens.

An adjuvanted, killed vaccine against *Microsporum canis*, the ringworm fungus, has been developed. The vaccine appears to reduce the incidence of infection in uninfected cats and to reduce the lesions found in infected cats. This is an infection in which many cats will eventually cure themselves. Nevertheless the disease seems to be refractory in a few individuals, especially long-haired breeds in which the disease becomes chronic, perhaps as a result of depressed immunity.

SOURCES OF ADDITIONAL INFORMATION

Amer AO, Swanson MS: A phagosome of one's own: a microbial guide to life in the macrophage, *Curr Opin Microbiol* 5:56-61, 2002.

Boschwitz JS, Timoney JF: Inhibition of C3 deposition on *Streptococcus equi* subsp. *equi* by M protein: a mechanism for survival in equine blood, *Infect Immun* 62:3515-3520, 1994.

Fenton MJ, Vermeulen MW: Immunopathology of tuberculosis: roles of macrophages and monocytes, *Infect Immun* 64:683-690, 1996.

Hondalus MK, Mosser DM: Survival and replication of *Rhodococcus equi* in macrophages, *Infect Immun* 62:4167-4175, 1994.

Hsieh C-S, Macatonia SE, Tripp CS, et al: Development of Th1 CD4+ T cells through IL-12 produced by *Listeria*-induced macrophages, *Science* 260: 547-549, 1993.

Lehmann PF: Immunology of fungal infections in animals, *Vet Immunol Immunopathol* 10:33-69, 1985.

Leveque G, Forgetta V, Morroll S, et al. Allelic variation in TLR4 is linked to susceptibility to *Salmonella enterica* serovar typhimurium infection in chickens. *Infect Immun* 71: 1116-1124, 2003.

Majury AL, Shewen PE: The effect of *Pasteurella hemolytica* A1 leukotoxic culture supernate on the in vitro proliferative response of bovine lymphocytes, *Vet Immunol Immunopathol* 29:57-68, 1991.

Malaviya R, Abraham SN: Mast cell modulation of immune responses to bacteria, *Immunol Rev* 179:16-24, 2001.

Narayanan SK, Nagaraja TG, Chengappa MM, Stewart GC: Leukotoxins of gram-negative bacteria, *Vet Microbiol* 84: 337-356, 2002.

Nathan C: Natural resistance and nitric oxide, *Cell* 82:873-876, 1995.

Nielsen K, Duncan JR: *Animal brucellosis*, Boca Raton, Fla, 1990, CRC Press.

Ozmen L, Pericin M, Hakimi J, et al. Interleukin 12, interferon γ, and tumor necrosis factor α are the key cytokines in the generalized Shwartzman reaction, *J Exp Med* 180: 907-915, 1994.

Pieters J, Gatfield J: Hijacking the host: survival of pathogenic mycobacteria inside macrophages, *Trends Microbiol* 3: 142-146, 2002.

Pisetsky DS: Immune activation by bacterial DNA: a new genetic code, *Immunity* 5:303-310, 1996.

Salyers AA, Whitt DD: *Bacterial pathogenesis: a molecular approach*, Washington, DC, 1994, ASM Press.

Thomas CB, Van Ess P, Wolfgram LJ, et al: Adherence to bovine neutrophils and suppression of neutrophil chemoluminescence by *Mycoplasma bovis*, *Vet Immunol Immunopathol* 27:365-381, 1991.

Tyler JW, Cullor JS, Spier SJ, Smith BP: Immunity targeting core antigens of gram-negative bacteria, *J Vet Intern* Med 4:17-25, 1990.

Wannemuehler MJ, Galvin JE: Bacterial immunogens and protective immunity in swine, *Vet Immunol Immunopathol* 43:117-126, 1994.

Wright SD: CD14 and innate recognition of bacteria, *J Immunol* 154:6-8, 1995.

Zhan Y, Cheers C: Differential induction of macrophage-derived cytokines by live and dead intracellular bacteria in vitro, *Infect Immun* 63:720-723, 1995.

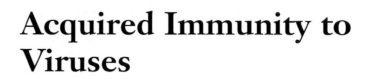

Acquired Immunity to Viruses

CHAPTER 24

Since viruses are obligate intracellular organisms, their very existence is threatened if they are destroyed by the immune system or by the death of their host. Because of these opposing factors, both viruses and their hosts have been subjected to rigorous selection and adaptation. Viruses are selected for their ability to evade the host's immune responses, while at the same time animals are selected for resistance to virus-induced disease. Virus diseases therefore tend to be lethal when the virus first encounters its host species or infects the wrong species. Once viruses and their hosts have interacted for a long period, however, any resulting disease tends to be relatively mild.

For example, in infections in which virus-host adaptation is poor, diseases tend to be acute and severe. Rabies is an excellent example of this. The virus is inevitably lethal in dogs, cats, horses, and cattle because they are unnatural hosts. On the other hand, in its natural hosts, especially bats and skunks, rabies virus persists and can be shed in saliva for a long period without causing disease. From the virus's "point of view," infection of dogs, cattle, or horses is unprofitable since those animals almost never transmit rabies to skunks. Other diseases of this type include feline panleukopenia, canine parvovirus-2, and the virulent forms of Newcastle disease. Vaccination is relatively successful in this type of infection since the virus has not adapted to the host's defenses.

When the virus and its host are more adapted, although disease may be severe, mortality may not be high and the virus may be persistent. In this type of disease, further attacks may occur as a result of infection by antigenic variants of the same virus. Examples of this type of virus infection include foot-and-mouth disease and influenza. Vaccination against diseases of this type is complicated by the antigenic diversity among viruses circulating in the population.

Even more adapted viruses can result in persistent infection, and the immune system is unable to eliminate the virus. Diseases of this type include the lentivirus infections, equine infectious anemia, maedi-visna of sheep, and AIDS in humans. The virus may even change during these infections and thus constantly evade the immune system. Vaccination against these diseases is essentially unsuccessful. As their adaptation increases, viruses may cause latent infections and relatively mild, nonlethal disease. Some herpesvirus infections fall into this category. The extreme examples of virus adaptation are those in which the viral genome becomes stably integrated into the host genome. These endogenous viruses are well recognized in domestic mammals such as the cat and pig.

In studying the nature of the host responses to viruses, it is well to recognize that this continuing selective pressure on both host and virus exists and profoundly influences the outcome of all viral infections.

VIRUS STRUCTURE AND ANTIGENS

Virus particles, called virions, consist of small segments of nucleic acid core surrounded by a layer of protein or lipoproteins (Figures 5-1 and 36-1). This protein layer is called the capsid; it is formed by subunits called capsomeres. An envelope containing lipoprotein derived in part from the host cell may also surround virions. The complexity of virions varies. Some, such as poxviruses, are complex, whereas others, such as foot-and-mouth disease viruses, are relatively simple. Antibodies can be produced against epitopes on all the proteins situated inside and on the surface of the virion. Antibodies against the nucleoprotein components are not usually significant from a protective point of view, but they may be of assistance in diagnosis.

PATHOGENESIS OF VIRUS INFECTIONS

Adsorption, the first step in the invasion of a cell by a virus, occurs when a virion binds to receptors on the cell surface. These receptors are not designed for the convenience of viruses but have some other physiological function in normal cells. Thus the rabies virus binds to the receptor for acetylcholine, a neurotransmitter. The Epstein-Barr virus (the cause of infectious mononucleosis) binds to a receptor for C3. Rhinoviruses that cause the common cold bind to cell-surface integrins. The bound virion is then taken into the cell through endocytosis. The nature, number, and distribution of host cell receptors determine the host range and tissue tropism of a virus.

Once inside a cell, the virus capsid breaks open so that its nucleic acid is released into the cell cytoplasm—a process called uncoating. Once the virus genome is uncoated, it begins the process of replication (Figure 24-1). First, the host cell DNA, RNA, and protein synthesis are inhibited so that only the viral genetic information is processed. The site within the cell where this happens differs among viruses and depends on their nucleic acid.

If the virus, for example, a herpesvirus, contains DNA, this viral DNA is replicated. The new viral DNA is then transcribed into viral messenger RNA, and this RNA is translated into new capsid proteins. The new capsid proteins are assembled into new virions. The host cell also replicates the viral nucleic acid so that large quantities of viral DNA are produced. This viral DNA is packaged inside the capsid so that complete new virions are formed. If the virus is unenveloped, the infected cells disintegrate and the virions are released into the environment. If the virions are enveloped, they leave the cell by budding through the cell surface. The cell membrane that encloses them serves as the new envelope. The released virions may then spread to nearby cells and invade them.

If a virus contains RNA rather than DNA, its replication takes a slightly different course. For most RNA viruses, such as Newcastle disease or foot-and-mouth disease virus (FMDV), viral DNA is not used. Thus in FMDV infection, the viral single-stranded RNA (the "plus strand") is used as a template to synthesize a complementary "minus strand" of RNA. These minus strands are then used to generate new plus strands that can be translated into viral proteins. Some viruses contain double-stranded RNA and use only one of the strands generated during replication. In other RNA viruses, the infecting virus RNA may be complementary to the newly synthesized viral RNA that will translate into viral proteins.

A different replication mechanism is employed in the case of some RNA tumor viruses and immunodeficiency viruses (Figure 24-2). These are called retroviruses since their RNA is first reversely transcribed into DNA. To do this, they use an enzyme called a reverse transcriptase. The new viral DNA moves into the cell's nucleus and is integrated into the host cell genome as a provirus. This proviral DNA can then be transcribed into RNA, as well

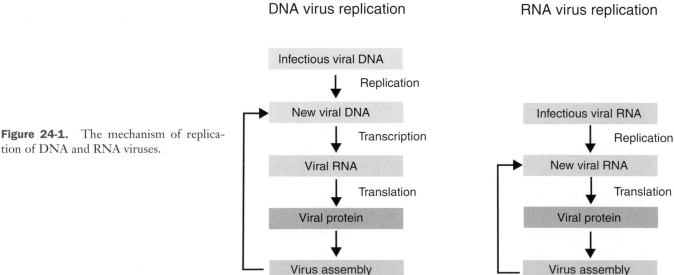

Figure 24-1.   The mechanism of replication of DNA and RNA viruses.

Retrovirus replication

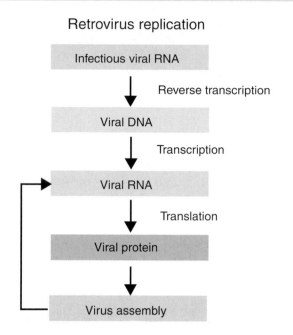

Figure 24-2. The mechanism of replication of retroviruses.

as being able to replicate itself. The proteins and RNA can then be packaged into a complete new virion.

Changes in virus-infected cells may be minimal, perhaps only detectable by the development of new proteins on the cell surface. Sometimes, however, the changes may be extensive and result in either cell lysis or malignant transformation and the development of tumors.

INNATE IMMUNITY

Innate immune responses influence the outcome of many viral infections by inhibiting viral replication early in infection. Interferons are especially important to viral

resistance. Lysozyme can destroy several viruses, as can many intestinal enzymes and bile. Collectins bind to viral glycoproteins and block virus interaction with host cells. For example, the collectins conglutinin, MBP, SP-A, and SP-D have all been shown to inactivate influenza viruses in this manner. Finally, cells invaded by viruses may undergo premature apoptosis, thus preventing successful viral invasion and replication.

Interferons

Interferons α/β are released from virus-infected cells within a few hours after viral invasion, and high concentrations of interferons may be achieved in vivo within a few days, long before acquired immunity has developed. For example, in cattle that receive bovine herpesvirus-1 intravenously, peak interferon levels in serum are reached 2 days later and then decline, but they are still detectable by 7 days (Figure 24-3). In contrast, antibodies are not usually detectable in serum until 5 to 6 days after the onset of a virus infection.

Interferons are glycoproteins with molecular weights of 20 to 34 kDa. They fall into two major types (Table 12-3). The type I interferons include interferon α (IFN-α), a family of molecules derived from virus-infected immature CD4+ DC2 cells (there are 18 different molecules in humans, 12 in pigs and cattle, 4 in horses, 2 in dogs); interferon β (IFN-β) derived from virus-infected fibroblasts (5 in cattle and pigs, 1 in dogs and humans); and interferon ω (IFN-ω), from the embryonic trophoblast (6 to 7 in pigs, 5 in humans, 2 in horses, 0 in dogs). (IFN-ω is also called IFN-αII). A distinct form of type I interferon, interferon τ (IFN-τ) has been isolated from the ruminant trophoblast, and interferon δ has been isolated from the pig trophoblast. Interferon κ is another name for interleukin 28. There is only one type II interferon, interferon γ (IFN-γ), a cytokine derived primarily from antigen-stimulated

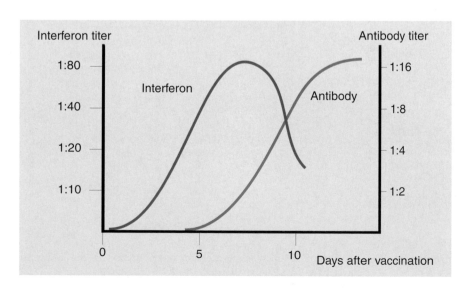

Figure 24-3. The sequential production of interferon and antibody following intranasal vaccination of calves with infectious bovine rhinotracheitis vaccine. (From data kindly provided by Dr. M Savan.)

BOX 24–1

Measuring Interferons

Interferons can be assayed by measuring their antiviral effects. For example, samples to be tested for interferon activity are added to fibroblast cultures at various dilutions and incubated for 18 to 24 hours. The fibroblast monolayers are then washed, and a standard quantity of bovine vesicular stomatitis virus (VSV) is added to each culture. After 48 hours of incubation, the monolayers are stained and virus plaques are seen as cleared areas in the monolayer. The presence of interferons reduces the number of plaques formed.

T cells. It is also produced in pig trophoblast cells. The type I interferons are stable at pH 2, whereas IFN-γ is not (Box 24-1).

Antiviral Activities

Production of interferons is triggered by the association between viral nucleic acid and host cell ribosomes, resulting in activation of the target-cell genes coding for interferon. This interferon is secreted by infected cells and binds to receptors on other nearby cells. The type I interferons use CDw118, whereas IFN-γ uses CDw119 (Figure 24-4). Receptor binding results in the development of resistance to virus infection within a few minutes and peaks 5 to 8 hours later. The interferons signal to the cell and stimulate the production of more than 100 new proteins, some of which have antiviral activity. For example, IFN-α/β upregulates transcription of 2'5'-oligoadenylate synthetase (2'5'OAS) genes. Expressed OAS enzymes are then converted from an inactive to an active form by exposure to dsRNA. The activated enzymes act on adenosine triphosphate (ATP) to form 2'5' adenylate oligomers. These oligomers in turn activate a latent ribonuclease called RNAase L (Figure 24-5). RNAase L degrades viral RNA and so inhibits viral growth.

Another enzyme induced by IFN-γ, especially in activated macrophages, is nitric oxide synthase. The nitric oxide produced by this enzyme prevents virus growth in interferon-activated macrophages. A third enzyme activated by interferon is a protein kinase. This protein kinase phosphorylates an initiation factor called eIF2, which then inhibits viral protein synthesis by preventing translation initiation of mRNA. A fourth set of new enzymes is called Mx proteins. These are GTPases that inhibit the translation of influenza virus mRNA by suppressing G-protein activity (Chapter 9).

The ability of cells to produce interferon varies. Virus-infected leukocytes, especially DC2 dendritic cells, produce large amounts of IFN-α; virus-infected fibroblasts produce IFN-β; and antigen-stimulated T cells are the major source of IFN-γ (Chapter 12). Kidney cells are poor interferon producers, and neutrophils produce no interferon. Although live or inactivated viruses are the most important stimulators of interferon production, interferons may also be induced by bacterial endotoxins, some plant lectins, and synthetic polymers that mimic viral RNA.

Lymphocytes from normal, unsensitized donors can kill virus-infected cells. This innate cytotoxicity is due to natural killer (NK) cells (Chapter 31). NK cell

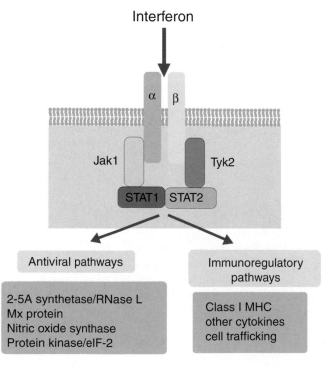

Figure 24-4. The receptor for the type I interferons. Ligand binding triggers both antiviral and immunoregulatory pathways.

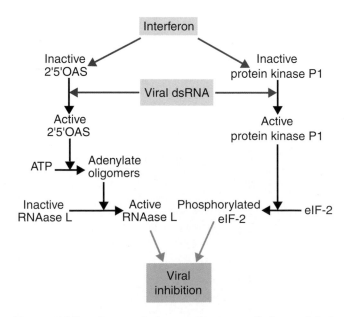

Figure 24-5. Some of the mechanisms of the antiviral activities of the interferons.

cytotoxicity is stimulated by IFN-α and, as a result, is rapidly enhanced early in a virus infection. NK cells also produce IFN-γ, and this too has a direct antiviral effect. NK cells can therefore reduce the severity of viral infections long before the development of acquired immunity and the appearance of specific cytotoxic T cells.

ACQUIRED IMMUNITY

Antibody-Mediated Immunity

Virus capsids are antigenic, and it is against these and the envelope proteins that antiviral immune responses are largely mounted (Figure 24-6). Antibodies can prevent cell invasion by blocking the adsorption of virions to target cells, by stimulating phagocytosis of viruses, by triggering complement-mediated virolysis, or by causing viral clumping and so reducing the number of infectious units available for cell invasion. The combination of antibody and virus does not destroy a virus, since the splitting of virus-antibody complexes may release infectious virions.

Antibodies are not only directed against proteins on free virions, but they are also directed against viral antigens expressed by infected cells. As a result, these infected cells may also be destroyed. Virus infections in which antibody-mediated destruction of infected cells occurs include Newcastle disease, rabies, bovine virus diarrhea, infectious bronchitis of birds, and feline leukemia. Antibodies may kill infected cells by complement-mediated cytolysis or by antibody-dependent cell-mediated

cytotoxicity (ADCC). These cytotoxic cells include lymphocytes, macrophages, and neutrophils with Fc receptors through which they can bind to antibody-coated target cells.

The immunoglobulins that neutralize viruses include IgG and IgM in serum and IgA in secretions. IgE may also play a protective role, since humans with an IgE deficiency suffer from severe respiratory infections. As in antibacterial immunity, IgG is quantitatively the most significant immunoglobulin, whereas IgM is qualitatively superior.

Although most viruses infect cells by binding directly to receptors on target cells, some use an intermediate molecule. For instance, some antibody-coated viruses bind to cells through Fc receptors. This, of course, facilitates endocytosis of the virus and may thus enhance virus infection. Complement may enhance some virus infections in a similar fashion. Examples of viruses whose infections are enhanced by antibodies include feline infectious peritonitis, Aleutian disease of mink, African swine fever, and human immunodeficiency virus.

Cell-Mediated Immunity

Although antibodies and complement can neutralize free virions and destroy virus-infected cells, cell-mediated immune responses are much more important in controlling virus diseases. This is readily seen in immunodeficient humans (Chapter 35). Those who cannot mount an antibody-mediated response suffer from overwhelming bacterial infections but tend to respond normally to smallpox vaccination and recover from the common viral

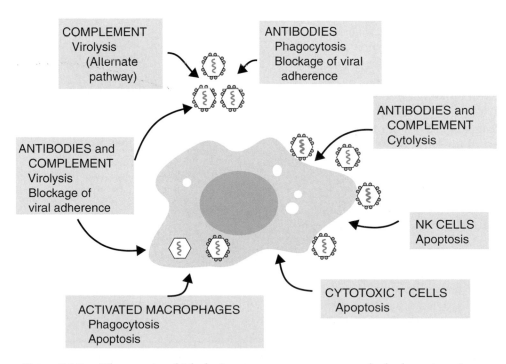

Figure 24-6. The ways in which the immune system can protect the body against viruses.

diseases. In contrast, humans with a deficiency of T cell–mediated immune responses are commonly resistant to bacterial infection but highly susceptible to virus diseases.

Viral antigens may be expressed on the surface of infected cells long before progeny viruses are produced. When this endogenous antigen is presented by MHC class I molecules, virus-infected cells are recognized as foreign and eliminated. Although antibody and complement or ADCC can play a role in this process, T cell–mediated cytotoxicity is the major destructive mechanism. Cytotoxic T cells recognize the peptide-MHC complexes and kill them. Under some circumstances, cytotoxic T cells may kill intracellular viruses without killing the infected cells. This antiviral effect is mediated by T cell–derived IFN-γ and TNF-α. These cytokines activate two virucidal pathways. One pathway eliminates viral nucleocapsid particles, including their contained genomes. The second pathway destabilizes viral RNA.

Some viral antigens may function as superantigens by binding directly to TCR V_β chains. For example, rabies virus nucleocapsid binds to mouse $V_\beta 8$ T cells. By stimulating helper T cell activity, rabies viruses can switch on Th2 cells. This in turn can result in an enhanced immune response to rabies viruses, as well as a polyclonal B cell response sometimes seen in this disease.

Macrophages also develop antiviral activity following activation. Viruses are readily endocytosed by macrophages and are usually destroyed. If the viruses are noncytopathic but can, however, grow inside macrophages, a persistent infection may result. Under these circumstances, the macrophages must be activated in order to eliminate the virus. Thus immunity mediated by IFN-γ is a feature of some virus diseases (Chapter 17). For example, macrophages from birds immunized against fowlpox show an enhanced antiviral effect against Newcastle disease virus and will prevent the intracellular growth of *Salmonella enterica gallinarum*, a feature that is not a property of normal macrophages.

The duration of immunological memory to viruses is highly variable. Thus, antibodies against viruses may persist for many years in the absence of the virus. On the other hand, because of the hazards of persistent cytotoxicity, cytotoxic T cells die soon after virus elimination. Memory T cells can, however, persist for many years.

EVASION OF THE IMMUNE RESPONSE BY VIRUSES

As discussed at the beginning of this chapter, during the millions of years they have coexisted with vertebrates, viruses have learned to manipulate host immune responses. As a result, the relationship between host and virus must be established on the basis of mutual accommodation so that the long-term survival of both is ensured. Failure to reach this accommodation will result in the elimination of either host or virus and death of the host automatically eliminates the virus.

Viruses in different families use different survival strategies. Thus RNA viruses have a very small genome with little room to spare for genes dedicated to suppressing immunity. The proteins of RNA viruses therefore tend to be multifunctional. On the other hand, DNA viruses have a larger genome and can afford to devote genes to immune control. In DNA viruses such as the poxviruses and herpesviruses, as much as 50% of the total genome may be devoted to immunoregulatory genes.

Inhibition of Humoral Immunity

One of the simplest mechanisms of evading destruction involves antigenic variation. The most significant examples of this occur among the type A influenza viruses and the lentiviruses.

Influenza A viruses possess envelope proteins called hemagglutinins and neuraminidases. There are 13 different hemagglutinins and 9 neuraminidases found among the type A influenza viruses; they are identified according to a standard nomenclature system. Thus the hemagglutinin of the swine influenza virus is called H1, and its neuraminidase is called N1. The two subtypes of the equine influenza viruses are typified by A/equine/Prague/56, which has H7 and N7, and A/equine/Hong Kong/92, which has H3 and N8 (Table 24-1).

As influenza viruses spread through a population, they undergo mutation and selection and gradually change the structure of their hemagglutinins and neuraminidases. These changes gradually lead to alterations in the antigenicity of the virus. This gradual change is called antigenic drift, and it permits the virus to persist in a population for many years. In addition to antigenic drift,

TABLE   **24-1**

Examples of Influenza A Viruses and Their Antigenic Structure

Species	Virus Strain	Antigenic Structure
Human	A/New Caledonia/20/99*	H1N1
	A/New Jersey/76 (swine flu)	H1N1
	A/Panama/2007/99	H3N2
Equine	A/Equine/Prague/1/56	H7N7
	A/Equine/Miami/1/63	H3N8
	A/Equine/Suffolk/89	H3N8
	A/Equine/Hong Kong/1/92	H3N8
Swine	A/Swine/Iowa/15/30	H1N1
Avian	A/Fowl Plague/Dutch/27	H7N7
	A/Duck/England/56	H11N7
	A/Turkey/Ontario/6118/68	H8N4
	A/Chicken/Hong Kong/258/97	H5N1

*The first number is the isolate number; the second is the year of isolation.

influenza viruses sporadically exhibit a sudden, major genetic change in which a new strain develops whose hemagglutinins show no apparent relationship to the hemagglutinins of previously known strains. Such a major change, called an antigenic shift, is not produced by mutation but results from recombination between two virus strains. It is the development of these influenza viruses with a completely new antigenic structure that accounts for the periodic major outbreaks of influenza in humans and poultry. In horses and pigs, in contrast, the rapid turnover of the population and the constant production of large numbers of susceptible young animals ensures the persistence of influenza viruses without the necessity for extensive antigenic drift. As a result, the antigenic structure of equine and swine influenza viruses has changed only slowly since they were first described. Nevertheless, the H3N8 equine influenza virus strains are evolving into two distinct lineages, one European and one American, based on the structure of the HA1 domain of their hemagglutinin. Viruses of both lineages can circulate in horse populations at the same time. Examples of the European strains include A/Suffolk/89 and A/Hong Kong/1/92. American strains include A/Kentucky/94 and A/Florida/93. All are distinctly different from the original strain A/Miami/1/63.

A similar, but much more rapid form of antigenic variation is observed in equine infectious anemia (EIA) caused by a lentivirus. Following recovery from the first attack of clinical disease characterized by anemia, fever, thrombocytopenia, weight loss, and depression, horses may remain healthy for weeks or months. However, three or four relapses commonly occur before the horse either develops a chronic wasting disease or becomes clinically normal. The cyclical relapses may occur at 2- to 8-week intervals. Each episode of disease tends to be milder than the previous one. The fevers are lower and the anemia less severe. The EIA virus, like other lentiviruses, undergoes rapid random mutation, and new, antigenically different variants are produced. The elimination of these variants is determined by the presence of neutralizing antibodies and cytotoxic T cells. As variant strains of the virus are produced, the infected horse makes neutralizing antibodies to that variant and, as a result, the viremia ends. Variants of the EIA virus, however, appear rapidly and randomly. The appearance of a new nonneutralizable variant leads to a clinical relapse. After the virus has undergone several of these mutations and the horse has responded to them all, the neutralizing antibody spectrum of the horse's serum becomes very broad and viremia drops to a low level. Large amounts of tissues may then have to be examined to isolate the virus.

A second form of immune evasion by viruses is seen in caprine arthritis-encephalitis (CAE), Aleutian disease (AD) of mink, and African swine fever. Although infected animals respond to these viruses, the antibodies formed are incapable of virus neutralization. Thus virus-antibody complexes from AD-infected mink are fully infectious.

Goats with CAE make large amounts of anti-envelope antibodies, but they develop negligible levels of neutralizing antibodies. In this case, goats fail to recognize and respond to the virus neutralizing epitopes. If rabbits are immunized with CAE virus, they can readily produce virus-neutralizing antibodies and even goats will produce these antibodies if immunized with large amounts of an adjuvanted viral antigen. The antibodies produced in these hyperimmunized goats are very specific and will react only with the immunizing strain of the virus. Notwithstanding the absence of neutralizing antibodies, other antibodies can bind to CAE virions, and the opsonized virions are endocytosed by macrophages. Unfortunately, this virus grows within macrophages so that opsonizing antibodies merely speed up virus replication, an example of antibody-mediated enhancement. Attempts to vaccinate goats against CAE lead only to more severe disease.

A third mechanism by which viruses can evade destruction by antibodies is seen in yet another lentiviral infection, maedi-visna, a complex disease of sheep (maedi is to a chronic pneumonia; visna is a chronic neurological disease caused by the same virus.) In maedi-visna infections, neutralizing antibodies are produced slowly. These neutralizing antibodies are unable to reduce the viral burden in infected sheep, and cyclical relapses do not occur. The antibodies have a low affinity for viral epitopes and take at least 20 minutes to bind to the virus and 30 minutes to neutralize it. In contrast, it takes only 2 minutes for this virus to infect a cell. Thus the virus can spread between cells much faster than it can be neutralized. The maedi-visna virus also invades monocytes and macrophages, where it stimulates GM-CSF production and its replication is stimulated by GM-CSF. In most of these cells the replication of the virus stops after its RNA has been reversely transcribed into proviral DNA. Cells are thus persistently infected by the virus without expressing viral antigens. The virus may therefore be disseminated without provoking immunological attack.

Maedi-visna is associated with extensive infiltration of the lungs, mammary gland, and central nervous system with MHC class II+ T cells (both CD4+ and CD8+) and macrophages. Immunosuppression reduces the severity of the lesions, whereas immunization against the virus increases their severity. It is suggested that persistently infected macrophages stimulate T cells to release cytokines. These cytokines delay the maturation of monocytes into macrophages and so restrict virus replication. They also enhance MHC class II expression on the macrophages and so trigger excessive T cell proliferation and chronic lymphoid hyperplasia.

Interference With Interferons

Viruses have available a number of techniques that block the effectiveness of antiviral interferons. These range from blocking interferon receptor signal transduction to synthesizing soluble interferon receptors. Some viruses inhibit IFN-γ production by blocking the activities of IL-18 and IL-12, both of which are required for its production. Herpesviruses and poxviruses express IL-10 homologs that suppress Th1 responses and hence reduce IFN-γ production.

For reasons unknown, some important viruses make chemokines or chemokine receptors. For example, equine herpesvirus makes CCR3, the receptor for CCL11. Marek's disease virus makes a protein related to CXCL8.

Inhibition of Apoptosis

One way by which animal cells fight virus infections is by dying. Apoptosis may be triggered directly by viral infection or, more commonly, by cytotoxic T cells. If a virus is to survive, therefore, it is logical for it to inhibit apoptosis. Viruses can inhibit T cell-mediated cytotoxicity in this way. They can, for example, interfere with the expression of cell-surface MHC class I molecules. Virus genes may encode caspase inhibitors that block caspase activity. Adenoviruses possess proteins that block the activities of granzyme B. Some viruses, such as foot-and-mouth disease viruses, can survive for significant periods on the surface of macrophages and for many hours after phagocytosis.

Inhibition of Cytotoxic T Cells and NK Cells

Many viruses can interfere with antigen processing and so prevent peptide expression on the surface of virus-infected cells. Thus bovine herpesvirus 1 downregulates the expression of MHC class I molecules by interfering with the transportation of peptides by the transporter proteins (TAP). BHV-1 also downregulates the expression of mRNA for MHC class I molecules. Other viruses may cause MHC class I molecules to be retained within a cell, they may prevent peptide binding to transporter proteins, they may prevent proteasomal degradation, or they may redirect MHC molecules to lysosomes for degradation. Some viruses can also block the killing activities of NK cells.

In contrast to the short-lived immune response against bacteria, antiviral immunity is, in many cases, very long-lasting. The reasons for this are unclear, but they are related to virus persistence within cells, perhaps in a slowly replicating or a nonreplicating form as typified by the herpesviruses. It is usually difficult to isolate viruses from an animal that has recovered from a herpesvirus infection. Some time later, however, especially when the individual is stressed, the herpesvirus may reappear and may even cause disease again. During the latent period, when it is present in the host but cannot be reisolated, the virus nucleic acid persists in host cells but its transcription is blocked and viral proteins are not made. The persistent virus may periodically boost the immune response of the infected animal and in this way generate long-lasting immunity to superinfection. The immune responses in these cases, although unable to eliminate viruses, may prevent the development of clinical disease and therefore serve a protective role. Immunosuppression or stress may permit disease to occur in persistently infected animals. The association between stress and the development of some virus diseases is well recognized. It is likely that the increased levels of steroid production in stressful situations may be sufficiently immunosuppressive to permit activation of latent viruses or infection by exogenous ones.

Sometimes viruses may interact with bacteria to overcome the immune system. For example, it is well recognized that *Mannheimia hemolytica* and bovine herpesvirus-1 interact to cause severe respiratory disease in cattle. It appears that BHV infection in the bovine lung increases expression of the β2-integrin CD11a/CD18 on lung neutrophils. The leukotoxin of *M. hemolytica* binds to this integrin and then kills the neutrophils, permitting growth of the invading bacteria.

ADVERSE CONSEQUENCES OF IMMUNITY TO VIRUSES

The immune response to viruses can, on occasion, be a disadvantage. Indeed, there are many virus diseases in which the major lesions develop as a result of inappropriate or excessive immune responses. For example, bovine respiratory syncytial viruses (RSV) induce a Th2 response in infected cattle with production of IL-4 and specific IgE antibodies in the lungs. This may result in a type I hypersensitivity reaction in the lungs since there is a direct correlation between this IgE level and the severity of clinical disease.

The destruction of virus-infected cells by antibody is classified as a type II hypersensitivity reaction (Chapter 27) and, although normally beneficial, may exacerbate virus diseases. Thus viruses are removed at the cost of some cell destruction. The severity and significance of this tissue damage depend on how widespread the infection becomes. In some diseases in which the virus causes little cell destruction, most of the tissue damage may result from immunological attack. A good example of this problem is seen in distemper encephalitis, in which neurons are demyelinated as a result of an antiviral immune response. Thus macrophages, which are numerous in these brain lesions, ingest immune-complexes and infected cells. As a result they release oxidants and other toxic products. These toxic products damage nearby cells, especially oligodendroglia and so cause demyelination. Old dog encephalitis, a disease of middle-aged dogs, is perhaps a variant of this postdistemper lesion.

It has been suggested that some cases of demyelinating encephalitis in canine distemper results from autoimmune attack. Thus most dogs with this syndrome make antibodies against myelin proteins, and it has been suggested that these cause tissue destruction. Their importance, however, is unclear. The level of antimyelin antibodies is unrelated to the course of the disease, and in general, the animals with the highest titers are those that recover. On the other hand, some sera from affected dogs can cause demyelination in canine cerebellum cultures.

Type III (immune-complex) lesions (Chapter 28) are commonly associated with viral diseases, especially those in which viremia is prolonged. For example, glomerulonephritis resulting from the deposition of immune-complexes is a common complication of equine infectious anemia, Aleutian disease of mink, feline leukemia, chronic hog cholera, bovine virus diarrhea-mucosal disease, canine adenovirus infections, and feline infectious peritonitis. A generalized vasculitis due to deposition of immune-complexes throughout the vascular system is seen in equine infectious anemia, Aleutian disease of mink, malignant catarrhal fever, and possibly, equine viral arteritis.

In dogs infected with canine adenovirus 1 (infectious canine hepatitis), an immune-complex–derived uveitis and a focal glomerulonephritis both develop. The uveitis, commonly called "blue-eye," is seen both in dogs with natural infections and in those vaccinated with live attenuated adenovirus vaccine (Figure 24-7). The uveitis results from the formation of virus-antibody complexes in the anterior chamber of the eye and in the cornea with complement activation and consequent neutrophil accumulation (Figure 24-8). The neutrophils release enzymes and oxidants that damage corneal epithelial cells leading to edema and opacity. The condition resolves spontaneously in about 90% of affected dogs.

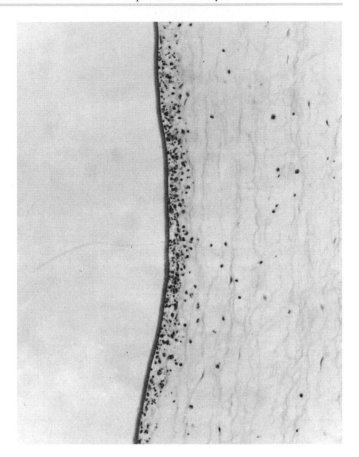

Figure 24-8. A section from the cornea of a dog with blue-eye. Note the neutrophil infiltration of the posterior surface of the cornea as a result of virus-antibody complex deposition in this region. (From Carmichael LE: *Pathol Vet* 1:73-95, 1964.)

Finally, many virus diseases are associated with the occurrence of rashes. The pathology of these is complex but may reflect type II, III, or IV hypersensitivity reactions occurring as the host responds to the presence of viral antigens in the skin.

Aleutian Disease of Mink

Although immune-complex–mediated lesions are usually only of passing interest in many infectious diseases, they generate the major pathological lesions in Aleutian disease of mink. Aleutian disease is a persistent parvovirus infection that was first recognized in mink with the Aleutian coat color. Although all strains of mink are susceptible to this virus, Aleutian mink are genetically predisposed to the development of severe lesions since they are also affected by the Chédiak-Higashi syndrome (Chapter 35). Persistently infected mink develop a slowly progressive lymphoproliferative disease with a plasmacytosis that has been compared to a myeloma, since it results in a marked polyclonal or monoclonal gammopathy (Figures 24-9 and 24-10). They also develop immune-complex lesions (Chapter 28), including glomerulonephritis and arteritis. They make

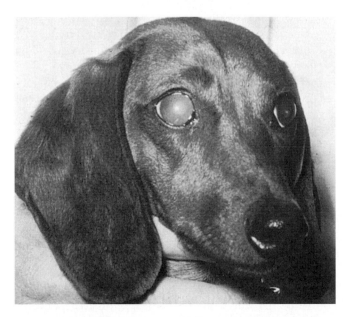

Figure 24-7. Blue-eye, a type III hypersensitivity reaction to canine adenovirus 1 (ICH) occurring in the cornea. (Courtesy of Dr. H Reed.)

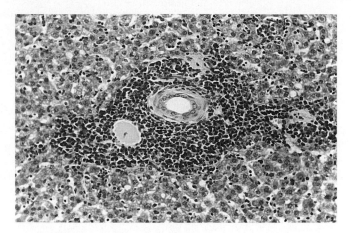

Figure 24-9. A section of liver from a mink infected with Aleutian disease. Note the marked plasma cell and mononuclear cell infiltration (×250). (From a specimen kindly provided by Dr. SH An.)

autoantibodies to their own immunoglobulins (rheumatoid factors) and to DNA (antinuclear antibodies). Their serum IgG concentration increases, sometimes to very high levels. On occasion these elevated immunoglobulins are monoclonal in origin. They are directed against the Aleutian disease virus. The virus transforms B cells so that they proliferate and differentiate excessively.

The immune-complex-mediated lesions of Aleutian disease include an arteritis, in which IgG, C3, and viral antigen are found within vessel walls, and a glomerulonephritis, in which deposits of immune-complexes containing virus and antibody are found. In addition, infected mink are anemic. Their red cells are coated with antiviral antibodies. It is likely, therefore, that the red cells of infected animals adsorb virus-antibody complexes from plasma. These coated red cells are then removed from the circulation by macrophages. As might be predicted, the use of immunosuppressive agents such as cyclophosphamide or azathioprine in infected mink prevents the development of many of these lesions and so prolongs survival, whereas experimental vaccination with inactivated Aleutian disease virus increases the severity of infections.

Feline Infectious Peritonitis

Feline infectious peritonitis (FIP) is a fatal disease of wild and domestic cats caused by a coronavirus. The FIP virus is closely related to feline enteric coronavirus, and viruses are found with properties intermediate between the two. However, feline enteric coronavirus prefers to replicate within intestinal epithelial cells, whereas FIP virus prefers to replicate within macrophages. Macrophages also spread the FIP virus throughout the body. FIP tends to infect relatively young cats between 6 months and 3 years of age. The disease presents in two major forms: an effusive ("wet") form with peritonitis (ascites) or pleuritis characterized by the presence of large amounts of proteinaceous fluid in the body cavities and associated with a vasculitis and a noneffusive ("dry") form characterized by multiple small granulomas on the surface of the major abdominal organs. Pleural lesions are uncommon in the noneffusive form of FIP. Some cats may show signs of central nervous system involvement and ocular lesions. Both forms of the disease are uniformly lethal, with affected cats dying between 1 week and 6 months.

The pathogenesis of FIP differs between the two forms of the disease. After invading a cat, the virus first replicates in intestinal epithelial cells. The virus shed by epithelial cells is then spread by monocytes and taken up by phagocytic cells in the target tissues. These target tissues include the serosa of the peritoneum and the pleura, as well as the meninges and the uveal tract. The course of the infection then depends on the nature of the immune response to the virus—a phenomenon also seen in several bacterial diseases (Chapter 23). Immunity to FIP virus is entirely cellular, and it is likely that a

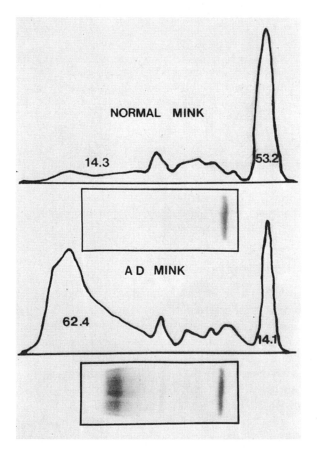

Figure 24-10. A comparison of the serum electrophoretic patterns seen in normal and Aleutian disease-infected mink. The serum of the infected animal shows a polyclonal gammopathy so that the gamma globulins account for 62.4% of the serum proteins in contrast to the normal level of 14.3%. (Courtesy of Dr. SH An.)

Th1 response is protective. Antibodies, on the other hand, may exacerbate the disease. A cat that mounts a good Th1 response will become immune, regardless of the amount of antibodies it makes. Some cats, however, probably make a Th2 response and fail to mount a cell-mediated immune response. In these animals, antibodies enhance virus uptake by macrophages in which it then replicates. Large numbers of virus-laden macrophages accumulate around the blood vessels of the omentum and serosa (Figure 24-11). These antibodies also form immune-complexes with the virus; these immune-complexes are deposited in the serosa, causing pleuritis or peritonitis, and in glomeruli, leading to glomerulonephritis. The serosal vasculitis is responsible for the effusion of fibrin-rich fluid into the serosal cavities. This massive production of immune-complexes may also be responsible for the disseminated intravascular coagulation seen in these cats. IL-1 and IL-6 are found in unusually high concentrations in the peritoneal fluid from cats with effusive FIP. Cats with high levels of antibodies against feline coronaviruses develop effusive FIP unusually rapidly on challenge. Administering antiserum to feline coronavirus before FIP challenge may also accelerate the peritonitis. The lesions in the non-effusive form of FIP probably result from a weak or partial Th1 immune response against the virus. Virus replication is not completely prevented in this case, and fewer macrophages with less virus are found in the lesions. It is possible that cats that mount a Th1 response to the coronavirus are protected, cats that mount a Th2 response develop effusive disease, and cats that have a mixed response develop noneffusive disease.

A modified live intranasal vaccine is available against FIP. The vaccine contains a temperature-sensitive mutant virus that replicates in the upper respiratory tract and induces a local IgA response in the mucosa. This local mucosal response should prevent coronavirus invasion without inducing high levels of serum antibodies. This vaccine will, however, only be effective if administered before FIP exposure. In highly endemic situations in which kittens are infected at a young age, vaccination at 16 weeks of age may be too late to prevent infection.

Equine Infectious Anemia

In addition to evading the immune response, the equine infectious anemia (EIA) virus is associated with significant immunologically mediated tissue damage. The red cells of viremic horses adsorb circulating EIA virus onto their surface. Antibodies and complement then bind to the virus, as a result of which the red cells are cleared from the circulation more rapidly than normal. In addition to anemia, infected horses may also develop a glomerulonephritis as a result of immune-complex deposition on glomerular basement membranes. Horses infected with EIA have unusually low levels of IgG3, although their circulating lymphocytes appear to be unaffected and respond normally to mitogens such as phytohemagglutinin.

SEROLOGY OF VIRAL DISEASES

Tests to Detect and Identify Viruses

Among the simplest and most widely employed tests for the detection of viruses are the direct and indirect fluorescent antibody tests, which may be used to identify virus in the tissues of infected animals. If these methods are not possible, it may be necessary to grow the virus in experimental animals, chick embryos, or tissue cultures to provide sufficient antigen for testing. Once sufficient virus has accumulated, it can be identified by its reaction with specific antiserum. The tests commonly employed for this purpose are fluorescent antibody tests, ELISA, hemagglutination inhibition, virus neutralization, complement fixation, and gel precipitation. The precise tests employed will depend on the nature of the unknown virus. Hemagglutination inhibition tests are technically simple and are preferred if available. They do, however, tend to be strain-specific. The complement fixation test and gel precipitation test, as a broad generalization, tend to be largely group-specific and thus lend themselves to attempts to identify the genus to which a virus belongs. In contrast, virus neutralization tests tend to be highly strain-specific, so much so that they are perhaps best employed in the classification of a virus into its subtypes rather than in identifying the specific genus of a particular organism. There are, of course, exceptions to these generalizations; for example, the New Jersey and Indiana strains of vesicular

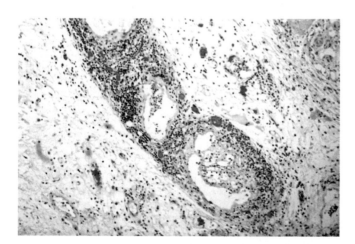

Figure 24-11. Granulomatous vasculitis of serosal blood vessels in a cat with feline infectious peritonitis. Note the marked cellular infiltration of the vessel adventitia and media. This reaction may be partially due to the deposition of virus-antibody complexes in the vessel walls. (Courtesy of Dr. RC Weiss.)

stomatitis virus do not cross-react in the complement fixation test.

A popular technique for the detection of viral antigen or antiviral antibodies is the membrane filter ELISA test (Chapter 16). This test has the advantage that both positive and negative controls can be incorporated with the test serum in one well. In addition to serum, whole blood, plasma, or saliva may be employed as a source of antigen or antibody.

Specific antibodies can be used to enrich virus suspensions before electron microscopy. For example, a fecal sample may be centrifuged, leaving a clear supernatant that contains a small number of many different viruses. After sonication to break up clumps, antibody specific for the virus of interest is added to the supernatant, and after a brief incubation, the fluid is centrifuged again. Virus particles clumped by antibody are spun to the bottom, where they can be removed and examined by electron microscopy after negative staining (Figure 24-12). The antibody, by clumping only the virus of interest, renders it much more visible in the electron microscope, and the presence of visible antibody within the virus clumps provides direct confirmation of the identity of the virus.

Tests to Detect and Identify Antiviral Antibodies

In general, the most widely employed techniques for detecting antibodies to viruses are hemagglutination inhibition, indirect ELISA, immunofluorescence, gel diffusion, Western blotting, complement fixation, and virus neutralization. The first four of these are technically simple and are thus preferred. The complement fixation test and the virus neutralization tests are complex, thus restricting the circumstances in which they may be used. The virus neutralization tests are also extremely specific, which as discussed earlier, tends to reduce their value as screening tests.

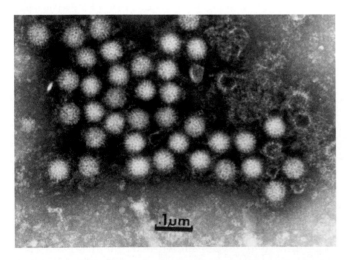

Figure 24-12. Immunoelectron microscopy of porcine rotavirus clumped by convalescent antiserum (×130,500). (Courtesy of Dr. L Saif.)

SOURCES OF ADDITIONAL INFORMATION

Aasted B, Leslie RGQ: Virus-specific B-lymphocytes are probably the primary targets for Aleutian disease virus, *Vet Immunol Immunopathol* 28:127-141, 1991.

Alcami A, Koszinowski UH: Viral mechanisms of immune evasion, *Trends Microbiol* 8:410-418, 2000.

Appel JMG, Mendelson SG, Hall WW: Macrophage Fc receptors control infectivity and neutralization of canine distemper virus-antibody complexes, *J Virol* 51:643-649, 1984.

Doherty PC: Immune memory to viruses, *ASM News* 61:68-71, 1995.

Goitsuka R, Ohashi T, Ono K, et al: IL-6 activity in feline infectious peritonitis, *J Immunol* 144:2599-2603, 1990.

Guidotti LG, Ishikawa T, Hobbs MV, et al: Intracellular inactivation of the hepatitis B virus by cytotoxic T lymphocytes, *Immunity* 4:25-36, 1996.

Haig DM: Subversion and piracy: DNA viruses and immune evasion, *Res Vet Sci* 70:205-219, 2001.

LaBonnardière C, Lefèvre F, Charley B: Interferon response in pigs: molecular and biological aspects, *Vet Immunol Immunopathol* 43:29-36, 1994.

Lachmann PJ: Microbial subversion of the immune response, *Proc Natl Acad Sci* 99:8461-8462, 2002.

Lentz TL: The recognition event between virus and host cell receptor: a target for antiviral agents, *J Gen Virol* 71:751-766, 1990.

McGuire TC, Fraser DG, Mealey RH: Cytotoxic T lymphocytes and neutralizing antibody in the control of equine infectious anemia virus, *Viral Immunol* 15:521-531, 2002.

Mims CA, ed: Virus immunity and pathogenesis, *Brit Med Bull* 41:1-102, 1985.

Pedersen NC: Animal virus infections that defy vaccination: equine infectious anemia, caprine arthritis-encephalitis, maedi-visna, and feline infectious peritonitis, *Adv Vet Sci Comp Med* 33:413-428, 1989.

Rigden RC, Carrasco CP, Summerfield A, McCullough KC: Macrophage phagocytosis of foot-and-mouth disease virus may create infectious carriers, *Immunology* 106:537-548, 2002.

Ringler SS, Krakowka S: Effect of canine distemper virus on natural killer cell activity in dogs, *Am J Vet Res* 46:1781-1786, 1985.

Scalzo AA: Successful control of viruses by NK cells—a balance of opposing forces? *Trends Microbiol* 10:470-474, 2002.

Sharma R, Woldehiwet Z: Cytotoxic T cell responses in lambs experimentally infected with bovine respiratory syncytial virus, *Vet Immunol Immunopathol* 28:237-246, 1991.

Thanawongnuwech R, Halbur PG, Thacker EL: The role of pulmonary intravascular macrophages in porcine reproductive and respiratory syndrome virus infection, *Anim Hlth Res Rev* 1:95-102, 2000.

Zhang Z, Harkiss GD, Hopkins J, Woodall CJ: Granulocyte macrophage colony-stimulating factor is elevated in alveolar macrophages from sheep naturally infected with maedi-visna virus and stimulates maedi-visna virus replication in macrophages *in vitro*, *Clin Exp Immunol* 129:240-246, 2002.

Zurbriggen A., Vandevelde M: The pathogenesis of nervous distemper, *Prog Vet Neurol* 5:109-116, 1994.

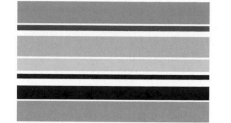

Acquired Immunity to Parasites

CHAPTER 25

Infectious disease is, as pointed out earlier, rarely a result of the activities of a malicious microorganism. In the vast majority of cases, it is a consequence of a microorganism being able to evade the immune defenses of an animal and exploit the resources of its host. Disease occurs as a result of the host's reaction to the infection or because the invader causes significant damage to its host.

Well-adapted parasites do not make these mistakes. They have evolved in such a way that their presence in the host is scarcely noticed. Thus they evade the immune defenses and then exploit the host's resources without causing irreparable damage. Ideally, they can continue to draw on their host's resources indefinitely.

Thus parasitic infections caused by protozoan parasites or helminths may be noticed only by production losses. Indeed, in many cases, the presence of parasites comes to our attention only when they are present in unusually large numbers or when they enter a critical organ by accident. Sometimes, of course, a parasite may deliberately cause disease. For instance, parasites such as *Toxoplasma*, transmitted by carnivorism, may benefit by causing their host to become slow or confused so that it can be more readily eaten by a predator.

The consistent feature of all parasite infestations, however, is that they block or significantly delay the innate and acquired defenses of their host so that they may persist for sufficient time to reproduce. Some parasites may simply delay their destruction until they complete a single life cycle. Other well-adapted parasites may contrive to survive for the life of their host protected from immunological attack by sophisticated and specific evasive strategies.

The success of any parasite is measured not by the disturbances it imposes on a host but by its ability to adapt and integrate itself within a host's internal environment. In contrast to the acute, short-lived infections caused by bacteria and viruses, infections by parasitic protozoa or helminths are long-lasting and in many cases not apparent. Ideally, the successful parasite will regulate a host's immune responses, suppressing these to permit parasite survival, while at the same time allowing other responses to proceed and so preventing the death of the host from other infections. In addition, many parasites make use of the host's metabolic or control pathways for their own purposes. For example protozoan parasites may make use of their host's growth factors to promote their own growth. Thus epithelial growth factor and interferon-γ can enhance the growth of *Trypanosoma brucei*, whereas IL-2 and GM-CSF can promote the growth of *Leishmania amazonensis*. The sharing of cytokines by parasites in this way reflects the long history of their association with their hosts and their success in adapting to a parasitic lifestyle. It is evident that they must have evolved very effective mechanisms to prevent immunological destruction.

IMMUNITY TO PROTOZOA

Innate Immunity

The mechanisms of innate resistance to protozoa appear to be similar to those that prevent bacterial and viral invasion. Thus the GPI anchor (Chapter 9) from

Trypanosoma cruzi activates TLR-2 and triggers the production of IL-12 and nitric oxide by macrophages. Species influences are of major significance. For example, *T. brucei*, *Trypanosoma congolense*, and *Trypanosoma vivax* do not cause disease in the wild ungulates of East Africa but will kill domestic cattle, presumably as a result of lack of mutual adaptation. Similarly, the coccidia are extremely host-specific; for example, *Toxoplasma gondii* tachyzoites can infect any species of mammal, but its coccidian stages affect only felids (cats, tigers, etc.).

Presumably, these species differences are but a reflection of more subtle genetic influences. Thus some breeds of African cattle, most notably N'Dama, show increased resistance to infection by pathogenic trypanosomes. This trypanotolerance results from natural selection of the most resistant animals over many years and reflects their greater ability to control infection, as well as their resistance to the pathological effects of the parasite. Analysis has shown that the γ/δ T cells of N'Dama are much more responsive to trypanosome antigens than are the γ/δ T cells of nonnative cattle. Trypanotolerant animals produce more IL-4 and less IL-6 than susceptible animals. At the same time trypanotolerant animals show neither the severe anemia nor the production loss seen in susceptible cattle. Trypanotolerant animals produce high levels of IgG against the trypanosome cysteine protease on infection with *T. congolense*. Since this enzyme contributes to the pathology of infection, these antibodies may partially account for trypanotolerance.

Perhaps the best analyzed example of genetically determined resistance to a protozoan infection is sickle cell anemia and its role in resistance to malaria in humans. Individuals who inherit the sickle cell trait possess hemoglobin S (HbS), in which a residue of valine has replaced a residue of glutamic acid present in normal hemoglobin. The changes in the sequence of the hemoglobin molecule cause deoxygenated hemoglobin molecules to precipitate when reduced, thus distorting the shape of the erythrocytes and resulting in increased erythrocyte fragility and clearance. Individuals who are homozygous for the sickle cell gene die from severe anemia when young. Heterozygous individuals are also anemic, but in west central Africa the fact that hemoglobin S kills *Plasmodium falciparum* ensures that affected individuals are resistant to malaria. As a result of this, more of these individuals tend to survive to reproductive age than do normal persons. The mutation is therefore maintained in the human population at a relatively high level.

Acquired Immunity

Like other organisms, protozoa stimulate both antibody- and cell-mediated immune responses. In general, antibodies control the numbers of parasites in blood and tissue fluids, whereas cell-mediated responses are directed largely against intracellular parasites.

Serum antibodies directed against protozoan surface antigens may opsonize, agglutinate, or immobilize them. Antibodies together with complement and cytotoxic cells may kill them, and some antibodies (called ablastins) may inhibit their division. In genital infections of humans due to *Trichomonas vaginalis*, a local IgE response is stimulated. The allergic reaction that ensues provokes intense discomfort; more important, by increasing vascular permeability, this reaction permits IgG antibodies to reach the site of infection and immobilize and eliminate the organisms.

In babesiosis the infective stages of the organisms (sporozoites) invade red blood cells. This invasion involves activation of the alternate complement pathway. Infected red cells incorporate *Babesia* antigens into their membranes. These in turn induce antibodies that opsonize the red cells and cause their removal by phagocytic cells. Infected red cells may also be destroyed by antibody-dependent cell-mediated responses. Macrophages and cytotoxic lymphocytes can recognize the *Babesia* antigen/opsonizing-antibody complex on the surface of infected erythrocytes. Cytotoxic T cells may play a role early in infection when the number of infected erythrocytes is small.

Protective immunity against apicomplexan protozoa such as *Cryptosporidia*, *Eimeria*, *Neospora*, *Plasmodia*, and *Toxoplasma* is generally mediated by Th1 responses. For example, *T. gondii* is an obligate intracellular parasite whose tachyzoites grow within cells (Figure 25-1). Eventually, the infected cell ruptures and the tachyzoites are released to invade other cells. They penetrate these cells by squeezing through a molecular junction in the cell membrane and so do not trigger proper phagosome formation and maturation. Toxoplasma tachyzoites are therefore not destroyed, since these phagosomes are unable to

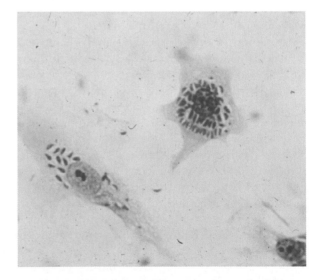

Figure 25-1. Mouse macrophages containing healthy, growing tachyzoites of *Toxoplasma gondii*. Once an immune response develops, these cells become activated and acquire the ability to destroy ingested tachyzoites. (Courtesy of Dr. CH Lai.)

mature and fuse with lysosomes. As a result, *Toxoplasma* tachyzoites can grow inside cells in an environment free of antibodies, oxidants, or lysosomal enzymes.

Normally, both Th1 and Th2 immune responses occur on exposure to *Toxoplasma*. The Th2 response involving antibodies together with complement destroys extracellular organisms and reduces the spread of the organism between cells (Figure 25-2). This response, however, has little or no influence on the intracellular forms of the parasite. The intracellular organisms are destroyed by an IL-12–dependent Th1 cell–mediated response. Sensitized Th1 cells secrete IFN-γ in response to *Toxoplasma* ribonucleoproteins. This IFN-γ activates macrophages, enabling them to kill the intracellular organism by permitting lysosome-phagosome fusion. Some T cells may also secrete cytokines that interfere directly with *Toxoplasma* replication. In addition, cytotoxic T cells can destroy *Toxoplasma* tachyzoites and *Toxoplasma*-infected cells. In these ways, both Th1 and Th2 immune responses act together to ensure the elimination of the tachyzoite stage of this organism. However, *T. gondii* tachyzoites can transform themselves into a cyst form containing bradyzoites. The cysts appear to be non-immunogenic and do not stimulate an inflammatory response. It is possible that this cyst stage is not recognized as foreign.

Th1-mediated responses involving activation of macrophages are important in many protozoan diseases in which organisms are resistant to intracellular destruction. One of the most significant destructive pathways in these activated cells is the production of nitric oxide. Nitrogen radicals formed by the interaction of NO with reactive oxidants are lethal for many intracellular protozoa. However, protozoa are also experts in surviving within macrophages, For example, some protozoa, such as *Leishmania*, *Toxoplasma*, and *Trypanosoma cruzi*, can migrate into safe intracellular compartments by stalling phagosome maturation. *Leishmania* and *T. cruzi* can suppress the production of oxidants or cytokine production, whereas *T. gondii* can promote macrophage apoptosis. *T. gondii* tachyzoites inhibit proinflammatory cytokine induction by preventing nuclear translocation of the transcription factor NF-κB.

In *Theileria parva* infection (East Coast fever) of cattle, sporozoites preferentially invade lymphocytes and induce uncontrolled cell proliferation. *T. parva* can invade α/β and γ/δ T cells, as well as B cells. The parasite then activates NF-κB by continuously phosphorylating its inhibitor proteins Iκ-Bα and Iκ-Bβ (Chapter 37). NF-κB thus persists, maintains the cell in an activated state, and prevents its apoptosis. The activated cells produce both IL-2 and IL-2R. As a result, an autocrine or paracrine loop is established, by which infected cells secrete IL-2, which in turn stimulates their growth. Cell growth ceases if IL-2 production is blocked. As *Theileria* shizonts develop within lymphocytes, the infected cells enlarge and proliferate. Since the parasite divides synchronously with its host cell, there is rapid growth of parasitized cells. In most cattle this results in overwhelming infection and death. Some animals, however, recover from infection and become solidly immune. In these animals, cytotoxic CD8+ T cells can kill infected lymphocytes by recognizing parasite antigens in association with MHC class I molecules. In other cases, the parasites interfere with MHC class I expression on infected cells.

Infection of chickens or mammals with *Eimeria* oocysts generally leads to strong, species-specific immunity that can prevent reinfection. This immune response inhibits the growth of trophozoites, the earliest invasive stage, within intestinal epithelial cells. This growth inhibition is reversible, since arrested stages can be transferred to normal animals and complete their development

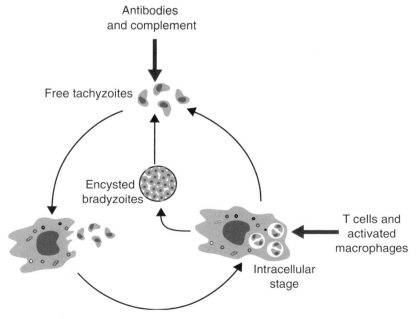

Antibodies and complement

Free tachyzoites

Encysted bradyzoites

Intracellular stage

T cells and activated macrophages

Figure 25-2. The points in the life cycle of *Toxoplasma gondii* at which the immune system can exert a controlling influence.

uneventfully. Studies in mice suggest that resistance to primary infection is mediated by multiple cell mediated mechanisms that include CD4+ T cells and their cytokines IL-12 and IFN-γ, macrophages and NK cells. In contrast, resistance to secondary challenge is mediated by CD8+ T cells. In chickens, IFN-γ, TNF-α, and TGF-β, as well as intraepithelial CD8+ α/β T cells, appear to be essential in host immunity.

Infections by coccidia in lambs and by *T. gondii* in cats effectively stimulate an immune response that can inhibit reinfection. In cats, the shedding of *Toxoplasma* oocysts, which ceases abruptly about 3 weeks after infection, coincides with the appearance of serum antibodies. It is not entirely clear, however, whether these antibodies are responsible for inhibiting oocyst production.

For many years it was thought that a common feature of many protozoan infections was *premunition*, a term used to describe resistance that is established after the primary infection has become chronic and is only effective if the parasite persists in the host. It was believed, for example, that only cattle actually infected with *Babesia* were resistant to clinical disease. If all organisms were removed from an animal, resistance was believed to wane immediately. Studies have shown that this is not entirely true. For example, cattle cured of *Babesia* infection by chemotherapy are resistant to challenge with the homologous strain of that organism for several years. Nevertheless, the presence of infection does appear to be mandatory for protection against heterologous strains. Babesiosis is also of interest since splenectomy of infected animals will result in clinical disease. The spleen not only serves as a source of antibodies in this disease but also removes infected erythrocytes. Loss of these functions by splenectomy permits the clinical disease to reappear.

Evasion of the Immune Response

Despite their antigenicity, parasitic protozoa manage to survive within their host for a long time by using multiple evasion mechanisms that have been acquired over many millions of years of evolution. Their survival depends on evading the host immune system. For example, *T. gondii* can avoid neutrophil attachment and phagocytosis. Many protozoa are immunosuppressive; for example, *T. parva* invades and destroys T cells. Other protozoa such as the trypanosomes may promote the development of suppressive regulatory cells or stimulate the B cell system to exhaustion. *Plasmodium falciparum* can suppress the ability of dendritic cells to process antigen.

Parasite-induced immunosuppression may promote parasite survival. For example, *Babesia bovis* is immunosuppressive for cattle. As a result, its host vector, the tick *Boophilus microplus*, is better able to survive on infected animals. Thus, infected cattle have more ticks than non-infected animals, and the efficiency of transmission of *B. bovis* is enhanced. It must be pointed out, however, that

parasite-induced immunosuppression can kill the host as a result of secondary infection, so it is not necessarily always beneficial to the parasite. Death in bovine trypanosomiasis is commonly due to bacterial pneumonia or sepsis following immunosuppression. In leishmaniasis the parasite can actively suppress transcription of the IL-12 gene. As a result, the host mounts an ineffective Th2 response rather than a protective Th1 response.

In addition to immunosuppression, protozoa have evolved two other effective evasive techniques. One involves becoming nonantigenic, and the other involves the ability to alter surface antigens rapidly and repeatedly. An example of a nonantigenic organism is the cyst stage of *T. gondii*, which, as mentioned previously, does not appear to stimulate a host response. Some protozoa can become functionally nonantigenic by masking themselves with host antigens. Examples of these include *Trypanosoma theileri* in cattle and *Trypanosoma lewisi* in rats, both nonpathogenic trypanosomes that survive in the blood of infected animals because they become covered with a layer of host serum proteins and so are not regarded as foreign. *T. brucei*, a pathogenic trypanosome of cattle, may also adsorb host serum proteins or red cell antigens and so reduce its antigenicity.

Although the absence of antigenicity may be considered the ultimate step in the evasive process, many protozoa, especially the trypanosomes, successfully employ repeated antigenic variation. If cattle are infected with the pathogenic trypanosomes *T. vivax*, *T. congolense*, or *T. brucei* and their parasitemia is measured at regular intervals, the numbers of circulating organisms are found to fluctuate greatly. Periods of high parasitemia alternate regularly with periods of low or undetectable parasitemia (Figure 25-3). Serum from infected animals contains antibodies against trypanosomes isolated before bleeding but not against those that develop subsequently. Each period of high parasitemia corresponds to the expansion of a population of trypanosomes with a new surface glycoprotein antigen. The elimination of this population by antibodies leads to a rapid fall in parasitemia. Among the survivors, however, some parasites express new surface glycoproteins and grow without hindrance. As a result, a fresh population arises to produce yet another period of high parasitemia (Figure 25-4). This cyclical fluctuation in parasite levels, with each peak reflecting the appearance of parasites with new surface glycoproteins, can continue for many months.

Variant surface glycoproteins (VSGs) are the major surface antigens of these trypanosomes. The VSGs produced early in trypanosome infections tend to develop in a predictable sequence. However, as the infection progresses, the production of VSGs becomes more random. Trypanosomes grown in tissue culture also show spontaneous antigenic variation demonstrating that the change in surface VSGs is not induced by antibody. The VSGs form a thick coat on the surface of the trypanosome. When antigenic change occurs, the VSGs

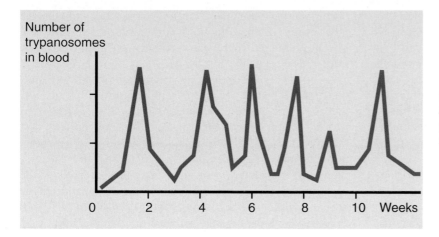

Figure 25-3. The time-course of *Trypanosoma congolense* parasitemia in an infected calf. Each parasitemic peak represents the development of a new, antigenically original population of organisms.

in the old coat are shed and replaced by an antigenically different VSG. Analysis of this process indicates that although the trypanosomes possess about 1000 VSG genes, only one VSG gene is active at a time. Antigenic variation occurs as a result of replacing an active VSG gene with one from the silent VSG gene pool. Since only a small part of the tightly packed VSG is exposed to host antibodies, it is not even necessary for the complete molecule to change. Replacement of exposed epitopes is sufficient for effective antigenic variation to occur. Early in infections, complete VSG gene replacement occurs. Later on, partial replacement and point mutations can create new antigenic specificities.

Trypanosomiasis is not the only protozoan infection in which variation of surface antigens is seen. It has also been recorded in infections by *Babesia bovis*, an intraerythrocyte organism that expresses a variant erythrocyte surface antigen. Presumably, the rapid variation of this polymorphic protein prolongs parasite survival. Other protozoa that show antigenic variation include the plasmodia and the intestinal parasite *Giardia lamblia*.

Since parasitic protozoa must evade the immune responses, it is not surprising that they preferentially invade immunosuppressed individuals. Organisms that are normally controlled by the immune response, such as the cyst forms of *T. gondii* or *Cryptosporidium bovis*, can grow and produce severe disease in immunosuppressed animals. For this reason, acute toxoplasmosis and cryptosporidiosis commonly occur in humans immunosuppressed for transplantation purposes, for cancer therapy, or with AIDS.

Adverse Consequences

The immune responses against protozoa may cause hypersensitivity reactions that contribute to the pathogenesis of protozoan diseases. Type I hypersensitivity is a feature of trichomoniasis and results in local irritation and inflammation in the genital tract. Type II cytotoxic reactions are of significance in babesiosis and trypanosomiasis, in which they contribute to the anemia. In babesiosis, parasitized red cells express parasite antigens

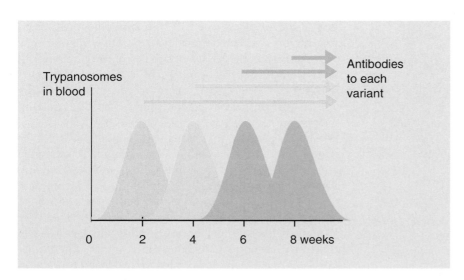

Figure 25-4. A schematic diagram showing how repeated antigenic variation accounts for the cyclical parasitemia observed in African trypanosomiasis. Each peak represents the growth of a new antigenic variant.

on their surfaces and are thus recognized as foreign and eliminated by hemolysis and phagocytosis. In trypanosomiasis, either fragments of disrupted organisms or possibly preformed immune-complexes bind to red cells and provoke their immune elimination, thus causing anemia. Immune-complex formation on circulating red cells is not the only problem of this type in trypanosomiasis. In some cases, excessive immune-complex formation can lead to vasculitis and glomerulonephritis (type III hypersensitivity; see Chapter 28).

Trypanosome infections also cause an enormous increase in the number of IgM-secreting cells, and very high levels of IgM are found in the blood of infected animals. Some of these antibodies are directed against autoantigens. These include rheumatoid factor–like molecules, and antibodies against thymocytes, ssDNA, red cells, and platelets. In *T. congolense*–infected cattle, these polyclonally stimulated B cells are BoCD5+. As pointed out earlier (Chapter 11) CD5+ B cells are of a different lineage to conventional B cells. The mechanism of this polyclonal B cell activation is unknown.

It is probable that a type IV hypersensitivity reaction contributes to the inflammation that occurs when *Toxoplasma* cysts break down and release fresh tachyzoites. Extracts of *T. gondii* (toxoplasmin), if administered intradermally to infected animals, will cause a delayed hypersensitivity response; this has been used as a diagnostic test for this infection (Figure 25-5).

Vaccination

Successful vaccination against protozoan infections of domestic animals is currently limited to coccidiosis, babesiosis, giardiasis, and theileriosis.

Several different live coccidial vaccines are currently used in poultry. These vaccines typically contain several species and strains of coccidia. Some consist of virulent,

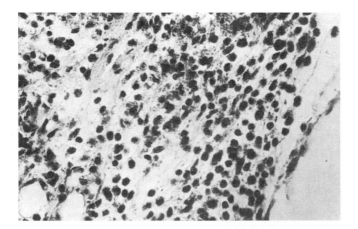

Figure 25-5. The characteristic mononuclear cell infiltration of a delayed hypersensitivity reaction in the skin of a mouse following an intradermal injection of an extract of *Toxoplasma gondii* (toxoplasmin). (Courtesy of Dr. Ch Lai.)

drug-sensitive organisms administered repeatedly in very low doses (trickle infection). Other vaccine strains have been attenuated by repeated passaging through eggs, or they have been selected for precocity. These precocious strains have a decreased prepatent time and, as a result, have a decreased ability to replicate and are thus less virulent. All of these vaccines provide solid immunity to coccidial infection when applied carefully under good rearing conditions. Nevertheless, the dose of coccidia vaccine must be carefully controlled, and the vaccines must be harvested from the feces of infected birds. Vaccinated birds shed oocysts that are transmitted to other birds in a flock. Because of regional strain variation, vaccination with a given suspension of live oocysts may not be effective in protecting against field strains in different locations.

A commercial vaccine is available to protect dogs and cats against *Giardia duodenalis*. The vaccine contains disrupted cultured *Giardia* trophozoite extracts administered subcutaneously and protects experimentally challenged dogs and cats against infection and clinical disease.

Babesia vaccines consist of tick-borne organisms that parasitize red cells and so cause anemia. Many factors contribute to the resistance of animals against babesiosis, including genetic factors (Zebu cattle are more resistant to disease than European cattle) and age (cattle show a significant resistance to babesiosis in the first 6 months of life). Animals that recover from acute babesiosis are resistant to further clinical disease, and this immunity has been considered to be a form of premunity. It is therefore possible to infect young calves when they are still relatively insusceptible to disease, and will become resistant to reinfection. The organisms employed for this procedure are first attenuated by repeated passage through splenectomized calves and then administered to recipient animals in whole blood. As might be anticipated, the side effects of this type of controlled infection may be severe, and chemotherapy is commonly required to control them. The transfer of blood from one calf to another may also trigger the production of antibodies against the foreign red cells. These antibodies complicate any attempts at blood transfusion in later life and may provoke hemolytic disease of the newborn (Chapter 27). In a slightly different approach, cattle can be made resistant to East Coast fever (*T. parva* infection) by infecting them with virulent sporozoites and treating them simultaneously with tetracycline.

Since a primary infection with *T. gondii* will confer strong protective immunity on an animal, protective immunization is a real possibility. Thus in New Zealand, a live *Toxoplasma* vaccine containing the S48 incomplete strain has been used successfully for the control of toxoplasmosis in sheep. The strain was developed by prolonged passage in laboratory mice and has lost the ability to develop bradyzoites or to initiate the sexual stages of the life cycle in cats. It produces protection against a severe challenge for at least 18 months. Unfortunately, the vaccine has a shelf life of only 7 to 10 days and can infect people.

IMMUNITY TO HELMINTHS

It is not surprising that the immune system is relatively inefficient in controlling helminth parasites. After all, these organisms have adapted to a parasitic existence and so, out of necessity, must have evolved to overcome or evade the immune responses. Parasitic helminths are therefore not maladapted pathogens but fully adapted obligate parasites whose very survival depends on reaching some form of accommodation with the host. Helminths do not replicate within a host; unlike protozoa, the number of helminths present in an individual will be no more than the number that has gained access to the host. Consequently, they usually cause only mild or subclinical disease. As a rule, they cause morbidity but not mortality. Only when helminths invade a host to which they are not fully adapted or in unusually large numbers does acute disease occur. Indeed, one consistent feature of intestinal nematode infestations is the very wide variation in parasite load within an animal population; it is not usually normally distributed but shows an overdispersed pattern. In other words, a minority of individuals may harbor the majority of parasites. Most animals harbor a few worms, but a few animals harbor a lot of worms. The size of the parasite burden in a host is controlled by genetic factors and by the host's response to these parasites. Some animals may be predisposed to a heavy infection as a result of genetic, behavioral, nutritional, or environmental factors. This predisposition may also reflect differences in exposure, susceptibility, or resistance.

Innate Immunity

Innate factors that influence helminth infestations include not only host-derived effects but also the influence of other parasites within the same host. The presence of adult worms in the intestine may delay the further development of larval stages of the same species within tissues. For example, calves infected with *Cysticercus bovis* show increased resistance to further infestation by this parasite. Similarly, lambs can acquire resistance to *Echinococcus granulosus* so that multiple dosing with large numbers of ova does not result in the development of massive worm burdens. The original dose of ova may stimulate rejection of subsequent doses. Interspecies competition among helminths for mutual habitats and nutrients in the intestinal tract will also influence the numbers, location, and composition of an animal's helminth population.

Innate factors of host origin that influence helminth burdens include the age, sex, and most important, the genetic background of the host. The influence of age and sex on helminth burdens appears to be largely hormonal.

In animals whose sexual cycle is seasonal, parasites tend to synchronize their reproductive cycle with that of their hosts. For instance, ewes show a spring rise in fecal nematode ova, which coincides with lambing and the onset of lactation. Similarly, the development of helminth larvae in cattle in early winter tends to be inhibited until spring in a phenomenon called hypobiosis. The larvae of *Toxocara canis* may migrate from an infected bitch to the liver of the fetal puppy, resulting in a congenital infection. Once born, the infected pups can reinfect their mother by the more conventional fecal-oral route.

An example of genetically mediated resistance to helminths is seen in the superior resistance of sheep with hemoglobin A to *Haemonchus contortus* and *Ostertagia circumcincta* as compared with sheep with hemoglobin B. The reasons for this are unclear, but sheep with HbA mount a more effective self-cure reaction and a better immune response to many other antigens as well. Another example is the enhanced resistance to *Cooperia oncophora* seen in Zebu cattle as compared with European cattle. In many cases resistance to parasites is linked to the MHC. Thus cattle possessing BoLA-Aw7 and A36 tend to have low fecal egg counts, whereas animals with Aw3 tend to have high fecal egg counts. Some BoLA haplotypes may also be associated with high antibody levels against *Ostertagia*. The SLA complex has been defined in certain lines of miniature swine, and the effects of the MHC on parasite immunity can be assessed in this species. Thus in one study there was a 50% lower muscle larval burden in *Trichinella spiralis*-infected *cc* minipigs as compared with pigs with the *dd* or *aa* haplotype. Minipigs carrying at least one copy of the *a* allele showed an enhanced ability to kill encysted muscle larvae—47% of pigs carrying the *a* allele responded to *Trichinella* as compared with 8% of pigs that lacked this allele. The response was characterized by a predominance of lymphocytes and macrophages in the cellular reaction around each larva.

Acquired Immunity

Helminths present the immune system with a challenge. Unlike bacteria or protozoa, parasitic worms have a thick extracellular cuticle that protects the nematode hypodermal plasma membrane. Some nematodes also have a loose coat that they can readily discard when attacked, ensuring that they cannot be severely damaged by conventional immune defenses. Helminth cuticles cannot be penetrated by the membrane attack complex of complement nor by T cell perforins. If the immune system is to successfully combat an invading helminth, it must either use cells that can destroy the intact cuticle or attack them through weak spots on their surface such as their digestive tract. Adult parasitic worms in the intestine are bathed in host enzymes, IgA, and mucin, while their feeding end and alimentary tract encounter effector cells, cytokines, antibodies, and complement.

The mechanisms of immunity to helminths are thus different from the mechanisms that control other pathogens.

In general parasitic worms elicit a very strong Th2 response characterized by production of high levels of IL-4, IgE antibodies, and large numbers of eosinophils and mast cells.

The immunodominant antigens of nematodes are the nematode polyprotein allergens/antigens (NPAs). These are lipid binding proteins that trigger Th2 responses and IgE formation. Helminth proteases are also potent inducers of allergic reactions and act directly on mast cells and basophils to induce their degranulation.

The best analyzed examples of acquired immunity to helminths are those in mice since inbred mouse strains differ widely in their ability to expel intestinal nematodes. This variability is a result of the relative activities of T cell subsets. For example, a consistent predisposition to infection is seen in outbred mice reinfected with *Trichuris trichiura* after their first infection is removed by anthelmintic treatment. Those mice that initially had low worm burdens reacquired low worm burdens, and those that had high worm burdens reacquired high worm burdens. These differences are a result of the type of helper cell response mounted by each animal. The expulsion of intestinal nematodes depends on helper T cells. Mice that expel their parasites mount a predominantly Th2 response. Those that cannot control their worm burden and become chronically infected mount a Th1 response. The Th2 response is associated with the production of IL-4, IL-10, and IL-13, leading to eosinophil mobilization, intestinal mast cell accumulation, and eventually the production of IgE. Expulsion of worms is accompanied by mucosal mast cell infiltration, intestinal eosinophilia, elevated serum IgE, and elevated parasite-specific IgG1 levels. Th2 cytokines also have a direct effect on worm populations. For example, mice whose genes for IL-4 or IL-13 have been knocked out are much more susceptible to *Trichuris muris* than normal mice. If IL-4 is neutralized by administration of specific antibodies or if the Th1 stimulator IL-12 is administered, mice lose their ability to expel worms and become chronically infected. Likewise, if TNF-α is neutralized, the mice also lose their ability to expel the worms. On the other hand, neutralization of the Th1 cytokines IFN-γ or IL-18 enables chronically infected mice to expel their parasites rapidly. Whether or not an animal mounts a Th1 or Th2 response depends on the dendritic cells that process the antigen. This in turn appears to depend on the way in which antigen encounters dendritic cells and the set of TLRs activated by the antigen.

Some inbred strains of mice show split resistance to *T. muris*. Some mount a Th2 response and expel their worms; others make a Th1 response and remain infected. Since inbred strains are genetically homogeneous, these variations must be due to differences among worms. Is it possible that some parasites can trigger DC1 responses

whereas others trigger DC2 responses? We know that strains of parasite differ in their ability to trigger Th1 and Th2 responses. This may be due to immune evasion by the parasites. Thus *T. muris* can produce a molecule related to IFN-γ that will suppress Th2 responses and enhance parasite survival. Alternatively, the differences may be due to parasite dose. Thus low level infestations of *T. muris* stimulate a Th1 response and the parasites persist. If higher doses of parasites are administered, this gradually changes to a Th2 response and the parasites are expelled. Therefore a threshold of infection is likely critical for the development of resistance.

γ/δ T cells in the intestinal epithelium may be activated by the presence of intestinal worms without the necessity of conventional antigen processing. In mice, these intraepithelial γ/δ T cells tend to produce IFN-γ in response to intracellular pathogens such as *Listeria monocytogenes*, whereas they produce IL-4 in response to the nematode *Nippostrongylus brasiliensis*.

Mammals will eventually develop immunity to most helminths after several months. In other words, the ability of the parasite to stave off immunological attack is limited, and eventually the host gains control. One parasite, *Ostertagia*, is an exception. Cattle remain susceptible to reinfection by *Ostertagia* for many months, and immunity that can inhibit the production of viable larvae is not seen until an animal is more than 2 years old. Thus it is no wonder that this is the most economically important bovine parasite.

Humoral Immunity

Because nematodes trigger Th2 responses, IgE levels and eosinophil numbers are usually elevated in parasitized animals. Many helminth infestations are associated with the characteristic signs of type I hypersensitivity, including eosinophilia, edema, asthma, and urticarial dermatitis. For example, pigs infested with *Ascaris suum* show cutaneous allergic reactions to injected parasite antigen, as well as degranulation of intestinal mucosal mast cells. In addition, many helminth infections, such as oesophagostomiasis, ancylostomiasis, strongyloidiasis, taeniasis, and fascioliasis, are accompanied by a positive passive cutaneous anaphylaxis (PCA) reaction to worm antigens (Chapter 26).

Th2-mediated IgE production is essential in controlling worm burdens. This is well seen in the self-cure reaction in sheep infected with gastrointestinal nematodes, particularly *H. contortus*. While embedded in the intestinal and abomasal mucosa, these worms secrete antigens (Figure 25-6). The combination of these helminth antigens with mast cell–bound IgE triggers mast cell degranulation and the release of vasoactive molecules and proteases. These molecules stimulate smooth muscle contraction and increase vascular permeability. The violent contractions of the intestinal muscles and the increase in the permeability of intestinal capillaries,

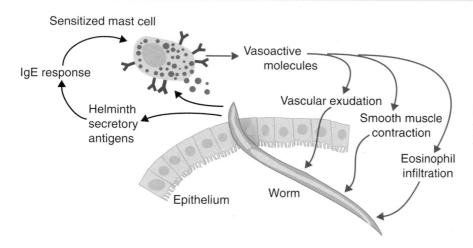

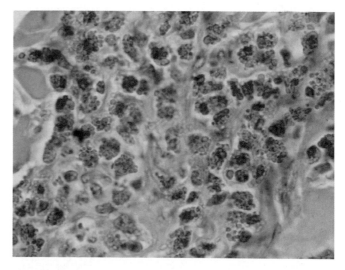

Figure 25-6. The mechanisms involved in the self-cure reaction against intestinal helminths.

leading to an efflux of fluid into the intestinal lumen (a leaky gut), can result in dislodgment and expulsion of many worms. In sheep that have just undergone self-cure, IgE antibody levels are high and experimental administration of helminth antigens will result in acute anaphylaxis, confirming the role of type I hypersensitivity in this phenomenon. A similar reaction is seen in fascioliasis in calves, in which peak PCA antibody titers coincide with expulsion of the parasite, as well as in rodent models.

Macrophages, platelets, and eosinophils possess FcεR (CD23). These cells can therefore bind to IgE-coated parasites, become activated, and kill them. Thus in cats infected with the filarial worm *Brugia pahangi*, those animals with high levels of parasite-specific IgE could kill adult worms. In contrast, cats that failed to mount a high IgE response permitted adult filaria to survive. Macrophages that bind to helminth larvae through IgE become activated with increased lysosomal enzymes, production of oxidants, IL-1, leukotrienes, prostaglandins, and platelet-activating factor. The net effect of this is enhanced parasite destruction.

Eosinophils are attracted to sites of helminth invasion by chemotactic molecules released by degranulating mast cells (Figure 25-7) (see Table 26-3). Cytokines such as IL-5 from Th2 cells also mobilize the bone marrow eosinophil pool, leading to the release of large numbers of eosinophils into the circulation. Other molecules chemotactic for eosinophils include many different chemokines (Figure 25-8). The eotaxins (CCL11, CCL24, and CCL26) have selective chemotactic activity for eosinophils. They act synergistically with IL-5. Parasites may induce two waves of eosinophil migration. The first is provoked by mast cell or parasite-derived products, the second by IL-5 and other cytokines from Th2 cells.

Eosinophils and Parasite Destruction

Eosinophils destroy parasitic worms. Because they have Fc receptors, eosinophils can bind to antibody-coated parasites, degranulate, and release their granule contents directly onto the worm cuticle (Figure 25-9). These contents include oxidants and nitric oxide generated by eosinophil peroxidase, and lytic enzymes such as lysophospholipase and phospholipase D. Major basic protein (MBP), the crystalline core of the specific granules, can damage the cuticles of schistosomula, *Fasciola*, and *Trichinella* at very low concentrations. Eosinophil cationic protein (ECP) and eosinophil neurotoxin are ribonucleases that are lethal for helminths. Given the diversity of parasitic worms, it is important to point out that eosinophils may not be effective against all parasites. They are probably most effective against larvae in tissues. However, even larval parasites may evade destruction. For example, larvae of *Toxocara canis*, exposed to eosinophils in vitro, simply shed their outer coat together with the attached cells.

Although the IgE-dependent eosinophil-mediated response is probably the most significant mechanism of

Figure 25-7. Photomicrograph of a lesion in horse skin caused by allergy to migrating parasitic helminth larvae. The granular cells are eosinophils, and their presence indicates the occurrence of a type I hypersensitivity reaction.

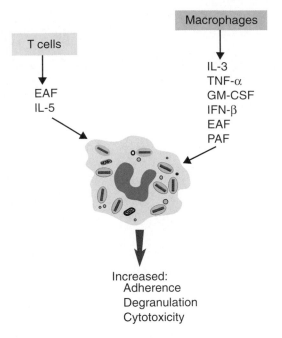

Figure 25-8. The factors involved in the activation of eosinophils. As a result of this activation, eosinophils gain enhanced antiparasite functions. *EAF,* Eosinophil activating factor; *PAF,* platelet-activating factor.

resistance to larval helminths, other immunoglobulins also play a protective role. The mechanisms involved include antibody-mediated neutralization of larval proteases, blocking of the anal and oral pores of larvae by immune-complexes (Figure 25-10), and prevention of ecdysis and inhibition of larval development by antibodies directed against exsheathing antigens. Antibodies to the enzyme glutathione-S-transferase protect against *Fasciola hepatica* in sheep. Other enzymes may be blocked by antibodies acting against adult worms, stopping egg production, or interfering with worm development (Figure 25-11). Thus female *Ostertagia ostertagi* worms fail to develop vulvar flaps when grown in immune calves. Similarly, spicule morphology may be altered in *Cooperia* males from immune hosts. The reduction in egg shedding is significant since it reduces parasite transmission within the herd.

Cell-Mediated Immunity

As pointed out previously, worm antigens preferentially stimulate Th2 responses, and Th1 responses may be of little protective benefit. Nevertheless, cytotoxic T cells may attack helminths that are deeply embedded in the intestinal mucosa or undergoing tissue migration. Cell-mediated immune reactions have been shown to occur in *Trichinella spiralis* and *Trichostrongylus colubriformis* infections. In the former, immunity can be transferred to normal animals by lymphoid cells, and infected animals show delayed hypersensitivity reactions to worm antigens. In vitro tests for cell-mediated immunity such as cytokine production and lymphocyte proliferation are also positive in these infections. In the case of *T. colubriformis,* immunity can be transferred to normal animals from immune ones by both cells and serum, and the site of worm attachment is subjected to a massive lymphocyte infiltration. Lymphocytes from sheep infected with *H. contortus* will release cytokines and divide in response to worm antigen, and it has been shown that immunity to this organism can be adoptively transferred to syngeneic sheep by using immune lymphocytes.

In infections with the tapeworm *Taenia solium,* live cysts trigger a Th2 response and thus IgE production. However, once the cysts die, they stimulate a Th1 response and granuloma formation. Biopsies show IL-12, IL-2, and IFN-γ associated with granulomas surrounding dying tapeworm cysts. Thus it may be that the Th1 response occurs only when the parasite can no longer modulate the host's immune response.

Sensitized T cells attack helminths by two mechanisms. First, the development of delayed hypersensitivity attracts mononuclear cells to the site of larval invasion and renders the local environment unsuitable for growth or migration. Second, cytotoxic lymphocytes may cause larval destruction. Thus treatment of experimental animals with BCG vaccine, a treatment that stimulates T cells (Chapter 37), inhibits the metastases of hydatid cysts (*E. granulosus*). In these treated animals the space that surrounds the cysts may be filled with large lymphocytes. It is also common to observe large lymphocytes adhering firmly to migrating nematode larvae in vivo.

In tapeworm infestations in which the parasite cyst (metacestode) grows within the host, the parasite must

Figure 25-9. Some of the molecules released from eosinophils that cause damage to parasitic helminths.

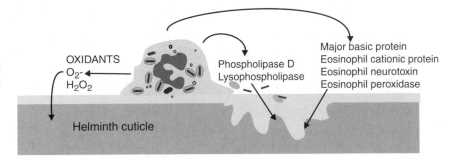

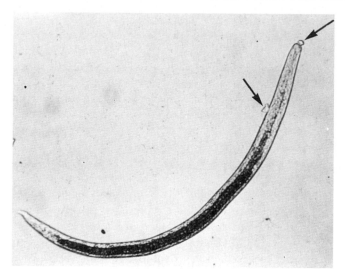

Figure 25-10. A *Toxocara canis* larva after incubation in specific antiserum. The immune precipitates at the oral and excretory pores are indicated by arrows. (Courtesy of Dr. DH DeSavigny.)

obtain protein for nourishment. However, the cysticerci of *Taenia ovis* actually grow larger in the presence of immune serum than in nonimmune serum. The parasites possess Fc receptors for host immunoglobulins, and it is possible that these immunoglobulins may serve as a food source for the parasite. Since cyst fluid contains lymphocyte mitogens, it has been suggested that these might stimulate immunoglobulin production that can then be ingested by the parasite.

The complexity of resistance to helminths is well demonstrated in sheep bred for resistance to *H. contortus*. Compared with susceptible sheep, there are differences in B cell function; resistant sheep have significantly more IgA- and IgG1-containing cells. There is also evidence for differences in T cell function, because resistant sheep respond better to a T-dependent antigen such as ovalbumin, and treatment of resistant lambs with a monoclonal antibody to CD4 completely blocks their resistance to *H. contortus*. Mucosal mast cell numbers and tissue eosinophilia are also reduced in these treated sheep. In contrast, depletion of CD8+ cells has no effect on resistance. In general, resistant sheep have higher eosinophil numbers, and curiously, these resistant sheep are calmer than susceptible sheep!

Evasion of the Immune Response

Although there are multiple mechanisms whereby animals resist helminth infection, it is obvious, even to a casual observer, that these responses are not very effective. Successfully adapted parasitic helminths can survive and function in the presence of a fully functional host immune system. Several strategies play a role in this adaptation, including loss of antigenicity by molecular mimicry or absorption of host antigens, antigenic variation, shedding of the glycocalyx, blocking of antibodies, and tolerance.

Helminths become progressively less antigenic as they evolve in the presence of a functioning immune system. Presumably, natural selection favors survival of parasites with reduced antigenicity. Thus *H. contortus* has become less antigenic for sheep, its natural host, than for rabbits, which it does not normally infect. Sheep therefore respond to fewer *H. contortus* antigens than do rabbits. In addition, helminths may synthesize and express nonpolymorphic MHC or blood group antigens on their surface in order to match those of their host.

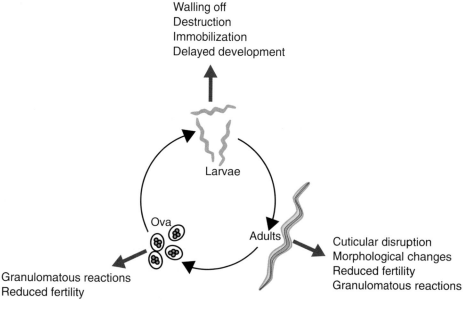

Walling off
Destruction
Immobilization
Delayed development

Larvae

Ova

Adults

Granulomatous reactions
Reduced fertility

Cuticular disruption
Morphological changes
Reduced fertility
Granulomatous reactions

Figure 25-11. Some effects of the immune responses on the stages of helminth development.

Helminths living within tissues may reduce their antigenicity by adsorbing host antigens onto their surface and so masking parasite antigens. This occurs in *Taenia solium* infestations in swine, in which the parasites are coated with IgG. It is not clear whether this IgG is synthesized by the worm or whether the worm synthesizes a receptor that binds host IgG. Cysticerci can also adsorb MHC molecules to their surface. Schistosomes can neutralize the alternative complement pathway by inserting functional decay accelerating factor (CD55) from their host into their outer lipid bilayer.

Other helminths interfere with antigen presentation. Thus macrophages from schistosome-infested animals are incompetent antigen-presenting cells. Filarial worms secrete inhibitors that block macrophage proteases. *Taenia taeniaeformis* secretes taeniastatin, a protease inhibitor that inhibits neutrophil chemotaxis, complement activation, T cell proliferation, and IL-2 production. Some parasites such as *F. hepatica* secrete proteases that destroy immunoglobulins. These proteases can generate Fab fragments that bind to parasite antigens and mask them. They may also generate Fc fragments that can block cellular receptors. Tapeworms can interfere with the complement system by secreting sulfated proteoglycans, which activate complement in the tissue fluid. *Brugia malayi* secretes serpins that inhibit neutrophil serine proteases. *E. granulosus* secretes an elastase inhibitor that blocks neutrophil attraction by C5a or PAF. Many helminths express surface antioxidants such as superoxide dismutase, glutathione peroxidase, and glutathione-S-transferase, which can neutralize the host's respiratory burst and protect surface structures against oxidation (Figure 25-12).

Another mechanism of evasion of the immune response involves sequential antigenic variation. Although helminths have not evolved a system similar to that seen in trypanosomiasis, gradual antigenic variation is recognized. Thus the cuticular antigens of *T. spiralis* larvae change following each molt. Even during their growth phase, these larvae change the expression of surface antigens. Some parasites such as *F. hepatica* shed their glycocalyx and hence their surface antigens when exposed to antibodies.

Immunosuppression may also contribute to the survival of parasitic worms. Sheep infected with *H. contortus* may become specifically suppressed so that they are unreactive to *H. contortus*, even though they remain responsive to unrelated antigens. *Ostertagia ostertagi* and *Trichostrongylus axei* infestations depress calf lymphocyte responses to mitogens. *Oesophagostomum radiatum* secretes molecules that inhibit the responses of lymphocytes to antigens and mitogens. Other immunosuppressive mechanisms may involve production of suppressor cells, as in filariasis or, alternatively, production of soluble immunosuppressive molecules as in fascioliasis. In other helminth infections, such as trichinosis, infected animals are nonspecifically immunosuppressed. This immunosuppression is reflected in a lowered resistance to other infections, a poor response to vaccines, and a prolongation of skin graft survival.

Vaccination

It is not surprising, considering the poor host response to parasitic worms and the availability of effective anthelmintics, that antihelminth vaccines are not widely available. Nevertheless, the emergence of anthelmintic resistance and environmental concerns raised by excessive chemical use have resulted in an increased interest in antiparasite vaccines. Vaccine use is predicated on the assumption that a host's immune response can control or prevent an infestation. This is not always obvious in helminth infestations, and traditional vaccines may be of little use. Despite this, a recombinant *T. ovis* vaccine has been produced that can induce protective immunity in sheep. This vaccine contains a cloned oncosphere antigen (To45W) with a saponin-based adjuvant. It stimulates a response that prevents parasite penetration of the intestinal wall. The vaccine provides protective immunity for at least 12 months, and up to 98% of naturally challenged lambs are protected. Similar single-antigen recombinant vaccines have been shown to be highly effective against *E. granulosus* in sheep.

Effective protection against some helminths has been obtained by the use of live irradiated organisms. The most important of these is the vaccine used to protect calves against pneumonia caused by the lungworm *Dictyocaulus viviparus*. In this vaccine, second-stage larvae hatched from ova in culture are exposed to 40,000 R X-irradiation, and two doses of these larvae are then fed to calves. The larvae can penetrate the calf's intestine, but since they are unable to develop to the third stage, they never reach the lung and are thus nonpathogenic. During their exsheathing process, the larvae stimulate the production of antibodies that can block reinfection.

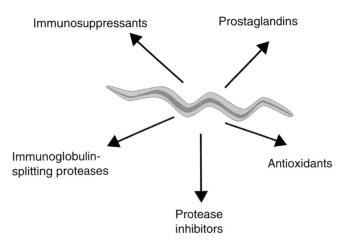

Immunosuppressants

Prostaglandins

Immunoglobulin-splitting proteases

Antioxidants

Protease inhibitors

Figure 25-12. Some methods by which migrating helminth larvae evade host defenses.

The efficiency of this vaccine, like other vaccines, depends very much on timing and on the size of the challenge dose, since even vaccinated calves may show mild pneumonic signs if placed on grossly infected pastures.

The major helminth antigens are of two types, soluble excretory/secretory products and antigens bound to the parasite surface (somatic antigens). Important somatic antigens include a common, 15 kDa polyprotein, and the enzyme γ-glutamyl transpeptidase. Some somatic antigens, such as those in the parasite gut, are hidden since they are not normally exposed to the host's immune response and may therefore be potential candidates for vaccines. For example, experimental vaccination of lambs and kids against the intestinal aminopeptidase of *H. contortus* (called H11) has resulted in significant drops in parasite numbers and fecundity.

Cattle are known to mount protective responses against *Fasciola* infections. This is especially effective against large infections but is less efficient against low-level trickle infections of the type likely to be encountered in the field. Thus immunity can be transferred from infected to naive cattle using either lymphocytes or serum. Irradiated parasites may induce immunity, as may crude parasite extracts. Animals may also be significantly protected against fascioliasis by the use of defined parasite antigens, including fatty-acid binding protein, glutathione-S-transferase, cathepsin L proteases, and liver fluke hemoglobin.

In general, the use of helminth vaccines has not been widely accepted. There appears to be reluctance on the part of farmers to change established control procedures, especially when the major financial burden of these infestations is borne by others.

IMMUNITY TO ARTHROPODS

When arthropods such as ticks or mosquitos bite an animal, they inject saliva, which contains molecules that assist the parasite in obtaining its blood meal. For example, arthropod saliva contains kininases that destroy bradykinin, which mediates pain and itch, histamine-binding proteins, and proteins that block complement activation. As a result, host scratching and grooming responses are minimized. Because some salivary molecules are antigenic, they induce immune responses. Because these immune responses may impair the parasite's ability to feed, the parasites have developed countermeasures that impair this response. Host responses to arthropod saliva are of three types. Some salivary components are of low molecular weight and cannot function as normal antigens. They may, however, bind to skin proteins such as collagen and then act as haptens, stimulating a Th1 response. On subsequent exposure, these haptens induce a delayed hypersensitivity reaction. Other salivary antigens may bind to epidermal Langerhans cells and induce

cutaneous basophil hypersensitivity, a Th1 response associated with the production of IgG antibodies and a basophil infiltration. If the basophils are destroyed by anti-basophil serum, resistance to biting arthropods is reduced. The third type of response to arthropod saliva is a Th2 response, leading to IgE production and type I hypersensitivity. This response may induce severe local inflammation in the skin, leading to pain or pruritus. Each of these three types of response may modify the skin in such a way that the feeding of the offending arthropod is impaired and the animal becomes a less attractive source of food. Unfortunately, it is also clear that these dermal immune responses to salivary antigens are not likely to be able to severely affect the parasite. Tick saliva impairs macrophage function and suppresses T cell responses to mitogens, as well as production of IL-1β and the Th1 cytokines IFN-γ and IL-2. In contrast, saliva from the ticks *Dermacentor andersonii* and *Ixodes ricinus* increases production of the Th2 cytokines IL-4 and IL-10. Natural selection and evolution ensure that the biting arthropod is well able to withstand such responses. (These hypersensitivities are discussed further in Chapter 26.)

Immune defenses may play a major role in preventing invasion of skin-penetrating arthropods. Thus body strike results from infestation of sheep skin with the larvae of the fly *Lucilia cuprina*. Sheep can be bred for low and high resistance to body strike. The resistant sheep have greater numbers of IgE+ B cells in their skin than do susceptible sheep. Resistant sheep also mount a greater inflammatory response and produce more fluid exudate when injected with larval excretory and secretory products. On the other hand, larval proteases inhibit complement activation and degrade immunoglobulins.

Demodectic Mange

The mange mite *Demodex folliculorum* appears to be a normal symbiont commonly present in hair follicles and only occasionally causes disease. When demodectic mange does occur, the reaction around mites and mite fragments is infiltrated by mononuclear cells with a few plasma cells. The infiltrating lymphocytes tend to be CD3+ and CD8+. Granuloma formation may occasionally occur. Thus the presence of cytotoxic T cells suggests that this is a type IV hypersensitivity reaction, perhaps a form of allergic contact dermatitis. The T cells may also be directed against mite antigens and reflect a defensive response by the host. The absence of eosinophils and edema in the lesion suggests that type I hypersensitivity is relatively unimportant. It is of interest to note that immunosuppressive agents such as antilymphocyte serum, azathioprine, or prolonged steroid therapy predispose animals to the development of demodectic mange. Animals with generalized demodicosis have normal neutrophil function and respond normally to vaccines or other foreign proteins. Nevertheless their

T cell response to mitogens such as phytohemagglutinin and concanavalin A is depressed. This is a progressive suppression, and it tends to become more severe as the disease progresses. If, however, the T cells of dogs with demodicosis are washed free of serum, they regain their ability to respond to mitogens. Serum from these animals is also able to suppress the proliferation of T cells from normal animals.

Flea Bite Dermatitis

Biting fleas secrete saliva into the skin wound. Some of the components of flea saliva are of low molecular weight and act as haptens by binding to dermal collagen. As a result, a local type IV hypersensitivity reaction characterized by a mononuclear cell infiltration occurs. In some sensitized animals, this type IV reaction is gradually replaced over a period of months by a type I reaction, and so the mononuclear cell infiltration gradually changes to an eosinophil infiltration. (A similar series of events has been recorded in sarcoptic mange in swine). The immune response mounted by flea-allergic animals may have a protective component. Thus female fleas produced fewer eggs on flea-allergic cats than on flea-naive cats. Flea-allergic cats also appear to remove more fleas by grooming than do flea-naive animals. Experimental vaccines containing the major antigens from the cat flea midgut have been able to reduce flea populations on dogs, and the female fleas recovered from these immunized animals produced significantly fewer eggs. This suggests that vaccination may eventually be a method of controlling flea populations.

Tick Infestation

It has been observed that ticks on nonimmune animals are larger than those on immune animals. Although the nature of this resistance is unclear, it has been suggested that local hypersensitivity reactions to tick saliva may restrict the blood flow to the tick, reduce its food supply, and stunt its growth. It is possible to immunize guinea pigs with tick homogenates and show that ticks feeding on these animals have reduced fertility and egg production. Although vaccination against salivary antigens is unlikely to be very effective in conferring effective immunity against blood feeding arthropods, there is an alternative approach. Since many of the arthropods of veterinary importance take the blood of their host into their digestive tract, it follows that they will also take up immunoglobulins, complement components, and cells. This suggests that if an animal were immunized with internal antigens from the parasite, this could lead to local damage. These internal antigens have been called "hidden" or "concealed" antigens since under normal circumstances the host would not usually encounter them. Vaccines made against antigens from the intestine of the tick *B. microplus* can inhibit tick reproduction.

Indeed, a recombinant tick vaccine based on such a recombinant antigen, Bm86, is available in Australia and Central America. The antibodies produced bind to the brush border of tick intestinal cells, inhibit endocytosis, and prevent the tick from engorging fully. Thus the digestive processes are impaired, and the tick experiences starvation, loss of fecundity, and weakness and may disengage from its host. This lowers the number of ticks found on vaccinated animals.

Hypoderma Infestation

Unlike the arthropods described above, the larvae of the warble flies (*Hypoderma bovis* and *Hypoderma lineatum*) actually migrate through body tissues. These larvae are therefore in somewhat the same position as migrating helminth larvae—they must effectively survive or evade the host's xenograft response. In fact, the first instar larvae of these flies do not trigger significant inflammation and are also immunosuppressive. Hypodermin A, the protease secreted by these larvae, can inhibit responses to mitogens and reduce IL-2 production, probably by destroying cell surface receptors. Vaccination with a cloned *Hypoderma* protein has effectively protected cattle against subsequent infestations.

SOURCES OF ADDITIONAL INFORMATION

Barbour AG, Restrepo BI: Antigenic variation in vector-borne pathogens, *Emerg Inf Dis* 6:449-456, 2000.

Barcinski MA, Costa-Moreira ME: Cellular response of protozoan parasites to host-derived cytokines, *Parasitol Today* 10:352-355, 1994.

Barriga OO: A review on vaccination against protozoa and arthropods of veterinary importance, *Vet Parasitol* 55:29-55, 1994.

Bogdan C, Röllinghoff M: How do protozoan parasites survive inside macrophages? *Parasitol Today* 15:22-27, 1999.

Brake DA: Vaccinology for control of apicomplexan parasites: a simplified language of immune programming and its use in vaccine design, *Int J Parasitol* 32:509-515, 2002.

Colditz IG, Lax J, Mortimer SI, et al: Cellular inflammatory responses in skin of sheep selected for resistance or susceptibility to fleece rot and fly strike, *Parasite Immunol* 16: 289-296, 1994.

Gasbarre LC, Leighton EA, Sonstegard T: Role of the bovine immune system and genome in resistance to gastrointestinal nematodes, *Vet Parasitol* 98:51-64, 2001.

Grencis RK: Enteric helminth infection: immunopathology and resistance during intestinal nematode infection. In Freedman DO, editor: *Immunopathogenetic aspects of disease induced by helminth parasites.* In Adorini L, Arai K, Berek C, et al, editors: *Chemical immunology,* vol 66, Basel, 1997, Karger.

Grencis RK: Cytokine regulation of resistance and susceptibility to intestinal nematode infection—from host to parasite, *Vet Parasitol* 100:45-50, 2001.

Heath AH, Arfsten A, Yamanaka M, et al: Vaccination against the cat flea *Ctenocephalides felis felis, Parasite Immunol* 16: 187-191, 1994.

Lillehof HS: Role of T lymphocytes and cytokines in coccidiosis, *Int J Parasitol* 28:1071-1081, 1998.

Maizels RM, Bundy DAP, Selkirk ME, et al: Immunological modulation and evasion by helminth parasites in human populations, *Nature* 365:797-805, 1993.

McDonald BJ, Foil CS, Foil LD: An investigation on the influence of feline flea allergy on the fecundity of the cat flea, *Vet Dermatol* 9:75-79, 1998.

Meeusen ENT, Balic A: Do eosinophils have a role in the killing of helminth parasites? *Parasitol Today* 16:95-101, 2000.

Mertens B, Taylor K, Muriuki C, Rocchi M: Cytokine mRNA profiles in trypanotolerant and trypanosusceptible cattle infected with the protozoan parasite *Trypanosoma congolense*: protective role for interleukin 4? *J Interferon Cytokine Res* 19:59-65, 1999.

Morrison WI, Taracha ELN, McKeever DJ: Contribution of T-cell responses to immunity and pathogenesis in infections with *Theileria parva*, *Parasitol Today* 11:14-18, 1995.

Olson ME, Ceri H, Morck DW: *Giardia* vaccination, *Parasitol Today* 16:213-217, 2000.

Phillips C, Coward WR, Pritchard DI, Hewitt CRA: Basophils express a type 2 cytokine profile on exposure to proteases from helminths and house dust mites, *J Leukoc Biol* 73:165-171, 2003.

Riding GA, Jarmey J, McKenna RV, et al: A protective concealed antigen from *Boophilus microplus*, *J Immunol* 153:5158-5166, 1994.

Spithill TW, Dalton JP: Progress in the development of liver fluke vaccines, *Parasitol Today* 14:224-227, 1998.

Wikel SK, Alarcon-Chaidez FJ: Progress toward molecular characterization of ectoparasite modulation of host immunity, *Vet Parasitol* 101:275-287, 2001.

Williams RB: Epidemiological aspects of the use of live anticoccidial vaccines for chickens, *Int J Parasitol* 28:1089-1098, 1998.

Zambrano-Villa S, Rosales-Borjas D, Carrero JC, Ortiz-Ortiz L: How protozoan parasites evade the immune response, *Trends Immunol* 18:272-278, 2002.

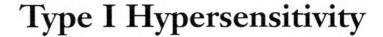

Type I Hypersensitivity

The importance of mast cells in inducing acute inflammation was discussed at the beginning of this book. Mast cells serve as sentinel cells that release inflammatory molecules in response to microbial invasion or tissue damage (Chapter 2). This release normally occurs in a controlled manner and ensures that the intensity of the inflammation is appropriate to the body's immediate needs. Type I hypersensitivity reactions, in contrast, are a form of acute inflammation resulting from the "explosive" release of mast cell granule contents. This type of response occurs when antigens bind to IgE bound to receptors on mast cells (Figure 26-1). The benefits of this type of acute inflammation are unclear, but it is of major clinical significance in veterinary medicine (Box 26-1).

INDUCTION OF TYPE I HYPERSENSITIVITY

All animals are exposed to many environmental antigens in food and in inhaled air. Most normal animals respond to these antigens by producing IgG or IgA antibodies, and there is no obvious clinical consequence. Some animals, however, may respond to environmental antigens by mounting an exaggerated Th2 response and produce IgE antibodies constantly and excessively. It is these animals that develop type I hypersensitivity reactions or allergies. The excessive production of IgE is called atopy, and affected individuals are said to be atopic. The origins of atopy and type I hypersensitivity depend on the interaction of multiple genes and environmental factors. The genetics of atopy and allergy are complex. Thus if both parents are atopic, most of their offspring will also be atopic and will suffer from allergies. If only one parent is atopic, the percentage of atopic offspring varies. There is also a breed predisposition to atopy in dogs. For example, atopic dermatitis is most commonly observed in terriers (Cairn, West Highland white, Scottish), Dalmatians, and Irish setters, although nonpurebred dogs may also be affected. In humans, some allergic individuals overexpress IL-4. This leads to excessive Th2 cell activity and enhanced IgE production.

Evidence also points to environmental factors such as childhood infections as influencing the development of atopy. Thus children who have had multiple infections when young appear to be less likely to develop allergies

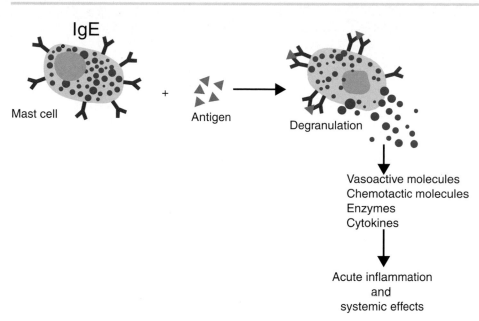

Figure 26-1. The mechanism of type I hypersensitivity reactions. Numerous biologically active molecules are released by mast cells and basophils when antigen cross-links two IgE molecules on the mast cell surface. Some are produced immediately. Others take several hours to synthesize.

than those not exposed to such infections. On the other hand, early contact with allergens (for example, on the first day of life) predisposes puppies to develop significantly higher IgE levels than puppies sensitized at 4 months of age (Box 26-2).

Normal animals infested by parasitic worms and insects also produce large amounts of IgE. It is believed that IgE may have evolved specifically to counteract these organisms. Indeed, the self-cure reaction seen in parasitized sheep has long been the only well-characterized beneficial feature of type I hypersensitivity (Chapter 25).

IMMUNOGLOBULIN E

IgE is an immunoglobulin of conventional four-chain structure with a molecular weight of about 200 kDa (Figure 13-7). It is found in serum in exquisitely small quantities (9 to 700 µg/ml in dogs), and its half-life there is only 2 days. Most of the body's IgE is not found in the

bloodstream but is firmly bound to Fcε receptors on tissue mast cells, where it has a half-life of 11 to 12 days. Some IgG subclasses may also bind to mast cell receptors and mediate type I hypersensitivity reactions. For example, IgG4 is associated with atopic dermatitis in the dog. However, the affinity of these subclasses for mast cells is much lower than that of IgE, and they are of much less clinical significance.

IgE Production

Irrespective of the predisposing factors, atopic individuals capture antigens using DC2 dendritic cells. These

---

BOX 26–1

Nomenclature

IgE mediates immediate hypersensitivity reactions, so called because they develop within seconds or minutes after exposure to antigen. This type of hypersensitivity reaction is also commonly called an allergy. Antigens that stimulate allergies may be called allergens. If an immediate hypersensitivity reaction is systemic and life-threatening, it is called anaphylaxis or anaphylactic shock. Sometimes an animal may have a reaction that is similar to anaphylaxis but is not immunologically mediated. This type of reaction is described as anaphylactoid.

BOX 26–2

Vertical Transmission of Allergies in Dogs!

There is growing evidence that the allergic status of parent animals, especially mothers, directly influences the development of allergies in their offspring. Thus in one experiment, two litters of newborn puppies from ragweed-allergic beagles were compared with two litters from nonallergic beagles. (The genetic differences between the parent animals were minimal.) The puppies were repeatedly exposed to ragweed pollen in their inhaled air beginning 1 week after birth. By 40 weeks of age, the puppies from allergic parents had produced high levels of total IgE and ragweed-specific IgE. The puppies from nonallergic parents had produced only IgG antibodies to ragweed. The puppies from allergic parents had eosinophils in their lung washings and developed asthmatic responses to inhaled ragweed pollen. The puppies from nonallergic parents did not. The mechanisms of this effect are unknown; however, it is believed that factors ingested with the mother's colostrum favor the switch to a Th2 response in the puppies from allergic mothers.

Data from Barrett EG, Rudolph K, et al: *Immunology* 110: 493-500, 2003.

dendritic cells generate Th2 cells. The Th2 cells produce the cytokines IL-4 or IL-13. These cytokines, together with costimulation from CD40, trigger B cell IgE synthesis. IL-4 is also produced in significant amounts by stimulated mast cells. This mast cell–derived IL-4 may alter the helper cell balance and enhance yet more Th2 cell production and IL-4 release (Figure 26-2).

IgE Receptors

There are two types of IgE receptors: high-affinity FcεRI and low-affinity FcεRII (CD23). There are two forms of FcεRI. One form is found on mast cells, basophils, neutrophils, and eosinophils. This form consists of one α, one β, and two γ chains ($\alpha\beta\gamma_2$) (Figure 26-3). The α chain binds IgE, the β chain stabilizes the complex, and the γ chains serve as signal transducers. (This same chain is also a signal transducer in FcγRI, FcγRIII, and γ/δ TCR.) The affinity of FcεRI for IgE is very high (10^{-10}M), so they bind almost irreversibly. The presence of FcεRI ensures that mast cells are constantly coated with IgE.

The second form of FcεRI is a trimer (it lacks a β chain) found on dendritic cells and monocytes. In allergic individuals this receptor binds IgE to antigen-presenting cells. When an antigen binds to this IgE it is directed into MHC class II presentation pathways. The expression of FcεRI is enhanced by IL-4 from Th2 cells. Thus a positive feedback loop (the allergy loop) develops (Figure 26-4). The antigen processing cells present

antigen more effectively to Th2 cells. The Th2 cells then secrete IL-4 and enhance IgE production.

The second type of IgE receptor, FcεRII (CD23), is a selectin found on B cells, NK cells, macrophages, dendritic cells, eosinophils, and platelets. In addition to acting as a receptor for IgE, FcεRII is also a ligand for the complement receptor CR2 (CD21) (Figure 26-5). Thus B cells expressing FcεRII will bind to CR2 on other B cells, T cells, and dendritic cells. By linking B cells to dendritic cells, FcεRII enhances B cell survival and promotes IgE production.

THE RESPONSE OF MAST CELLS TO ANTIGEN

When IgE binds to FcεRI on the surface of a mast cell it has no obvious immediate effect on the cell. The mast cell is now, however, primed to bind antigen. The mast cell can reside in tissues with its attached IgE acting like a mine in a minefield. If an antigen enters the tissue, encounters the mast cell, and cross-links two of these bound IgE molecules, the mast cell will be triggered to suddenly release all its granule contents and inflammatory mediators into the surrounding tissues (Figure 26-6).

This triggering is initiated because antigen cross-linking of two FcεRI causes activation of tyrosine kinases. These, in turn, activate phospholipase C, leading to the production of diacylglycerol and inositol triphosphate. These mediators then increase intracellular calcium and

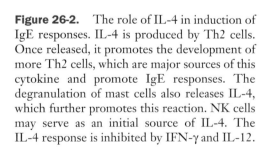

Figure 26-2. The role of IL-4 in induction of IgE responses. IL-4 is produced by Th2 cells. Once released, it promotes the development of more Th2 cells, which are major sources of this cytokine and promote IgE responses. The degranulation of mast cells also releases IL-4, which further promotes this reaction. NK cells may serve as an initial source of IL-4. The IL-4 response is inhibited by IFN-γ and IL-12.

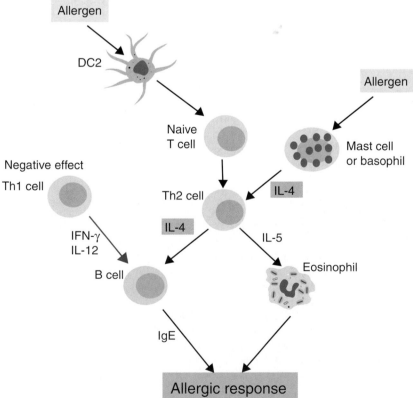

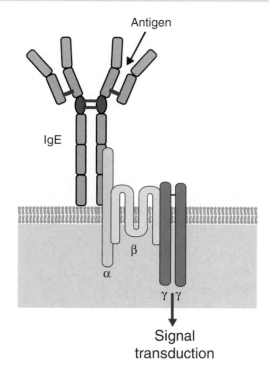

Figure 26-3. The structure of FcεRI. The tetrameric form containing two γ chains is found on mast cells and basophils.

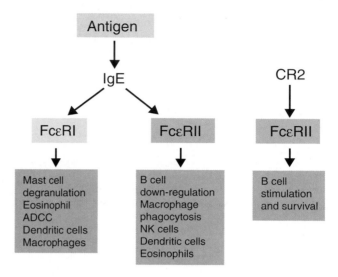

Figure 26-5. The combination of the Fcε receptors with their ligands stimulates a variety of different responses in mast cells depending on the combination of stimuli.

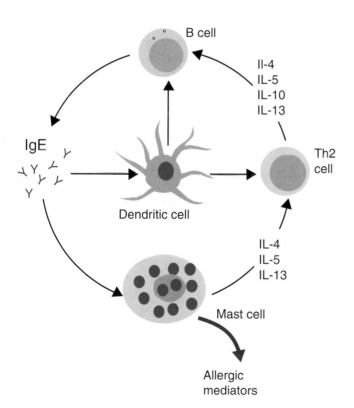

Figure 26-4. The allergy loop. Dendritic cells express trimeric FcεRI and as a result can bind antigen bound to IgE. This antigen, once processed, stimulates Th2 responses. These Th2 cells in turn secrete cytokines, which further promote the IgE response.

activate protein kinases. The protein kinases phosphorylate myosin in intracellular filaments and make the granules move to the cell surface, fuse with the plasma membrane, and release their contents into the extracellular fluid.

Cross-linking of two FcεRI also activates phospholipase A, which acts on membrane phospholipids to produce arachidonic acid. Other enzymes then convert the arachidonic acid to leukotrienes and prostaglandins. Finally, the protein kinases promote transcription and expression of genes coding for many different cytokines.

These mast cell responses are extremely rapid. For example, granules are released within seconds after antigen binds to IgE (Figure 26-7). Because the release is rapid and extensive, sudden acute inflammation develops. Degranulated mast cells do not die but, given time, will regenerate their granules.

Mast Cell–Derived Mediators

Mast cells are loaded with a complex mixture of inflammatory mediators, enzymes, and cytokines. Triggering of receptor-bound IgE by antigen causes the mast cells to release all these molecules and triggers the productions of many others. All these molecules (both preformed and newly synthesized) generate the acute inflammation characteristic of type I hypersensitivity response (Figure 26-8). These molecules have been described in detail in Chapter 2.

Regulation of Mast Cell Degranulation

Mast cells express two types of surface receptor for catecholamines (α and β adrenoceptors), that regulate their activity. These G-protein–linked adrenoceptors have opposing effects. Thus molecules that stimulate

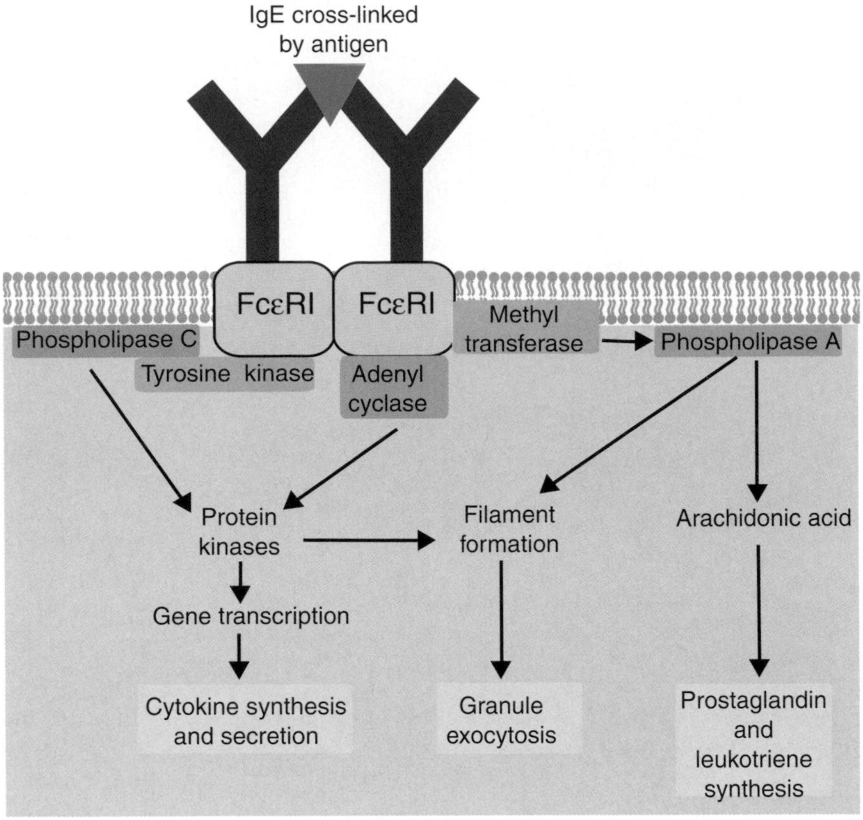

Figure 26-6. A simplified view of mast cell signal transduction. The process is triggered by cross-linking two bound IgE molecules with antigen. The combined signal eventually leads to degranulation (granule exocytosis), leukotriene and prostaglandin synthesis, and cytokine production.

β receptors (such as norepinephrine and phenylephrine) or block β receptors (such as propranolol) enhance mast cell degranulation (Table 26-1). In contrast, molecules that stimulate β receptors inhibit mast cell degranulation. These beta agonists include isoproterenol, epinephrine, and salbutamol and are widely used in the treatment of allergies. β-receptor blockers, in contrast, by enhancing mast cell degranulation, promote allergies. For example, some respiratory tract pathogens such as *Bordetella pertussis* or *Haemophilus influenzae* cause β blockage. As a result, the airways of infected animals are more likely to become severely inflamed because of mast cell degranulation. These infections may also predispose animals to the development of respiratory allergies.

Regulation of the Response to Mast Cell Mediators

The α and β adrenoceptors are found not only on mast cells but also on secretory and smooth muscle cells throughout the body. Alpha agonists mediate vasoconstriction and may be of use treating severe allergic reactions, reducing edema and raising blood pressure. Beta agonists mediate smooth muscle relaxation and may therefore reduce the severity of smooth muscle contraction. Pure α and β agonists are of only limited use in the treatment of allergic diseases because each alone is insufficient to counteract all the effects of mast cell–derived factors. Epinephrine (or adrenaline), on the other hand, has both

α and β adrenergic activity. In addition to causing vasoconstriction in skin and viscera, its β effects cause smooth muscle to relax. This combination of effects is well suited to combat the vasodilation and smooth muscle contraction produced in type I hypersensitivity. Ideally, epinephrine solution should be available whenever potential allergens are administered to animals.

The Late-Phase Reaction

When antigen is injected into the skin of an allergic animal, two distinct inflammatory reactions occur. There is an immediate acute inflammatory reaction that occurs within 10 to 20 minutes as a result of mast cell degranulation. This is followed several hours later by a late-phase reaction, which peaks at 6 to 12 hours and then gradually diminishes. This late-phase reaction is characterized by redness, edema, and pruritus. The reaction is especially obvious if large doses of antigen are administered. It is believed that the late reaction results from the release of inflammatory mediators by eosinophils and neutrophils attracted by mast cell–derived chemotactic factors.

BASOPHILS

The least numerous granulocyte, the basophils, are so called because their cytoplasmic granules stain intensely with basophilic dyes, such as hematoxylin (Figure 26-9).

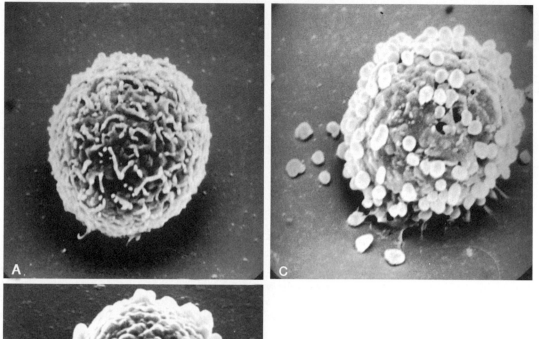

Figure 26-7. Scanning electron micrographs. **A,** A normal rat mast cell. **B,** A sensitized mast cell fixed 5 seconds after exposure to antigen. **C,** A sensitized mast cell fixed 60 seconds after exposure to antigen (×3000). (From Tizard IR, Holmes WL: *Int Arch Allergy Appl Immunol* 46:867-879, 1974.)

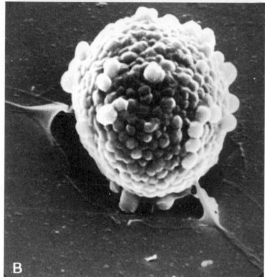

Granule exocytosis - seconds, minutes
Histamine
Serotonin
Tryptase
Kallikreins
Proteases
Proteoglycans

Eicosanoid synthesis and secretion - minutes
Leukotrienes
Prostaglandins
Platelet-activating factor

Cytokine synthesis and secretion - hours
IL-4
IL-5
IL-6
IL-13
TNF-α
MIP-1α

Figure 26-8. The soluble mediators released from degranulating mast cells. These fall into three categories: molecules released from exocytosed granules, lipids (eicosanoids) synthesized within minutes, and proteins synthesized over several hours.

TABLE 26-1
Effects of Stimulating α and β Adrenoceptors

System	α Receptor Stimulation or β Blockade	β Receptor Stimulation or α Blockade
Mast cells	Enhances degranulation	Suppresses degranulation
Smooth muscle	Contracts	Relaxes
Blood vessels	Constricts	Dilates

Basophils constitute about 0.5% of blood leukocytes. They are not normally found in extravascular tissues but may enter tissues under the influence of some T cell–derived chemokines. Basophils are terminally differentiated granulocytes. They are not mast cell precursors, but the precise relationship of basophils to mast cells is unclear. Basophil granules contain a complex mixture of vasoactive molecules similar to those found in mast cells.

EOSINOPHILS

Tissues undergoing type I hypersensitivity reactions characteristically contain large numbers of eosinophils. These cells are attracted to sites of mast cell degranulation, where they degranulate and release their own biologically active molecules.

Eosinophils are polymorphonuclear cells, slightly larger than neutrophils, with cytoplasmic granules that stain intensely with the red dye eosin (Figure 26-10). They originate in the bone marrow and spend about 30 minutes circulating in the bloodstream before migrating into the tissues, where they have a half-life of about 12 days. The proportion of eosinophils among the blood leukocytes varies greatly since it is affected by the presence of parasites. Normal values range from 2% in dogs to about 10% in cattle.

Eosinophils contain two types of granule (Figures 26-11 and 26-12). Their small, primary granules contain arylsulfatase, peroxidase, and acid phosphatase. Their large crystalloid granules have a core of major basic protein (MBP) surrounded by a matrix containing eosinophil cationic protein (ECP), eosinophil peroxidase (EPO), and eosinophil-derived neurotoxin (EDN).

Eosinophil Activation

The presence of eosinophils is characteristic of type I hypersensitivity reactions. Two mechanisms are involved in mobilizing eosinophils (Figure 26-13). First, Th2 cells and mast cells produce molecules that stimulate the release of eosinophils into the bloodstream. These include cytokines, such as IL-5, and the chemokines known as eotaxins. Thus Th2 cells mobilize eosinophils at the same time that they stimulate IgE responses. Second, these eosinophils are attracted to sites of mast cell degranulation by other molecules. These include the eotaxins, as well as mast cell products such as histamine and its breakdown product imidiazoleacetic acid, leukotriene B$_4$, and platelet-activating factor. Activated eosinophils are especially attracted by CXCL8 (IL-8) complexed to IgA (Table 26-2).

Once they reach sites of mast cell degranulation, the eosinophils are activated by these same molecules. The mobilization and activation of eosinophils enhances their ability to kill parasites and supports the contention that the major role of the IgE mediated responses is the control of helminth parasites. (Chapter 25).

Eosinophil Degranulation and Mediators

Although eosinophils can phagocytose small particles, they are much more suited to extracellular destruction of large parasites since they can degranulate into the surrounding fluid. Eosinophils undergo a process called piecemeal degranulation. In this process small vesicles bud off the secondary granules and are released into the tissues (Figure 26-14). This degranulation occurs in response to IgE-coated parasites, antigen-bound IgE, many chemokines, PAF, and C5a.

Eosinophil granules contain a mixture of inflammatory and toxic mediators, including cationic proteins, peroxidase, and major basic protein. Eosinophils can

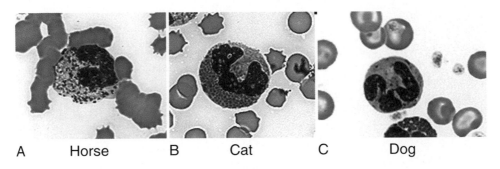

A Horse   B Cat   C Dog

Figure 26-9. Light photomicrographs of peripheral blood basophils from a horse (**A**), a cat (**B**), and a dog (**C**). These cells are about 10 μm in diameter; all were photographed at the same magnification. Giemsa stain. (Courtesy of Dr. MC Johnson.)

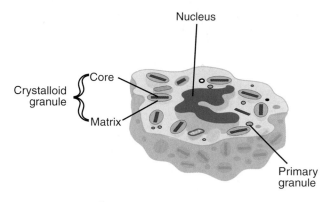

Figure 26-10. The major structural features of an eosinophil.

produce their own CCL5 and CCL11 so that additional eosinophils can be attracted to the inflammatory focus. Eosinophils also produce lipid mediators such as leukotrienes and PAF. Particles bound to eosinophil receptors trigger a powerful respiratory burst. The eosinophil peroxidase uses bromide in preference to chloride, thus producing OBr⁻. The peroxidase also has a role in generating nitric oxide. Eosinophils also release nitrotyrosine, a potent oxidizing agent.

The toxic granule contents released by degranulation include major basic protein, cationic protein, and peroxidase. All of these can kill helminths and bacteria and are important mediators of tissue pathology in allergic diseases. The proteins, for example, all damage respiratory epithelium. Eosinophils also synthesize and secrete

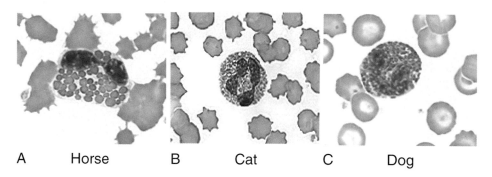

Figure 26-11. Light photomicrographs of peripheral blood eosinophils from a horse (**A**), a cat (**B**), and a dog (**C**). Each cell is about 12 μm in diameter. Giemsa stain. (Courtesy of Dr. MC Johnson.)

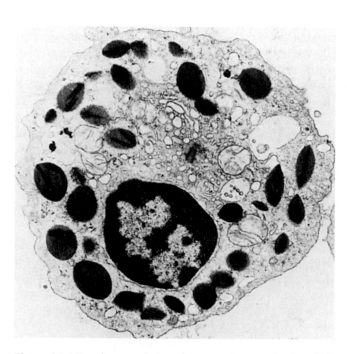

Figure 26-12. A transmission electron micrograph of a rabbit eosinophil. (Courtesy of Dr. S Linthicum.)

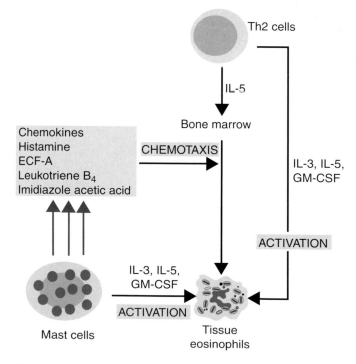

Figure 26-13. The regulation of eosinophil mobilization, chemotaxis, and activation.

TABLE 26-2	
Chemotactic Factors for Mast Cells, Eosinophils, and Basophils	
Chemotactic Factor	**Cell Type**
CCL11, CCL26, CCL7, CCL13, CCL28	Mast cells, basophils, and eosinophils
CCL3, CCL5, CXCL12, C3a, C5a, PAF	Eosinophils and basophils
CCL20	Eosinophils
CXCL1, CXCL8, CCL2	Basophils

many different cytokines, including IL-1α, IL-3, IL-4, IL-5, IL-6, GM-CSF, TNF-α, TGF-α, and TGF-β.

Regulation of Eosinophil Degranulation

Mast cells and eosinophils interact extensively in allergic reactions. Thus eosinophil-derived basic proteins activate mast cells to release histamine. Mast cells in turn release eosinophil chemotactic agents, activate eosinophils, and enhance the expression of eosinophil receptors. Mast cells can synthesize and secrete IL-3, IL-5, and GM-CSF, all of which promote eosinophil degranulation, growth, and survival.

CLINICAL TYPE I HYPERSENSITIVITY

The clinical signs of type I hypersensitivity result from the abrupt and excessive release of inflammatory mediators from mast cells, eosinophils, and basophils. The severity and location of these responses depend on the number and location of these cells; this, in turn, depends on the degree of sensitization of an animal, the amount of antigen involved, and its route of administration. In its most extreme form, antigen administered rapidly to a sensitized animal will cause generalized mast cell degranulation and massive mediator release. If the rate of release of

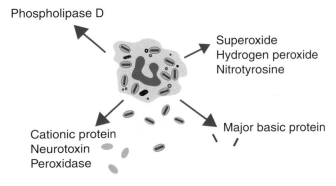

Figure 26-14. The principal inflammatory mediators released by degranulation of eosinophils.

vasoactive molecules from these mast cells exceeds its ability to respond to the rapid changes in the vascular system, an animal will undergo acute anaphylaxis and may die.

ACUTE ANAPHYLAXIS

The clinical course of acute anaphylaxis, or anaphylactic shock (Table 26-3), is determined by organ system involvement, which differs among the major domestic animal species. Many of the symptoms are a result of vasoactive molecules binding to their receptors and making smooth muscle contract in the bronchi, gastrointestinal tract, uterus, and bladder.

In cattle the major shock organ is the lung. Acute anaphylaxis is characterized by profound systemic hypotension and pulmonary hypertension. The pulmonary hypertension results from constriction of the pulmonary vein and leads to pulmonary edema and severe dyspnea. The smooth muscle of the bladder and intestine contract, causing urination, defecation, and bloating. The main mediators of anaphylaxis in cattle are serotonin, kinins, and the leukotrienes. Histamine is of much less importance. Dopamine acts in bovine anaphylaxis by enhancing histamine and leukotriene release from the lung, thus exerting a form of positive feedback. Because of the anticoagulant properties of heparin from mast cells, blood from animals experiencing anaphylaxis may fail to coagulate.

In cattle, in contrast to the other species, beta agonists such as isoproterenol potentiate histamine release from leukocytes, whereas alpha agonists, such as norepinephrine, inhibit histamine release. In addition, epinephrine potentiates histamine release in the bovine. The significance of these anomalous effects is unclear.

In sheep, pulmonary signs predominate in acute anaphylaxis as a result of constriction of the bronchi and pulmonary vessels. Smooth muscle contraction also occurs in the bladder and intestine with predictable results. The major mediators of type I hypersensitivity in sheep are histamine, serotonin, leukotrienes, and kinins.

The major shock organs of horses are the lungs and the intestine. Bronchial and bronchiolar constriction leads to coughing, dyspnea, and eventually apnea. On necropsy, severe pulmonary emphysema and peribronchiolar edema are commonly seen. In addition to the lung lesions, edematous hemorrhagic enterocolitis may cause severe diarrhea. The major mediators of anaphylaxis in horses are probably histamine and serotonin.

In pigs, acute anaphylaxis is largely the result of systemic and pulmonary hypertension, leading to dyspnea and death. In some pigs the intestine shows signs of involvement, whereas in others no gross intestinal lesions are observed. The most significant mediator identified in this species is histamine.

Dogs differ from the other domestic animals in that the major shock organ is not the lung but the liver, specifically the hepatic veins. Dogs undergoing

TABLE 26-3
Anaphylaxis in the Domestic Species and Humans

Species	Shock Organs	Symptoms	Pathology	Major Mediators
Ruminants	Respiratory tract	Cough Dyspnea Collapse	Lung edema Emphysema Hemorrhage	Serotonin Leukotrienes Kinins Dopamine
Horse	Respiratory tract Intestine	Cough Dyspnea Diarrhea	Emphysema Intestinal hemorrhage	Histamine Serotonin
Swine	Respiratory tract Intestine	Cyanosis Pruritus	Systemic hypotension	Histamine
Dog	Hepatic veins	Collapse Dyspnea Diarrhea Vomiting	Hepatic engorgement Visceral hemorrhage	Histamine Leukotrienes Prostaglandins
Cat	Respiratory tract Intestine	Dyspnea Vomiting Diarrhea Pruritus	Lung edema Intestinal edema	Histamine Leukotrienes
Human	Respiratory tract	Dyspnea Urticaria	Lung edema Emphysema	Histamine Leukotrienes
Chicken	Respiratory tract	Dyspnea Convulsions	Lung edema	Histamine Serotonin Leukotrienes

anaphylaxis show initial excitement followed by vomiting, defecation, and urination. As the reaction progresses, the dog collapses with muscular weakness and depressed respiration, becomes comatose, convulses, and dies within an hour. On necropsy, the liver and intestine are massively engorged, perhaps holding up to 60% of the animal's total blood volume. All these signs result from occlusion of the hepatic vein due to a combination of smooth muscle contraction and hepatic swelling. This results in portal hypertension and visceral pooling, as well as a decrease in venous return, cardiac output, and arterial pressure. H3 receptors appear to be involved in canine anaphylaxis. Identified mediators include histamine, prostaglandins, and leukotrienes.

In cats, the major shock organ is the lung. Cats undergoing acute anaphylaxis show vigorous scratching around the face and head as histamine is released into the skin. This is followed by dyspnea, salivation, vomiting, incoordination, and collapse. Necropsy reveals bronchoconstriction, emphysema, pulmonary hemorrhage, and edema of the glottis. The major pharmacological mediators in the cat are histamine and the leukotrienes.

SPECIFIC ALLERGIC CONDITIONS

Although acute anaphylaxis is the most dramatic and severe type I hypersensitivity reaction, it is more common to observe local allergic reactions, the sites of which are referable to the route of administration of antigens. For example, inhaled antigens (allergens) provoke inflammation in the upper respiratory tract, trachea, and bronchi, resulting in fluid exudation from the nasal mucosa (hay fever) and tracheobronchial constriction (asthma). Aerosolized antigen will also contact the eyes and provoke conjunctivitis and intense lacrimation. Ingested antigens may provoke diarrhea and colic as intestinal smooth muscle contracts violently. If sufficiently severe, the resulting diarrhea may be hemorrhagic. Antigen reaching the skin causes local dermatitis. The reaction is erythematous and edematous and is described as an urticarial type (*urtica* is Latin, meaning "stinging nettle") (Figure 26-15). Urticarial lesions are extremely irritating because of the histamine released; consequently, scratching may mask the true nature of the lesion.

Milk Allergy

Jersey cattle may become allergic to the α casein of their own milk. Normally, this protein is synthesized in the udder, and provided that the animals are milked regularly, nothing untoward occurs. If milking is delayed, however, the increased intramammary pressure forces milk proteins back into the bloodstream. In allergic cattle, this may result in reactions ranging from mild discomfort with urticarial skin lesions to acute anaphylaxis and death. Prompt milking can treat the condition, although some seriously affected animals may have to go

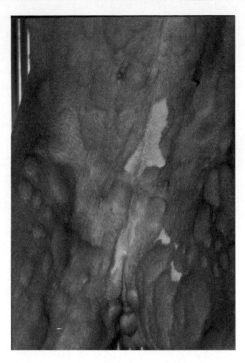

Figure 26-15. Severe urticaria in a boxer stung by three wasps. (Courtesy of Dr. G Elissalde.)

BOX 26–3

Terminology

It is important not to confuse *food allergy*, an immunologically mediated reaction to food allergens, with *food intolerance*. The American Academy of Allergy and Immunology has defined *food intolerance* as "those adverse reactions to foods that are not immunologically mediated." These reactions can include food idiosyncrasies, in which an animal responds abnormally to a food; metabolic reactions, in which a food component affects the metabolism of the animal; pharmacological reactions, in which some food components may act like drugs; and food poisoning, in which the adverse reaction is caused by a toxin or organism.

for several lactations without drying-off because of the severe reactions that occur on cessation of milking.

Food Allergy

About 2% of ingested protein is absorbed as peptide fragments large enough to be recognized as foreign. This antigen can travel in the blood and reach mast cells in the skin within a few minutes. It has been claimed that up to 30% of skin diseases in dogs are due to allergic dermatitis and that responses to ingested allergens may account for 1% of cutaneous disease in dogs and cats, although its true prevalence is unknown. The clinical consequences of food allergies are seen both in the digestive tract and on the skin (Box 26-3).

Adverse reactions to foods have many causes. These include not only food allergies but also food idiosyncrasy or intolerance and food poisoning, as well as "dietary indiscretion." About 10% to 15% of dogs with food allergies have gastrointestinal problems. The intestinal reaction may be mild, perhaps showing only as an irregularity in the consistency of the feces, or it may be severe, with vomiting, cramps, and violent, sometimes hemorrhagic diarrhea occurring soon after feeding. About half of affected dogs have a nonseasonal pruritic dermatitis. The skin reactions are usually papular and erythematous and may involve the feet, eyes, ears, and axillae or perianal area. The lesion itself is highly pruritic and is commonly masked by self-inflicted trauma and secondary bacterial or yeast infections. This pruritus tends to respond poorly to corticosteroids. In chronic cases the skin may be hyperpigmented, lichenified, and infected, leading to a pyoderma. A chronic pruritic otitis externa may also develop. The foods involved vary but are usually protein-rich foods such as dairy products, wheat meal, fish, chicken, beef, or eggs. In pigs, fishmeal and alfalfa have been incriminated. Food allergies have been reported in the horse but are uncommon. Wild oats, white clover, and alfalfa have been recognized as allergens in this species. The most reliable test for suspected food allergies is to remove all potential allergens and then feed a hypoallergenic diet. These elimination diets usually contain meat and carbohydrates from sources to which the animal is unlikely to have been exposed. Examples include mutton, duck, venison, or rabbit with brown rice or potato. Several commercial hypoallergenic diets are available to facilitate this diagnosis. The diet may be supplemented by adding other ingredients until the allergen is identified by a recurrence of clinical signs. Intradermal skin testing and RAST or ELISA are of limited usefulness in diagnosing food allergies (p. 321). Treatment involves elimination of the responsible food after correctly identifying it.

Allergic Inhalant Dermatitis

In dogs and cats, inhalant allergy most commonly leads to an atopic dermatitis with intense pruritus. Terriers and Dalmatians appear to be predisposed to this, but any breed may be affected. Animals may present with the allergic triad: face rubbing, axillary pruritus, and foot licking, although allergic skin lesions can be found anywhere on the body. The specific lesions are secondary to the pruritus and vary from acute erythema and edema to more chronic secondary changes including crusting, scaling, hyperpigmentation, lichenification, and pyoderma. Some animals may have otitis externa or conjunctivitis. The cutaneous inflammatory infiltrate contains mast cells, γ/δ T cells, dendritic cells, low numbers of eosinophils and neutrophils, and few B cells. The allergens implicated include molds; tree, weed and grass pollens (especially pollens that are small and light and are produced in very large quantities); house dust mites (*Dermatophagoides farinae* and *D. pteronyssinus*); animal danders; and fabrics such as wool. Depending on the source of allergen, the atopy may be seasonal. Hypersensitivity to a single allergen is uncommon, and most animals develop multiple sensitivities. Diagnosis is based on history and identification of the offending antigens by direct skin testing. Canine allergic dermatitis may be treated by corticosteroids or by hyposensitization therapy. Antihistamines and nonsteroidal antiinflammatory drugs seem to help some of the time.

Nasolacrimal urticaria (hay fever) is an uncommon manifestation of respiratory allergy in dogs and cats. Pollens usually provoke a rhinitis and conjunctivitis characterized by a profuse watery nasal discharge and excessive lacrimation. If the offending allergenic particles are sufficiently small, they may reach the bronchi or bronchioles, where the resulting reaction can cause bronchoconstriction, wheezing, and recurrent asthma-like paroxysmal dyspnea. It should be noted that Basenji dogs have unusually sensitive airways and experience a condition similar to that seen in humans with asthma. Cats are also recognized as suffering from asthma manifested by paroxysmal wheezing, dyspnea, and coughing. Although its pathogenesis has not been clarified, asthmatic cats respond well to corticosteroids and inhaled bronchodilators.

A familial allergic rhinitis characterized by extreme nasal pruritus, violent sneezing, dyspnea, mucoid nasal discharge, and excessive lacrimation has been observed in cattle. Depending on the allergen, it may be seasonal. The antigens involved are inhaled and come from a variety of plant and fungal sources. Diagnosis may be confirmed by skin testing. Nasal granulomas may form in chronically affected cattle. These consist of numerous polypoid nodules, 1 to 4 mm in diameter, situated in the anterior nasal mucosa. The nodules contain large numbers of mast cells, eosinophils, and plasma cells.

Atopic Dermatitis

Atopic dermatitis is a chronic, multifactorial syndrome characterized by chronically inflamed and itchy skin. It is very common in dogs (as many as 15% are affected) and has been recognized in cats, horses, and goats. Canine AD has a major breed predilection, being most common in retrievers, setters, terriers, beagles, cocker spaniels boxers, bulldogs, and Shar-Peis. It is commonly associated with reactions to environmental allergens such as house dust mites, pollens, and molds, such as the yeast *Malassezia pachydermatis*. However, the etiology of atopic dermatitis is complex and it is unlikely to be a pure type I hypersensitivity reaction of the conventional type. Certainly not all affected dogs have raised IgE levels.

Affected dogs commonly present with pruritus. Initially there may be no skin lesions, but this progresses to diffuse erythema. Chronic licking and scratching leads to hair loss, papules, scaling, and crusting. Hyperpigmentation and lichenification may occur. Skin lesions occur most commonly on the ventral abdomen and in the inguinal and axillary regions. About half of affected dogs have otitis externa. Dogs may develop focal "hot spots." The cellular infiltrate within the lesions contains mast cells, Langerhans cells, and γ/δ T cells. There are low numbers of eosinophils and neutrophils and very few B cells. Secondary bacterial or yeast infections complicate the disease Depending on the inducing allergen, the disease may be seasonal and relapsing. Once it starts, it tends to get progressively worse unless treated. Control of both allergies and secondary infection is critical.

Atopic dermatitis is provoked by environmental, food, and respiratory allergens that enter animals by the oral, respiratory, or percutaneous routes. The importance of the latter route is reflected by the frequency of lesions on contact areas such as the face, feet, and ears. Affected animals commonly show positive skin test responses to intradermally injected allergens. However, serologic assays such as the ELISA or RAST, which measure IgE antibodies to the offending allergens, rarely correlate with disease severity or the levels of IgE in the skin and are of limited usefulness. Blood IgE levels may drop to undetectable levels while levels in skin and skin reactivity remain high. There is thus little correlation between circulating and cell-bound IgE. The many false positive results probably reflect the fact that the immunologic reactions such as the presence of reactive Th2 cells and elevated IL-4 levels are largely restricted to affected skin. Affected skin contains more IL-4, IFN-γ, TNF-α, and IL-2 and less TGF-β compared with healthy skin. Allergen avoidance is the best treatment. Specific desensitization therapy gives good responses in up to 80% of cases, but secondary problems such as bacterial or yeast (*Malassezia*) infections or flea infestations must also be controlled. It may take several months before the benefits of immunotherapy become apparent. Topical therapy such as bathing with emollient shampoos helps considerably. Antihistamines are of limited usefulness but may be of benefit in mild cases. Essential fatty acids such as n(Ω)3 (fish oil) and n(Ω)6 (evening primrose oil) help some cases of atopic dermatitis, possibly by affecting lipid synthesis in the skin and promoting the synthesis of antiinflammatory eicosanoids. Glucocorticoids, such as prednisolone, produce rapid remission but may cause significant side effects. They should be used only as a last resort and given, preferably, by the oral route. Treatment with the prostaglandin analog misoprostol has given encouraging results. The immunosuppressive agents, cyclosporine and azathioprine, have also been effective in some cases of nonseasonal atopic dermatitis, as has the phosphodiesterase-inhibitor pentoxifylline.

Allergies to Vaccines and Drugs

An IgE response may result from the administration of any antigen, including vaccines. It is most likely to occur in vaccines that employ aluminum adjuvants. This must always be taken into account when animals are vaccinated. Severe allergies have been associated with the use of killed foot-and-mouth disease vaccines, rabies vaccines, and contagious bovine pleuropneumonia vaccines in cattle. IgE responses may also occur following administration of drugs. Most drug molecules are too small to be antigenic, but many can bind to host proteins and then act as haptens. Penicillin allergy, for example, may be induced in animals either by therapeutic exposure or by ingestion of penicillin-contaminated milk. The penicillin molecule is degraded in vivo to several compounds; the most important of these contains a penicilloyl group. This penicilloyl group can bind to proteins and provoke an immune response. In sensitized animals, injection of penicillin may cause acute systemic anaphylaxis or milder forms of allergy. Feeding of penicillin-contaminated milk to these animals can lead to severe diarrhea.

Allergies to many drugs, especially antibiotics and hormones, have been reported in the domestic animals. Even substances contained in leather preservatives used in harnesses, in catgut sutures, or compounds such as methylcellulose or carboxymethylcellulose used as stabilizers in vaccines may provoke local allergies.

Allergies to Parasites

The beneficial role of the IgE-mast cell–eosinophil system in immunity to parasitic worms was first observed in the self-cure phenomenon. Helminths preferentially stimulate IgE responses, and helminth infestations are commonly associated with many of the signs of allergy and anaphylaxis; for example, animals with tapeworms may show respiratory distress or urticaria. Anaphylaxis may be provoked by rupture of a hydatid cyst during surgery or through transfusion of blood from a dog infected with *Dirofilaria immitis* to a sensitized animal.

Allergies are also commonly associated with exposure to arthropod antigens. Insect stings account for many human deaths each year as a result of acute anaphylaxis following sensitization to venom. Anaphylaxis can also occur in cattle infested with the warble fly (*Hypoderma bovis*). The pupae of this fly develop under the skin on the back of cattle after the larvae have migrated through the tissues from the site of egg deposition on the hind leg. Because the pupae are so obvious, it is tempting to remove them manually. Unfortunately, if they rupture during this process, the release of coelomic fluid into the sensitized animal may provoke an anaphylaxis-like response that may kill the animal.

In horses and cattle, hypersensitivity to insect bites may cause an allergic dermatitis variously called Gulf Coast itch, Queensland itch, or sweet itch. The insects involved include midges (*Culicoides* spp.), black flies (*Simulium* spp.), stable flies (*Stomoxys calcitrans*), mosquitoes, and stick-tight fleas (*Echidnophaga gallinacea*). If animals are allergic to antigens in the saliva of these insects, biting results in the development of urticaria accompanied by intense pruritus. The itching may provoke severe self-mutilation with subsequent secondary infection that may mask the original allergic nature of the lesion.

In mange due to *Sarcoptes scabiei* in dogs and due to *Otodectes cynotis* in cats, allergies may contribute to the development of skin lesions. The infested dermis is infiltrated with mast cells, lymphocytes, and plasma cells, and an intradermal injection of an antigen leads to an immediate wheal-and-flare response. Infested animals may also make precipitating antibodies to mite antigens so that immune-complexes may contribute to the development of lesions.

Animals do not inevitably respond to arthropod allergens with a type I hypersensitivity. Thus, responses to *Demodex* mites and to components of flea saliva may be cell-mediated (type IV hypersensitivity, Chapter 29). Flea-bite allergic dermatitis is the single most important allergic skin disease. There is no breed or gender predisposition, but atopic animals as well as those exposed to fleas on an intermittent basis tend to get more severe disease. (This occurs, for example, in pets whose flea infestation is partially controlled.) Continual exposure to fleas at an early age appears to result in a form of hyposensitization. Pruritus is a consistent feature, as is a history of flea infestation. Affected animals, in addition to the characteristic clinical signs, show a reaction to intradermally injected flea antigen. Most positive animals will respond within a few minutes, but up to 30% may show a delayed reaction at 24 to 48 hours. Flea allergy is treated by total flea control. Hyposensitization therapy has not been shown to be successful in treating flea allergy.

The Eosinophilic Granuloma Complex

This is a confusing group of clinical conditions associated with various types of skin lesions (ulcer, plaque, granuloma) in cats. Although their cause is unknown, these conditions have been associated with flea or food allergies or inhalant dermatitis. It has been suggested that they are an allergic response to a feline autoantigen. A seasonal form has clearly been associated with mosquito bites. The eosinophilic plaques in the skin are intensely pruritic. As a result, the lesions may be masked by self-inflicted trauma. Histologically they are associated with a local mast cell and eosinophil infiltration, as well as an eosinophilia. Eosinophilic granulomas, in contrast, are not pruritic, and they present as a line of raised pink plaques. Some may present as scattered individual crusted papules. Eosinophilic ulcers are commonly located in the oral cavity or on the lips. Removal of the offending allergen may result in clinical improvement, and corticosteroid treatment is also of benefit. An idiopathic hypereosinophilic syndrome has been described in humans, cats, and dogs. It is characterized by a prolonged, unexplained eosinophilia, the infiltration of many organs with eosinophils, organ dysfunction (affecting especially the heart, but also the lungs, spleen, liver, skin, bone marrow, GI tract, and central nervous system), and death. An eosinophilic enteritis may result from canine hookworm infestation.

Lymphocytic-Plasmacytic Enteritis

The most common cause of chronic intestinal disease in the dog is associated with extensive infiltration of the lamina propria of the small intestine with lymphocytes and plasma cells. The disease presents with a history of chronic vomiting, diarrhea, and weight loss. Its cause is unknown, and it has been speculated that it might be autoimmune in nature. It is more likely, however, that it represents a local hypersensitivity reaction to dietary or microbial antigens. A similar condition is lymphocytic-plasmacytic colitis. This is a diarrheal disease in which weight loss or vomiting are infrequent. A hypoallergenic diet may result in significant clinical improvement and strongly suggests that the disease results from a food hypersensitivity. The condition may also respond well to glucocorticoids and the immunosuppressive drug, aza-thioprine. A monoclonal gammopathy has been associated with this condition. Lymphocytic-plasmacytic enteritis has also been described in cats, horses, and a cow.

DIAGNOSIS OF TYPE I HYPERSENSITIVITY

The term *hypersensitivity* is used to denote inflammation that occurs in response to normally harmless material. For example, animals normally do not react to antigens injected intradermally. If however, a hypersensitive animal is given an intradermal inoculation of antigen, this provokes local inflammation. Vasoactive molecules are released within minutes to produce redness (erythema) as a result of capillary dilation, as well as circumscribed edema (a wheal) due to increased vascular permeability. The reaction may also generate an erythematous flare due to arteriolar dilation caused by a local axon reflex. This "wheal and flare" response to antigen reaches maximal intensity within 30 minutes and then fades and disappears within a few hours. A late-phase reaction sometimes occurs 6 to 12 hours after injection of antigen as a result of the release of mediators by eosinophils and neutrophils.

Direct skin testing using very dilute aqueous solutions of various allergens has been widely used for the diagnosis of allergies in animals, especially those with allergic inhalant dermatitis. Following careful intradermal inoculation of an allergen solution, the site is examined for a local inflammatory response. The results obtained must be interpreted carefully since both false-positive and false-negative responses may occur. For example, the concentration of antigen in commercial skin testing solutions may be too low. Dogs may be up to 10 times less sensitive than humans to intradermal allergens such as pollens, fungi, or danders. Other problems may be due to the presence of preservatives in the allergen solutions. Results of skin testing are affected by steroid treatment. The precise set of allergens used for intradermal skin testing varies among different locations. However they commonly include an assortment of allergens from trees, grasses, fungi, weeds, danders, feathers, house dust mites, and insects. Intradermal skin testing is less commonly performed in cats because they fail to develop a significant wheal and the reaction is therefore difficult to evaluate.

An experimental technique used to detect IgE antibodies is called the passive cutaneous anaphylaxis (PCA) test. In this test, dilutions of test serum are injected at different sites into the skin of a normal animal. After waiting 24 to 48 hours, the antigen solution is administered intravenously. In a positive reaction, each injection site shows an immediate inflammatory response. The injected antibodies may remain fixed in the skin for a very long period. In the case of the calf, this may be up to 8 weeks. In the PCA test, it is sometimes difficult to detect very mild inflammatory responses. One way to make them more visible is to inject the test animal intravenously with Evans blue dye. The dye binds to serum albumin and does not normally leave the bloodstream. In sites of acute inflammation in which vascular permeability is increased, the dye-labeled albumin enters the tissue fluid and forms a striking blue patch (Figure 26-16). The size of this patch may be used as a measure of the intensity of the inflammatory reaction.

Serological methods of measuring the level of specific IgE in body fluids include the radioallergosorbent test (RAST), western blotting, and the ELISA (Chapter 16).

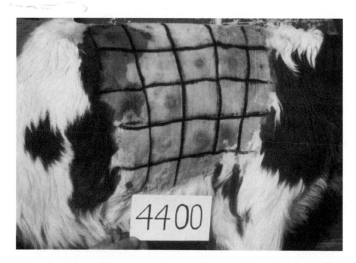

Figure 26-16. Passive cutaneous anaphylaxis (PCA) reactions in a calf. Several different sera were tested for PCA activity on the flank of a normal calf. (Courtesy of Dr. P Eyre.)

These are not subject to clinical bias, but there has been a poor correlation between the results obtained by serology or skin testing and clinical severity. There is also a poor correlation between ELISA results and intradermal testing. Serological assays are especially prone to a high level of false-positive results (low specificity). A negative ELISA will generally rule out atopy. Best results are obtained by testing for individual allergens rather than for groups of allergens. The reasons for this poor correlation between direct IgE measurements and in vivo methods such as skin testing are debatable. It may be that IgE itself is heterogeneous and may vary in its biological activity. It may also be that animals also differ in the properties of their mast cell receptors. Circulating IgE levels may drop very rapidly in the absence of allergen exposure. Heavily parasitized dogs may have elevated IgE levels, and this may result in false-positive serological results. It is also possible that immunoglobulins of other classes such as IgG4 may contribute to the development of allergic dermatitis in the dog and not be detected by an ELISA employing anti-IgE. For these reasons many veterinary dermatologists prefer skin testing, despite its drawbacks. It is of interest to note that atopic and parasitized dogs may have reduced IgA levels, an observation supporting the concept that a deficiency of IgA may predispose to increased IgE production (Chapter 20).

TREATMENT OF TYPE I HYPERSENSITIVITY

In practical terms, by far the most satisfactory treatment of allergic disease is avoidance of exposure to the allergen. Except for food allergies, however, avoidance may be difficult or impossible. Other treatments such as desensitization therapy may be used (see below). This has the potential to induce stable, long-term remissions, but immunotherapy of this type is not a substitute for avoidance. The principal indications for drug therapy include short-term temporary relief either while waiting to begin immunotherapy or while waiting for it to take effect. Drugs may also be useful for relief of transient recurrences or in animals in which immunotherapy is not possible. Many different drugs are available to treat type I hypersensitivity, although veterinarians tend to employ only a few of these. Corticosteroids are most commonly used to reduce the irritation and inflammation associated with the acute allergic response. These drugs can suppress all aspects of inflammation by inhibiting NF-κB activity and so blocking the production of prostaglandins and leukotrienes (Chapter 37). Corticosteroids have a considerable palliative effect on chronic type I hypersensitivities, but it is important to remember that these drugs can have serious side effects. They can be immunosuppressive and increase an animal's susceptibility to infection (Chapter 37).

The β agonists include epinephrine, isoprenaline, and salbutamol; α antagonists include methoxamine and phenylephrine. All have been used extensively in humans and are available for use in animals. Epinephrine is the most important drug used to treat anaphylaxis. It is rapidly absorbed following intramuscular injection and thus can rapidly reverse the clinical signs of shock. Another group of drugs widely employed in the treatment of type I hypersensitivity reactions are the specific pharmacological inhibitors. These drugs, by mimicking the structure of the active mediators, competitively block specific receptors. Thus H1 antihistamines such as diphenhydramine can effectively inhibit the activities of histamine. However, since histamine is but one of a large number of mast cell–derived mediators, antihistamines possess limited effectiveness in controlling hypersensitivity diseases in animals.

Desensitization Therapy

In many animals, allergic disease may be controlled though the use of allergy shots—injections of the offending allergen. These injections promote IgG rather than IgE production and reduce the recruitment of inflammatory cells. In humans, immunotherapy of this type reduces mast cell and eosinophil numbers in the lung, as well as the infiltration of CD4+ T cells and eosinophils in the skin. Allergy shots induce a shift in the dominant helper cell response from Th2 to Th1 cells (Figure 26-17). The resulting changes in cytokine production are the reason for the subsequent shift in allergen specific immunoglobulin production from IgE to IgG. It is also probable that allergy shots stimulate Th1 cells to release IFN-γ. This IFN-γ blocks the stimulation of IgE antibody synthesis by IL-4 from Th2 cells. Specific immunotherapy also induces the appearance of regulatory T cells, producing IL-10. IL-10 inhibits IgE production, mast cell activation, histamine and leukotriene

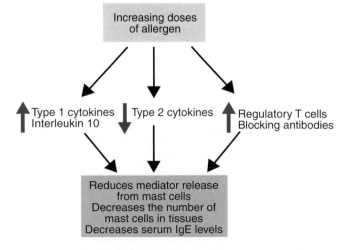

Figure 26-17. The principles of desensitization therapy. Increasing doses of allergen promote a Th1 response, while at the same time reducing the Th2 response and regulating antibody production.

release, and mediator production by neutrophils and eosinophils.

In desensitization therapy, small amounts of dilute aqueous solutions of antigen are administered. The first injections contain very little allergen. Over a number of weeks, the dose is gradually increased. If an animal's allergy is of the seasonal type, the course of injections should be timed to reach completion just before the anticipated antigen exposure. It has been estimated that up to 80% of dogs have a good to excellent response to desensitization. Cats may respond even better. On the other hand, horses with hypersensitivity to biting flies have a poor response to this form of therapy (although, paradoxically, they may show clinical improvement following immune stimulation).

SOURCES OF ADDITIONAL INFORMATION

Anderson GP, Coyle AJ: Th2 and Th2-like cells in allergy and asthma: pharmacological perspectives, *TIPS* 15:324-332, 1994.

Bochner BS, Schleimer RP: Mast cells, basophils and eosinophils: distinct but overlapping pathways for recruitment, *Immunol Rev* 179:9-15, 2001.

Borish L, Mascali JJ, Rosenwasser J: IgE-dependent cytokine production by human peripheral blood mononuclear phagocytes, *J Immunol* 146:63-67, 1991.

Chen T, Halliwell R, Pemberton A, Hill P: Identification of major allergens of *Malassezia pachydermatis* in dogs with atopic dermatitis and *Malassezia* overgrowth, *Vet Dermatol* 13:141-150, 2002.

Chesney CJ: Food sensitivity in the dog: a quantitative study, *J Small Anim Pract* 43:203-207, 2002.

Chrusch C, Sharma S, Unruh H, Bautista E, et al: Histamine H3 receptor blockade improves cardiac function in canine anaphylaxis, *Am J Resp Crit Care Med* 160:1142-1149, 1999.

Cocoran BM, Foster DJ, Fuentes VL: Feline asthma syndrome: a retrospective study of the clinical presentation in 29 cats, *J Small Anim Pract* 36:481-488, 1995.

Conrad DH: FcεRII/CD23, the low affinity receptor for IgE, *Ann Rev Immunol* 8:623-645, 1990.

Fadok VA: Diagnosing and managing the food-allergic dog, *Compend Contin Educ Pract Vet* 16:1541-1545, 1994.

Gröne A: Keratinocytes and cytokines, *Vet Immunol Immunopathol* 88:1-12, 2002.

Hill PB, Martin RJ: A review of mast cell biology, *Vet Dermatol* 9:145-166, 1998.

Hill PB, Moriello KA, DeBoer DJ: Concentrations of total serum IgE, IgA, and IgG in atopic and parasitized dogs, *Vet Immunol Immunopathol* 44:105-113, 1995.

Hillier A, Cole LK, Kwochka KW, McCall C: Late-phase reactions to intradermal testing with *Dermatophagoides farinae* in healthy dogs and dogs with house dust mite-induced atopic dermatitis, *Am J Vet Res* 63:69-73, 2002.

Jain NC: A brief review of the pathophysiology of eosinophils, *Compend Contin Educ Pract Vet* 16:1212-1218, 1994.

Kemp SF, Lockey RF: Anaphylaxis: a review of causes and mechanisms, *J Allergy Clin Immunol* 110:341-346, 2002.

Lindén A: Role of interleukin-17 and the neutrophil in asthma, *Int Arch Allergy Appl Immunol* 126:179-184, 2001.

Martin LB, Kita H, Leiferman KM, Gleich GJ: Eosinophils in allergy: role in disease, degranulation, and cytokines. *Int Arch Allergy Immunol* 109:207-215, 1996.

McEwen BJ: Eosinophils: a review, *Vet Res Comm* 16: 11-44, 1992.

McGorum BC, Dixon PM, Halliwell REW: Responses of horses affected with chronic obstructive pulmonary disease to inhalation challenges with mould antigens *Equine Vet* J 25: 261-267, 1993.

Mueller DL, Noxon JO: Anaphylaxis: pathophysiology and treatment, *Compend Contin Educ Pract Vet* 12:157-171, 1990.

Noli C, Miolo A: The mast cell in wound healing, *Vet Dermatol* 12:303-313, 2001.

Olivry T, Steffan J, Fisch R, Prélaud P, et al: Randomized controlled trial of the efficacy of cyclosporine in the treatment of atopic dermatitis in dogs, *JAVMA* 221:370-377, 2002.

Padrid P: Feline Asthma, *Vet Clin NA: Small Anim Pract* 30:1279-1292, 2000.

Schiessl B, Zeman B, Hodgin-Pickart LA, et al: Importance of early allergen contact for the development of a sustained immunoglobulin E response in a dog model, *Int Arch Allergy Immunol* 130:125-134, 2003.

Strait RT, Morris SC, Smiley K, et al: IL-4 exacerbates anaphylaxis, *J Immunol* 170:3835-3842, 2003.

Wisselink MA, van Ree R, Willemse T: Evaluation of *Felis domesticus* allergen I as a possible autoallergen in cats with eosinophilic granuloma complex, *Am J Vet Res* 63:338-341, 2002.

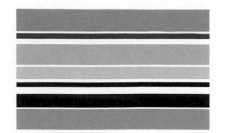

Red Cell Antigens and Type II Hypersensitivity

CHAPTER 27

Red cells, like nucleated cells, have many characteristic cell surface molecules that can act as antigens. However, unlike the major histocompatibility complex (MHC) molecules, red cell surface antigens are not involved in antigen processing, although they do influence graft rejection. (Grafts between blood group–incompatible animals are rapidly rejected.) Most red cell surface antigens are either glycoproteins or glycolipids and are integral components of the cell membrane that serve key cellular functions. For example, the ABO antigens in humans are anion and glucose transporter proteins, whereas the antigens of the M and C systems of sheep red cells are associated with the membrane potassium pump and amino acid transport, respectively.

If blood is transfused from one animal to another, genetically different individual, the red cell antigens will stimulate an antibody response. These antibodies will cause the rapid elimination of the transfused red cells as a result of intravascular hemolysis by complement and of extravascular destruction through opsonization and removal by the mononuclear phagocyte system. Cell destruction by antibodies in this way is classified as a type II hypersensitivity reaction.

BLOOD GROUPS

The antigens expressed on the surface of red blood cells are called blood group antigens or erythrocyte antigens (EAs). There are many different blood group antigens, and they vary in their antigenicity, some being more potent and therefore of greater importance than others. The expression of blood group antigens is controlled by genes and inherited in conventional fashion. Thus for each blood group system there exists a variable number of alleles. (If blood group alleles are invariably inherited together in groups of two or more, they are called phenogroups.) The alleles, in turn, control a variable number of erythrocyte antigens. The complexity of erythrocyte blood group systems varies greatly. They range from simple systems like the L system of cattle, which consists of two alleles controlling a single antigen, to the highly complex B system of cattle. The B system contains several hundred alleles or phenogroups that, together with the other cattle blood groups, may yield millions of unique blood group combinations. Although most blood group antigens are integral cell membrane components, some are soluble molecules found free in serum, saliva, and other body fluids and passively adsorbed onto red cell surfaces. Examples of such soluble antigens include the J antigens of cattle, the R antigens of sheep, the A antigens of pigs, and the DEA 7 antigens of dogs.

Animals can make antibodies against foreign blood group antigens even though they may never have been exposed to foreign red cells. For example, J-negative cattle have anti-J antibodies in their serum, and A-negative pigs have anti-A antibodies. These "natural" antibodies (or isoantibodies) are derived not from previous contact with foreign red cells but from exposure to similar or identical epitopes that commonly occur in nature (Figure 5-8). Thus many blood group antigens are also common structural components of other organisms, including plants, bacteria, protozoa, and helminths. However, the presence of these natural antibodies is not a uniform phenomenon, and not all blood group antigens are accompanied by the production of natural antibodies to their alternative alleles.

BLOOD TRANSFUSION AND INCOMPATIBLE TRANSFUSIONS

Blood is easily transfused from one animal to another. If the donor red cells are identical to those of the recipient, no immune response results. If, however, the recipient possesses preexisting antibodies to donor red cell antigens, they will be attacked immediately. These preexisting antibodies are usually (but not always) of the IgM class. When these antibodies bind red cell antigens, they may cause agglutination or hemolysis, or stimulate opsonization and phagocytosis of the transfused cells. In the absence of preexisting antibodies, foreign red cells stimulate an immune response in the recipient. The transfused cells then circulate until antibodies are produced and immune elimination occurs. A second transfusion with identical foreign cells results in their immediate destruction.

The rapid destruction of large numbers of foreign red cells can lead to serious illness, ie, a type II hypersensitivity reaction. The severity of transfusion reactions varies from a mild febrile response to death and depends on the amount of incompatible blood transfused. Early recognition of a problem may avert the most severe consequences. The most severe reactions occur when large amounts of incompatible blood are transfused to a sensitized recipient. This results in complement activation and massive hemolysis. The hemolysis releases large amounts of free hemoglobin, resulting in hemoglobinemia and hemoglobinuria. Large numbers of lysed red cells may trigger blood clotting and disseminated intravascular coagulation. Complement activation also results in anaphylatoxin release, mast cell degranulation, and the release of vasoactive molecules and cytokines. These molecules provoke circulatory shock with hypotension, bradycardia, and apnea. The animal may show sympathetic responses such as sweating, salivation, lacrimation, diarrhea, and vomiting. This may be followed by a second stage in which the animal is hypertensive, with cardiac arrhythmias as well as increased heart and respiratory rates.

If a reaction is suspected the transfusion must be stopped immediately. It is important to maintain urine flow with fluids and a diuretic because accumulation of hemoglobin in the kidney may cause renal tubular destruction. Recovery follows elimination of the foreign red cells.

Transfusion reactions can be prevented by prior testing of the recipient for antibodies against the donor's red cells. The test is called cross-matching. Blood from the donor is centrifuged and the plasma discarded. The red cells are then resuspended in saline and recentrifuged. This washing procedure is repeated (usually three times), and eventually a 2% to 4% suspension of red cells in saline is made. These donor red cells are mixed with recipient serum and then incubated at 37° C for 15 to 30 minutes. If the red cells are lysed or agglutinated by the recipient's serum, then no transfusion should be attempted with those cells. It is occasionally found that the donor's serum may react with the recipient's red cells. This is not of major clinical significance because transfused donor antibodies are rapidly diluted within the recipient. Nevertheless, blood giving such a reaction is best avoided.

HEMOLYTIC DISEASE OF THE NEWBORN

Female animals may become sensitized to foreign red cells not only by incompatible blood transfusions given for clinical purposes but also by leakage of fetal red cells into the bloodstream through the placenta during pregnancy. In sensitized females, these anti-red cell antibodies may then be concentrated in their colostrum. When the newborn animal suckles, these colostral antibodies are absorbed through the intestinal wall and so reach its circulation. These antibodies, directed against the blood group antigens of the newborn, cause rapid destruction of red cells. The resulting disease is called hemolytic disease of the newborn (HDN) or neonatal isoerythrolysis.

Four conditions must be met for HDN to occur. Thus the young animal must inherit a red cell antigen from its sire that is not present in its mother. The mother must be sensitized to this red cell antigen. The mother's response to this antigen must be boosted repeatedly by transplacental hemorrhage or repeated pregnancies. Finally, a newborn animal must ingest colostrum containing high-titered antibodies to its red cells.

BLOOD GROUPS, BLOOD TRANSFUSION, AND HEMOLYTIC DISEASE IN DOMESTIC ANIMALS

All mammals possess characteristic red cell antigens that can interfere with blood transfusions and on occasion cause hemolytic disease in newborn animals (Table 27-1). Although historically they were named alphabetically in order of their discovery, there is a growing tendency to add the prefix EA (erythrocyte antigen) to reduce confusion with MHC antigens.

Cattle

Eleven blood group systems—A, B, C, F, J, L, M, S, T', Z, and R'—have been identified in cattle. Two of these (B and J) are of the greatest importance. The B blood group system is one of the most complex systems known,

TABLE 27-1
Domestic Animal Blood Groups

Species	Blood Group Systems	Serology
Bovine	A, B, C, F, J*, L, M, R*, S, Z, T'	Hemolytic
Sheep	A, B, C, D, M, R*	Hemolytic Agglutination (D only)
Pig[†]	A*, B, C, D, E, F, G, H, I, J, K, L, M, N, O, P	Agglutination Hemolytic Antiglobulin
Horse[†]	A, C, D, K, P, Q, U	Agglutination Hemolytic
Dog	DEA 1.1, 1.2, 3, 4, 5, 6, 7*, 8	Agglutination Hemolytic Antiglobulin
Cat	AB	Agglutination Hemolytic

*Soluble blood group substances.

[†]In these species there is growing acceptance of the convention to denote red cell antigens with the prefix "EA" (erythrocyte antigen).

since it is estimated to contain more than 60 different alleles. These alleles are not inherited independently but in combinations called phenogroups. Because of the complexity of the B system, it is practically impossible to obtain absolutely identical blood from any two unrelated cattle. Indeed, it has been suggested that the complexity of the B system is such that there exist sufficient different antigenic combinations to provide a unique identifying character for each bovine in the world. Naturally, such a system provides an ideal method for the accurate identification of individual animals, and many breed societies use blood grouping as a check on the identity of registered animals. The C system is also complex, with 10 alleles combining to form about 90 phenogroups.

The J antigen is a lipid found free in body fluids and passively adsorbed onto red cells. It is absent from the red cells of newborn calves but is acquired within the first 6 months of life. J-positive cattle are of two types. Some possess J antigen in high concentration, and this may be detected both on their red cells and in serum. Other animals may have low levels of J antigen in serum, and it is only with great difficulty detected on red cells. (It is probable that a secretor gene controls the expression of J in cattle). J-negative cattle, lacking the J antigen completely, may possess natural anti-J antibodies, although the level of these antibodies shows a marked seasonal variation being highest in the summer and fall. Because of the presence of these antibodies, transfusion of J-positive red cells into J-negative recipients may result in a transfusion reaction even in the absence of known previous sensitization.

HDN in calves is rare but has resulted from vaccination against anaplasmosis or babesiosis. Some of these vaccines contain red cells obtained from infected calves.

In the case of *Anaplasma* vaccines, for example, the blood from a large number of donor animals is pooled, freeze-dried, and mixed with adjuvant before being administered to cattle. The vaccine against babesiosis consists of fresh, infected calf blood. Both vaccines cause infection and, consequently, the development of immunity in the recipient animals. They may also stimulate the production of antibodies against blood group antigens of the A and F systems. Cows sensitized by these vaccines and then mated with bulls carrying the same blood groups can transmit colostral antibodies to their calves, which may then develop hemolytic disease.

The clinical signs of HDN in calves are related to the amount of colostrum ingested. Calves are usually healthy at birth but begin to show symptoms from 12 hours to 5 days later. In acute cases, death may occur within 24 hours after suckling, with the animals developing respiratory distress and hemoglobinuria. On necropsy these calves have severe pulmonary edema, splenomegaly, and dark kidneys. Less severely affected animals develop anemia and jaundice and may die during the first week of life. The red cells of affected calves have antibodies on their surface (detected by an antiglobulin test) and may sometimes be lysed by the addition of complement in the form of fresh normal rabbit serum. Death is due to disseminated intravascular coagulation as a result of activation of the clotting system by red cell ghosts.

Serological testing. Bovine blood groups are detected by hemolytic tests. Washed red cells are incubated in specific antisera, and rabbit serum is used as a source of complement.

Sheep

The blood groups of sheep resemble those of cattle. Six blood group systems (A, B, C, D, M, R) are currently recognized. The ovine equivalent of bovine B is also termed B and, like the bovine system, is relatively complex, containing at least 52 different alleles. Sheep also possess an ovine equivalent of the bovine J system, called the R system. Two soluble antigens are found in this system, R and O, coded for by alleles R and r. The production of R and O substances is controlled by a gene called I and its recessive allele i. If a sheep is homozygous for i it possesses neither R nor O antigens. This interaction between the I/i genes and the R-O system is called an epistatic effect (Figure 27-1). R and O antigens are soluble antigens found in the serum of II or Ii sheep and are passively adsorbed onto red cells. Natural anti-R antibodies may be found in R-negative sheep. Sheep also fall into two groups according to whether their red cells have high or low potassium levels. This is regulated by the M blood group system. The Mb antigen acts as an inhibitor of potassium transport.

Serological testing. Sheep blood groups are detected by hemolytic tests. The only exception to this rule is the D system, which is detected by agglutination.

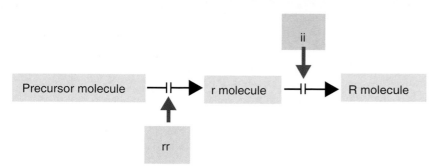

Figure 27-1. Regulation of expression of R blood group antigens in sheep. The I gene controls expression of the R system.

Pigs

Sixteen pig blood group systems have been identified (EAA-EAP). Of these the most important is the EAA system. The EAA system controls the expression of two antigens, A and O. Their expression is regulated by a gene called S (secretor) with two alleles S and s. In the homozygous recessive state (ss) this gene can prevent the production of the A and O substances (Figure 27-2). As a result, the amount of these antigens bound to red cells in these animals is reduced to an undetectable level (Box 27-1). A and O, like J in cattle and R and O in sheep, are not true red cell antigens but soluble molecules found in serum and passively adsorbed onto red cells after birth. Natural anti-A antibodies may occur in A-negative pigs, and transfusion of A-positive blood into such an animal may cause transient collapse and hemoglobinuria.

HDN in piglets formerly occurred as a result of the use of hog cholera vaccine containing pig blood. This vaccine consisted of pooled blood from viremic pigs inactivated with the dye crystal violet. Sensitization of sows by this vaccine led to the occasional occurrence of hemolytic disease of their offspring. There appeared to be a breed predisposition to this disease, which was most commonly seen in the offspring of Essex and Wessex sows. Affected piglets did not necessarily show clinical disease, although their red cells were sensitized by antibody. Other piglets showed rapidly progressive weakness and pallor of mucous membranes preceding death, and those animals that survived longest showed hemoglobin-

uria and jaundice. The severity of the reaction did not appear to be directly related to the anti-red cell antibody titer in the piglet serum. Since the withdrawal of all live hog cholera virus vaccines, the problems associated with their use have disappeared.

True HDN has also been recorded in the pig. The antibodies responsible are usually directed against antigens of the very complex EAE system. In addition to the development of hemolytic anemia in newborn piglets, the presence of antibodies to platelet antigens may cause a thrombocytopenia. This is seen clinically as a bleeding problem on tail docking and a tendency to bruise easily (neonatal purpura). On blood smears, the platelets may be clumped, and antiglobulin testing of them will yield a positive result. Deprivation of colostrum in an attempt to prevent piglets from absorbing anti-red cell antibodies may result in the newborn animals being highly susceptible to infection.

Serological testing. Pig blood groups are detected by agglutination, hemolytic, and antiglobulin tests.

Horses

Horses possess seven internationally recognized blood group systems (EAA, EAC, EAD, EAK, EAP, EAQ, and EAU.) Some, such as EAC, EAK, and EAU, are simple, one-factor, two-allele, two-phenotype systems. On the other hand, the EAD system is very complex with at least 25 alleles identified to date. Their major significance lies in the fact that HDN in foals is relatively common (Figure 27-3). In mules, in which the antigenic differences between dam and sire are great, about 8% to 10% of foals may be affected. In thoroughbreds and standardbreds the prevalence is considerably less, ranging from 0.05% to 2% of foals. This is true in spite of the fact that in up to 14% of pregnancies the mare and the stallion have incompatible red cells.

HDN may occur in foals from mares that have been sensitized by previous blood transfusions or by administration of vaccines containing equine tissues. Most commonly, however, mares are sensitized by exposure to fetal red cells through repeated pregnancies. The mechanism of this sensitization is unclear, but fetal red cells are assumed to gain access to the maternal circulation as a result of transplacental hemorrhage. Mares have been shown to respond to fetal red cells as early as day 56 after

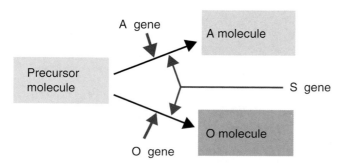

Figure 27-2. Production of A or O blood group substances by a pig requires the presence of the S gene. Pigs that lack this gene (ss animals) produce neither of these blood group substances.

BOX 27–1

The Inheritance of the A Blood Group System in Pigs

In pigs, the expression of the A blood groups is under the control of two loci. One, the A locus, contains two alleles, A and O, of which A is dominant. The other, the S locus, also contains two alleles, S and its recessive allele s. The S locus controls the expression of the A system so that A or O blood group factors will only be expressed if the animal carries at least one S gene.

Possible genotypes are therefore

AA   AO   OO   and SS, Ss, and ss

These may be combined thus:

Animals that are	AASS AASs AOSS AOSs	will all have A red cells
Animals that are	OOSS OOSs	will all have O red cells
Animals that are	AAss AOss OOss	will have neither A nor O red cells, i.e., – red cells

If we cross an animal of blood group O whose genotype is OOSs with an animal of blood group – whose genotype is AOss, the offspring may be either

AOSs   with blood group A
OOSs   with blood group O
AOss ⎱
OOss ⎰ with blood group –

---

conception. The greatest leakage probably occurs during the last month of pregnancy and during foaling as a result of the breakdown of placental blood vessels.

Maternal sensitization is usually minimal following a first pregnancy. However, if repeated pregnancies result in exposure to the same red cell antigens, then the maternal response will be boosted. Hemolytic disease is therefore usually only a problem in mares that have had several foals. The most severe form of the disease results from the production of antibodies directed against the Aa antigen of the EAA system. Anti-Qa (EAQ system) produces a less severe disease of slower onset. All in all, 90% of clinical cases are attributable to anti-Aa and -Qa although other minor antigens, such as Pa, Ab, Qc, Ua, Dc, and Db, have also been implicated. Mares that lack Aa and Qa are therefore most likely to produce affected foals. Pregnant mares may also produce antibodies to Ca

(EAC system), but these are rarely associated with clinical disease. Indeed preexisting antibodies to Ca may reduce sensitization by Aa. The presence of this anti-Ca in a mare may cause the rapid elimination of any foal red cells that enter its bloodstream and so prevent further sensitization. A red cell antigen that is found in donkeys and mules but not horses causes hemolytic disease in mules. Thus horse mares can readily make antibodies to this donkey antigen.

Antibodies produced by mares do not cross the placenta but reach the foal through the colostrum. Affected foals are therefore born healthy but sicken several hours after suckling. The severity of the disease is determined by the amount of antibody absorbed and by the sensitizing antigen. The earliest signs are weakness and depression. The mucous membranes of affected foals may be pale and may eventually show a distinct jaundice. Some foals

Figure 27-3. Pathogenesis of hemolytic disease of the newborn in foals. In the first stage, fetal lymphocytes leak into the mother's circulation and sensitize her. In the second stage, these antibodies are concentrated in colostrum and are then ingested by the suckling foal. These ingested antibodies enter the foal's circulation and cause red cell destruction.

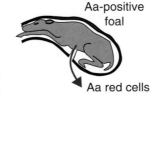
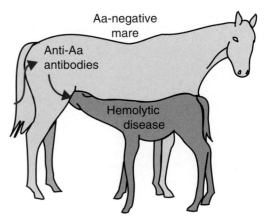

sicken by 6 to 8 hours and die from shock so rapidly that they do not have time to develop jaundice. More commonly the disease presents as lethargy and weakness between 12 and 48 hours of age, although it may be delayed for as long as 5 days. Icterus of the mucous membranes and sclera is consistent in foals that survive for at least 48 hours. Hemoglobinuria, although uncommon, is pathognomonic in a newborn foal. As a result of anoxia, some foals in the terminal stages of the disease may convulse or become comatose.

Hemolytic disease is readily diagnosed by clinical signs alone. Hematological examination is of little diagnostic use but may be of assistance in indicating appropriate treatment. Definitive diagnosis requires that immunoglobulin be demonstrated on the surface of the red cells of the foal. In the case of anti-Aa or anti-Qa, addition of a source of complement (fresh normal rabbit serum) causes rapid hemolysis. If hemolytic disease is anticipated, the serum of a pregnant mare can be tested for antibodies by an indirect antiglobulin test. By using red cells from horses with a major sensitizing blood group it is possible to show that the antibody titer increases significantly in the month before parturition when sensitization is occurring.

A test that has may be useful for detecting the presence of antierythrocyte antibodies in colostrum is the jaundiced foal agglutination test. This involves making serial dilutions of colostrum in saline. A drop of anticoagulated foal blood is added to each tube and the tubes are centrifuged so that the red cells form pellets at the bottom. In the presence of antibodies, the pellets clump together and remain intact when the tubes are emptied. Unagglutinated red cells, in contrast, flow down the side of the tube. Concentrated colostrum is viscous and tends to induce rouleaux formation that mimics agglutination. However, if the mare's blood is used as a negative control, this can be accounted for. The foal's blood should also be diluted in saline to ensure that the foal has not already absorbed antibodies and that false-positive results are not obtained.

Mildly affected foals [with a packed cell volume (PCV) of 15% to 25% and a red cell count greater than 4×10^6 µL] will continue to nurse. Those with a PCV of less than 10% will stop nursing and become recumbent. Marked icterus is suggestive of HDN in foals, but mild icterus may be seen in septicemia despite the fact that septic foals are not anemic.

The prognosis of uncomplicated hemolytic disease is good provided the condition is diagnosed sufficiently early and the appropriate treatment instituted rapidly. Management of HDN includes prevention of further antibody absorption, adequate nutrition, oxygen therapy, fluid and electrolyte therapy, and maintenance of the acid-base balance. Warmth, adequate hydration, and antimicrobial therapy are also critically important. In acute cases, blood transfusion is necessary. A red cell count less than 3×10^6/µL or a PVC less than 15%

warrants a blood transfusion. Transfused equine red cells have a half-life of only 2 to 4 days, so that transfusion is only a temporary life-saving measure. Compatible blood may be difficult to find because of the high prevalence of Aa and Qa in the normal equine population. A donor should not only be Aa or Qa negative but should also lack antibodies to these antigens. Exchange transfusion, though efficient, requires a donor capable of providing at least 5 L of blood as well as a double intravenous catheter and an anesthetized foal. A much simpler technique that avoids many difficulties is transfusion of washed cells from the mare. About 3 to 4 L of blood is collected in sodium citrate and centrifuged, after which the plasma is discarded. The red cells are washed once in saline and transfused slowly into the foal. The blood is usually given in divided doses about 6 hours apart. Milder cases of hemolytic disease may require only careful nursing.

If hemolytic disease is anticipated as a result of either a rising antibody titer or the previous birth of a hemolytic foal, stripping off the mare's colostrum and giving the foal colostrum from another mare may prevent its occurrence. The foal should not be allowed to suckle its mare for 24 to 36 hours. Once suckling is permitted, the foal should only be allowed to take small quantities at first and should be observed carefully for adverse side effects.

Neonatal thrombocytopenia has been recorded in the foal. Immunoglobulins can be identified on the foal's platelets, and antibodies to these platelets can be found in the mare's serum.

Serological testing. Horse blood groups may be identified by agglutination, hemolytic, and antiglobulin tests. As in the pig, each blood group system has a preferred test system. The complement used in the hemolytic test comes from rabbits but it must be absorbed before use to remove any antihorse antibodies.

Dogs

In dogs, eight red cell antigens are internationally recognized [dog erythrocyte antigen (DEA) 1.1, 1.2, 3, 4, 5, 6, 7, 8], but five others have been described. (An older nomenclature called them by the traditional alphabetic system, A, Tr, B, C, D, F, J, K, L, M, and N). The majority of these appear to be inherited as simple Mendelian dominants. Only the DEA 1 antigens are sufficiently antigenic to be of clinical significance. These include the alleles 1.1, 1.2, and 1.3. About 60% of dogs express a DEA 1 antigen. Naturally occurring antibodies to DEA 1.1 and 1.2 do not occur. Antibodies to DEA 7 may occur in 20% to 50% of DEA 7–negative dogs. Antibodies to DEA 1.3, 3, and 5 are found in about 10% of negative dogs, but these are usually of low titer and not of clinical significance. Therefore, it is recommended that canine blood donors be negative for DEA 1.1, 1.2, 3, 5, and 7. More than 98% of the canine population is DEA 4 positive. A universal donor would be an animal negative for all the DEA groups except DEA 4. Unless the blood type of the recipient is known, universal donor blood should only be used and a cross match performed on all recipients, even if universal blood is used. In practice, the most important canine blood type is DEA 1.1. About 33% to 45% of the dog population are DEA 1.1 positive and in general can be considered to be universal recipients. Dogs that are DEA 1.1 negative can also be considered to be universal donors. DEA 1.1–positive blood should never be transfused into a DEA 1.1–negative dog. If so, the recipient will become sensitized to DEA 1.1 blood and high titered antibodies produced. Subsequent transfusion of positive blood into such an animal could lead to a severe reaction. Similarly, if a negative bitch is sensitized by incompatible transfusions and mated to a positive dog, hemolytic disease may occur in her puppies. Natural HDN in dogs is extremely rare. It occurs when a DEA 1.1–negative breeding bitch is transfused with DEA 1.1–positive blood and subsequently bred to a DEA 1.1–positive male. The puppies develop a hemolytic anemia after 3 to 10 days.

The DEA 7 system (Tr system) is a soluble antigen system antigenically related to the human A, cattle J, sheep R, and pig A systems. Two antigens belong to the system Tr and O. An epistatic secretor gene controls their expression. Anti-DEA 7 occurs naturally in some DEA 7–negative dogs.

Serological testing. Agglutination at 4° C, hemolytic, and antiglobulin tests have all been used for the detection of canine blood groups. The source of complement can be either fresh dog or rabbit serum.

Cats

In cats, only one major blood group system, the AB system, has been reported. The AB antigens are glycolipids. Cats may be A, B, or AB. A is completely dominant over B. About 75% to 95% of cats are A positive, about 5% to 25% are B positive, and less than 1% are AB. However, this distribution differs among countries and among different purebred cat breeds. Thus in the United States more than 99% of domestic short-hair and long-hair cats are type A, whereas in the British short-hair breed only about 40% are type A. Severe transfusion reactions have been described in group B cats that received very small quantities of group A blood since 95% of B cats possess IgM anti-A. (Interestingly, only about 35% of A cats possess anti-B, and it is of the IgG and IgM classes and of much lower titer.) If completely matched blood is transfused into cats, its half-life is about 4 to 5 weeks. If, however, group B blood is transfused into cats of blood group A, its half-life is only a few days. If group A blood is transfused into a cat of blood group B, its half-life is just over 1 hour. It is this very rapid destruction that results in severe clinical reactions. Thus a group B cat given as little as 1 mL of group A blood will go into shock, with hypotension, apnea, and atrioventricular block, within a few minutes. Cross-matching is therefore essential in this species.

Hemolytic disease of the newborn has been recorded in Persian and related (Himalayan) breeds but is very rare. It occurs in kittens from queens of blood group B bred to sires of blood group A. The queens subsequently develop high-titered anti-A antibodies. Although healthy at birth, these kittens develop severe anemia as a result of intravascular hemolysis. Affected kittens show depression and possibly hemoglobinuria. Necropsy may reveal splenomegaly and jaundice. Antibodies to the sire's and the kitten's red cells are detectable in the queen's serum.

Serological testing. Agglutination and hemolytic tests are used for feline blood typing.

Chickens

Chickens have at least 12 different blood group systems with multiple alleles. The red cell B system is also the major histocompatibility system in the chicken. A hemolytic disease may be artificially produced in chicken embryos by vaccinating the hen with cock red cells.

Humans

In humans, HDN is due almost entirely to immunization of the mother against the antigens of the Rhesus (Rh) system (now classified as CD240). The condition is, or should be, of historical interest only because a very simple but effective technique is available for its prevention. This depends on preventing an Rh-negative mother from reacting to the Rh-positive fetal red cells that escape from the placenta into her circulation at birth. Strong human anti-Rh globulin is obtained from male volunteers and given to mothers at risk soon after birth. It acts by specifically inhibiting the B-cell response to that antigen (Chapter 18). Routine use of this material therefore prevents maternal sensitization, antibody production, and hemolytic disease. The use of a similar system is unnecessary in the domestic mammals where deprivation of colostrum is sufficient to prevent the disease.

PARENTAGE TESTING

Under some circumstances it is necessary to confirm the parentage of an animal. One way of doing this is by examining the blood group antigens of an animal and its alleged parents (Table 27-2). The method is based on the principle that since blood group antigens are inherited, they must be present on the red cells of one or both parents. If a blood group antigen is present in a tested animal but absent from both its putative parents, then parentage must be reassigned. Similarly, if one parent is homozygous for a specific blood group antigen, then this antigen must inevitably appear in the offspring. However, it must be recognized that blood typing procedures can only exclude, never prove, parentage.

TABLE 27-2
The Use of Blood Groups to Assign Paternity

	Blood group				
	1.1	1.2	6	7	8
Sire 1 ?	+	+	−	+	−
Sire 2 ?	+	+	−	−	+
Dam	−	−	+	+	−
Puppy 1	+	+	−	−	−
2	+	+	−	+	−
3	−	−	−	+	+*
4	−	−	+	+	−

Courtesy of Dr. D Colling.

*This puppy possesses DEA 8, which could not have come from sire 1 or its dam. Sire 1 could not have sired this litter.

TYPE II HYPERSENSITIVITY REACTIONS TO DRUGS

Red cells may be destroyed in drug hypersensitivities by three mechanisms. First, the drug and antibody may combine directly and activate complement, and red cells will be destroyed in a bystander effect as activated complement components bind to nearby cells.

Second, some drugs may bind firmly to cells, especially those in the blood. For example, penicillin, quinine, L-dopa, aminosalicylic acid, and phenacetin may adsorb onto the surface of red cells. Since these cells are then modified, they may be recognized as foreign and eliminated by an immune response, resulting in hemolytic anemia. Penicillin-induced hemolytic anemia is not uncommon in horses. These conditions can be suspected based on recent treatment with penicillin and improvement when its use is discontinued. It may also be possible to detect antibodies against penicillin or penicillin-coated red cells in these animals. Sulfonamides, phenylbutazone, aminopyrine, phenothiazine, and possibly chloramphenicol may cause agranulocytosis by binding to granulocytes, and phenylbutazone, quinine, chloramphenicol, and sulfonamides may provoke thrombocytopenia. If the cells from animals experiencing these reactions are examined using a direct antiglobulin test, antibody may be demonstrated on their surface. If these antibodies are eluted, they can be directed not against the blood cells but against the offending drug.

Third, drugs such as the cephalosporins may modify red cell membranes in such a way that the cells passively adsorb antibodies and then are removed by phagocytic cells.

TYPE II HYPERSENSITIVITY IN INFECTIOUS DISEASES

Just as drugs can adsorb onto red cells and render them immunologically foreign, so also can bacterial antigens such as the lipopolysaccharides, viruses such as equine infectious anemia virus and Aleutian disease virus, rickettsia such as *Anaplasma*, and protozoa such as the trypanosomes and *Babesia*. These altered red cells are regarded as foreign, and are either lysed by antibody and complement or phagocytosed by mononuclear phagocytes. Clinically severe anemia is, therefore, characteristic of all these infections.

SOURCES OF ADDITIONAL INFORMATION

Auer L, Bell K, Coates S: Blood transfusion reactions in the cat, *J Am Vet Med Assoc* 180:729-730, 1982.

Bailey E: Prevalence of anti-red blood cell antibodies in the serum and colostrum of mares and its relationship to neonatal isoerythrolysis, *Am J Vet Res* 43:1917-1921, 1982.

Becht JL: Neonatal isoerythrolysis in the foal, I, Background, blood group antigens and pathogenesis, *Compend Contin Educ Pract Vet* 5:591-599, 1983.

Bell K: The blood groups of domestic mammals, in Agar NS, Board PG (eds): *Red blood cells of domestic mammals*, Amsterdam, 1983, Elsevier Science.

Blue JT, Dinsmore RP, Anderson KL: Immune-mediated hemolytic anemia induced by penicillin in horses, *Cornell Vet* 77:263-276, 1987.

Bücheler J, Giger U: Alloantibodies against A and B blood types in cats, *Vet Immunol Immunopathol* 38:283-295, 1993.

Buechner-Maxwell V, Scott MA, Godber L, Kristensen A: Neonatal alloimmune thrombocytopenia in a quarter horse foal, *J Vet Intern Med* 11:304-308, 1997.

Colling DT, Saison R: Canine blood groups I Description of new erythrocyte specificities, *Anim Blood Groups Biochem Genet* 11:1-12, 1980.

Dimmock CK, Webster WR, Shiels IA, Edwards CL: Isoimmune thrombocytopenic purpura in piglets, *Aust Vet J* 59:157-159, 1982.

Harrell K, Parrow J, Kristensen A: Canine transfusion reactions, *Compend Contin Educ Pract Vet* 19: 181-199, 1997.

Jonsson NN, Pullen C, Watson ADJ: Neonatal isoerythrolysis in Himalayan kittens, *Aust Vet J* 67:416-417, 1990.

McClure JJ, Kohn C, Traub-Dargatz JL: Characterization of a red cell antigen in donkeys and mules associated with neonatal isoerythrolysis, *Anim Genet* 25:119-120, 1994.

McConnico RS, Roberts MC. Tompkins M: Penicillin-induced immune-mediated hemolytic anemia in a horse, *J Am Vet Med Assoc* 201:1402-1403, 1992.

Norsworthy GD: Clinical aspects of feline blood transfusions, *Compend Contin Educ Pract Vet* 14:469-475, 1992.

Symons M, Bell K: The occurrence of feline A blood group antigens on lymphocytes, *Anim Blood Grps Biochem Gen* 16:77-84, 1985.

Symons M, Bell K: Canine blood groups: description of 20 specificities, *Anim Genet* 23:509-515, 1992.

Wagner R, Oulevey J, Thiele OW: The transfer of bovine J blood group activity to erythrocytes: evidence of a transferable and of a non-transferable J in serum, *Anim Blood Groups Biochem Genet* 15: 223-225, 1984.

Whiting JL, David JB: Neonatal isoerythrolysis, *Compend Contin Educ Pract Vet* 22:968-976, 2000.

Yamamoto F, Clausen H, White T, et al: Molecular genetic basis of the histo-blood group ABO system, *Nature* 345: 229-223, 1990.

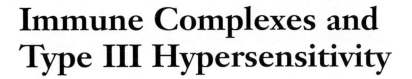

Immune Complexes and Type III Hypersensitivity

Acute inflammation can be triggered by the presence of immune complexes in tissues. Immune complexes formed by the combination of antibodies with antigen activate complement. When these immune complexes are deposited in tissues, they generate chemotactic peptides that attract neutrophils. The accumulated neutrophils may then release oxidants and enzymes into tissues, causing acute inflammation and tissue destruction. Lesions generated in this way are classified as type III or immune complex–mediated hypersensitivity reactions.

CLASSIFICATION OF TYPE III HYPERSENSITIVITY REACTIONS

The severity and significance of type III hypersensitivity reactions depend, as might be expected, on the amount and site of deposition of immune complexes. Two major forms of reaction are recognized. One form includes local reactions that occur when immune complexes form within tissues. The second form results when large quantities of immune complexes form within the bloodstream. This can occur, for example, when an antigen is administered intravenously to an immune recipient. Immune complexes generated in the blood may eventually be deposited in the walls of blood vessels. Local activation of complement then leads to neutrophil accumulation and the development of inflammation (vasculitis). Circulating immune complexes are also deposited in glomeruli in the kidney, and the development of glomerular lesions is characteristic of this type of hypersensitivity. If the complexes bind to blood cells, anemia, leukopenia or thrombocytopenia may also result.

It might reasonably be pointed out that the combination of an antigen with antibody always produces immune complexes. However, the occurrence of clinically significant type III hypersensitivity reactions results from the formation of excessive amounts of these immune complexes. For example, several grams of an antigen may be needed to sensitize an animal, such as a rabbit, in order to produce experimental type III reactions. Minor immune complex–mediated lesions probably develop relatively frequently following an immune response to many antigens, without causing clinically significant disease.

LOCAL TYPE III HYPERSENSITIVITY REACTIONS

If an antigen is injected subcutaneously into an animal that already has precipitating antibodies, then acute inflammation will develop at the injection site within several hours. This is called an Arthus reaction after the scientist who first described it. It starts as a red, edematous

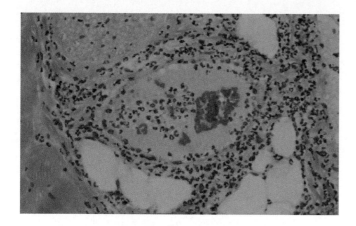

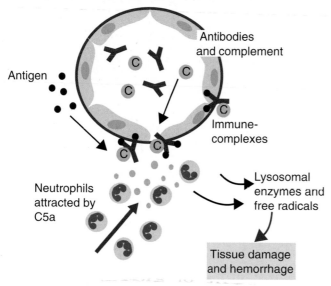

Figure 28-1. Diagram depicting the mechanisms of an Arthus reaction, as well as a histological section of an Arthus reaction in the skin of a cat 6 hours after intradermal inoculation of chicken red blood cells. (Courtesy of Dr A Kier.)

swelling; eventually local hemorrhage and thrombosis occur and, if severe, culminates in local tissue destruction.

The first histological changes observed following antigen injection are neutrophil adherence to vascular endothelium followed by their emigration through the walls of small venules into the tissues. By 6 to 8 hours, when the reaction has reached its greatest intensity, the injection site is densely infiltrated by large numbers of these cells (Figure 28-1). As the reaction progresses, destruction of blood vessel walls results in hemorrhage and edema, platelet aggregation, and thrombosis. By 8 hours, mononuclear cells appear in the lesion, and by 24 hours or later, depending on the amount of antigen injected, they become the predominant cell type. Eosinophils are not a significant feature of this type of hypersensitivity.

The fate of the injected antigen can be followed using a direct fluorescent antibody test. The antigen first diffuses away from the injection site through tissue fluid. When small blood vessels are encountered, the antigen diffuses into the vessel walls, where it encounters circulating

BOX 28-1

Antibodies Cause Tissue Damage

It has long been assumed that immunoglobulin molecules do not themselves damage antigens. The elimination of antigenic microorganisms and the tissue damage associated with this defense has been believed to result from complement activation or the activities of phagocytic cells. Recent evidence however has shown that antibodies alone can kill microorganisms and cause tissue damage. When provided with singlet oxygen from phagocytic neutrophils, antibodies can catalyze the production of oxidants including ozone. This ozone not only kills bacteria but can also cause significant tissue damage. Biopsies from Arthus reactions contain detectable amounts of ozone!

From Babior BM, Takeuchi C, Ruedi J, et al: *Proc Natl Acad Sci USA* 100: 3031-3034, 2003.

antibodies. Provided the antibodies involved are both precipitating and complement activating (and are therefore usually IgG), immune complexes form and are deposited between and beneath vascular endothelial cells.

The immune complexes act on two major cell types: mast cells and neutrophils. The relative contribution of each varies among tissues.

Immune complexes formed in tissues bind to mast cells through several FcγRs, especially FcγRIII. This binding triggers the mast cells to release their vasoactive molecules. Among the molecules released by mast cells are neutrophil chemotactic factors and proteases that activate complement.

The immune complexes activate complement to generate the chemotactic factor C5a (Figure 28-2). The neutrophils, attracted by C5a as well as mast cell–derived chemotactic factors, emigrate from the blood vessels, adhering to immune complexes and promptly phagocytosing them. Eventually the immune complexes are eliminated. During this process, however, proteases and oxidants are released into the tissues (Box 28-1). When neutrophils attempt to ingest immune complexes attached to a structure such as a basement membrane, they secrete their granule contents directly into the surrounding tissues. Neutrophils may also release their enzymes into the tissues before immune complexes are completely enclosed. These proteases disrupt collagen fibers and destroy ground substances, basement membranes, and elastic tissue. Normally tissues contain antiproteinases that inhibit neutrophil enzymes. However, neutrophils can subvert these inhibitors by secreting OCl⁻. The OCl⁻ destroys the inhibitors and allows tissue destruction to proceed. Neutrophil proteases also act on C5 to generate C5a, which stimulates neutrophil degranulation and enzyme release and so promotes further neutrophil accumulation and degranulation. Other enzymes released by neutrophils make mast cells degranulate or generate kinins. As a result of all this, inflammation and destruction of tissues (especially of blood vessel walls) results in the development of the edema, vasculitis, and hemorrhage characteristic of the Arthus reaction.

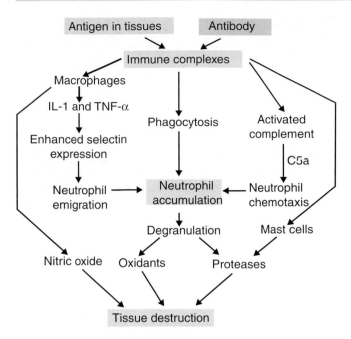

Figure 28-2. Some of the mechanisms involved in the pathogenesis of the Arthus reaction.

Although the classical direct Arthus reaction is produced by local administration of an antigen to hyperimmunized animals, any technique that permits immune complexes to be deposited in tissues will stimulate a similar response. A reversed Arthus reaction can therefore be produced if antibodies are administered intradermally to an animal with a high level of circulating antigen. Injected preformed immune complexes, particularly those containing a moderate excess of an antigen, will provoke a similar reaction, although, as might be anticipated, there is less involvement of blood vessel walls and the reaction is less severe. A passive Arthus reaction can be produced by giving antibody intravenously to a nonsensitized animal followed by an intradermal injection of an antigen, and real enthusiasts can produce a reversed passive Arthus reaction by giving antibody intradermally followed by intravenous antigen.

Although it is unusual for pure hypersensitivity reactions of only a single type to occur under natural conditions, there are some diseases in the domestic animals in which type III reactions play a major role. The classical Arthus reaction is usually produced in the skin, since that is the most convenient site at which to inject the antigen. However, local type III reactions can occur in many tissues, with the precise site depending on the location of the antigen.

Blue Eye

Blue eye is a condition seen in a small proportion of dogs that have been either infected or vaccinated with live canine adenovirus type 1 (Figures 24-7 and 24-8). The lesion in blue eye is an anterior uveitis leading to corneal edema and opacity. The cornea is infiltrated by neutrophils, and virus–antibody complexes can be detected in the lesion. Blue eye develops about 1 to 3

weeks after the onset of infection and usually resolves spontaneously as virus is eliminated.

Hypersensitivity Pneumonitis

Type III hypersensitivity reactions may occur in the lungs when sensitized animals inhale antigens. For example, cattle housed during the winter are usually exposed to dust from hay. Normally, these dust particles are relatively large and are deposited in the upper respiratory tract, trapped in mucus, and eliminated. If, however, hay is stored when damp, bacterial growth and metabolism will result in heating. As a result of this warmth, thermophilic actinomycetes will grow. One of the most important of these thermophilic actinomycetes is *Saccharopolyspora rectivirgula* (*Micropolyspora faeni*), an organism that produces large numbers of very small spores (1 μm in diameter). On inhalation, these spores can penetrate to the alveoli (Figure 28-3). If cattle are fed moldy hay for long periods, constant inhalation of *S. rectivirgula* spores will result in sensitization and in the development of high-titered precipitating antibodies to *S. rectivirgula* antigens in serum. Eventually inhaled spore antigens will encounter antibodies within the alveolar walls, and the resulting immune complexes and complement activation will cause a pneumonia (or pneumonitis), the basis of which is a type III hypersensitivity reaction.

The lesions of this hypersensitivity pneumonitis consist of an acute alveolitis together with vasculitis and exudation of fluid into the alveolar spaces (Figure 28-3). The alveolar septa may be thickened, and the entire lesion is infiltrated with inflammatory cells. Since many of these cells are eosinophils and lymphocytes, it is obvious that the reaction is not a pure type III reaction. Nevertheless, examination of the lungs of affected cattle by immunofluorescence demonstrates deposits of immunoglobulin, complement, and antigen. In animals inhaling low levels

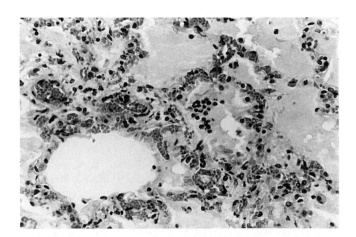

Figure 28-3. Histological section of the lung from a cow that died suddenly 24 hours after being fed moldy hay. The alveoli are full of fluid and the alveolar walls are thickened and inflamed. This acute alveolitis is probably due to a hypersensitivity reaction to inhaled actinomycete spores. Original magnification ×400. (Courtesy of Dr. BN Wilkie.)

of an antigen over a long period, proliferative bronchiolitis and fibrosis may be observed. Clinically, hypersensitivity pneumonitis presents as a pneumonia occurring between 5 and 10 hours after exposure to grossly moldy hay. The animal may have difficulty breathing and develop a severe cough. In chronically affected animals, the dyspnea may be continuous. The most effective method of managing this condition is by removing the source of the antigen. Administration of steroids may be beneficial.

A hypersensitivity pneumonitis also occurs in farmers chronically exposed to *S. rectivirgula* spores from moldy hay and is called farmer's lung. Many other syndromes in humans have an identical pathogenesis and are usually named after the source of the offending antigen. Thus pigeon breeder's lung arises following exposure to the dust from pigeon feces, mushroom grower's disease is due to hypersensitivity to inhaled spores from actinomycetes in the soil used for growing mushrooms, and librarian's lung results from inhalation of dusts from old books! Hay sickness is a form of hypersensitivity pneumonitis seen in horses in Iceland that is probably an equine equivalent of farmer's lung.

Two forms of chronic respiratory disease occur in horses. Recurrent airway obstruction (RAO) is seen in middle-aged horses and inflammatory airway disease in younger horses. RAO occurs in horses that inhale large amounts of organic dusts. It includes chronic obstructive pulmonary disease seen in stabled horses and summer pasture–associated obstructive pulmonary disease. Both are forms of bronchiolitis associated with chronic mold exposure. Horses with these syndromes may show positive skin reactions to intradermal inoculation of actinomycete and fungal extracts (such as *Rhizopus nigricans, Candida albicans, S. rectivirgula, or Geotrichum deliquescens*). They may also respond to aerosol challenge with extracts of these organisms by developing respiratory distress. Clinical signs may resolve on removal of the moldy hay and reappear on reexposure. However, there is little correlation between skin test results and severity of disease. Affected animals usually have large numbers of neutrophils or eosinophils in their small bronchioles, and high titers of antibodies to equine influenza in their bronchial secretions. The significance of the latter is unclear. However, levels of the chemokine CXCL8 (IL-8) are elevated in the bronchoalveolar washings of affected animals. Removal of clinically affected horses to air-conditioned stalls results in improvement of the disease, but this is reversed if the horses are returned to dusty stables. It has been suggested that continuous prolonged activation of bronchoalveolar macrophages by dust particles and air-borne endotoxins leads to excessive production of neutrophil chemotactic chemokines such as CXCL8 and CXCL2. These neutrophils then cause lung damage as a result of secretion of proteases, peroxidases, and oxidants.

Inflammatory airway disease affects up to 30% of young horses in training. Although commonly linked to bacterial or viral infections, in many cases no infectious agent can be isolated. Affected animals have airway inflammation associated with a neutrophil infiltration, but occasionally eosinophils and mast cells may be increased.

Staphylococcal Hypersensitivity

Staphylococcal hypersensitivity is a pruritic pustular dermatitis of dogs. Skin testing with staphylococcal antigens suggests that types I, III, and IV hypersensitivity may be involved. The histological findings of neutrophilic dermal vasculitis suggest that the type III reaction may predominate in some cases.

GENERALIZED TYPE III HYPERSENSITIVITY REACTIONS

If an antigen is administered intravenously to animals with a high level of circulating antibodies, then immune complexes form in the bloodstream. These immune complexes are normally removed either by binding to erythrocytes or to platelets, (Figure 28-4) or, if large,

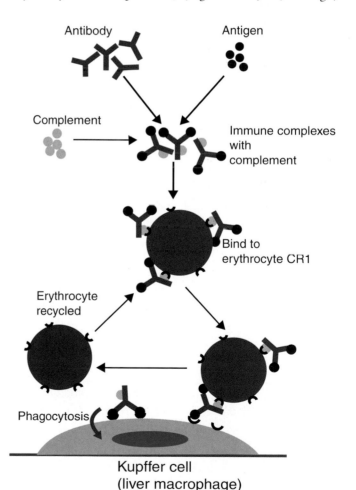

Figure 28-4. In primates, the normal process of removal of immune complexes involves their first binding to red cells. They are then carried to the liver where they are transferred to Kupffer cells for phagocytosis. In the absence of complement components significant accumulation of immune complexes occurs in tissues. In other mammals immune complexes bind to platelets.

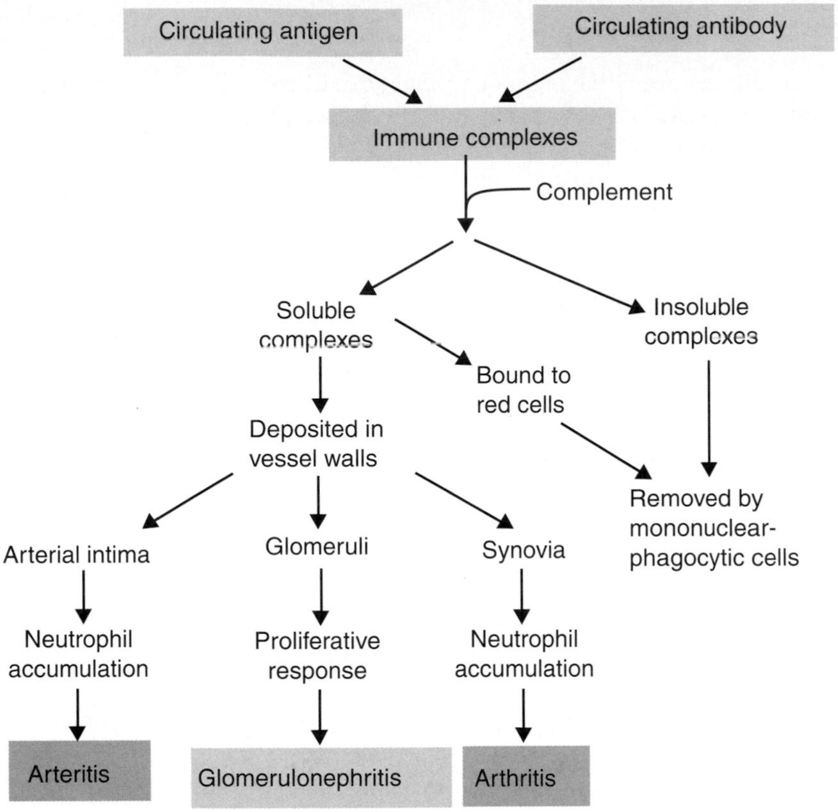

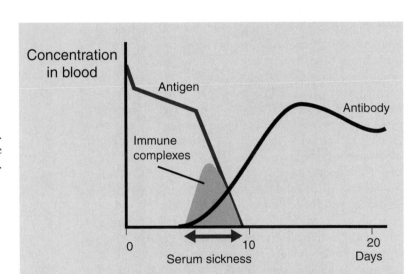

Figure 28-5. Mechanisms involved in the pathogenesis of acute serum sickness.

Figure 28-6. Time course of acute serum sickness. The appearance of the disease coincides with the generation of immune complexes in the bloodstream.

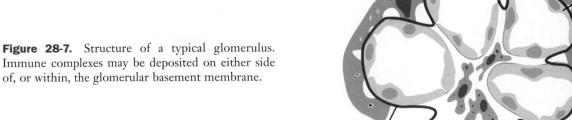

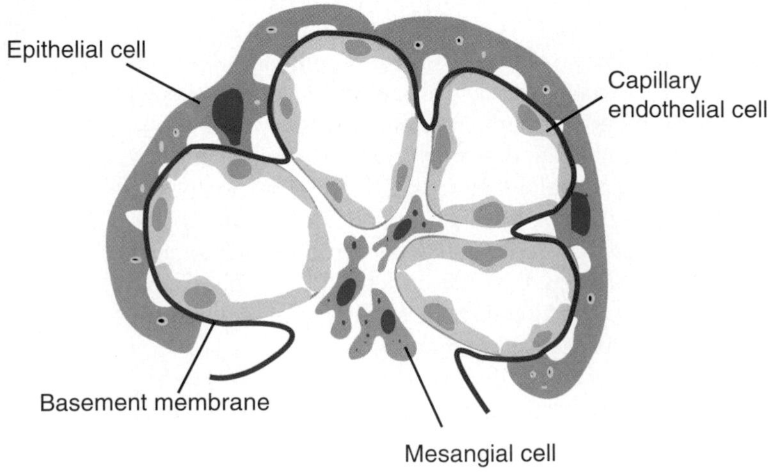

Figure 28-7. Structure of a typical glomerulus. Immune complexes may be deposited on either side of, or within, the glomerular basement membrane.

they are removed by the cells of the mononuclear phagocyte system. However, if complexes are produced in excessive amounts they may be deposited in the walls of blood vessels, especially medium-sized arteries, and in vessels where there is a physiological outflow of fluid such as glomeruli, synovia, and the choroid plexus (Figure 28-5). An excellent example of this type of hypersensitivity is serum sickness.

Serum Sickness

Many years ago, when the use of antisera for passive immunization was in its infancy, it was observed that human patients who had received a very large dose of equine antitetanus serum developed a characteristic reaction about 10 days later. This reaction, called serum sickness, consisted of a generalized vasculitis with erythema, edema, and urticaria of the skin, neutropenia, lymph node enlargement, joint swelling, and proteinuria. The reaction was usually of short duration and subsided within a few days. A similar reaction can be produced experimentally in rabbits by administration of a large intravenous dose of antigen. The development of lesions coincides with the formation of large amounts of immune complexes in the circulation as a result of the immune response to circulating antigens (Figure 28-6). The experimental disease may be acute if it is caused by a single, large injection of an antigen; or chronic, if caused by multiple small injections. In either case, animals develop a glomerulonephritis (Figure 28-7) and an arteritis.

Glomerulonephritis

When immune complexes are deposited in the glomeruli they cause basement membrane thickening and stimulate glomerular cells to proliferate. Any or all of the three glomerular cell populations—epithelial cells, endothelial cells, and mesangial cells—can undergo proliferation. The lesion is therefore called membranoproliferative glomerulonephritis (MPGN). If immune complexes are deposited only in the mesangium, then mesangial cell proliferation will result in a mesangioproliferative glomerulonephritis. MPGN lesions are classified into three major types based on their histopathology (Figure 28-8).

Type I Membranoproliferative Glomerulonephritis

Type I MPGN is caused by immune complex deposition in glomerular vessels. These complexes usually penetrate the vascular endothelium but not the basement membrane, and are therefore trapped on the endothelial side, where they stimulate endothelial cell swelling and proliferation (Figure 28-9). If an animal is given repeated injections of small doses of an antigen over a long period, continued damage to the glomerular cells by immune complexes leads to production of transforming growth factor-β (TGF-β). This cytokine stimulates nearby cells to produce fibronectin, collagen, and proteoglycans. This results in a thickening of the basement membrane to form the so-called wire loop lesion (also called a membranous glomerulonephritis). Alternatively, the immune complexes may be deposited in the mesangial region of glomeruli. Mesangial cells are modified smooth muscle cells. As such they can release cytokines and prostaglandins and take up immune complexes. They respond to the immune complexes by proliferation and release of IL-6 and TGF-β. The IL-6 stimulates autocrine growth of the mesangial cells. The TGF-β stimulates production of extracellular matrix. This mesangioproliferative glomerulonephritis eventually interferes with glomerular function. By immunofluorescence it can be shown that lumpy aggregates of immune

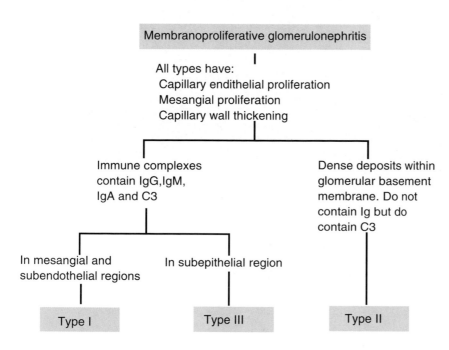

Membranoproliferative glomerulonephritis

All types have:
Capillary endithelial proliferation
Mesangial proliferation
Capillary wall thickening

Immune complexes contain IgG, IgM, IgA and C3

Dense deposits within glomerular basement membrane. Do not contain Ig but do contain C3

In mesangial and subendothelial regions

In subepithelial region

Type I

Type III

Type II

Figure 28-8. Classification of different forms of membranoproliferative glomerulonephritis.

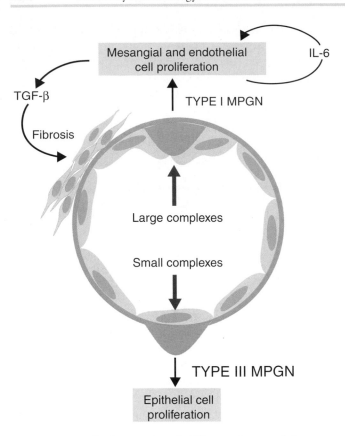

Figure 28-9. Pathogenesis of different forms of immune complex–mediated glomerulonephritis. Remember, however, that more than one type of lesion may be present in an animal at the same time.

complexes are deposited in capillary walls and on the epithelial side of the glomerular basement membrane (Figure 28-10).

Type II Membranoproliferative Glomerulonephritis

Type II MPGN (or dense deposit disease) is similar to the type I disease in that there is endothelial and mesangial proliferation. However, it is characterized by the presence of homogeneous, dense deposits within the glomerular basement membrane (in the lamina densa) rather than on its surface (Figure 15-16). The deposits may contain C3 but not immunoglobulin. Type II MPGN results from uncontrolled complement activation and is seen in factor H deficiency in pigs (Chapter 15).

Type III Membranoproliferative Glomerulonephritis

Type III MPGN is a variant of type I MPGN. It differs from typical type I disease by the presence of immune complexes on both the endothelial and epithelial sides of the basement membrane. It is believed that very small immune complexes penetrate the basement membrane and are deposited where they stimulate epithelial cell swelling and proliferation. If excessive, these proliferating cells may fill the glomerular space to form epithelial crescents. A single case of unknown cause has been described in a cat.

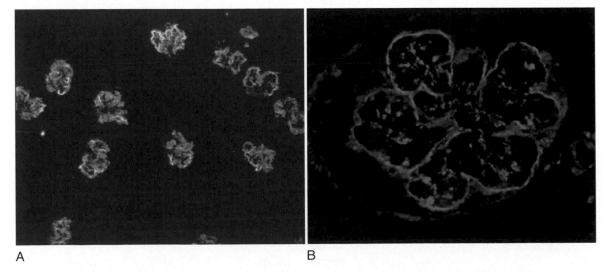

A   B

Figure 28-10. Fluorescent micrographs of a section of glomerulus from a Finnish-Landrace lamb with immune complex–mediated glomerulonephritis. The labeled antisheep globulin reveals the presence of "lumpy-bumpy" deposits characteristic of type I membranoproliferative glomerulonephritis in many glomeruli. **A,** Low-power micrograph showing multiple glomeruli. **B,** High-power micrograph. (From Angus KW, Gardiner AC, Morgan KT, et al: *J Comp Pathol* 84:319-330, 1974.)

CLINICAL FEATURES OF GLOMERULONEPHRITIS

Type I MPGN develops when prolonged antigenemia persists in the presence of antibodies. It is therefore characteristic of chronic viral diseases such as equine infectious anemia, infectious canine hepatitis, Aleutian disease of mink, and African swine fever; parasitic diseases such as leishmaniasis; and chronic bacterial diseases such as Lyme disease and ehrlichiosis (Table 28-1). Clinically it should be suspected in an animal with proteinuria without evidence of infection although definitive diagnosis requires a renal biopsy and histological evaluation. Type I MPGN has also been reported in dogs with pyometra, chronic pneumonia, distemper encephalitis, acute pancreatic necrosis, and bacterial endocarditis. In 17% to 40% of animals with tumors, large amounts of antigen may be shed into the bloodstream and give rise to a type I MPGN. This is, for example, a feature of feline leukemia. It has also been reported in animals with lymphosarcoma, osteosarcoma, and mastocytoma. Circulating immune complexes and renal lesions have been found in dogs with systemic lupus erythematosus (Chapter 34), discoid lupus, generalized demodicosis, and recurrent staphylococcal pyoderma. Some cases are due to deficiencies of complement components. As a result of these deficiencies, removal of immune complexes is impaired and they accumulate in glomeruli. Many cases of type I MPGN develop in the absence of an obvious predisposing cause.

The presence of immune complex lesions within glomeruli stimulates cells such as neutrophils, mesangial cells, macrophages, and platelets to release thromboxanes, nitric oxide, and platelet-activating factor. These act on the basement membranes to increase their permeability to macromolecules; as a result, plasma proteins, especially albumin, are lost in the urine. This loss, if severe, may exceed the ability of the body to replace the protein. As a result, albumin levels drop, the plasma colloid osmotic pressure falls, fluid passes from blood into tissue spaces, and the animal may become edematous and ascitic. The loss of fluid into tissues results in a reduction of blood volume, a compensatory increase in secretion of antidiuretic hormone, increased sodium retention, and accentuation of the edema. The decreased blood volume also results in a drop in renal blood flow, reduction in glomerular filtration, retention of urea and creatinine, azotemia, and hypercholesterolemia. Although all these may occur as a result of immune complex deposition in glomeruli, the development of this nephrotic syndrome is not inevitable. In fact, the clinical course of these conditions is extremely unpredictable, with some animals showing a progressive deterioration in renal function and others showing spontaneous remissions. Many animals may be clinically normal in spite of the presence of immune complexes in their glomeruli, and immune complexes are commonly observed in old, apparently healthy dogs, horses, and sheep. The most common initial signs are anorexia, weight loss, and vomiting. Polyuria and polydipsia occur when about 66% of glomeruli are destroyed. Azotemia occurs when 75% are destroyed. Development of nephrotic syndrome (proteinuria, hypoproteinemia, edema or ascites) only occurs in about 15% of affected dogs but in up to 75% of affected cats. Some dogs become hypertensive. Thromboembolic disease may also develop. Because of the unpredictable occurrence of spontaneous remissions, it is difficult to judge the effects of treatment. It has been usual to treat affected animals with corticosteroids and immunosuppressive drugs, but the rationale and effectiveness of this treatment is open to question except when the glomerulonephritis is associated with concurrent autoimmune disease such as systemic lupus erythematosus. Recently encouraging responses have been obtained with angiotensin-converting enzyme inhibitors and thromboxane synthase inhibitors. Protein restriction may help reduce the clinical signs of renal failure. If the glomerulopathy is secondary then clearly the underlying cause should be treated. The glomerular lesion is not inflammatory, and although the lesion in primary immune complex glomerulonephritis contains immunoglobulins, there is no evidence to suggest that it is caused by hyperactivity of the immune system. Steroid treatment of rabbits with experimental immune complex disease has been shown to exacerbate the condition.

TABLE 28-1

Infectious Diseases With a Significant Type III Hypersensitivity Component

Organism or Disease	Major Lesion
Erysipelothrix rhusiopathiae	Arthritis
Mycobacterium johnei	Enteritis
Streptococcus equi	Purpura
Staphylococcus aureus	Dermatitis
Borrelia burgdorferi	Glomerulonephritis
Ehrlichiosis	Glomerulonephritis
Canine adenovirus 1	Uveitis, glomerulonephritis
Canine adenovirus 2	Glomerulonephritis
Feline leukemia	Glomerulonephritis
Feline infectious peritonitis	Peritonitis, glomerulonephritis
Aleutian disease	Glomerulonephritis, anemia, arteritis
Hog cholera	Glomerulonephritis
African swine fever	Glomerulonephritis
Bovine virus diarrhea	Glomerulonephritis
Equine viral arteritis	Arteritis
Equine infectious anemia	Anemia, glomerulonephritis
Leishmaniasis	Glomerulonephritis
Dirofilaria immitis	Glomerulonephritis

IgA Nephropathy

By far the most important cause of renal failure in humans is IgA nephropathy. In this form of type I MPGN, patients have elevated serum IgA and deposits of IgA-containing immune complexes form in the mesangial region. The resulting glomerulonephritis can frequently lead to renal failure. The cause of IgA nephropathy is unknown. IgA deposits can be found in the glomeruli of up to 35% of some human populations and up to 47% of dogs. In these dogs, the IgA is deposited in the mesangial and paramesangial areas and is associated with mesangial proliferation. Dogs with enteritis or liver diseases showed the highest incidence of glomerular IgA deposition. A slightly different condition has also been described in dogs aged 4 to 7 years. The animals developed a type III MPGN with mild hematuria, proteinuria, and hypertension. IgA-containing immune complexes formed in both the subepithelial and subendothelial locations.

Swine Glomerulopathy

Spontaneous type I MPGN is observed in pigs. It is especially common in Japan where it appears to be due to deposition of immune complexes containing IgG (and IgA) antibodies against *Actinobacillus pleuropneumoniae*. In other cases, it may be secondary to chronic virus infections such as hog cholera or African swine fever. Occasionally, however, a proliferative glomerulonephritis develops spontaneously. In most cases epithelial crescent formation suggests that the proliferating cells are epithelial in origin. However, occasional mesangioproliferative lesions are observed as well. On immunofluorescence there is usually strong staining for C3 and weaker staining for IgM. Rarely pigs may have IgG or IgA deposits. Affected pigs are relatively young (less than 1 year). There is a high prevalence of gastric ulcers in affected animals but whether this is related is unclear. An inherited complement factor H deficiency in Yorkshire pigs results in the development of a lethal type II MPGN called porcine dense deposit disease (Chapter 15).

Porcine Dermatitis and Nephropathy Syndrome

Porcine dermatitis and nephropathy syndrome is mainly seen in nursery and growing animals between 2 and 7 months of age. The clinical signs include weight loss, skin lesions, and, most commonly, sudden death. Clinically affected pigs may have high mortality although this is highly variable. Skin lesions are seen in most cases. They present as flat or slightly raised multiple, reddish areas affecting the skin over the hamstrings, perineum, and ventral abdomen. In surviving animals, these lesions resolve in 2 to 3 weeks. The kidneys are enlarged, congested, and may show multiple red spots. The skin lesions are associated with a widespread vasculitis involving medium and small arteries in the dermis and subdermis. Infarction leads to epidermal necrosis. The kidney lesions consist of a glomerulonephritis that may be acute and necrotizing or may be proliferative. Vasculitis is also seen in vessels in the kidney, lymph nodes, spleen, and liver. Some pigs may have renal lesions or skin lesions alone. This syndrome appears to be an immune complex disease affecting vascular epithelium. Immunoglobulins (IgG and IgM) and complement are deposited in and around the necrotic vessels in the early stages of the disease. The cause of the syndrome is unknown but both bacteria and viruses have been implicated. Thus *Pasteurella multocida*–specific antigen has been isolated from affected kidney tissue. On the other hand, the lesions may be secondary to infections by porcine reproductive and respiratory system virus or by porcine circovirus 2 (PCV2). The syndrome is commonly associated with porcine postweaning multisystemic wasting syndrome, a disease that may also be caused by PCV2 infection (Chapter 36). Pigs suffering from the combined syndromes have higher morbidity and mortality.

Dirofilariasis

Some dogs heavily infected with the heartworm *Dirofilaria immitis* develop glomerular lesions and proteinuria. The lesions include thickening of the glomerular basement membrane with minimal endothelial or mesangial proliferation. Since IgG1-containing deposits may be found on the epithelial side of the basement membrane (type III MPGN), it has been suggested that immune complexes formed by antibodies to heartworm antigens provoke these lesions. Other investigators dispute the immune complex nature of this condition and claim that the lesions develop in response to the physical presence of microfilariae in glomerular blood vessels. The fact that infected dogs may develop amyloidosis (Chapter 4) suggests that they mount a significant immune response to the worms.

Finnish-Landrace Glomerulopathy

Some lambs of the Finnish-Landrace breed die when about 6 weeks of age as a result of renal failure due to a type I MPGN. The glomerular lesions are similar to those seen in chronic serum sickness, with mesangial cell proliferation and basement membrane thickening (Figure 28-11). In extreme cases epithelial cell proliferation may result in epithelial crescent formation. Neutrophils may be present in small numbers within glomeruli, and the rest of the kidney may exhibit diffuse interstitial lymphoid infiltration and necrotizing vasculitis. Deposits containing IgM, IgG, and C3 are found in the glomeruli and choroid plexus, and serum C3 levels are low. The lesions are therefore probably produced as a result of immune complex deposition within these organs, although the nature of the inducing antigen is unknown.

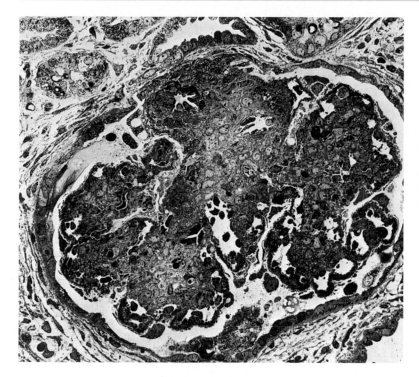

Figure 28-11.   A thin section of glomerulus from a Finnish-Landrace lambs with type I membranoproliferative glomerulonephritis. The primary lesion in this case is mesangial proliferation with some basement membrane thickening. (From Angus KW, Gardiner AC, Morgan KT, et al: *J Comp Pathol* 84:319-330, 1974.)

Canine Glomerulopathy

C3 deficiency inherited as an autosomal recessive condition has been described in Brittany Spaniels (Chapter 15). Many of these dogs develop type I MPGN, which may result in renal failure. The lesions are typical with mesangial proliferation, thickening of the glomerular capillary wall, and deposition of electron-dense deposits in the mesangium and subendothelial space. The deposits contain both IgG and IgM. A familial glomerulopathy has been observed in Bernese mountain dogs. It is associated with MPGN and interstitial nephritis.

OTHER IMMUNE COMPLEX–MEDIATED LESIONS

Purpura Hemorrhagica

Two to four weeks after an acute *Streptococcus equi* infection (or vaccination against *S. equi*), horses may develop an acute disease characterized by an initial urticaria, followed by severe subcutaneous edema, especially involving the limbs, and the development of hemorrhages in the mucosa and subcutaneous tissues. Affected horses are anorexic and depressed and have a high fever. Immune complexes containing *S. equi* antigens (M-protein or R-protein) may be found in the bloodstream of affected animals. These immune complexes cause an acute vasculitis, as well as a type I MPGN with resulting proteinuria and azoturia. Other triggers of purpura hemorrhagica in the horse include infections with *Corynebacterium*

pseudotuberculosis, equine influenza virus, equine herpesvirus type 1, and *Rhodococcus equi*. In some cases it develops in the absence of any obvious infection. Horses usually recover if aggressively treated with systemic glucocorticosteroids.

Pigs may also suffer from sporadic cases of an immune complex–mediated thrombocytopenic purpura syndrome. The animals have thrombocytopenia, anemia, excessive bleeding, with membranoproliferative lesions in their glomeruli. The cause is unknown.

Dietary Hypersensitivity

If an antigenic milk replacer, such as soy protein, is fed to very young calves before the development of ruminal function, the foreign antigen may be absorbed and stimulate antibody formation and a type III hypersensitivity. As a result, the calves become unthrifty and lose weight. However, the precise pathogenesis of this condition is unclear. A small proportion of calves develop an IgE response and a type I hypersensitivity.

Polyarthritis

Immune complexes can be readily found in the blood and synovial fluid of animals with rheumatoid arthritis and in many with osteoarthritis. In rheumatoid arthritis they are believed to have a major role in the etiologic progression of disease. Their role in osteoarthritis is unclear, but they may be a secondary result of local trauma. Important examples of this type of arthritis are the nonerosive polyarthritides seen in foals and puppies and described in Chapter 34.

Drug Hypersensitivities

In the previous chapter, it was pointed out that if a drug attached itself to a cell such as an erythrocyte, then the immune response against the drug could lead to elimination of the cell. A similar reaction may occur through type III hypersensitivity reactions if immune complexes bind directly to host cells. In this case, the cells are recognized as opsonized and are removed by phagocytosis. As might be predicted, if immune complexes bind to erythrocytes, anemia results; if they bind to platelets, thrombocytopenia and purpura result. Binding to granulocytes leads to a granulocytopenia and, consequently, recurrent infection. Severe skin reactions may follow deposition of antibody–drug complexes in the blood vessels of the dermis. However, in many cases it is difficult to distinguish between the toxic effects of a drug and type III hypersensitivity unless specific antibodies can be eluted from affected cells.

SOURCES OF ADDITIONAL INFORMATION

Bauman U, Chouchakova N, Gewecke B, Kohl J, et al: Distinct tissue site-specific requirements of mast cells and complement components C3/C5a receptor in IgG immune complex-induced injury of skin and lung, *J Immunol* 167: 1022-10027, 2001.

Bourgault A, Drolet R: Spontaneous glomerulonephritis in swine, *J Vet Diag Invest* 7:122-126, 1995.

Carrasco L, Madsen LW, Salguero FJ, et al: Immune complex-associated thrombocytopenic purpura syndrome in sexually mature Gattingen minipigs, *J Comp Pathol* 128:25-32, 2003.

Choi C, Kim J, Kang IJ, Chae C: Concurrent outbreak of PMWS and PDNS in a herd of pigs in Korea, *Vet Rec* 151:484-485, 2002.

Cork LC, Morris JM, Olson JL, et al: Membranoproliferative glomerulonephritis in dogs with a genetically determined deficiency of the third component of complement, *Clin Immunol Immunopathol* 60:455-470, 1991.

Darwich L, Segalés J, Domingo M, Mateu E: Changes in CD4+, CD8+, CD4+ CD8+, and immunoglobulin M-positive peripheral blood mononuclear cells of postweaning multisystemic wasting syndrome-affected pigs and age-matched uninfected wasted and healthy pigs correlate with lesions and porcine circovirus type 2 load in lymphoid tissues, *Clin Diag Lab Immunol* 9:236-242, 2002.

Divers TJ, Timoney JF, Lewis RM, Smith CA: Equine glomerulonephritis and renal failure associated with complexes of Group-C streptococcal antigen and IgG antibody, *Vet Immunol Immunopathol* 32:93-102, 1992.

Fearon DT: Complement, C receptors and immune complex disease, *Hosp Pract* 23:63-72, 1988.

Grant DC, Forrester SD: Glomerulonephritis in dogs and cats: glomerular function, pathophysiology, and clinical signs, *Compendium Contin Educ Prac Vet* 23:739-743, 2001.

Harris CH, Krawiec DR, Gelberg HB, Shapiro SZ: Canine IgA glomerulopathy, *Vet Immunol Immunopathol* 36:1-16, 1993.

Hélie P, Drolet R, Germain M-C, Bourgault A: Systemic necrotizing vasculitis and glomerulonephritis in grower pigs in southwestern Quebec, *Can Vet J* 36:150-154, 1995.

Inoue K, Kamieie J, Ohtake S, et al: Atypical membranoproliferative glomerulonephritis in a cat, *Vet Pathol* 38:468-470, 2001.

Jansen JH: Porcine membranoproliferative glomerulonephritis with intramembranous dense deposits (porcine dense deposit disease), *APMIS* 101:281-289, 1993.

Kier AB, McDonnell JJ, Stern A, et al: The Arthus reaction in domestic cats, *Vet Immunol Immunopathol* 18:229-235, 1988.

Kohl J, Gessner JE: On the role of complement and Fc gamma-receptors in the Arthus reaction, *Mol Immunol* 36:893-903, 1999.

Ladekjaer-Mikkelsen A, Nielsen J, Stadejek T, et al: Reproduction of postweaning multisystemic wasting syndrome (PMWS) in immunostimulated and non-immunostimulated 3-week-old piglets experimentally infected with porcine circovirus type 2 (PCV2), *Vet Microbiol* 89:97-114, 2002.

Lainson FA, Aitchison KD, Donachie W, Thomson JR: Typing of *Pasteurella multocida* isolated from pigs with and without porcine dermatitis and nephropathy syndrome, *J Clin Microbiol* 40:488-593, 2002.

Monteiro RC, Moura EC, Launay P, et al: Pathogenic significance of IgA receptor interactions in IgA nephropathy, *Trends Mol Med* 8:464-468, 2002.

Pusterla N, Watson JL, Affolter VK, et al: Purpura haemorrhagica in 53 horses, *Vet Rec* 153:118-121, 2003.

Shirota K, Ohtake S, Inoue K, et al: Reactivity of immunoglobulins eluted from the isolated renal glomeruli of nephritic pigs with *Actinobacillus pleuropneumoniae* antigen, *Vet Rec* 151: 390-392, 2002.

Smith WJ, Thomson JR, Done S: Dermatitis/nephropathy syndrome of pigs, *Vet Rec* 132:47, 1993.

Thibault S, Drolet R, Germain MC, et al: Cutaneous and systemic necrotizing vasculitis in swine, *Vet Pathol* 35: 108-116, 1998.

Thomson JR, Higgins RJ, Smith WJ, Done SH: Porcine dermatitis and nephropathy syndrome: clinical and pathological features of cases in the United Kingdom (1993–1998), *J Vet Med* 49:430-437, 2002.

Wright NG, Mohammed NA, Eckersall PD, Nash AS: Experimental immune complex glomerulonephritis in dogs receiving cationised bovine serum albumin, *Res Vet Sci* 38: 322-328, 1985.

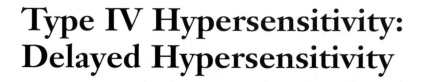

Type IV Hypersensitivity: Delayed Hypersensitivity

Certain antigens when injected into the skin of sensitized animals provoke slowly developing inflammation at the injection site. Since this "delayed" hypersensitivity reaction can only be transferred from sensitized to normal animals by lymphocytes, it must be cell mediated. Delayed hypersensitivity reactions are classified as type IV hypersensitivities and result from interactions among the injected antigen, antigen-presenting cells, and T cells. An important example of a delayed hypersensitivity reaction is the tuberculin response, which is the skin reaction in an animal with tuberculosis that results from an intradermal injection of tuberculin. Delayed hypersensitivity reactions can be considered to be specialized forms of inflammation directed against organisms that are resistant to elimination by conventional acute inflammatory processes.

THE TUBERCULIN REACTION

Tuberculin is the name given to extracts of *Mycobacterium tuberculosis*, *M. bovis*, or *M. avium*, used to skin-test animals for the purpose of identifying those suffering from tuberculosis. Several types of tuberculin have been employed for this purpose. The most important is purified protein derivative (PPD) tuberculin, which is prepared by growing organisms in synthetic medium, killing them with steam, and filtering. The PPD tuberculin is precipitated from this filtrate with trichloroacetic acid, washed, and resuspended in buffer ready for use. Thus PPD tuberculin is a poorly defined complex antigen mixture. Its major antigenic component is probably the heat-shock protein HSP 65. Many of its proteins are shared among

different mycobacterial species, thus ensuring that tests using PPD tuberculin are relatively nonspecific.

When tuberculin is injected into the skin of a normal animal there is no apparent response. On the other hand, if it is injected into an animal infected with mycobacteria, a delayed hypersensitivity response occurs. Following intradermal injection into a sensitized animal, a red, indurated (hard) swelling develops at the injection site. The inflammation begins between 12 and 24 hours, reaches its greatest intensity by 24 to 72 hours, and may persist for several weeks before fading gradually. In very severe reactions, tissue destruction and necrosis may occur at the injection site. Histological examination of the lesion shows that it is infiltrated with mononuclear cells (lymphocytes, macrophages), although neutrophils are present in the early hours of the reaction (Figure 29-1).

The tuberculin reaction is a hypersensitivity reaction mediated by T cells. When an animal is invaded by *M. tuberculosis*, the organisms are readily phagocytosed by macrophages. Some of this mycobacterial antigen triggers a Th1 cell–mediated response and generates memory cells. These memory T cells can respond to mycobacterial antigen entering the body by any route. Since delayed hypersensitivity can be elicited many years after exposure to an antigen, some of these memory T cells must be very long lived.

When tuberculin is injected intradermally, it is taken up by Langerhans cells, which then migrate to the draining lymph node (Figure 29-2). Here they present antigen to memory T cells that respond by generating Th1 effector cells. The circulating Th1 cells recognize the antigen when they encounter it in the skin and accumulate around the antigen deposit. By 12 hours in cattle, the

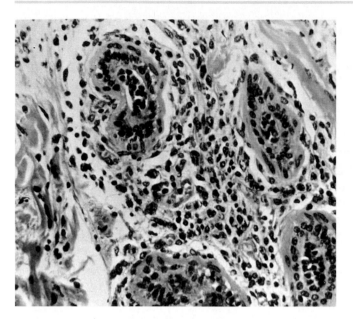

Figure 29-1. Histological section of a positive tuberculin reaction in bovine skin. Note the perivascular mononuclear cell infiltration as well as the lack of neutrophils or edema. (From Thomson RG: *General veterinary pathology*, Philadelphia, 1978, WB Saunders.)

injection site is mainly infiltrated with γ/δ^+, WC1$^+$ T cells. (In humans and mice, α/β T cells tend to predominate, whereas in sheep and cattle, γ/δ T cells predominate.) There are no B cells in the lesion.

The γ/δ T cells help to recruit other Th1 lymphocytes and macrophages to the site. The Th1 cells secrete IFN-γ, IL-2, and IL-16. The first two act on endothelial cells to increase expression of adherence molecules. IL-2 stimulates production of the chemokines CXCL8, CCL5, and XCL1, which attract and activate more T cells. IL-16 attracts CD4$^+$ T cells. The macrophages also release serotonin and chemokines such as CXCL1 and CCL2, which attract basophils. Basophil-derived serotonin (in rodents) or histamine (in humans) causes yet more inflammation and enhances migration of mononuclear cells into the lesion. The T-cell-derived chemokines CCL2 and CCL3 can induce mast cell degranulation whereas some CD4$^+$ T cells can activate mast cells through major histocompatibility complex II (MHC II)–bound antigen.

T-cell-derived chemokines cause inflammation and attract even more T cells. Most of these new T cells are not specifically sensitized for the inducing antigen. Only a very small proportion, perhaps 5%, of the lymphocytes seen in a delayed hypersensitivity reaction are specific for the antigen. The vast majority are attracted nonspecifically by XCL1. By 60 to 72 hours, the predominant lymphocytes are α/β^+, CD4$^+$, and CD8$^+$. Macrophages accumulate in the lesion as a result of the production of CXCL8 and may be locally activated by IFN-γ. Some of the tissue damage in intense delayed hypersensitivity reactions may be due to the release of proteases and oxidants from these activated macrophages. The macrophages ingest and eventually destroy the injected antigen. This, plus the appearance of regulatory cells in the lesion, permits the tissues to return eventually to normal.

Figure 29-2. Schematic diagram depicting the mechanism of a delayed hypersensitivity reaction

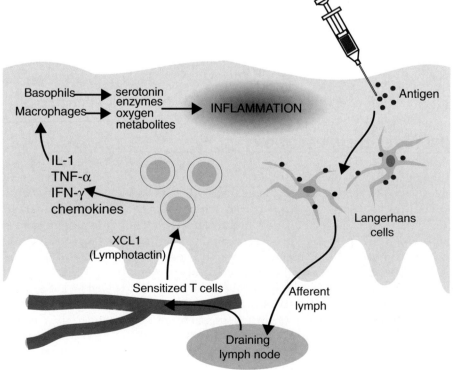

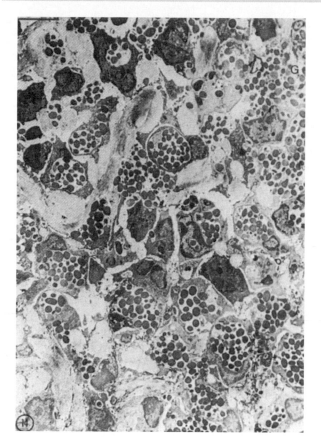

Figure 29-3. A section of guinea pig skin 18 hours after attachment of a tick in an animal sensitized by prior infestation with tick larvae. The skin is infiltrated with large numbers of basophils. (From McLaren D, Worms MJ, Askenase PW: *J Pathol* 139:299, 1983.)

Cutaneous Basophil Hypersensitivity

Under some circumstances, basophils may become the predominant cells in a delayed hypersensitivity reaction (Figure 29-3). This type of reaction, called cutaneous basophil hypersensitivity (CBH), can be transferred between animals with antibody, with purified B cells, or even with T cells. CBH is therefore a reaction mediated by several different mechanisms. CBH occurs in chickens in response to intradermal Rous sarcoma virus, in rabbits in response to schistosomes, and in humans with allergic contact dermatitis and renal allograft rejection. CBH reactions may contribute to the development of lesions in flea allergy dermatitis in dogs.

TUBERCULIN REACTIONS IN CATTLE

Because a positive tuberculin reaction occurs only in animals that have, or have had, tuberculosis, skin testing may be used to identify animals affected by this disease. Indeed, the tuberculin test has provided the basis for all tuberculosis eradication schemes that involve the detection and subsequent elimination of infected animals.

Skin testing of cattle may be performed in several ways (Table 29-1). The simplest is the single intradermal (SID) test. In this test, 0.05 mL of PPD tuberculin derived from *M. tuberculosis* or *M. bovis* is injected into one anal fold and the injection site is examined 72 to 96 hours later. A comparison is easily made between the injected and the uninjected folds, and a positive reaction consisting of a diffuse hard lump at the injection site is readily detected.

In the United States, two separate tests are performed. Thus two injections of tuberculin are made, one into the mucocutaneous junction of the vulva and the other into an anal fold; in other countries, tuberculin is normally injected into the skin on the side of the neck. The neck site is more sensitive than the anal folds, but restraint of the animal may be more difficult and good injection technique is critical.

The advantage of the SID test is its simplicity. Its main disadvantage is that because of the complex nature of tuberculin it cannot distinguish between tuberculosis and infection by other mycobacteria such as *M. avium, M. avium paratuberculosis*, or the related *Nocardia* group of organisms. A second disadvantage is that some animals react positively to the test but on necropsy do not have detectable tuberculosis lesions. The reasons for this are unclear but may be a result of exposure to nonpathogenic mycobacteria such as *M. phlei*.

False-negative SID tests may occur in animals with advanced tuberculosis, in animals with very early infection,

TABLE 29-1			
Tuberculin Tests Used in Cattle			
Test	**Usage**	**Advantages**	**Disadvantages**
Single intradermal	Routine testing	Simple	Prone to false positives Poor sensitivity
Comparative	When avian TB or Johne's disease is prevalent	More specific than SID	More complex than SID
Short thermal	Use in postpartum animals and in infected animals	High efficiency	Time consuming Risk of anaphylaxis
Stormont	Use in postpartum animals and in advanced cases	Very sensitive and accurate	Three visits required May sensitize an animal

in animals that have calved within the preceding 4 to 6 weeks, in very old cows, and in animals tested during the preceding 1 to 10 weeks. The lack of reaction (anergy) seen in advanced cases of tuberculosis is also observed in clinical Johne's disease and appears to be due to the presence of a blocking factor in the serum of these animals. This factor may be an antibody that prevents T cells from reacting with antigen. There is also evidence for the involvement of regulatory cells. Because of these defects in the SID, several modifications of this test have been developed. The comparative test, for example, involves intradermal inoculation of both avian and bovine tuberculins. Each tuberculin is injected into the side of the neck at separate sites, and these sites are examined 72 hours later. In general, if the avian tuberculin site shows the greatest reaction, the animal is considered to be infected with *M. avium* or *M. avium paratuberculosis*. On the other hand, if the *M. bovis* site shows the greatest reaction, then it is believed that the animal is infected with *M. tuberculosis* or *M. bovis*. This test is useful when a high prevalence of avian tuberculosis or Johne's disease is anticipated. PPD from *M. bovis* is more specific in cattle than *M. tuberculosis*, giving less cross-reaction with *M. avium* as well as being more appropriate for use in cattle and is therefore preferred. In practice, recent evidence suggests that the comparative test has a sensitivity of 90% (10% false negatives) and a specificity of greater than 99% (less than 1% false positives); however, this depends on the criteria used to read the results.

Anther modified tuberculin test is the short thermal test, in which a large volume of tuberculin solution is given subcutaneously and the animal examined for a rise in temperature between 4 and 8 hours later. (Presumably the tuberculin acts on T cells that then provoke the release of IL-1 from macrophages.) The Stormont test relies on the increased sensitivity of a test site, which occurs after a single injection; it is performed by giving two doses of tuberculin at the same injection site 7 days apart. Both tests are relatively sensitive. As a result, they may be used in postpartum cows as well as for the testing of heavily infected animals. Repeated tuberculin testing results in a period of decreased reactivity and the induction of antibodies against *M. bovis* antigen HSP 70.

TUBERCULIN REACTIONS IN OTHER ANIMALS

Tuberculin skin testing has never been a widely employed procedure in domestic animals other than cattle, so information on these is scanty. Nevertheless, it appears that the ability of different species to mount a classic tuberculin reaction varies greatly. In pig and cat, for example, the tuberculin test is unreliable, being positive for only a short period following infection. In pig and dog, the best test is an SID test given in the skin behind the ear, whereas in the cat the short thermal test is probably best. In sheep and goat, the antigen is usually given in the anal fold, but the results are usually unreliable in these species as well. Horses appear to be unusually sensitive to tuberculin, and the dose used must be reduced accordingly. Nevertheless, the results obtained do not always correlate well with the disease status of the animal. In birds, good reactions may be obtained by inoculating tuberculin into the wattle or wing web.

JOHNIN REACTIONS

Animals infected with *M. avium* var. *paratuberculosis*, the cause of Johne's disease, may develop a delayed hypersensitivity reaction following intradermal inoculation of an extract of this organism called johnin. Johnin can be used in a single intradermal test but, like tuberculin, may give a negative result in animals with clinical disease. An intravenous johnin test is positive in these cases and may be a preferable alternative to the SID test. In this test the antigen is administered intravenously and the animal's temperature is noted at intervals. A rise in temperature of 1° C or neutrophilia after 6 hours is considered a positive result. These tests are probably of limited usefulness in individual animals but may be employed for the identification of infected herds.

OTHER SKIN TESTS

Positive delayed hypersensitivity skin reactions may be obtained in any infectious disease in which cell-mediated immunity has a significant role. Thus, extracts of *Brucella abortus* have been used from time to time in attempts to diagnose brucellosis. These include brucellin, a filtrate of a 20-day broth culture, and brucellergen, a nucleoprotein extract. Because these preparations may stimulate production of antibodies to brucella, they cannot be employed in areas where eradication is monitored by serological tests. In glanders of horses, a culture filtrate of the organism *Pseudomonas mallei*, termed mallein, is used for skin testing. Mallein can be used in either a short thermal test or an ophthalmic test. An ophthalmic test, also occasionally employed in tuberculosis, is performed by dropping the antigen solution into an eye. Transient conjunctivitis develops if the test is positive. Another and perhaps preferable method of testing for glanders is the intrapalpebral test. In this test, mallein is injected into the skin of the lower eyelid where a positive reaction results in swelling and ophthalmia.

Intradermal skin testing with microbial extracts is also employed in the diagnosis of many fungal diseases; thus histoplasmin is used for histoplasmosis, coccidioidin in coccidioidomycosis, and so on. In these cases, the tests are not very specific, and the test procedure may effectively sensitize the tested animal, causing it to become serologically positive. This problem also arises when toxoplasmin is used in attempts to diagnose toxoplasmosis (Chapter 25).

PATHOLOGICAL CONSEQUENCES OF TYPE IV HYPERSENSITIVITY

Tubercle Formation

Although the tuberculin reaction induced by intradermal inoculation is artificial in that antigen is administered by injection, a similar inflammatory response occurs if living tubercle bacilli lodge in tissues and cause sensitization of an animal. However, *M. tuberculosis* is resistant to intracellular destruction until macrophages are activated by Th1 cells (Chapter 17), and dead organisms are very slowly removed because they contain large quantities of poorly metabolized waxes. As a result, the reaction to whole organisms is prolonged, and macrophages accumulate in very large numbers. Many of these macrophages ingest the bacteria but fail to prevent its growth and so die. Other macrophages fuse to form multinucleated giant cells. After 4 to 5 weeks of infection, microscopic granulomas enlarge and coalesce. The lesion that develops around invading tubercle bacilli therefore consists of a mass of necrotic debris containing both living and dead organisms surrounded by a layer of fibroblasts, lymphocytes, and macrophages, which in this location are called epithelioid cells (Chapter 4). The entire lesion is called a tubercle (Figure 29-4). The Mycobacteria are unable to multiply within the caseous tissue because of its low pH and lack of oxygen. Nevertheless some bacteria may survive in a dormant state. If the host mounts an adequate immune response of the correct (Th1) type, this may be sufficient to control the infection. However, if immunity is insufficient or inappropriate (Th2), the organisms may escape from the tubercle and spread to local lymph nodes and nearby tissues. When the response is inadequate, the multiplying organisms continue to spread, and the resulting lung damage together with liquefaction of the caseous center of the tubercle leads to rapidly progressive disease. Granuloma formation is also a common result of persistent chronic inflammation. This inflammation may be of immunological origin, as in tuberculosis or brucellosis in some species, or it may occur as a result of the presence in tissues of other chronic irritants. For example, granulomas may arise in response to the prolonged irritation caused by talc or asbestos particles.

Allergic Contact Dermatitis

If reactive chemicals are painted onto the skin they may bind to skin proteins, and the resulting complexes are processed by Langerhans cells in the dermis (Figure 29-5). Depending on the antigen the Langerhans cells may bind the antigen directly to MHC molecules on the cell surface or process the hapten internally into a complete antigen. The Langerhans cells then migrate to draining lymph nodes through afferent lymphatics and present the antigen to T cells. While presenting the antigen, the Langerhans cells secrete large amounts of IL-12 and IL-18; as a result, a Th1 cell response ensues. These cells in turn produce large amounts of IFN-γ and promote the activities of cytotoxic T cells. Following exposure to an antigen in sensitized animals, macrophages and lymphocytes infiltrate the dermis by 24 hours. Eventually, the cytotoxic T cells destroy and remove the altered cells, resulting in the development of intraepithelial vesicles. This inflammatory reaction presents as an intensely pruritic skin disease called allergic contact dermatitis. In addition to α/β T cells, other cell types, such as γ/δ T cells, B-1 cells, and natural killer T cells, may be involved in the reaction.

The chemicals that induce allergic contact dermatitis are usually very reactive molecules that can combine chemically with skin proteins; they include formaldehyde, picric acid, aniline dyes, plant resins and oils, organophosphates, some topical medications such as neomycin, and salts of metals such as nickel and beryllium (Figure 29-6). Thus, allergic contact dermatitis can occur on pathologists' fingers as a result of exposure to formaldehyde; on the ears of dogs treated with neomycin for otitis externa; on the foot pads, scrotum, and ventral abdomen of dogs on exposure to some carpet dyes and deodorizers; on parts of the body exposed to the oils (urushiol) of the poison ivy plant (*Rhus radicans*); and around the neck of animals as a result of exposure to dichlorvos (2,2-dichlorovinyldimethylphosphate) in flea collars (Table 29-2). Allergic contact dermatitis involving the muzzle of dogs has been reported to result from sensitivity to components of plastic food bowls. Some dogs, instead of developing the more usual type I hypersensitivity to

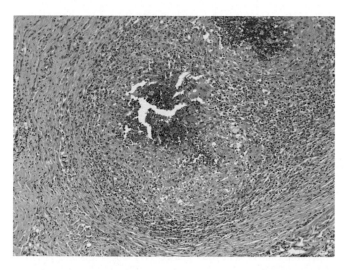

Figure 29-4. Histological section from the lymph node of a cow infected with *Mycobacterium bovis* showing a small tubercle. The dark central mass is caseous material. It is surrounded by layers of macrophages and lymphocytes and walled off by fibroblasts. (Courtesy of Dr. John Edwards.)

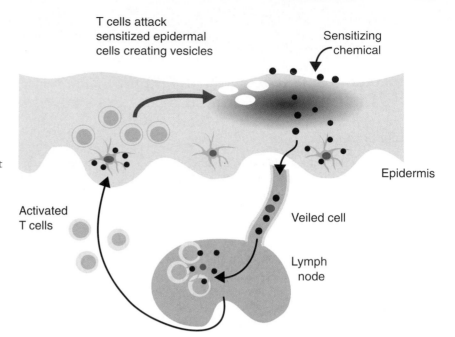

Figure 29-5. Pathogenesis of allergic contact dermatitis.

pollen proteins, experience an allergic contact dermatitis as a result of a type IV hypersensitivity to pollen resins. It is unusual for allergic contact dermatitis to affect the haired areas of the skin unless the allergen is in a liquid. Thus allergic contact dermatitis to shampoo components may result in total-body involvement. The period required for sensitization ranges from 6 months to several years.

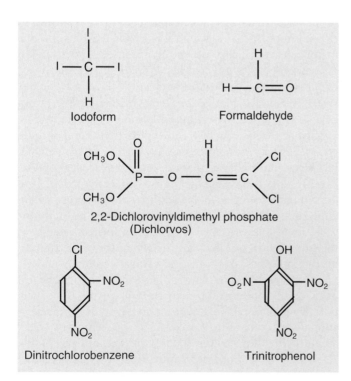

Figure 28-6. Some of the simple chemicals that can cause allergic contact dermatitis.

The lesions of allergic contact dermatitis vary in severity, ranging from a mild erythema to a severe erythematous vesiculation. However, because of the intense pruritus, self-trauma, excoriation, ulceration, and secondary staphylococcal pyoderma often mask the true nature of the lesion. If the exposure to the allergen persists, hyperkeratosis, acanthosis, and dermal fibrosis may eventually occur. Histologically, the lesion is marked by a mononuclear cell infiltration and vacuolation of skin cells under attack by cytotoxic T cells (Table 29-3).

Allergic contact dermatitis is diagnosed by removal of the suspected antigen and by patch testing. In closed patch tests, suspected allergens are used to impregnate gauze swabs that are then attached to the shaved skin with tape. After 48 to 72 hours the dressing may be removed and the areas in contact with the swabs examined. A positive reaction is indicated by local erythema and vesiculation. Closed patch tests may be impractical for some dogs and cats. An open patch test may therefore be employed. In this procedure, a solution of the suspected allergen is applied to shaved normal skin and the area examined daily for up to 5 days. Identification of the offending allergen and its avoidance by the animal are the optimal therapies for allergic contact dermatitis. Hyposensitization therapy is not effective. Steroids are used in acute cases, with antibiotics to control secondary infections.

MEASUREMENT OF CELL-MEDIATED IMMUNITY

Although diagnostic immunology is based largely on the detection of antibodies, measurement of cell-mediated immune responsiveness in animals may be desirable

---

TABLE 29-2
Sources of Contact Allergens in Animals

Insecticides in flea collars
In sprays
In dips
Wood preservatives
Floor waxes
Carpet dyes
Some pollens
Dermatological drugs (creams, ointments)
Leather products
Paints
House plants

---

under some circumstances. Currently, both in vivo and in vitro techniques are used for this purpose.

In Vivo Techniques

The simplest in vivo test of cell-mediated immunity is an intradermal skin test such as the tuberculin test. The inflammatory response to intradermally administered antigens may be considered cell mediated, provided that it has the characteristic time-course and histological features of a type IV reaction. Intradermal skin tests are not always convenient, and injection of an antigen into an animal may effectively sensitize it, thus preventing further testing.

It is sometimes useful to measure the ability of an animal to mount cell-mediated immune responses in general rather than to one specific antigen. One way to do this is to give the animal a small skin allograft and measure its survival time. A much simpler technique is to paint a small area of the animal's skin with a sensitizing chemical such as dinitrochlorobenzene. The intensity of the resulting allergic contact dermatitis provides a rough estimate of the animal's ability to mount a cell-mediated immune response.

If the lectin phytohemagglutinin is injected intradermally, it provokes a local tissue reaction with many features of a delayed hypersensitivity response. In pigs

this reaction is characterized by infiltration with γ/δ^+ CD4$^-$ CD8$^-$ T cells. This is a very convenient and rapid method of assessing an animal's ability to mount a cell-mediated response without the need for first sensitizing the animal to an antigen. However, the response to phytohemagglutinin is nonspecific and its interpretation may be difficult.

In Vitro Techniques

In vitro tests are designed to measure the proliferation of T cells in response to an antigen, their cytotoxic activities, or their production of cytokines. All of these tests require that T cells be grown in cell culture; therefore none is useful for use in the field.

To measure T-cell proliferation in response to an antigen, a suspension of purified peripheral blood lymphocytes from the animal to be tested is mixed with the antigen and cultured for 48 to 96 hours. Twelve hours before harvesting, thymidine labeled with the radioactive isotope tritium is added to the cultures. Normal, nondividing lymphocytes do not take up thymidine, but dividing cells do because they are actively synthesizing DNA. Thus, if the T cells are proliferating, they will take up the tritiated thymidine and their radioactivity provides a measure of the amount of proliferation. The greater the response of the cells to an antigen, the greater will be their radioactivity. The ratio of the radioactivity in the stimulated cultures to the radioactivity in the controls is called the stimulation index. A related technique is to measure the proliferation of lymphocytes in response to mitogenic lectins (Chapter 9). The intensity of the lymphocyte proliferative response, as measured by tritiated thymidine uptake, provides an estimate of the reactivity of an animal's lymphocytes.

Radioactive tritium is being replaced in some assays with a simple colorimetric enzyme assay. Methylthiazoldiphenyltetrazolium bromide (MTT) is a pale yellow compound that serves as a substrate for active mitochondrial enzymes. The enzymes change the MTT color to dark blue. The intensity of this color change is a measure of the number of living cells in a culture. Thus in proliferation assays, the number of living cells increases, and this

---

TABLE 29-3		
Comparison of the Major Forms of Allergic Dermatitis		
	Atopic Dermatitis	**Allergic Contact Dermatitis**
Pathogenesis	Type I hypersensitivity	Type IV hypersensitivity
Clinical signs	Hyperemia, urticaria, pruritus	Hyperemia, vesiculation, alopecia, erythema
Distribution	Face, nose, eyes, feet, perineum	Hairless areas, usually ventral abdomen and feet
Major allergens	Foods and pollens, fleas, inhaled allergens	Reactive chemicals, dyes in contact with skin
Diagnosis response	Intradermal testing, immediate testing	Delayed response on patch
Pathology	Eosinophilic infiltration edema	Mononuclear cell infiltration, vesiculation
Treatment	Steroids, antihistamines, hyposensitization	Steroids

can be measured colorimetrically. The test is sufficiently sensitive to quantify the increase in T-cell numbers mediated by antigen or mitogens.

To measure T-cell-mediated cytotoxicity it is necessary to have a simple method of measuring cell death. This is usually based on the fact that living cells take up sodium chromate but if the cell dies the chromium is released into the extracellular fluid. Radioactive chromium 51 (^{51}Cr) may be used in this way to label target cells. Lymphocytes from an immune animal are mixed in an appropriate ratio with ^{51}Cr-labeled target cells. The mixture is then incubated for 4 to 24 hours at 37° C. At the end of this time, the cell suspension is centrifuged and the presence of ^{51}Cr in the supernatant measured. The amount of chromium released is related directly to the number of target cells killed. The amount of chromium released in the absence of cytotoxic cells must also be measured and subtracted from that released in the presence of cytotoxic cells in order to get a true reading.

A third in vitro assay is the measurement of cytokine release by T cells. One such technique involves assaying the release of IFN-γ by peripheral blood lymphocytes on exposure to tuberculin or to purified mycobacterial proteins. This technique has been developed as an alternative to the tuberculin test for the diagnosis of tuberculosis in cattle and deer. It involves adding tuberculin PPD to heparinized blood and incubating the mixture for 24 to 48 hours at 37° C. The plasma is then removed and assayed for any interferon produced either by means of a simple bioassay or preferably by use of a sandwich ELISA using monoclonal antibodies. Three "antigens" are used: no antigen (negative control), *M. bovis* PPD, and *M. avium* PPD. The *M. avium* PPD is used to detect false-positive cross-reactions. This technique has advantages over conventional tuberculin tests in that it does not compromise the immune status of the animal under test by injection of antigen. In addition, the animal does not have to be held for several days for the test to be read. It is also much simpler than other in vitro tests for cell-mediated immunity. The assay is at least as sensitive as the single intradermal test and, if purified recombinant mycobacterial proteins are employed, is highly specific. (Its sensitivity is about 85% and its specificity is as high as 90% to 99%). However, it does appear to detect a slightly different population of animals than the skin test. It has also been successfully used to diagnose Johne's disease in sheep.

Although all of the assays described above can be used to measure at least some aspects of cell-mediated immunity, none provides a complete picture. The investigator may of course be simply interested in the response to a single antigen or organism. In these cases either a skin test or an in vitro assay may be appropriate. This is best exemplified by the tests available for the diagnosis of tuberculosis. In vitro tests are also useful if the time course of a cell-mediated immune response is to be examined. Repeated testing can be performed simply by obtaining more lymphocytes. If, on the other hand, an investigator wishes to obtain an overview of an animal's abilities in this area, then one of the nonspecific in vivo assays may be more appropriate. These can be useful, for example, in assessing immune function in young animals thought to be immunodeficient. However, it is important to point out that in these animals a complete hematological examination should be performed before more complex assays are considered. It is also prudent to measure the important lymphocyte subpopulations by flow cytometry. An animal that has no T cells is unlikely to mount any sort of cell-mediated response.

SOURCES OF ADDITIONAL INFORMATION

Askenase PW: The role of basophils in health and disease, *Res Staff Phys* 32:33-41, 1986.

Askenase PW, Van Loveren M: Delayed-type hypersensitivity: activation of mast cells by antigen-specific T-cell factors initiates the cascade of cellular interactions, *Immunol Today* 4:259-264, 1983.

Chambers WH, Klesius PH: Direct bovine leukocyte migration inhibition assay: standardization and comparison with skin testing, *Vet Immunol Immunopathol* 5:85-95, 1983.

Coe Clough NE, Roth JA: Methods for assessing cell-mediated immunity in infectious disease resistance and in the development of vaccines, *J Am Vet Med Assoc* 206:1208-1216, 1995.

Dannenberg AM: Delayed-type hypersensitivity and cell-mediated immunity in the pathogenesis of tuberculosis, *Immunol Today* 12:228-233, 1991.

Doherty ML, Monaghan ML, Bassett HF, et al: The sequential cellular changes which characterize the tuberculin reaction in cattle, *Vet Immunol Immunopathol* 35 (Suppl):70-71, 1993.

Godfrey MP, Phillips ME, Askenase PW: Histopathology of delayed-onset hypersensitivities in contact-sensitive guinea pigs, *Int Arch Allerg Appl Immunol* 70:50-58, 1983.

Halliwell REW, Schemmer KR: The role of basophils in the immunopathogenesis of hypersensitivity to fleas (*Ctenocephalis felis*) in dogs, *Vet Immunol Immunopathol* 15:203-213, 1987.

Kelner GS, Kennedy J, Bacon KB, et al: Lymphotactin: a cytokine that represents a new class of chemokine, *Science* 266:1395-1397, 1994.

Kennedy HE, Welsh MD, Bryson DG, et al: Modulation of immune responses to *Mycobacterium bovis* in cattle depleted of WC1+ γδ T cells, *Infect Immun* 70:1488-1500, 2002.

Larsen CG, Thomsen MK, Gesser B, et al: The delayed type hypersensitivity reaction is dependent on IL-8, *J Immunol* 155:2151-2157, 1995.

Lens JW, Drexhage HA, Benson W, Balfour BM: A study of cells present in lymph draining from a contact allergic reaction in pigs sensitized to DNFB, *Immunology* 49:415-422, 1983.

Morrison WI, Bourne FJ, Cox DR, et al: Pathogenesis and diagnosis of infections with *Mycobacterium bovis* in cattle, *Vet Rec* 146:236-242, 2000.

Pollock JM, Girvin RM, Lightbody KA, et al: Assessment of defined antigens for the diagnosis of bovine tuberculosis in skin test reactor cattle, *Vet Rec* 146:659-665, 2000.

Schultz KT, Maguire HC: Chemically-induced delayed hypersensitivity in the cat, *Vet Immunol Immunopathol* 3:585-590, 1982.

Toews GB, Bergstresser PR, Streilein JW, Sullivan S: Epidermal Langerhans cell density determines whether contact hypersensitivity or unresponsiveness follows skin painting with DNFB, *J Immunol* 124:445-453, 1980.

Wang B, Feliciani C, Howel BG, Freed I, et al: Contribution of Langerhans cell-derived IL-18 to contact hypersensitivity, *J Immunol* 168:3303-3308, 2002.

Whipple DL, Bolin CA, Davis AJ, et al: Comparison of the sensitivity of the caudal fold skin test and a commercial γ-interferon assay for diagnosis of bovine tuberculosis, *Am J Vet Res* 56:415-419, 1995.

Whyte A, Haskard DO, Binns RM: Infiltrating γδ T-cells and selectin endothelial ligands in the cutaneous phytohemagglutinin-induced inflammatory reaction, *Vet Immunol Immunopathol* 41:31-40, 1994.

Wong MM, Fish EN: Chemokines: attractive mediators of the immune response, *Semin Immunol* 15:5-14, 2003.

Wood PR, Corner LA, Plackett P: Development of a simple, rapid in vitro cellular assay for bovine tuberculosis based on the production of γ-interferon, *Res Vet Sci* 49:46-49, 1990.

Wood PR, Corner LA, Rothel JS, et al: Field comparison of the interferon-gamma assay and the single intradermal tuberculin test for the diagnosis of bovine tuberculosis, *Aust Vet J* 68:286-290, 1991.

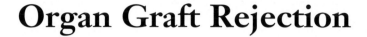

Organ Graft Rejection

Although the immune response first attracted the attention of scientists because of the body's ability to fight infections, the observation that animals reject foreign organ grafts led to a much broader view of the function of the immune system as a whole in that it indicated that the immune system had a surveillance function. The rejection of a foreign organ graft simply reflects the role of the immune system in identifying and destroying "abnormal" cells.

GRAFTING OF ORGANS

Advances in surgery have permitted the transfer of many tissues or organs between different parts of the body or between different individuals. When moved to a different part of an animal's own body such transplants do not trigger an immune response. This type of graft within an individual is called an autograft (Figure 30-1). Good examples of autografting include the grafting of skin to cover a burn in plastic surgery and the use of a segment of vein to bypass blocked cardiac arteries. Since autografts do not express foreign antigens, they do not trigger an immune response.

Isografts are grafts transplanted between two genetically identical individuals. Thus a graft between identical (monozygotic) twins is an isograft. Similarly, grafts between two inbred mice of the same strain are isografts and present no immunological difficulties. Since the animals are identical, the immune system of the recipient cannot differentiate between the graft and normal body cells.

Allografts are transplanted between genetically different members of the same species. Most grafts performed on animals or humans for therapeutic reasons are of this type because tissues are obtained from a donor who is usually unrelated to the graft recipient. Because the major histocompatibility complex (MHC) and blood group molecules on the allograft are different from those of their host, allografts induce a strong immune response that causes graft rejection. This rejection process must be suppressed if the grafted organ is to survive.

Xenografts are organ grafts transplanted between animals of different species. Thus, the transplant of a baboon heart into a human infant is a xenograft. Xenografted tissues differ from their host both biochemically and immunologically. As a result, they can provoke a rapid, intense rejection response that is very difficult to suppress.

Clinical grafting in domestic animals is a very recent procedure. However, renal allografting is now routine in dogs and cats, and bone marrow allografting promises to be a very useful contributor to some forms of tumor therapy. It is highly unlikely that cadaveric allografting will become important in veterinary medicine. Most current organ grafts are obtained from healthy donor animals. This raises significant ethical issues as to whether it is appropriate to subject a donor animal to major surgery in order to provide an organ for another animal. While the benefits of allografting to the recipient are obvious, it is unclear how the donor animal might benefit. Unlike human donors driven by altruism, the donor is given no choice in the matter. It is possible,

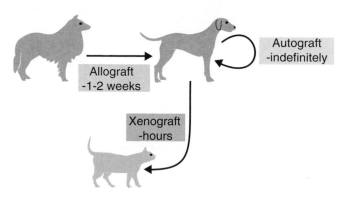

Figure 30-1. Differences among autografts, allografts, and xenografts.

however, to justify organ donation if thereby an animal would be saved from inevitable euthanasia and if the donor could be provided with a good home. For this reason, many animal transplantation centers require that the donor animal be adopted and cared for by the owner of the recipient animal.

ALLOGRAFT REJECTION

The identification and destruction of foreign molecules are central to the body's defense. Allografted organs represent a major source of these foreign molecules. They include not only antigens such as the foreign blood group glycoproteins and MHC molecules expressed on the grafted cells, but also any endogenous antigens presented on the MHC class I molecules of these same cells. The mechanisms of allograft rejection are basically the same irrespective of the organ grafted, and both antibodies and T cells participate in the rejection of allografts.

Renal allograft rejection is of major clinical importance in humans and has been widely studied in animals. It therefore serves as a good example of the allograft response. In dogs receiving renal allografts, rejection may be acute or chronic. Acute rejection should be suspected when the recipient shows a rapidly rising blood creatinine associated with an enlarged, painful kidney accompanied by signs of depression, anorexia, vomiting, proteinuria, hematuria, and ultrasonography showing an enlarged, hypoechoic kidney. In contrast, chronic rejection should be suspected if the creatinine and urea levels rise gradually and this is associated with proteinuria, microscopic hematuria and a small, hyperechoic kidney. Renal biopsy is necessary to confirm the diagnosis. In humans where a great deal of experience with transplantation has been gained, four distinct clinical rejection syndromes are recognized. *Hyperacute rejection* occurs within 48 hours following grafting. Rejection occurring up to 7 days after grafting is called *accelerated rejection*. Rejection after 7 days is called *acute rejection*. *Chronic*

rejection develops several months after grafting. It is unclear whether a similar classification is useful in animals.

Histocompatibility Antigens

When an organ is transplanted into a genetically dissimilar animal, the recipient will mount an immune response against many different antigens in and on the cells of the allograft. These are called histocompatibility antigens. Three types of histocompatibility antigens are of major importance in stimulating graft rejection. These are the MHC class I and class II molecules, and the major blood group molecules. All are expressed on the surface of the graft cells but their distribution varies. Thus, MHC class I antigens are found on almost all nucleated cells. The major blood group antigens are found both on red cells and nucleated cells. MHC class II antigens, in contrast, have a restricted distribution that varies among mammals. For example, in rats and mice, MHC class II molecules are expressed only on the professional antigen-presenting cells: macrophages, dendritic cells, and B cells. In other species, such as humans and pigs, MHC class II molecules are also expressed on the endothelium of renal arteries and glomeruli, the sites where host cells first make contact with the graft. These MHC class II molecules are recognized as foreign and trigger the rejection process. It is interesting to note that, as a result of these differences, it is much easier to prolong renal allograft survival in laboratory rodents than in humans or pigs.

As would be expected, grafts that differ minimally from the recipient will generally survive longer than grafts that are highly incompatible. Thus when blood group A-O–compatible pigs are given renal allografts, median survival is about 12 days for completely unmatched grafts, 25 days for grafts compatible for MHC class I alone, 30 days for grafts compatible for MHC class II alone, and 80 days for grafts compatible for both class I and class II (Figure 30-2). When dogs are given MHC-unmatched renal allografts, the grafts survive for about 10 days. Completely matched allografts in dogs survive for about 40 days. A more impressive result is obtained with canine liver grafts, which survive for about 8 days in unmatched animals and for 200 to 300 days in DLA-matched recipients.

The failure of MHC and blood group–compatible grafts to survive indefinitely is a result of the cumulative effects of many minor histocompatibility differences. For example, skin grafts from male donors placed on histocompatible females are usually rejected, although the reverse is not the case. This is because male cells carry an antigen coded for by genes on the Y chromosome called the H-Y molecule. Antibodies to H-Y can be used to selectively kill male sperm or male embryos and so alter the sex ratio of laboratory or farm animals. In one mouse experiment, 86% of the embryos surviving after such treatment were female. It is possible, by labeling with

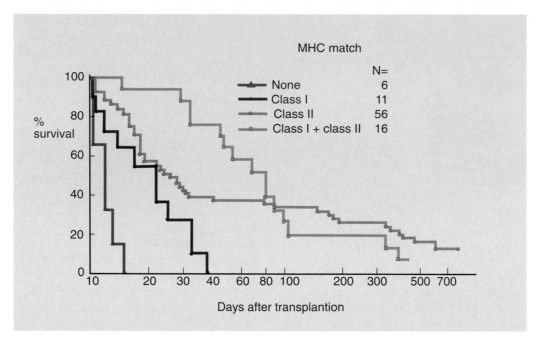

Figure 30-2. Survival time of organ allografts between SLA-incompatible minipigs clearly depends on the degree of MHC compatibility between donor and host. (From Pescovitz MD, Sachs DHJ: *J Exp Med* 160:1493, 1994.)

fluorescent anti-H-Y, to identify the gender of bovine embryos correctly before embryo transfer.

In practice it is usually not difficult to ensure that the donor and recipient have identical major blood group antigens. MHC compatibility is much harder to achieve because the extreme polymorphism of MHC molecules ensures that individuals differ widely in their MHC haplotype. In general, the more closely donor and recipient are related, the less will be their MHC difference. For this reason it is preferable that grafts be obtained from a recipient's parents or siblings. If this is not possible then a donor must be selected at random and the inevitable rejection responses overcome by the use of drugs such as cyclosporine or tacrolimus (Chapter 37).

RENAL ALLOGRAFTS

Pathology of Allograft Rejection

When kidneys are allografted, the blood supply to the transplanted kidney is established at the time of transplantation. Thus, the graft and host cells come into contact almost immediately. Damage to the graft through oxidant stress and surgical trauma causes the release of chemokines that attract inflammatory cells such as neutrophils and macrophages into the graft. In an unsensitized host, a primary immune response (first-set reaction) is mounted and renal allografts are only rejected after at least 10 days and possibly much longer. In sensitized animals where the immune system is already primed, hyperacute rejection occurs and the graft is destroyed within days or even hours without ever becoming functional.

During the rejection process, the whole organ gradually becomes infiltrated with mononuclear cells, especially cytotoxic T cells, that cause progressive damage to the endothelial cells lining small intertubular blood vessels (Figure 30-3). T-cell-mediated damage releases chemokines that attract more T cells into the graft. Tubular destruction, stoppage of blood flow, hemorrhage, and death of the grafted kidney follow thrombosis of these vessels. The blood vessels of second kidney grafts rapidly become blocked as a result of the action of antibodies and complement on the vascular endothelium. This leads to decreased urine production and stoppage of renal function. This "second-set" reaction is specific for any graft from the original donor or from a donor syngeneic with the first. It is not restricted to any particular site or to any specific organ since MHC and blood group molecules are present on most nucleated cells.

Mechanisms of Allograft Rejection

The allograft rejection process is directed against the dominant antigens on the cells of the graft. The MHC molecules tend to trigger a T-cell-mediated rejection response whereas the blood group antigens tend to trigger antibody formation. The rejection process may be divided into two stages. First, the antigens of the graft encounter the host's antigen-sensitive cells and trigger a

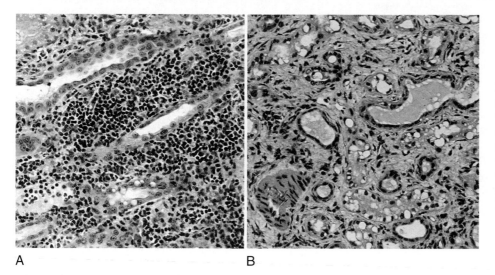

Figure 30-3. A, Section of a canine kidney that had been acutely rejected and as a consequence is densely infiltrated with lymphocytes. **B,** Section of a kidney that has undergone chronic allograft rejection. In this case the section shows interstitial fibrosis with tubular atrophy and a mild lymphocytic infiltration. (Courtesy of Dr AE Kyles.)

response. Second, cytotoxic T cells and antibodies from the host enter the graft and destroy those graft cells that they encounter (Figure 30-4).

Cytotoxic, CD8⁺ T cells recognize and respond to foreign or abnormal proteins synthesized in cells (endogenous antigens). Cells automatically send peptides from newly synthesized proteins to their surface locked in the groove of an MHC class I molecule. Normal proteins presented in this way are not recognized by T cells and do not therefore trigger an immune response. However, abnormal proteins, such as those synthesized by viruses, can bind to the T-cell receptor and trigger a cytotoxic T-cell response. The T-cell receptors of CD8⁺ T cells recognize the complex formed by the foreign peptide bound to the antigen-binding groove of an MHC class I molecule. If either the peptide or the MHC molecule is foreign a cytotoxic T-cell response will be triggered. Cytotoxic T cells therefore attack not only virus-infected cells but also cells bearing foreign class I MHC molecules on their surface.

MHC class II molecules trigger graft rejection in two ways. First, as foreign proteins made by graft cells they

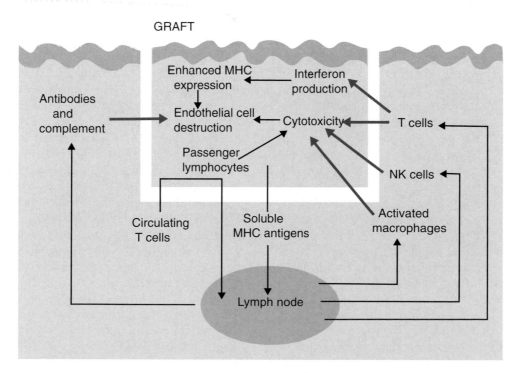

Figure 30-4. Some of the mechanisms involved in the rejection of an allograft (see text for details).

are processed as endogenous antigens and so trigger a cytotoxic response. More important, these molecules can stimulate host T-helper cells (Th1 cells) to release interleukin-2 (IL-2) and interferon-γ (IFN-γ). These cytokines stimulate cytotoxic T-cell activity and enhance the expression of MHC molecules on the cells of the graft. During allograft rejection, therefore, MHC expression is increased and the graft becomes an even more attractive target for cytotoxic T cells.

Blood group antigens mainly stimulate B cells. Released by the graft cells, they are processed as exogenous antigens and so trigger B-cell responses and antibody formation. Since animals may have preexisting antibodies to some of these blood group antigens, they can trigger hyperacute rejection.

Sensitization of the Recipient

Allograft recipients may be sensitized either directly as their T cells enter the graft or indirectly as soluble foreign antigens leak into the recipient. In the direct pathway, recipient T cells pass into the blood vessels of the graft, encounter foreign MHC class I and class II molecules on endothelial cell surfaces, and respond to them. Some graft antigens may also be processed and presented by donor antigen presenting cells or by host dendritic cells that invade the graft.

Alternatively, soluble antigens may be released from the grafted organ and sensitize the recipient indirectly. Thus graft cells can release soluble MHC peptides that enter the host, and are processed and recognized in the conventional manner. In humans, the direct pathway is responsible for the vigorous immune response that occurs in acute rejection whereas the indirect pathway is important in chronic rejection.

In laboratory rodents, MHC class II molecules are expressed on professional antigen-presenting cells. In these species therefore the intensity of graft rejection is related to the number of donor lymphocytes, macrophages, and dendritic cells transplanted within the graft. Previous removal of these cells by careful flushing of the graft before surgery or by pretreatment of the donor with cytotoxic drugs greatly reduces the intensity of the rejection process. In other mammals where MHC class II molecules are also expressed on vascular endothelial cells, these passenger cells are of less significance.

The cells that recognize the MHC molecules on graft cells move to the draining lymph node and activate other T cells. The paracortical regions of lymph nodes draining a graft therefore contain increased numbers of lymphoblasts. The number of these cells is greatest about 6 days after grafting and declines rapidly once the graft has been rejected. In addition to these signs of an active T-cell-mediated immune response, it is usual to observe germinal center formation in the cortex and plasma cell accumulation in the medulla, indicating that antibody formation is occurring.

Destruction of the Graft

Once activated by exposure to antigen, CD8+ T cells leave the node in the efferent lymph and reach the graft through the blood. When these T cells enter the graft, they bind and destroy vascular endothelium and other accessible cells. As a result of this damage, hemorrhage, platelet aggregation, thrombosis, and stoppage of blood flow occur. The grafted tissue dies because of the failure of its blood supply. CD4+ T cells that enter the graft may also kill graft cells by releasing cytotoxic cytokines such as TNF-α. If renal allografts are biopsied and the lymphocytes within them examined, host CD8+ T cells are seen to predominate early in the allograft response whereas CD4+ T cells tend to dominate later in the response.

Although cytotoxic T cells are of major importance in destroying allografts, antibodies also play a significant role in hyperacute and chronic rejection (Figure 30-5). Antibody formation is especially important when the donor and recipient differ in their major blood groups. Antibodies also have a major role in the second-set reaction where they may be directed against MHC class I molecules on the graft. These antibodies activate the classical complement pathway leading to target cell lysis. They also act through neutrophils and other cells with Fc receptor to mediate antibody-dependent cytotoxic cell activity.

Prevention of Allograft Rejection

In preventing allograft rejection, the transplantation surgeon is seeking to cause sufficient immunosuppression while at the same time not making the recipient any more susceptible than necessary to infectious agents. Dogs mount very strong allograft responses, and kidney allografts are rejected in 6 to 14 days in untreated animals. Unrelated dogs with renal allografts show about 50% 1-year survival when treated with azathioprine, prednisolone, and cyclosporine. Survival is considerably enhanced by a simultaneous bone marrow allograft from the donor animal or by treatment with rabbit antidog thymocyte serum. In practice, median survival times of 8 months can be achieved, with some animals surviving for longer than 5 years. Dogs have significant perioperative mortality, and two thirds experience recurrent acute infections, especially respiratory tract infections with *Bordetella bronchiseptica* and urinary tract infections. Newer immunosuppressive agents such as leflunamide show promise of vastly improving the prognosis for canine renal allografting.

Cats that have been given renal allografts receive immunosuppressive therapy with prednisolone and cyclosporine possibly supplemented with ketoconazole. (The ketoconazole suppresses cyclosporine metabolism in the liver and significantly prolongs its half-life.) The therapy can be begun 2 days before surgery so that cyclosporine levels are optimal when the graft is

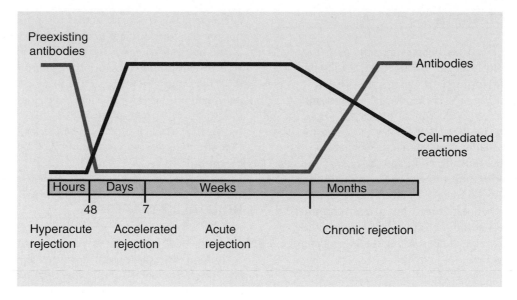

Figure 30-5. Role of antibodies and cell-mediated immunity in different allograft rejection syndromes.

introduced. Six-month survival ranges from 59% to 70%, whereas 3-year survival ranges from 40% to 50%. The longest survival time reported for cats receiving renal allografts is 81 months. These figures are gradually improving as experience grows. Long-term complications include acute or chronic rejection and opportunistic infections. Acute rejection can occur at any time, especially if cyclosporine levels fall below the therapeutic range. Chronic allograft rejection (graft vascular disease) due to progressive arterial arteriosclerosis may cause ischemic graft destruction. It is not responsive to immunosuppressive therapy.

In some circumstances, such as when a dog has maintained functioning renal allografts for several years, immunosuppressive therapy may be reduced gradually and eventually discontinued as graft acceptance becomes complete. It is probable that the immunosuppressive drugs gradually eliminate antigen-sensitive cells. Once their numbers are sufficiently low, the large mass of grafted tissue may be sufficient to establish and maintain tolerance.

SKIN ALLOGRAFTS

Although the mechanisms of rejection are similar among different tissues, minor differences are observed in the process. For example, if a skin graft is placed on an animal, it takes several days for blood vessels and lymphatic connections to be established between the graft and the host. Only when these connections are made can host cells enter the graft and commence the rejection process. The first sign of rejection is a transient neutrophil accumulation around the blood vessels at the base of the graft. This is followed by infiltration with mononuclear cells (lymphocytes and macrophages) that eventually extends throughout the grafted skin. The first signs of tissue damage are observed in the capillaries of the graft, whose endothelium is destroyed. As a result, the blood clots, blood flow stops, and tissue death follows rapidly. The presence of Langerhans cells in the epidermis significantly enhances the antigenicity of skin allografts. Skin allograft rejection is delayed if the graft is prevented from developing lymphatic connections with the host. In a second-set reaction, host blood vessels usually do not have time to grow into a skin graft, since a destructive mononuclear cell and neutrophil infiltration rapidly develops in the graft bed.

LIVER ALLOGRAFTS

It was originally reported that a high percentage of liver allografts between outbred pigs were accepted without immunosuppression. However, these pigs were not genetically defined, and the degree of MHC mismatching was unclear. When liver allografts are made between genetically defined miniature pigs with known MHC differences, it is found that their speed of rejection is similar to that observed with kidney or skin allografts. Liver graft rejection in dogs tends to occur fairly slowly. This inhibition of liver allograft rejection appears to be due to the presence of the enzyme indolamine dioxygenase (IDO). IDO destroys the amino acid tryptophan. Since tryptophan is essential for T-cell responses, its elimination within the grafted liver is highly immunosuppressive.

CARDIAC ALLOGRAFTS

Acute rejection of canine heart allografts is associated with massive lymphocytic infiltration and myocyte damage leading to rapid graft destruction. If, however, the rejection process is slowed for some reason, the pathologic process of the chronically rejected organ may change. In these cases, lymphocytes and antibodies directed against vascular endothelial cells stimulate them to proliferate. The resulting cell growth leads to obliteration of the blood vessel lumen and eventually cardiac failure (Figure 30-6). This graft arteriosclerosis (or graft vascular disease) results from the growth-stimulating effects of T-cell-derived cytokines and antibodies. A similar lesion is sometimes seen in renal allografts undergoing chronic rejection.

CORNEAL ALLOGRAFTS

Certain areas of the body, such as the anterior chamber of the eye, the cornea, the thymus, the testes, and the brain, are immune-privileged sites. As a result, grafts made into these sites may not be rejected. In humans, for example, 90% of first-time corneal allografts survive without tissue typing or immunosuppressive drugs. These sites are privileged because the body rigorously controls inflammation in their critical tissues. Several mechanisms are involved in this. Thus they have an impermeable blood–tissue barrier, lack dendritic cells, express low levels of MHC class I and II molecules, and may contain high levels of immunosuppressive molecules such as transforming growth factor-β (eyes and testes), neuropeptides (eyes), complement inhibitors (eyes), and corticosteroids (testes). Factors found in normal aqueous humor also block innate immune mechanisms. Thus they block natural killer (NK) cell lysis, inhibit neutrophil activation by CD95L, suppress nitric oxide production by activated macrophages, and interfere with alternative complement activation. The eye and testes are also unique in that they express very high levels of CD95L (fas ligand). As a result, any CD95$^+$ (fas)–activated T cells that enter these organs will bind to CD95L and be killed by apoptosis.

BONE ALLOGRAFTS

Bone cortical allografts are used to repair severe nonreconstructible diaphyseal fractures as well as to reconstruct defects created by the resection of tumors. Rejection of bone allografts is rarely a problem, probably because of the absence of soft tissues in the graft. Unfortunately, long-term bone allografts have a high incidence of mechanical failure because the graft is resorbed before it is replaced. Joints may be successfully transplanted in horses provided that such joints have been previously frozen.

BONE MARROW ALLOGRAFTS

Bone marrow allografts are given to dogs as a component of the treatment for leukemia or lymphoma (Figure 30-7). The recipient dog must first be conditioned by total-body irradiation or chemotherapy with cyclophosphamide. This creates space for the growing transplanted cells, reduces the intensity of the rejection process, and,

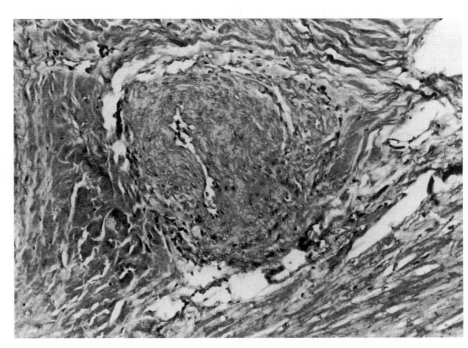

Figure 30-6. A section of coronary artery from a canine cardiac allograft. There is severe narrowing of the lumen as a result of endothelial proliferation, an example of graft vascular disease. Original magnification ×100. (From Penn OC, McDicken I, Leicher F, Bos E: *Transplantation* 22:313, 1976.)

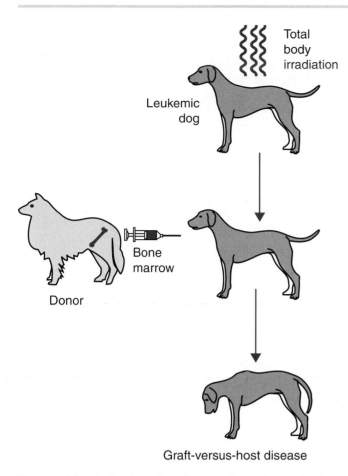

Total body irradiation

Leukemic dog

Donor

Bone marrow

Graft-versus-host disease

Figure 30-7. Induction of graft-versus-host disease in dogs that have received a bone marrow allograft.

in leukemic animals, destroys all tumor cells. Marrow is aspirated from the long bones of the donor and administered intravenously to the recipient. Hematopoietic stem cells migrate from the blood to the bone marrow. An optimal dose is about 2×10^8 allogeneic bone marrow cells per kilogram of body weight for matched recipients. The success rate of this procedure is relatively low. Thus there was a 20% success with untreated mismatched canine marrow allografts but a 90% success with treated matched allografts. In a successfully engrafted dog it takes about 30 days for the granulocytes to return to normal but the lymphocytes take about 200 days to recover. Marrow survival is not generally enhanced by treatment with single immunosuppressive agents, but combinations such as mycophenolate mofetil plus cyclosporine or methotrexate plus cyclosporine can result in the development of stable canine bone marrow chimeras.

Graft-versus-Host Disease

If healthy lymphocytes are injected into the skin of an allogeneic recipient, the lymphocytes attack the host cells and cause local acute inflammation. Provided the recipient has a functioning immune system, this graft-versus-host (GVH) reaction is not serious because the recipient is able to destroy the foreign lymphocytes and thus terminate the reaction. If, however, the recipient cannot reject the grafted lymphocytes because it has been immunosuppressed or is otherwise immunodeficient, then these grafted cells may cause uncontrolled destruction of the host's tissues and, eventually, death. Thus GVH disease occurs in bone marrow allograft recipients who have been effectively immunosuppressed by total-body irradiation or cyclophosphamide treatment.

The lesions generated in GVH disease depend on the MHC disparity between graft and host. When the difference is only in the MHC class I molecules, then the disease is caused by cytotoxic T cells that attack all the nucleated cells of the host. This leads to a wasting syndrome characterized by bone marrow destruction leading to pancytopenia, aplastic anemia, loss of T and B cells, and hypogammaglobulinemia. There is a lymphocyte infiltration of the intestine, skin, and liver. These lymphocytes secrete TNF-α, which causes mucosal destruction and diarrhea, skin and mouth ulcers, liver destruction, and jaundice. (Cytokines of the Th1 type are produced in this condition and it can be treated by antibodies to IFN-γ or TNF-α.)

If there is only an MHC class II disparity between the host and graft antigen-presenting cells, then the graft and host CD4+ T helper cells will be stimulated. The production of Th2-derived cytokines may lead to immunostimulation, autoantibody formation, and even clinical signs resembling systemic lupus erythematosus and polyarthritis (Chapter 34). (This is called autoimmune GVH disease and can be treated with antibodies against IL-4.)

In practice, pure class I or class II disparities rarely occur naturally. Thus in dogs GVH disease can either be an acute disease causing death within 4 weeks of transplantation or it can be prolonged and chronic. The major target organs are the skin, liver, gastrointestinal tract, and lymphoid system. The first clinical signs seen are exudative ear lesions, scleral injection, hyperkeratosis, alopecia, skin atrophy, and generalized erythema seen by 10 days (Figure 30-8). Jaundice and diarrhea frequently occur as does inflammation of the eyes, nose, and oral mucus membranes. An antiglobulin-positive hemolytic anemia may also occur. Good tissue matching and administration of the immunosuppressive drug methotrexate, together with monoclonal antilymphocyte antibodies may be used to suppress GVH disease.

It is of interest to note that bone marrow transplantation in cats who previously received immunosuppressive X radiation or cyclosporine is a very successful procedure and GVH disease is not a major problem in this species.

XENOGRAFTS

Although humans currently receive organs from other, dead, human donors, the demand for organ grafts greatly exceeds the supply. It is possible that xenografting from

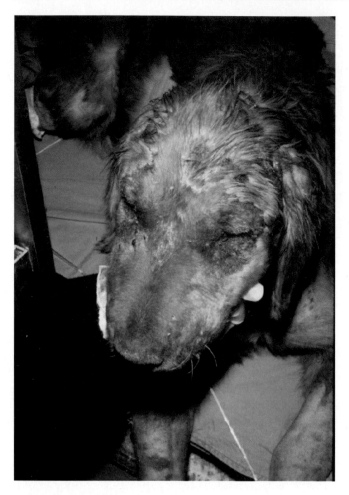

Figure 30-8. Very severe cutaneous erythematous lesions on the face of a dog suffering from graft-versus-host disease as a result of a bone marrow allograft. (From Harris CK, Beck ER, Gasper PW: *Compend Contin Educ Prac Vet* 8:337, 1986.)

nonhuman donors would eliminate this shortage. Unfortunately, xenografts are usually rejected within a few hours. The pathology of hyperacute xenograft rejection includes widespread hemorrhage and thrombosis brought about by massive destruction of endothelial cells. This allows blood cells to escape while at the same time exposing the underlying matrix to platelets.

Concordant xenografts are those between two closely related species such as between a chimpanzee and a human. In these cases rejection is largely mediated by cellular reactions. In discordant xenografts (those between unrelated species such as from a pig to a human), rejection is mediated largely by humoral mechanisms. In practice, concordant human xenografting from other primates such as chimpanzees or baboons is impractical because of the difficulty in providing large numbers of donor animals.

Pigs, however, may be more practical sources of organs. They breed rapidly and their organs are of an appropriate size. Unfortunately pig organs trigger a severe discordant xenograft rejection response in humans

mediated by natural anticarbohydrate antibodies. Humans and Old-World monkeys lack the enzyme α1-3 galactosyltransferase and do not therefore make carbohydrates or glycoproteins with the α1-3 galactosyl linkage. Because humans are exposed to this structure on many bacteria, we make high levels of antibodies to the Gal α1-3Gal epitope. Indeed more than 2% of total human IgM and IgG consists of antibodies to this αGal epitope. αGal, on the other hand, is a major component of pig glycoproteins. Thus if a pig organ is grafted into a human, these antibodies bind to graft cells, activate the classical complement pathway, and induce rapid cell lysis. A second mechanism that contributes to the hyperacute rejection process is activation of the alternate complement pathway. This activation results from the failure of human factor H to prevent assembly of the alternate C3 convertase on the surface of pig cells. A third mechanism involved in the xenograft rejection process is the species-specific activity of complement control proteins. Thus the natural inhibitors of complements such as CD46, CD55, and CD59 on pig cells cannot control the activation of human complement. Transgenic pigs have been produced that express these human complement inhibitors on their cells. When grafted into nonhuman primates, hyperacute rejection did not occur. Should the xenograft survive attack by these natural antibodies and complement, it is still susceptible to attack from induced antibodies and from antibody-dependent, cell-mediated cytotoxicity mediated through NK cells and monocytes, which together induce a delayed xenograft rejection. Thus many difficult barriers are yet to be overcome if pig organs are ever to be routinely used as human organ transplants.

One other point relevant to xenografting is that donor animals may carry viruses that could cause disease in a severely immunosuppressed recipient or, even worse, recombine with human viruses to create new and potentially hazardous pathogens. These xenograft-derived infections (xenozoonoses) are of special concern if primates are used as organ donors. These animals are known to carry viruses such as simian immunodeficiency virus and herpes B virus that can infect humans. Pigs possess an endogenous retrovirus that has the ability to infect some human cell lines in tissue culture.

ALLOGRAFTS AND THE REPRODUCTIVE SYSTEM

Sperm

Allogeneic sperm can successfully and repeatedly penetrate the female reproductive tract without provoking a significant immune response. The reason for this is that seminal plasma is immunosuppressive. Sperm exposed to this fluid are nonimmunogenic, even after washing. Prostatic fluid, one of the immunosuppressive components of seminal plasma, also inhibits complement-mediated hemolysis. In cattle, the immunosuppressive components of seminal plasma are proteins of less than 50 kDa and 150 kDa. Nevertheless, occasional cases of infertility resulting from the production of antisperm antibodies in the uterus do occur.

Pregnancy

When mammals evolved to become viviparous and the fetus developed inside its mother, a significant immunological problem had to be overcome. The fetus could not be rejected like an allograft. After all, the fetus possesses paternal MHC molecules, and its trophoblast lodges deep in the uterine wall. Nevertheless, in a normal pregnancy the fetus establishes and maintains itself in spite of these MHC differences. The uterus is not a privileged site, since grafts of other tissues, such as skin, in the uterine wall are readily rejected. Likewise, a mother may make antibodies against fetal blood group antigens and these can destroy fetal red blood cells either in utero, as in primates, or following ingestion of colostrum, as occurs in other mammals (Chapter 27). Nevertheless, allograft rejection does not occur.

We know that a mother may mount an immune response to her fetus. For example, in the pregnant mare placental cells invade the uterine wall to form structures called endometrial cups. These in turn stimulate a strong immune response by the mare against paternal MHC antigens around day 60 of gestation. As a result, the cups are surrounded by large numbers of CD4+ and CD8+ lymphocytes, macrophages, and plasma cells. Virtually all mares carrying an MHC-incompatible fetus produce strong antibody responses to paternal MHC class I antigens by day 60 of pregnancy. This eventually leads to degeneration of the endometrial cups around 120 days of pregnancy. At the same time, the ability of the pregnant mare to mount cytotoxic T-cell responses is reduced. Despite these responses, the pregnancy is unaffected. It is possible that these interactions lead to a Th2 immune response dominated by IL-10 production that does not threaten the pregnancy rather than a Th1 response that could lead to fetal rejection. In general, pregnancy is associated with a strong skewing of the mother's immune system in favor of Th2 responses and a reduction in Th1 responses. (This raises the interesting concept that infections that promote a strong Th1 response might reverse this skewing, compromise pregnancy, and lead to abortion. Thus would certainly apply to protozoan infections such as toxoplasmosis, *Neospora caninum* infection, and brucellosis.)

The immunological destruction of the fetus and its trophoblast is prevented by the combined activities of many different immunosuppressive mechanisms (Figure 30-9). First, no MHC class Ia or class II molecules are expressed on preimplantation embryos or oocytes, and these cannot be induced by exposure to

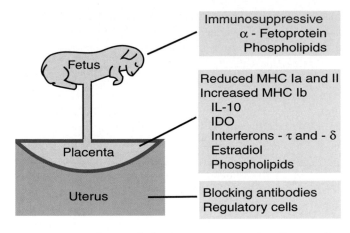

Figure 30-9. Some of the immunosuppressive factors that prevent rejection of the fetus by the mother's immune system.

interferon. Likewise MHC class Ia or class II molecules are not expressed on the cell layer of the trophoblast in contact with maternal tissues. Cytokines that usually enhance MHC expression, such as IFN-γ, have no effect on trophoblast cells. Instead, in humans these cells make the nonpolymorphic class Ib molecules human leukocyte antigens G and E. These molecules probably prevent attack on the trophoblast by NK cells while the NK cells control invasion of the uterine wall by the trophoblast. Thus there is a balance between MHC class Ib expression on the trophoblast and NK cells in the uterine wall that together regulates trophoblast growth and invasion. NK-like cells called endometrial gland cells have been described in rodents, bats, and horses. NK cells invade the pregnant porcine uterus in large numbers.

Although the trophoblast minimizes maternal sensitization by allogeneic fetal cells, cytotoxic T cells or antibodies can develop during pregnancy. For example, up to 90% of pregnant mares make antibodies to foal MHC class I molecules. Similar antibodies frequently develop in multiparous sheep and cattle. In some mouse strains, up to 95% of pregnant animals make antibodies against fetal MHC molecules. Up to 40% of women make antibodies to fetal MHC molecules after giving birth. The presence of these antibodies has no adverse effect on the course of the pregnancy. On the contrary, the maternal immune response may actually stimulate placental function. Thus in mice, hybrid placentas are larger than the placentas of inbred animals and females tolerant to paternal antigens have smaller placentas than intolerant females. Other studies show that mothers sensitized to paternal MHC molecules have better fetal survival. It appears that this effect is due to the stimulatory effect of IL-3 and granulocyte-macrophage colony-stimulating factor (GM-CSF) from maternal T cells on trophoblast growth. It is of interest to note that in cattle there is a clear association between retention of the placenta and its MHC class I molecules. In general, MHC class I compatibility between a mother and her calf increases the risk of a retained placenta. MHC class II compatibility had no effect. It has been suggested that the expulsion of the placenta after birth may be due, at least in part, to an allograft response.

Some antibodies made by the mother against fetal antigens may coat placental cells, thus preventing their destruction by maternal T cells. This blocking antibody can be eluted from the placenta and shown to suppress other cell-mediated immune reactions against paternal antigens, such as graft rejection. Absence of this blocking antibody accounts for some cases of recurrent abortion in women. Nevertheless it can also be shown that totally immunodeficient mice can have successful pregnancies. Mouse trophoblast cells are protected against complement-mediated damage by high levels of expression of a complement inhibitory protein called Crry on their surface. In its absence, fetal rejection appears inevitable.

The fetus does not depend entirely on maternal mechanisms for its protection. The placenta is a source of many immunosuppressive factors, including the hormones estradiol and progesterone and possibly also chorionic gonadotropin. Some isoforms of α-fetoprotein, the major protein in fetal serum, are immunoregulatory. In addition, some pregnancy-associated glycoproteins, including $\alpha2$-macroglobulin, a molecule related to TGF-β (possibly derived from suppressor cells infiltrating the placenta) and placental interferons, have immunosuppressive properties. In mammals, unique interferons (interferon-ω in humans, horses and dogs, interferon-τ in ruminants, and interferon-γ and interferon-δ in pigs) from the embryonic trophoblast act as signaling proteins between the embryo and mother during early development. These interferons can also inhibit lymphocyte proliferation. Amniotic fluid is rich in immunosuppressive phospholipids. CD55 (DAF) is incorporated in the trophoblast at the fetomaternal interface and so protects it against complement attack.

Recently it has been demonstrated that cells in the placenta manufacture indolamine 2,3-dioxygenase (IDO), which mediates the catabolism of tryptophan. Tryptophan is required for T cells to grow and respond to antigen. T cells cannot make their own tryptophan, and tryptophan starvation blocks T-cell division and promotes apoptosis. Inhibitors of IDO permit maternal rejection of allogeneic fetuses in mice. IDO+ cells appear in the trophoblast soon after implantation and are of maternal origin.

Despite the previous discussion, if the antigenic differences between the mother and her fetus are very great, then pregnancy may not go to completion. Thus experiments on xenogeneic combinations of two mouse species show that the embryos develop until midgestation and are then attacked and destroyed by maternal lymphocytes. Similarly, donkey embryos transferred to horse mares are destroyed by large numbers of maternal lymphocytes.

Mild immunosuppression is a consistent feature of late pregnancy and the early postpartum period. Pregnant animals may have minor deficiencies in cell-mediated immune reactivity to nonfetal antigens. Dairy cows experience a periparturient depression in neutrophil function and reduced T-cell cytotoxicity and cytokine production. This suppression appears to be mediated by CD8+ T cells. Blood lymphocyte responses to mitogens drop in the mare from 4 weeks before to 5 weeks after parturition. NK cell activity in pigs drops at the end of gestation to reach a low point 2 to 3 weeks after parturition. Ewes in late pregnancy may show a reduction of some immunoglobulin classes such as IgG1. This may be due to alterations in T helper cell function or, more plausibly, to diversion of the IgG1 into the mammary gland to produce colostrum. This suppression may be significant in parasitized animals, where the immune response barely controls the parasite. Similarly, immunosuppression may permit *Demodex* mite populations to rise in pregnant or lactating bitches and aid in the transmission of mites to their puppies.

SOURCES OF ADDITIONAL INFORMATION

Brown J, Matthews AL, Sandstrom PA, Chapman LE: Xenotransplantation and the risk of retroviral zoonosis, *Trends Microbiol* 6:411-415, 1998.

Carpenter CB: Immunosuppression in organ transplantation, *N Engl J Med* 322:1224-1226, 1990.

Cooper DKC, Kemp E, Platt JL, White DJG: *Xenotransplantation*, ed 2, Berlin, 1997, Springer-Verlag.

Ferrara JLM, Deeg HJ: Graft-versus-host disease, *N Engl J Med* 324:667-674, 1991.

Finco DR, Rawlings CA, Barsanti JA, Crowell WA: Kidney graft survival in transfused and nontransfused Beagle dogs, *Am J Vet Res* 46:2327-2331, 1985.

Gregory CR, Gourley IM, Kochin EJ, Broaddus TW: Renal transplantation for treatment of end-stage renal failure in cats, *J Am Vet Med Assoc* 201:285-291, 1992.

Harris CK, Beck ER, Gasper PW: Bone marrow transplantation in the dog, *Compend Contin Educ Prac Vet* 8:337-345, 1986.

Jacoby DR, Olding LB, Oldstone MBA: Immunologic regulation of fetal-maternal balance, *Adv Immunol* 35:157-208, 1984.

Joosten I, Sanders MF, Hensen EJ: Involvement of major histocompatibility complex class I compatibility between dam and calf in the aetiology of bovine retained placenta, *Anim Gen* 22:455-463, 1991.

Katayama M, McAnulty JF: Renal transplantation in cats: techniques, complications, and immunosuppression, *Compend Contin Educ Prac Vet* 24:874-882, 2002.

Kenmochi T, Mullen Y, Miyamoto M, Stein E: Swine as an allotransplantation model, *Vet Immunol Immunopathol* 43:177-183, 1994.

Krensky AM, Weiss A, Crabtree G, et al: T-lymphocyte-antigen interactions in transplant rejection, *N Engl J Med* 312: 510-517, 1990.

Lu CY, Khair-el-din TA, Dawidson IA, et al: Xenotransplantation, *FASEB J* 8:1122-1130, 1994.

Lunn P, Vagnoni KE, Ginther OJ: The equine immune response to endometrial cups, *J Reprod Immunol* 34:203-216, 1997.

Mathews KA, Gregory CR: Renal transplants in cats: 66 cases (1987–1996), *J Am Vet Med Assoc* 211:1432-1436, 1997.

Mathews KA, Holmberg DL, Miller CW: Kidney transplantation in dogs with naturally occurring end-stage renal disease, *J Am Anim Hosp Assoc* 36:294-301, 2000.

Mellon AL, Munn DH: Extinguishing maternal immune responses during pregnancy: implications for immunosuppression, *Semin Immunol* 13:213-218, 2001.

Munn DH, Zhou M, Attwood JT, et al: Prevention of allogeneic fetal rejection by tryptophan catabolism, *Science* 281:1191-1193, 1998.

Reynolds GE, Griffin JFT: Humoral immunity in the ewe. 2. The effect of pregnancy on the primary and secondary antibody response to protein antigen, *Vet Immunol Immunopathol* 25:155-166, 1990.

Skopets B, Li J, Thatcher WW, et al: Inhibition of lymphocyte proliferation by bovine trophoblast protein-1 (type I trophoblast interferon) and bovine interferon-αI1, *Vet Immunol Immunopathol* 34:81-96, 1992.

Xu C, Mao D, Holers VM, et al: A critical role for murine complement regulator Crry in fetomaternal tolerance, *Science* 287:498-502, 2000.

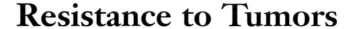

Resistance to Tumors

CHAPTER 31

Normal body processes depend on careful regulation of cell division. If cells are permitted to multiply, it is essential that they do so only as and when required. Unfortunately, as a result of exposure to certain chemicals, virus infection, or mutation, cells may occasionally break free of the constraints that regulate cell division. A cell that is proliferating in an uncontrolled fashion will give rise to a growing clone of cells that eventually develops into a tumor or neoplasm. If these cells remain clustered together at a single site, the tumor is said to be benign. Benign tumors can usually be removed through surgery. In some cases, however, tumor cells break off from the main tumor mass and are carried by the blood or lymph to distant sites where they lodge and continue to grow. This form of tumor is said to be malignant. The secondary tumors that arise in these distant sites are called metastases. Treatment for malignant tumors may be very difficult because it may be impossible to remove all metastases surgically. Malignant tumors are

subdivided according to their tissue of origin. Tumors arising from epithelial cells are called carcinomas; those arising from mesenchymal cells, such as muscle, lymphoid, or connective tissue cells, are called sarcomas. A leukemia is a tumor derived from hematopoietic cells.

The essential difference between a normal cell and a tumor cell is a loss of control of cell growth as a result of multiple mutations. These mutations may also result in the tumor cells' expressing abnormal proteins on their surface. These proteins may, under some circumstances, be recognized by the immune system and so trigger immunological attack.

TUMORS AS ALLOGRAFTS

When organ transplantation became a common procedure as a result of the development of potent immunosuppressive drugs, it was found that patients with prolonged graft survival were many times more likely to develop certain cancers than were nonimmunosuppressed individuals. It was also observed that some immunodeficient patients had an increased tendency to develop some malignant tumors. For example, patients with acquired immune deficiency syndrome (AIDS) may develop Kaposi's sarcoma. It was therefore suggested that the immune system was responsible for the prevention of cancer. From this suggestion the immune surveillance theory emerged. This theory held that the body constantly produces neoplastic cells but that in a healthy individual the immune system rapidly recognizes and eliminates these cells through cell-mediated mechanisms. The theory suggested that progressive cancer would result if the cancer cells somehow evaded recognition by T cells.

The immune surveillance theory soon ran into problems. Common human cancers such as those of the lung or breast did not develop more frequently in immunodeficient people. Likewise nude (*nu/nu*) mice, although deficient in T cells, are no more susceptible than normal mice to chemically induced or spontaneous tumors (Chapter 35). Finally, by using transgenic mice in which specific T cells for tumor-associated antigens were carefully monitored, it became clear that many tumor antigens induce tolerance in a manner similar to normal self-antigens. Thus all evidence has supported the idea that the immune system does not normally distinguish between tumor cells and normal, healthy cells.

Notwithstanding this, there are some situations where the immune system appears to recognize and kill cancer cells. For example, some immunodeficient mouse strains, which are "cleaner" subjects than nude mice, show an increased prevalence of spontaneous cancer. (Nude mice have some persistent T- and B-cell function and intact innate defenses). These include recombinase-activating gene (RAG) knockout mice that cannot produce functional T or B cells and signal transducer and activator of transcription 1 (STAT-1) knockout mice that lack both acquired and innate responses by being unresponsive to interferon-γ (IFN-γ). RAG knockout mice suffer from an increased incidence of spontaneous tumors of the intestinal epithelium whereas RAG/STAT-1 knockout mice develop mammary cancers. Thus the role of the immune system in affecting tumors, while relatively minor, is still somewhat significant. Whether or not cancer cells induce immunity is probably determined in part by whether they also cause inflammation. Thus if a metastasizing tumor does not invade lymphoid organs it may be ignored by the immune system. On the other hand, tumors that invade lymph nodes can be divided into strongly and weakly immunogenic types. Strongly immunogenic tumors elicit a strong T-cell response following processing by dendritic cells. Weakly immunogenic tumors tend to grow as walled-off nodules that may not be processed in sufficient amounts to trigger immune responses. These are the commonest tumors in humans. It is possible that tumor cells that trigger inflammation in tissues trigger dendritic cell activation and processing. On the other hand, tumors that fail to generate inflammation may simply be ignored by the immune system. Alternatively, it is possible that the antigens of the tumor may be tolerated by the immune system. If successful tumor therapy is to be achieved, then these two states must be distinguished.

Most animals that develop cancer have normal immune systems, and immunosuppressed individuals such as allograft recipients and AIDS victims develop a very different spectrum of cancers from that of the general population. The only cancers to which they are at greater risk are those caused by viruses, such as Kaposi's sarcoma. They are no more likely than the general population to develop the common cancers, such as those of breast, lung, or colon.

Although the original surveillance hypothesis has had therefore to be drastically modified, it is clear that under some circumstances the immune system destroys tumor cells and that this response may be enhanced to protect an individual against some cancers. However, there is a great difference between the strong and effective cell-mediated immune response triggered by foreign organ grafts and the much weaker responses to the antigens associated with tumor cells.

Tumor-Associated Antigens

Cancer may sometimes be diagnosed based on the production of new proteins by tumor cells. These may simply be normal proteins produced in excessive amounts. A good example is the production of prostate-specific antigen (PSA) in prostate carcinomas of humans. PSA is a protease exclusively produced by the prostate epithelium. Increased blood levels of this protein indicate excessive prostate activity. One cause of this is the growth of a carcinoma.

Alternatively, some tumors may express the products of developmental genes that are turned off in adult cells and are normally only expressed early in an individual's development. These proteins are called oncofetal antigens. For example, tumors of the gastrointestinal tract may produce a glycoprotein called carcinoembryonic antigen (CEA; also called CD66e), normally found only in the fetal intestine. The presence of detectable amounts of CEA in serum may therefore indicate the presence of a colon or rectal adenocarcinoma. α-Fetoprotein produced by hepatoma cells is also an example of an oncofetal antigen since it is normally found only in the fetal liver. Likewise, squamous cell carcinoma cells may possess antigens normally restricted to fetal liver and skin. These oncofetal antigens are poor immunogens and do not provoke protective immunity. However, measurement of their level in blood may be useful in diagnosis and in monitoring the progress of the tumor.

Tumor cells rarely develop completely new antigens; they simply express normal antigens in unusual quantities or produce abnormal proteins. Many of these molecules

Tissue-specific antigens

Normal proteins found in both normal and cancer cells

Reactivated gene products

Normal proteins not normally expressed after fetal development

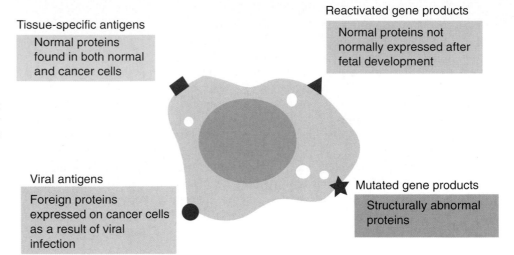

Figure 31-1. Some of the great variety of new antigens that may appear on the surface of tumor cells and provoke an immune response.

Viral antigens

Foreign proteins expressed on cancer cells as a result of viral infection

Mutated gene products

Structurally abnormal proteins

are those associated with cell division. Some of the tumor antigens are recognized because they are abnormally glycosylated. For example, melanoma cells may express the products of mutated oncogenes on the cell surface (Figure 31-1). Melanomas express characteristic gangliosides and many carcinomas express mucins.

Tumors induced by oncogenic viruses tend to gain new antigens characteristic of the inducing virus or of other endogenous retroviruses. These antigens, although coded for by a viral genome, are not part of a virion. Examples include the FOCMA antigens found on the neoplastic lymphoid cells of cats infected with feline leukemia virus and Marek's tumor-specific antigens found on Marek's disease tumor cells in chickens. (Both of these are virus-induced, naturally occurring, T-cell tumors.)

Chemically induced tumors may express mutated surface antigens unique to the tumor and not to the inducing chemical (Figure 31-2). Because carcinogenic chemicals can produce many different mutations, tumors induced by a single chemical in different animals may be antigenically different. Even within a single chemically induced tumor mass, antigenically distinct subpopulations of cells exist. As a result, resistance to one chemically induced tumor does not prevent growth of a second tumor induced by the same chemical.

IMMUNITY TO TUMORS

If tumor cells express different antigens from normal cells, then why are they not regarded as foreign and attacked by the immune system? The main problem appears to be that the abnormal molecules are not appropriately presented to the cells of the immune system, especially cytotoxic T cells. Nevertheless on occasion tumor cells may be attacked by natural killer (NK) cells, cytotoxic T cells, activated macrophages, or antibodies (Figure 31-3). It is likely that the most important of these are NK cells.

NATURAL KILLER CELLS

About 15% of mammalian blood lymphocytes are neither T nor B cells but belong to a third population of lymphocytes called natural killer cells. Unlike T and B cells that circulate as resting cells and require several days in order to be activated, NK cells can be activated almost immediately by interferons from virus-infected cells and by IL-12 from macrophages. As a result, NK cells enter tissues and rapidly attack abnormal cells. They can participate in innate defenses long before antigen-specific T or B cells are generated. Unlike T and B cells, NK cells do not rearrange TCR or immunoglobulin genes to produce a repertoire of antigen receptors. Indeed, they do not express antigen-specific receptors at all. Instead they use different combinations of receptors to bind abnormal cells. By using multiple receptors in this way, NK cells can discriminate between normal and abnormal cells.

Oncogenic virus   Chemical carcinogen

Malignant transformation

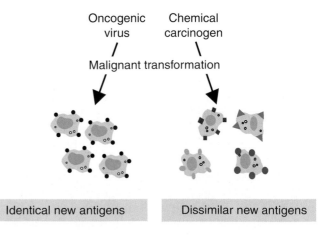

Identical new antigens   Dissimilar new antigens

Figure 31-2. Although oncogenic viruses induce tumor cells with identical new antigens, chemical carcinogens induce tumor cells with a great variety of new antigens.

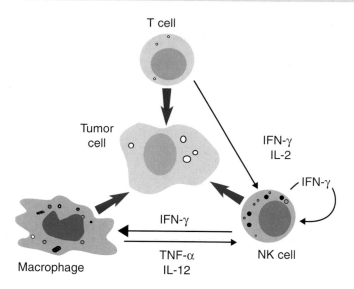

Figure 31-3. The three major cell types that participate in tumor cell destruction and the role of interferon in stimulating that activity.

NK cells in most mammals are large, granular, nonphagocytic lymphocytes (Figure 31-4). They probably arise from the same bone marrow precursor as T cells. However, T cells depend on thymus processing for their full development whereas NK cells do not. NK cells are concentrated mainly in the secondary lymphoid organs, a few are found in the bone marrow, and none is found in the thymus. They do not recirculate.

Surface Markers

NK cells do not express conventional antigen receptors like B-cell receptors or T-cell receptors, nor do they express a CD3 complex. Therefore they cannot recognize conventionally processed antigen. On the other hand, they do express a characteristic major surface antigen called CD56. Thus an NK cell can be defined as a lymphocyte that expresses CD56 on its surface rather than CD3. They also express CD2, CD16 (FcγRIII, the low-affinity receptor for immunoglobulins), CD178 (CD95L or fas ligand), and the CD40 ligand, CD154. Some NK cells express CD8. Those NK cells that express CD154 may have regulatory functions. (In humans, there is evidence of two subsets of NK cells. NK1 cells produce IFN-γ but almost no IL-4, IL-10, or IL-13. NK2 cells do not secrete IFN-γ but produce IL-13. It is not known whether such subsets occur in domestic mammals.)

Target Cell Recognition

NK cells can recognize and kill abnormal cells using a totally different mechanism than do T cells. Triggering of NK cell cytotoxicity results from a change in the balance between activating and inhibitory signals. When NK cells encounter normal body cells, inhibitory signals predominate. When they encounter infected, damaged, or malignant cells, the activating signals prevail. Thus MHC class I molecules on the surface of healthy normal cells provide inhibitory signals sufficient to block NK cell killing If, however, a target cell does not express MHC class I molecules, then the NK will not receive the inhibitory signal and the target cell will be killed (Figure 31-5). Viruses may suppress MHC class I expression in an attempt to hide within infected cells, and metastatic tumor cells often fail to express MHC class I. These cells are therefore targets for NK cell attack.

NK cells use two different receptors to bind MHC class I molecules. These are totally unrelated molecules

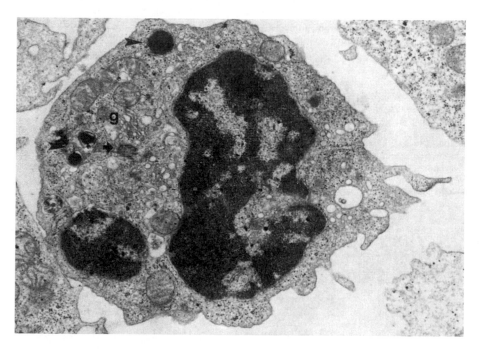

Figure 31-4. A transmission electron micrograph of a human NK cell. The nucleus is indented and rich in chromatin. The cytoplasm is abundant and contains many granules. Numerous mitochondria, centrioles, and a Golgi are visible. Original magnification ×17,000. (From Carpen O, Virtanen I, Saksela E: *J Immunol* 128:2691, 1982.)

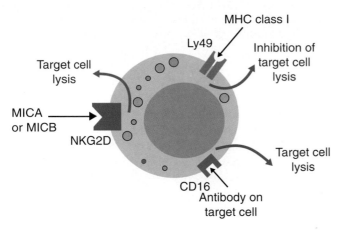

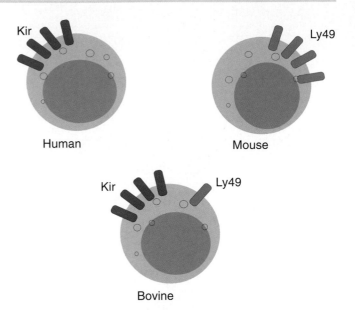

Figure 31-5. Three of the receptors found on mouse NK cells. Ly49 recognizes MHC class I molecules and suppresses NK cytotoxicity. CD16 binds immunoglobulins and triggers cytotoxicity by antibody-dependent cellular cytotoxicity. NK cells also express NKG2D, a receptor for molecules such as MICA and MICB. These molecules are commonly expressed on tumor cells.

Figure 31-6. Species difference between the MHC class I receptors on NK cells. Humans possess a single, nonfunctional Ly49 gene. Thus they rely totally on KIR molecules whereas mice rely totally on Ly49 molecules for recognition of their MHC ligands.

in primates (humans) and mice. For example, the human NK receptors belong to a highly polymorphic, Ig-like, killer cell inhibitory receptor (KIR or CD158) family of proteins. The KIR genes are clustered together with the genes of many other Ig-like transcripts (ILTs) in the leukocyte receptor complex. The KIR and ILT families contain not only receptors with activating potential but also inhibitors and receptors with no known ligand.

In contrast, in mice the NK cell MHC class I receptors are C-type lectins belonging to the highly polymorphic Ly49 family of proteins. Mice have no homologs of KIR. The genes for 15 of these Ly49 molecules are located in the "NK cell gene complex." These genes are also present in multiple copies in the rat and the horse. Only one Ly49 gene has been found in humans and it is probably not functional. Cattle possess multiple KIR genes but only a single copy of a functional Ly49 gene. The dog, cat, and pig have only a single functional Ly49 gene. This suggests that the use of multiple Ly49 genes by mice, rats, and horses is not typical of mammals in general. Since the single Ly49 molecule cannot serve as a receptor for all the polymorphic MHC class I molecules, it is likely that the KIR molecules are the major NK cell receptors in cattle (Figure 31-6). However, sequence analysis has also suggested that some bovine KIR molecules have an inhibitory function whereas others have an opposite effect.

The reasons for these species differences are unclear. However, it is recognized that with their short life span rodents have been subjected to severe infectious disease pressure and as a result exhibit very unique MHC polymorphisms. It is possible that during their evolution the mouse Ly49 molecules became better adapted to bind these ligands than the KIR molecules.

A second mechanism that triggers NK cell cytotoxicity involves the recognition of proteins on the target cell surface called MICA (*m*ajor histocompatibility complex, class *I* chain-related *A*) and MICB. These two molecules are expressed during cell stress and are up-regulated in tumor cells and virus-infected cells. They are not expressed on normal, healthy cells. Natural killer cells have a receptor called NKG2D that binds to MICA and MICB. Several homologs of this receptor have been identified in cattle. When engaged, NKG2D overrides the inhibitory effects of MHC class I molecules and permits the NK cells to kill their target. MICA and MICB are not found in mice. NKG2D is also expressed on activated γ/δ and α/β T cells. Thus these cells also recognize MICA and MICB, suggesting that they too have a role in both acquired and innate immunity. It may be that on surfaces, the combination of γ/δ T cells and NK cells kills tumors while within the body a combination of α/β T cells and NK cells is most effective. These mechanisms may be especially effective against precancerous cells when they begin to express these new ligands.

NK cells also recognize target cells by a third, antibody-dependent process using CD16. CD16 is an Fc receptor (FcγRIII) expressed on NK cells, granulocytes, and macrophages. The form on macrophages and NK cells is a 36- to 38-kDa transmembrane protein linked to either the gamma chain of FcεRI (in macrophages) or the zeta chain (in NK cells). Triggering of NK cells by antigen and antibody through CD16 results in production of IFN-γ, CD25, and TNF-α. NK cells may spontaneously release CD16 so that the NK cell may detach from an antibody-coated target cell after delivering the lethal hit.

Effector Mechanisms

Once triggered, NK cell killing is mediated, like T cells, through perforins and granzymes as well as through the death receptor pathway involving CD95L, TNF-α, and TNF-β. Perforins and granzymes are constitutively expressed in NK cells. Their expression is increased by exposure to interleukin-2 (IL-2) and IL-12. The NK cell perforin is a molecule of 70 to 72 kDa (slightly larger than that produced by T cells). It produces characteristic small (5 to 7 nm) lesions in target cell surfaces. Presumably granzymes are injected into the target cells in association with the perforin channels. NK cells also secrete a protease called fragmentin that can induce DNA fragmentation and apoptosis in target cells. CD178 (CD95L) on NK cells can induce apoptosis in target cells by binding to CD95 on the target cell surface. These targets can include tumor cells, virus-infected cells, and some immature T-cell populations.

Function

Initially, it was believed that NK cells functioned only as an innate antitumor surveillance system. However, we now recognize that they are active against other targets such as xenografted cells and virus-infected cells (Figure 31-7). Some Ly49 molecules on the surface of mouse NK cells can recognize viruses. NK cells can kill bacteria such as *Staphylococcus aureus* and *Salmonella enterica typhimurium* as well as some fungi.

Most of the evidence that supports a role for NK cells in innate immunity to tumors is derived from studies on tumor cell lines grown in vitro. Thus NK cells destroy cultured tumor cell lines, and a correlation exists between the level of NK activity measured in vitro and resistance to tumor cells in vivo. It is possible to increase resistance to tumor growth in vivo by passive transfer of NK cells.

NK cells destroy human leukemia, myeloma, and some sarcoma and carcinoma cells in vitro, and this activity is enhanced by IFN-γ. NK cells can also invade small primary mouse tumors. Some carcinogenic agents, such as urethane, dimethylbenzanthracene, and low doses of radiation, can inhibit NK activity. It is also interesting to note that certain stresses, such as surgery, may depress NK activity and so promote tumor growth.

Regulation

NK cells are regulated by cytokines. For example, both IL-2 and IFN-γ stimulate NK cell growth. Culture of NK cells in the presence of IL-2 enhances their cytotoxic activity so that they can lyse normally resistant tumor targets. IL-4 also stimulates NK function and enhances cytotoxicity, whereas IL-3 prevents the death of cultured NK cells. Although NK cells are active in the nonimmunized animal, virus infections or interferon inducers stimulate NK activity above normal levels. In these diseases, macrophages phagocytose the invading organisms and produce TNF-α and IL-12. These cytokines induce IFN-γ production by NK cells. This IFN-γ then enhances NK activity by promoting the rapid differentiation of pre-NK cells. It also activates more macrophages so that production of TNF-α is augmented by IFN-γ. The NK cell/interferon system probably has a role in resistance to tumors since neutralization of interferon by specific antisera enhances tumor growth in mice, presumably by depressing NK cell activity. IFN treatment may be useful in the therapy of some human cancers. For example, IFN-α is of significant benefit in the treatment of hairy cell leukemia (a B-cell tumor) and Kaposi's sarcoma in humans. IL-21 from activated CD4+ T cells also regulates NK cell function. It blocks activation of uninvolved NK cells, it promotes IFN-γ secretion of activated NK cells, and it initiates a delayed apoptosis of activated NK cells while stimulating T- and B-cell proliferation. Thus IL-21 appears to terminate NK cell innate immunity by optimizing their function, triggering their elimination, and initiating T- and B-cell-mediated acquired immunity.

SPECIES DIFFERENCES

Cattle

Bovine NK cells are CD2+, CD5+, WC1+, MHC class II+, and asialo-GM1+. (GM$_1$ is a ganglioside, which is a glycolipid molecule composed of a fatty ceramide residue buried in the lipid bilayer of a cell with at least three sugar groups projecting into the extracellular fluid. One of these is normally a sialic acid group. This is lacking in asialo-GM$_1$). Bovine NK cells are found in highest concentrations in the spleen and peripheral blood. In cattle, NK cells are large cells although they may not contain

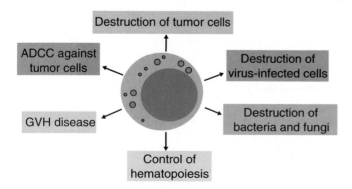

Figure 31-7. Schematic diagram showing the many functions of NK cells. *GVH*, Graft-versus-host; *ADCC*, antibody-dependent cellular cytotoxicity.

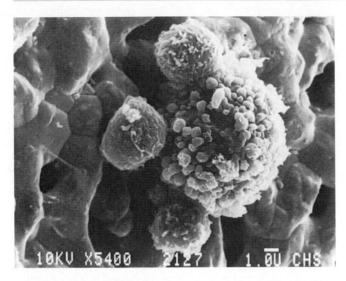

Figure 31-8. Scanning electron micrograph of NK cells from a pig (small round cells) attached to a target cell (a human tumor cell). Original magnification ×5400. (From Yang WC et al: *Vet Immunol Immunopathol* 14:345-356, 1987.)

large intracytoplasmic granules. Bovine NK cells can attack human cancer cell targets and bovine cells infected with parainfluenza-3, bovine leukemia virus (BLV), and bovine herpesvirus type 1 (BHV-1). They are activated by IL-2, IFN-α, and IFN-γ.

Pigs

Pig NK cells are CD2+, CD8+, MHC class II+, and LFA-1+. They are found in spleen and peripheral blood but very few are found in lymph nodes or thymus (Figure 31-8). There is a debate about their morphology. Some investigators claim that they are large granular lymphocytes whereas others claim that they are small lymphocytes without obvious cytoplasmic granules. Porcine NK cells can lyse human cancer cells, as well as cells infected with transmissible gastroenteritis virus or pseudorabies virus.

Cats

Feline NK cells are large granular lymphocytes found in the blood and spleen. They are active against feline target cells infected with feline leukemia virus, herpesvirus, or vaccinia.

Dogs

Canine NK cells can lyse distemper-infected target cells, as well as cancer cells from melanomas, osteosarcomas, and mammary carcinomas.

Horses

Equine NK cells are activated by recombinant human IL-2 and are active against human tumor cell targets.

Chickens

Chicken NK cells are asialo-GM$_1$+ and may share determinants with T cells. Their morphology is unclear but they are probably large granular lymphocytes. NK activity is found in the thymus, bursa, spleen, and intestinal epithelium. These cells can attack human cancer cells, lymphoid leukosis, leukemia virus, and Marek's disease virus–infected cells.

OTHER CELLULAR DEFENSES

Natural Killer T Cells

NK T cells are lymphocytes that share features with both T cells and NK cells. Thus they express α/β T-cell receptors in addition to the NK cell receptor NK1.1 and members of the Ly49 family. However, their T-cell receptor repertoire is restricted since they use an invariant α chain together with polyclonal β chains. Like conventional T cells, they originate in the thymus. NK T cells probably recognize glycolipids in association with the MHC class Id molecule CD1d. Binding of these glycolipids stimulates NK T cells whereas binding to the Ly49 ligand inhibits their activity. During maturation these cells initially secrete predominantly IL-4 and thus have a Th2 phenotype. As they mature they increase their secretion of IFN-γ and assume a Th1 phenotype. NK T cells have a role in antitumor immunity, in autoimmunity, and in antimicrobial immunity, especially that to *Mycobacterium*. Thus they serve to link the T-cell system with the innate NK cell system.

Conventional T Cells

It is occasionally possible to detect a cell-mediated response to tumor antigens by skin testing. Lymphocytes from some tumor-bearing animals may kill tumor cells cultured in vitro. Nevertheless, responses by T cells are probably significant only in the management of virus-induced tumors.

Macrophage-Mediated Immunity

In some experimental systems macrophages may have an antitumor function. This is especially true of macrophages activated by exposure to IFN-γ. These activated macrophages release cytotoxic molecules such as arginase and oxidants. Nonspecific activation of macrophages by bacillus Calmette-Guerin (BCG) or *Propionibacterium acnes* results in enhanced production of IL-1 or TNF-α and subsequent activation of T helper cell and NK cell activity. IL-1 has a cytostatic effect on some tumors, and TNF-α may have potent antitumor activity. Unfortunately, malignant tumors may inhibit macrophage activation, and the macrophages of tumor-bearing animals may show defective mobilization and chemotaxis.

Antibody-Mediated Immunity

Antibodies to tumor cells are found in many tumor-bearing animals; for instance, about 50% of sera from dogs with lymphosarcomas contain precipitating antitumor antibodies. These antibodies may be of some protective significance since together with complement they may lyse free tumor cells. Antibodies are not effective in destroying the cells in solid cancers.

FAILURE OF IMMUNITY TO TUMOR CELLS

The fact that neoplasia are so readily induced and are so relatively common testifies to the inadequacies of the immunological protective mechanisms. Studies of tumor-bearing animals have indicated several mechanisms by which immune systems fail to reject tumors.

Immunosuppression

It is commonly observed that tumor-bearing animals are immunosuppressed. This suppression is most clearly seen in animals with lymphoid tumors; thus tumors of B cells tend to suppress antibody formation, whereas tumors of T-cell origin generally suppress cell-mediated immune responses and NK cell activity. In contrast, immunosuppression in animals with chemically induced tumors appears to be due in part to production of immunosuppressive molecules, such as prostaglandins, from the tumor cells or from tumor-associated macrophages. The presence of actively growing tumor cells represents a severe protein drain on an animal. This protein loss may also be immunosuppressive.

Some tumor-derived molecules may redirect macrophage activities so that they promote tumor development. Thus tumor-derived IL-4, IL-6, IL-10, transforming growth factor β_1, prostaglandin E_2, and macrophage colony-stimulating factor can deactivate or suppress the activation of macrophages and suppress Th1 responses. Tumor cells can suppress macrophage cytokine production and circumvent macrophage cytotoxicity.

Suppressor Cells

Much of the immunosuppression seen in tumor-bearing individuals may be due to the activities of suppressive regulatory cell populations. These suppressor cells may be CD8+ T cells, IL-10-secreting Th2 cells or macrophages, or even B cells. Enhanced suppressor cell activity can be detected in humans with osteogenic sarcomas, thymomas, myelomas, and Hodgkin's disease, and in many tumor-bearing animals.

An excellent example of the role of suppressor cells is seen in skin cancer induced by ultraviolet (UV) light in mice. Thus when UV radiation–induced skin cancer cells are transferred to the skin of normal allogeneic mice they are rejected. When transferred to chronically UV-irradiated mice they grow successfully. This is because immunosuppressive cells develop in the UV-irradiated skin before tumors appear. If adoptively transferred to normal mice, these suppressor cells prevent rejection of a subsequent tumor challenge. These suppressor cell populations are a mixture of T cells and macrophages secreting IL-10.

Conventional cancer therapy may influence suppressor cell activity. Thus cyclophosphamide can inhibit suppressor-cell function whereas immunostimulants such as *P. acnes* and BCG enhance suppressor cell activity in some patients, and this may account for the inconsistent results obtained with their use.

CD95 Ligand Expression

CD95 ligand (CD95-L) is normally expressed on cytotoxic T cells and NK cells. When it binds to CD95 on target cells it triggers apoptosis. CD95-L has been detected on some leukemic T cells and NK cells, on colon adenocarcinoma cells, melanomas, and hepatocellular carcinomas. At the same time, these cells may down-regulate CD95 so that they become resistant to cell-mediated cytotoxicity and cannot be killed by their own or a neighbor's CD95-L. Since cytotoxic T cells may also express CD95, it is possible that these tumor cells may kill T cells. It is interesting to note that the anticancer drug doxorubicin enhances expression of both CD95 and CD95-L on tumor cells and may permit these molecules to interact with T cells, thus killing themselves by apoptosis. Some tumor cells such as those in lung carcinomas may secrete decoy receptors for CD95-L. These decoy receptors can bind to CD95-L and block its binding to CD95. Thus tumor cells that down-regulate CD95 while up-regulating their decoy receptor expression can become resistant to cytotoxic cells.

Blocking Antibodies

Although tumor cells are antigenic and may stimulate a protective cell-mediated immune response, antibodies may have an opposite effect. Thus the serum of a tumor-bearing animal may cause the tumors of other animals to grow even faster—a phenomenon called enhancement. This serum may also inhibit T-cell cytotoxicity. Many tumors release large quantities of cell surface antigen into serum, and this may bind to cytotoxic T cells, saturating their antigen receptors and so blocking their ability to bind to target cells. Alternatively, blocking antibodies may be produced. These are non–complement-activating, antitumor antibodies that can mask tumor antigens and thus protect the tumor cells from attack by cytotoxic T cells. In general, the presence or absence of these blocking factors correlates well with the state of progression of a tumor.

Tumor Cell Selection

Tumor cells don't usually become malignant in one step. Rather they gradually become malignant over a long period, going from benign to malignant in a process called tumor progression. The process occurs through a series of mutations that switch genes on and off. These mutations do not necessarily alter the immunogenicity of tumor cells or do so in small steps. Immunogenicity may not alter until the cells are irreversibly committed to malignancy. Thus there are two selection mechanisms by which tumor cells can evade the host's immune response and so enhance their own survival. One is "sneaking through," the process by which malignant cells may not trigger an immune response until the tumor has reached a size at which it cannot be controlled by the host. Thus in experimental tumors, small numbers of tumor cells may grow after subcutaneous inoculation although large numbers may not. It may be that the tumor cells may not reach lymph nodes and trigger an immune response until the tumor burden is too large to be controlled. Even a very small tumor may contain an enormous number of cells. For example, a 10-mm tumor contains about 10^9 cells. Second, tumor cells that have mutated in such a way as to be antigenically different from the host will induce a strong immune response and be eliminated without leading to disease. Those tumors cells that survive must therefore be selected for their lack of antigenicity and their inability to stimulate the host's immune system. To this extent, therefore, tumors that do develop have by definition already beaten the immune system.

TUMOR IMMUNOTHERAPY

Immunotherapy may be either active or passive. In active immunotherapy the patient's own immune system is stimulated to respond to the tumor. In passive immunotherapy immune cells or their products are administered.

Active Immunotherapy

Two general approaches have been used in attempts to cure or modify tumor growth through immunotherapy (Box 31-1). The simplest is to stimulate the immune system nonspecifically (Figure 31-9). Any improvement in an animal's immune abilities will tend to enhance its resistance to tumors, although a cure may be expected only if the tumor mass is small or is surgically excised. The most widely used immune stimulant is the attenuated strain of *Mycobacterium bovis*, BCG. This organism activates macrophages and stimulates cytokine release, thus promoting T-cell activity. It may be given systemically or injected directly into the tumor mass. Most positive results from the use of BCG have come from studies on patients with melanomas or bladder cancer. Direct injection of BCG into skin melanoma metastases may cause complete regression, not only of the injected lesion but also, occasionally, of uninjected skin metastases. However, visceral metastases usually remain unaffected. BCG enhances survival or remission length in some

---

BOX 31–1

Some of the Approaches to Tumor Immunotherapy

NONSPECIFIC IMMUNE STIMULATION
Microbial products (bacille Calmette-Guérin, *Propionibacterium acnes*, yeast glucans, levamisole, etc.)
Complex carbohydrates (acemannan)
Cytokines (interferons, tumor necrosis factor, interleukin-2, interleukin-4)
Cytokine-activated cells (natural killer cells, T cells, tumor-infiltrating lymphocytes)

PASSIVE IMMUNIZATION
Monoclonal antibodies (alone or conjugated to toxins)

ACTIVE IMMUNIZATION
Chemically modified tumor cells
Vaccination against oncogenic viruses (feline leukemia, Marek's disease)

---

leukemias, and its direct intravesicular application in human bladder cancer gives complete or partial response rates of up to 70%. However, BCG can cause severe lesions at the site of injection and, occasionally, systemic hypersensitivity. Other immunostimulants that have been employed include *P. acnes*, levamisole, and various mixed bacterial vaccines.

Many investigators have also studied the effects of immunizing a patient with tumor cells or antigens. This approach has worked best in human melanoma patients where several different antigen preparations are undergoing clinical trials. Because many tumors can evade the immune response, it is usual to treat the tumor cells in an attempt to enhance their antigenicity. Thus, X-irradiated, neuraminidase-, or glutaraldehyde-treated

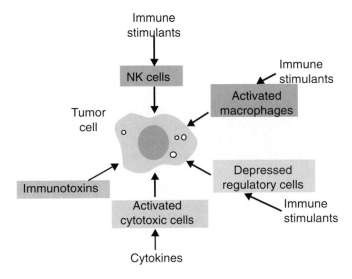

Figure 31-9. Some of the ways in which the immune system can be stimulated to mount a protective response to tumors.

cells have been used in tumor vaccines. The results obtained with these vaccines so far have been erratic and unsatisfactory.

Passive Immunotherapy

Cytokine Therapy

Many attempts have been made to treat human cancer patients with isolated cytokines but with limited success. Interferons, for example, are only effective against certain selected tumors. Thus 70% to 90% of patients with hairy cell leukemia treated with IFN-α show complete or partial remission. The antitumor activities of TNF-α are synergistic with the interferons. On the other hand, administration of IL-2 to melanoma and renal cell cancer patients induces partial or complete remission in 15% to 20% of cases.

One major difficulty in cytokine therapy has been their toxicity. For example, when given at pharmacological doses, TNF produces clinical signs similar to those induced by endotoxin. IL-2 is extremely toxic when administered alone. In low doses it induces fever, chills, nausea, and weight gain as well as a capillary leak syndrome resulting in massive pulmonary edema. IL-2 also produces anemia, thrombocytopenia, and eosinophilia. Patients may develop a severe, very itchy rash, neuropsychiatric changes, and endocrine abnormalities. Thus IL-2 is a hazardous protein and has limited usefulness when used alone. Preliminary trials of IL-4 have indicated that toxic effects similar to those seen with IL-2 occur in treated patients. Nevertheless it is important to note that local application of IL-2 may produce useful results. For example, relatively low doses of recombinant human IL-2 when injected locally into papillomas or carcinomas of the vulva in cattle induced significant remissions in 83% of treated animals. Some complete regressions were observed.

Activated Cytotoxic Cell Therapy

If NK cells or NK-like (CD4⁻CD8⁻) T cells are incubated in the presence of IL-2 for 4 days they develop cytotoxic properties. These cells are called lymphokine-activated killer (LAK) cells. Injection of LAK activated cells into mice with experimental lung tumors can lead to cancer remission. A combination of LAK cells and IL-2 has given encouraging results when administered to cancer patients.

LAK cells from blood include about 40% NK cells; the remainder are T cells. The activated NK cells are mainly CD3⁺, CD16⁺, and CD56⁺. They release LAK-1, a cytotoxic protein, as their effector molecule. IL-4 and IL-7 also activate cytotoxic cells. LAK cells have been induced in both cat and dog (Figure 31-10). Cell supernatants rich in IL-2 derived from concanavalin A–stimulated feline blood lymphocytes kill feline leukemia virus–transformed tumor cells. Recombinant human IL-2 activated the antitumor cytotoxic activity of canine blood lymphocytes.

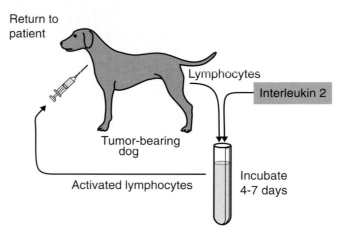

Figure 31-10. Production of LAK cells by incubation of blood lymphocytes in the presence of IL-2 for 4 to 7 days.

In an attempt to obtain even better results in humans, tumors were surgically removed from cancer-bearing patients; then the lymphocytes in these tumors were removed and cultured in the presence of IL-2 for 4 to 6 weeks so that their numbers would grow significantly. These tumor-infiltrating lymphocytes recognize and infiltrate only the tumors from which they come. Given together with IL-2 back to the donor patients, they have produced remissions in about one third of patients. The most encouraging results have been obtained in patients with melanomas, and those with colorectal and kidney cancer. Experimental injection of anti-CD152 (CTLA-4) into tumors in mice has caused tumor regression. By blocking the suppressive receptor CD152, these antibodies permit T-cell clones to expand and attack the tumor cells.

Antibody Therapy

Despite the risk of tumor enhancement by antibodies, some successes have been achieved by the use of monoclonal antibodies for tumor therapy. Monoclonal antibodies can be used to destroy tumors, either when given alone or when complexed to highly cytotoxic drugs or potent radioisotopes, which they carry directly to the tumor cells. Thus a monoclonal antibody against canine T cells (CL/MAb231) has yielded encouraging results when used to manage lymphomas in dogs. It greatly increased life expectancy following two cycles of L-asparaginase/vincristine/cyclophosphamide/doxorubicin chemotherapy to bring the lymphoma into remission. The monoclonal antibody is given for 5 days, beginning 3 weeks after the conclusion of chemotherapy.

Successful Antitumor Vaccines

In contrast to the techniques described above (most of which have met with only limited success), there are established successful techniques for vaccination against tumor viruses. The most important of these are the vaccines against feline leukemia in cats. These vaccines usually contain high concentrations of the major viral antigens, and immunity is almost entirely directed against viral glycoproteins. Another important vaccine is that directed against Marek's disease, a T-cell tumor of chickens caused by a herpesvirus. The immune response evoked by this vaccine has two components. First, humoral and cell-mediated responses act directly on the virus to reduce the quantity available to infect cells. Second, an immune response is provoked against virus-coded antigens that are generated by the virus on the surface of tumor cells. Both the antiviral and antitumor immune responses act synergistically to protect the birds.

SOME SPECIFIC TUMORS

Transmissible Venereal Sarcoma

Transmissible venereal sarcoma is a neoplasm transmitted between dogs during copulation by transplantation of tumor cells. To colonize a new host, these cells must be capable of establishing themselves in allogeneic hosts. This is not always successful, and after an initial growth phase the tumor eventually regresses and is eliminated. Nevertheless lethal metastases do occur in immunosuppressed dogs. When growing aggressively, these tumor cells fail to express β_2-microglobulin and, as a result, MHC class I antigens are not assembled on the cell surface. Exposed dogs, whether or not they develop progressive neoplasia, develop antibodies to tumor cells, although the serum of dogs with regressive tumors is most effective in inhibiting tumor growth. Thirty to forty percent of cells in the regressive phase express MHC class I and II. Dogs whose tumors regress also develop cytotoxic T cells. If recipient dogs are immunosuppressed, the tendency to malignant growth is enhanced. These tumor cells appear to secrete a cytotoxic factor that kills B cells.

Papillomas

Warts are self-limiting neoplasia of epidermal cells induced by papillomaviruses. The wart virus invades epidermal cells in the basal cell layer but these cells do not express viral antigen. Since no viral antigen is expressed in this area where the blood supply is good, the cells are not attacked by lymphocytes. As the infected cells move away from the basal layer toward the skin surface they also move away from blood vessels and the chances of immunological attack are minimized. Increasing amounts of virus are shed as the cells move toward the surface into a region devoid of antibodies or lymphocytes. Wart vaccines containing inactivated papillomavirus are available.

Equine Sarcoids

Equine sarcoids are locally aggressive fibroblastic neoplasms of horse skin associated with infection by bovine papillomavirus. Equine sarcoids are remarkably amenable to immunotherapy. If BCG vaccine is infiltrated into the region between the tumor and normal skin the tumor regresses in about two thirds of cases. The rate of regression depends on the size of the tumor (surgical debulking is required to remove most of the tumor mass), and multiple treatments are usually necessary for a complete cure. Mycobacterial cell walls may also be used to eradicate this tumor. They possess the advantage of not rendering an animal tuberculin positive. Sarcoids are also responsive to other immunostimulants such as acemannan or killed *P. acnes*.

Ocular Squamous Cell Carcinoma

Ocular squamous cell carcinoma is a common and economically important tumor of cattle that responds to several forms of immunotherapy. One successful treatment involves inoculation of affected animals with a phenol-saline extract of allogeneic carcinomas. This suggests that these neoplasia possess characteristic tumor-associated antigens. Indeed sera from affected cattle can react with cancer cells (but not normal cells) obtained from the eyes of other cattle. It is also of interest to note that sera from some cattle with ocular squamous cell carcinoma also react with equine sarcoid and bovine papilloma cells, implying that all three may have a common cause.

Swine Melanoma

The Sinclair melanoma-bearing swine is a line of animals that spontaneously develop melanotic tumors. Most such tumors are benign and regress spontaneously. However, some are malignant and lethal. The tumor regression seen in most of these pigs is immunologically mediated. The tumors are invaded by macrophages, and at the same time the animals generate non–MHC-restricted cytotoxic T cells that are CD4$^-$CD8$^-$, γ/δ^+. The pigs may also generate antibodies against melanoma antigens.

LYMPHOID TUMORS

The immune response requires that antigen-sensitive cells stimulated by exposure to antigen respond by division and differentiation. Much of the complexity of the immune system is due to the need for rigid control of this cellular response. A failure in this control system may result in uncontrolled lymphoid cell proliferation and the development of lymphoid tumors. Surveillance was originally proposed as a function of the immune system when it was observed that immunosuppressed animals and humans had an increased prevalence of tumors.

However, analysis shows that an unusually high proportion of these tumors are of lymphoid origin. Therefore it is likely that at least some of the lymphoid tumors that develop in immunosuppressed individuals result from a failure in the immunological control systems rather than from a failure of surveillance.

Normal immune responses, whether antibody or cell mediated, involve a burst of rapid proliferation in lymphocytes. This burst of proliferation must be carefully controlled (Chapter 18). Although uncontrolled lymphocyte function may induce autoimmunity, uncontrolled lymphocyte proliferation may result in the development of a lymphoma or lymphosarcoma. It is no accident that individuals with autoimmune disease are more likely than normal individuals to develop lymphoid cell tumors.

Several important viruses stimulate nonspecific lymphocyte proliferation. These include the maedi-visna virus, the Aleutian disease parvovirus, and the herpesvirus responsible for malignant catarrhal fever (MCF). MCF is a fatal lymphoproliferative disease of cattle and sheep characterized by lymphadenopathy with widespread tissue accumulations of lymphocytes. Lymphocytes from MCF-infected animals show prolonged growth in tissue culture.

Neoplastic transformation may occur in lymphoid cells of both branches of the immune system at almost any stage in their maturation process. Providing that the tumor cells have not dedifferentiated as a result of very rapid growth (as in acute lymphatic leukemia of calves), it is possible to identify the cells present in a lymphoid tumor by their surface antigens. For example, the presence of cell surface immunoglobulin is characteristic of B cells, whereas the ability to form rosettes with sheep erythrocytes through CD2 is an identifying feature of T cells.

Bovine Lymphosarcoma

Bovine lymphosarcoma is one of the most common cancers of cattle. It occurs in two main forms: an enzootic form and a sporadic form. The enzootic form of the disease is caused by bovine leukemia virus (BLV), a delta retrovirus. BLV is transmitted by infected lymphocytes. Thus it can be spread by contaminated instruments, by vaccines containing blood, or by biting flies; or calves may be infected in utero. The primary target of the virus is the B cell. Early in infection the proportion of B cells in peripheral blood increases before there is a significant increase in the number of blood lymphocytes. Eventually some infected animals develop a persistent lymphocytosis (PL). Not all BLV-infected cattle develop PL although 95% of cattle with this condition are infected with BLV. These lymphocytes may be enlarged, are CD5+, express increased levels of IgM, and show altered glycosylation. Cells in PL are not malignant and can occasionally return to the normal state. BLV becomes stably integrated into these B lymphocytes. Some T cells may also contain the BLV provirus. Susceptibility to tumor development differs among species. Sheep are very sensitive, cattle have intermediate sensitivity, and goats are the least sensitive. The virus is essential for neoplastic transformation but not for the continued growth of tumor cells.

The mechanism by which BLV leads to tumor development is unclear, and there is no rearrangement of any known oncogenes. It may be that a viral gene *Tax* could initiate tumorigenesis. Tax is a transactivating protein that can turn on many different cellular genes. Animals with advanced clinical bovine leukosis may be immunosuppressed as a result of the presence in their serum of a suppressor factor (Table 31-1). This suppression is reflected by reduced numbers of T cells and lowered serum IgM levels. Occasionally the neoplastic cells in bovine leukosis may be sufficiently differentiated to secrete immunoglobulin in a manner similar to that seen in myelomas. One to five percent of BLV-infected cattle develop a multicentric lymphosarcoma 1 to 8 years after infection. In the sporadic form of bovine leukosis it is generally considered that the tumor cells are of T-cell lineage. However, some originating from pre-B cells have also been identified.

Lymphomas in Other Species

In sheep, lymphomas are divided fairly evenly between T and B cells, and about 15% are unclassifiable (null cells). Some of these may be due to BLV infection. A B-cell lymphoma inherited as an autosomal recessive condition is recognized in swine. Horses carrying lymphosarcomas are commonly immunosuppressed. This usually involves T-cell functions, but B-cell function may also be impaired. A case of a horse with a lymphosarcoma with suppressor cell activity has been described. The animal presented with signs of immunodeficiency and was found to be deficient in IgM. The tumor cells grew in the presence of IL-2, possessed many T-cell markers, and were noncytotoxic.

In dogs, leukemias may be classified on the basis of the cell type involved (lymphoid or myeloid) and on the basis of the clinical course and cytology (acute or chronic). Chronic lymphoid leukemia (CLL) is most frequently diagnosed. It is characterized by the presence of large numbers of mature lymphocytes in the blood. Animals may be asymptomatic and the course of the disease is slow. About 70% of these cases involve T cells (CD3+), and most are large granular lymphocytes (LGLs). Of these LGLs, about 65% are α/β T cells and the remainder are γ/δ T cells. The non-LGL T-cell CLL cases involve α/β T cells. B-cell CLLs identified as CD21+, CD79a+ account for about 30% of canine CLL cases. Chronic myeloid leukemias are extremely rare in the dog.

Acute leukemias, which are less common in dogs, may be of lymphoid (B cell) origin (20%), or myeloid origin (70%). The remainder of these acute leukemias are difficult to classify and are considered undifferentiated. Many of these tumor cells, both myeloid and lymphoid, express

TABLE   31-1
Immunosuppressive Effects of Lymphoid Tumors

Tumor	Cell Type	Evidence for Immunosuppression	Mechanisms
Feline leukemia	T cell	Lymphopenia Prolonged skin grafts Increased susceptibility to infection Lack of response to mitogens	Suppressive viral protein, pl5E Suppressor cells
Marek's disease	T cell	Lack of response to mitogens Depressed cell-mediated cytotoxicity Depressed IgG production	Suppressor macrophages
Avian lymphoid leukosis	B cell	Increased susceptibility to infection	Suppressor lymphocytes
Bovine leukosis	B cell	Depressed serum IgM	Soluble suppressor factor
Myeloma	B cell	Increased susceptibility to infection factor	Soluble tumor-cell Negative feedback
Canine malignant lymphoma	B cell	Predisposition to infection associated with autoimmune disorders	Unknown
Equine lymphosarcoma	T cell	Increased susceptibility to infection	Tumor of suppressor cells

CD34. The prognosis of these acute leukemias is usually very poor.

Lymphosarcomas account for 5% to 7% of canine malignancies. There is no evidence to suggest that these tumors are virus induced. They may be classified according to their apparent site of origin (such as multicentric, alimentary, or anterior mediastinal) or, alternatively, by their cell type (such as histiocytic, lymphocytic, lymphoblastic, or plasmacytic). The lymphocytic forms are usually of T-cell origin. In many cases of canine lymphoma, affected dogs produce antibodies against crude tumor antigens. These antigens are not found on normal lymphoid cells.

Cutaneous T-cell lymphomas (mycosis fungoides) are common in old dogs. The lesions consist of CD3+ cells. Eighty percent are CD8+, and the remainder are double negative. Most (70%) have γ/δ T-cell receptors, especially if the tumor is confined to the epidermis.

Avian Lymphoid Tumors

Marek's disease is a herpesvirus-induced tumor of T-cell origin. Birds with this disease are usually immunosuppressed. Thus their antibody responses, rejection of allografts, and delayed hypersensitivity responses are all depressed. This depression results from several factors including virus-induced lymphoid destruction and the development of suppressor macrophages. These macrophages restrict the replication of the tumor cells, but in doing so they suppress the resistance of birds to other infections. Lymphoid leukosis is a tumor of B-cell origin. Affected birds normally have a depressed antibody response and reduced responses to mitogens. Nevertheless some cases of this disease may present with hypergammaglobulinemia.

SOURCES OF ADDITIONAL INFORMATION

Arase H, Arase N, Saito T: Fas-mediated cytotoxicity by freshly isolated natural killer cells, *J Exp Med* 181:1235-1238, 1995.

Belardelli F, Ferrantini M: Cytokines as a link between innate and adaptive antitumor immunity, *Trends Immunol* 23: 201-208, 2002.

Boise LH, Thompson CB: Hierarchical control of lymphocyte survival, *Science* 274:67-68, 1996.

Büttner M, Wanke R, Obermann B: Natural killer (NK) activity of porcine blood lymphocytes against allogeneic melanoma target cells, *Vet Immunol Immunopathol* 29:89-103, 1991.

Coussens LM, Werb Z: Inflammation and cancer, *Nature* 420: 860-867, 2002.

Elgert KD, Alleva DG, Mullins DW: Tumor-induced immune dysfunction: the macrophage connection, *J Leukoc Biol* 64:275-287, 1998.

Evans DL, Jaso-Friedmann L: Natural killer (NK) cells in domestic animals: phenotype, target cell specificity and cytokine regulation, *Vet Res Commun* 17:429-447, 1993.

Govaerts MM, Goddeeris BM: Homologues of natural killer cell receptors NKG2-D and NKR-P1 expressed in cattle, *Vet Immunol Immunopathol* 80:339-344, 2001.

Hill FWG, Klein WR, Hoyer MJ, et al: Antitumor effect of locally injected low doses of recombinant human interleukin-2 in bovine vulval papilloma and carcinoma, *Vet Immunol Immunopathol* 41:19-29, 1994.

Jardine JH, Jackson HJ, Lotzová E, et al: Tumoricidal effect of interleukin-2-activated killer cells in canines, *Vet Immunol Immunopathol* 21:153-160, 1989.

Jensen J, Schultz RD: Bovine natural cell-mediated cytotoxicity (NCMC): activation by cytokines, *Vet Immunol Immunopathol* 24:113-123, 1990.

Li W, Splitter GA: Bovine NK and LAK susceptibility is independent of class I expression on B lymphoblastoid variants, *Vet Immunol Immunopathol* 41:189-200, 1994.

McConkey DJ, Chow SC, Orrenius O, Jondal M: NK cell induced cytotoxicity is dependent on a Ca^{++} increase in the target, *FASEB J* 4:2661-2664, 1990.

McQueen KL, Wilhelm BT, Harden KD, Mager DL: Evolution of NK receptors: a single Ly49 and multiple KIR genes in the cow, *Eur J Immunol* 32:810-817, 2002.

Misfeldt ML, Grimm DR: Sinclair miniature swine: an animal model of human melanoma, *Vet Immunol Immunopathol* 43: 167-175, 1994.

Pardoll DM: Stress, NK receptors, and immune surveillance, *Science* 294, 534-536, 2001.

Pardoll DM: T cells and tumours, *Nature* 411:1010-1012, 2001.

Raulet DH, Heid W: Natural killer cell receptors: the offs and ons of NK cell recognition, *Cell* 82:697-700, 1995.

Robertson MJ: Role of chemokines in the biology of natural killer cells, *J Leukoc Biol* 71:173, 2002.

Rutten VPMG, Misdorp W, Gauthier A, et al: Immunological aspects of mammary tumors in dogs and cats: a survey including own studies and pertinent literature, *Vet Immunol Immunopathol* 26:211-226, 1990.

Schwartz I, Lévy D: Pathobiology of bovine leukemia virus, *Vet Res* 25:521-536, 1994

Storset AK, Slettedal IO, Williams JL, et al: Natural killer cell receptors in cattle: a bovine killer cell immunoglobulin-like receptor multigene family contains members with divergent signaling motifs, *Eur J Immunol* 33:980-990, 2003.

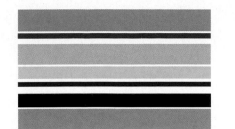

Autoimmunity: General Principles

CHAPTER 32

One inescapable hazard associated with the acquired immune system is the development of autoimmunity. The random generation of antigen-binding receptors ensures that lymphocytes capable of binding and responding to self-antigens are produced. These self-reactive cells are rigorously suppressed. Nevertheless, despite an extensive array of regulatory processes and pathways, autoimmune diseases still occur. Indeed, autoimmune diseases are common in humans and in companion animals. However, the "causes" of many of these autoimmune diseases are still unclear. We know that many factors influence susceptibility to these diseases. Such factors include sex and age, genetic background, and virus infections. We also know that the development of autoantibodies is a relatively common event and by itself does not inevitably lead to autoimmune disease. Indeed, some autoantibodies serve a physiological function.

Because we do not know precisely what causes autoimmune disease, this chapter looks at some of the many different predisposing causes that have been identified or proposed as well as the mechanisms by which autoimmunity causes tissue damage and disease.

As with other immune functions, either B or T cells can mediate autoimmunity. Thus in some autoimmune diseases the disease is mediated by autoantibodies alone. In others, the damage may be mediated by T cells alone or by some combination of autoantibodies and T cells.

INDUCTION OF AUTOIMMUNITY

Autoimmune diseases appear to develop spontaneously and predisposing causes are rarely obvious. Nevertheless they fall into two major categories. They can either result from a normal immune response to an unusual or abnormal antigen, or they can result from an abnormal immune response to a normal antigen (Figure 32-1). The second category is probably the most significant from the perspective of clinical disease. In these cases, the mechanisms that normally prevent the development of self-responsive T cells fail. Many different environmental factors and genes contribute to this failure, and the failure may not always be complete. Autoimmune diseases may result from an aberrant response to a single specific antigen or, alternatively, they may be due to a general defect in the regulation of B- or T-cell functions.

NORMAL IMMUNE RESPONSES

Many autoimmune responses simply reflect a normal immune response to an antigen that has been previously hidden or, alternatively, are a result of cross-reactivity between an infectious agent and a normal body component. Some may be a result of abnormal antigen processing.

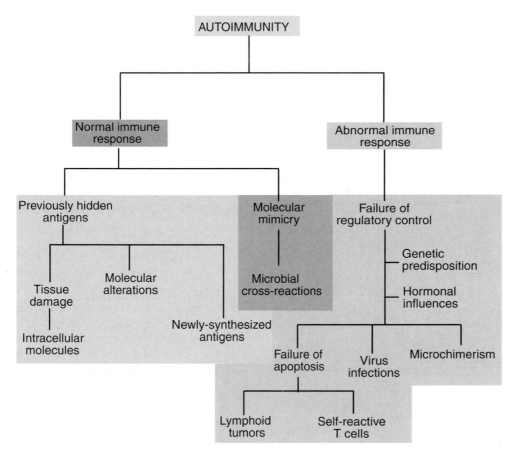

Figure 32-1. Simplified scheme for the pathogenesis of autoimmune diseases.

Antigens Hidden in Cells or Tissues

Many autoimmune responses appear to be triggered when nontolerant T cells meet previously hidden autoantigens. After all, T cells can only be made tolerant to autoantigens if the T cells are first exposed to these antigens. There are many autoantigens that cannot induce tolerance because they are hidden within cells or tissues.

Although the control of the immune system requires that most self-reactive cells be eliminated, one should not assume that all autoimmune responses are bad or even cause disease. Indeed, some autoimmune responses have physiological functions. For example, red blood cells must be removed from the blood once they reach the end of their life span. This process is accomplished by autoantibodies. As red cells age, an anion transport protein called CD233 (or band 3 protein) is cleaved and a new epitope is exposed. This new epitope is recognized by IgG autoantibodies. These autoantibodies thus bind to aged red cells and trigger their phagocytosis by macrophages in the spleen. CD233 is also found on many other cell types, and it may be that its cleavage in aged cells and their subsequent opsonization constitutes a major mechanism for their elimination.

Many autoantigens are found in places where they never encounter circulating lymphocytes. For example, in the testes, new antigens may only appear at puberty—long after the T-cell system has developed and become tolerant to autoantigens. Injury to the testes may permit proteins released by damaged tissues to reach the bloodstream, encounter antigen-sensitive cells, and stimulate autoimmunity. Hidden antigens may also be found inside cells. For example, after a heart attack, autoantibodies may be produced against the mitochondria of cardiac muscle cells. In chronic hepatitis in dogs, animals develop antibodies to liver membrane proteins. In diseases such as trypanosomiasis or tuberculosis in which widespread tissue damage occurs, autoantibodies to many different tissue antigens may be detected in serum.

Antigens Generated by Molecular Changes

The production of some autoantibodies may be triggered by the development of completely new epitopes on normal proteins. Two examples of autoantibodies generated in this way are the rheumatoid factors (RFs) and the immunoconglutinins (IKs, after the German spelling).

RFs are autoantibodies directed against other immunoglobulins. When an antibody binds to an antigen, the antibody conformation is changed in such a way that new epitopes are exposed on its Fc region. These new epitopes may stimulate RF formation. RFs are produced in diseases in which large amounts of immune complexes are generated. These include the autoimmune disease of joints called rheumatoid arthritis and a disease called systemic lupus erythematosus (SLE), in which B cells respond to many different autoantigens.

IKs are autoantibodies directed against the complement components C2, C4, and especially C3. The epitopes that stimulate IK formation are found on sites that are exposed when complement is activated. The level of IK in serum reflects the amount of complement activation; this, in turn, is a measure of the antigenic stimulation to which an animal is subjected. IK levels are thus nonspecific indicators of the prevalence of infectious disease within an animal population. Their physiological role is unclear, but they may enhance complement-mediated opsonization.

Minor structural changes in normal proteins may be generated artificially and used to induce autoantibodies. For example, chemically modified thyroglobulin can be used to induce autoantibodies against normal thyroglobulin.

Molecular Mimicry

Autoimmunity may result from molecular mimicry, a term used to describe the sharing of epitopes between an infectious agent or parasite and an autoantigen (Figure 32-2). Thus B cells may bind a foreign epitope that cross-reacts with an autoantigen. However, they will only respond to this epitope if they receive T-cell help. If T cells recognize nearby microbial epitopes as foreign, they may trigger a helper T-cell response that permits the self-reactive B cells to make autoantibodies. Once a B-cell response is triggered in this way, the infectious agent may be removed while the autoimmune response continues—a "hit-and-run" process.

Many examples of molecular mimicry are now recognized. For example, the parasite *Trypanosoma cruzi* contains antigens that cross-react with mammalian neurons and cardiac muscle. Individuals infected with this parasite make autoantibodies that can cause nervous system and heart disease. Molecular mimicry may also cause the heart lesions of rheumatic fever in children. Antibodies to the cell wall M protein of group A streptococci cross-react with cardiac myosin. Children infected with certain strains of group A streptococci produce antimyocardial antibodies and so develop heart disease. Other strains of streptococci can cause acute glomerulonephritis in children as a result of the production of antibodies cross-reacting with glomerular basement membranes. Other examples of molecular mimicry that may be significant include the Epstein-Barr virus DNA polymerase that cross-reacts with myelin basic protein and may be involved in the induction of multiple sclerosis, and poliovirus capsid protein VP2 that cross-reacts with the acetylcholine receptor and may induce myasthenia gravis.

The integrin CD11a/18 (LFA-1) shares an antigenic determinant with the outer surface protein of the causal agent of Lyme disease, *Borrelia burgdorferi*. Thus patients

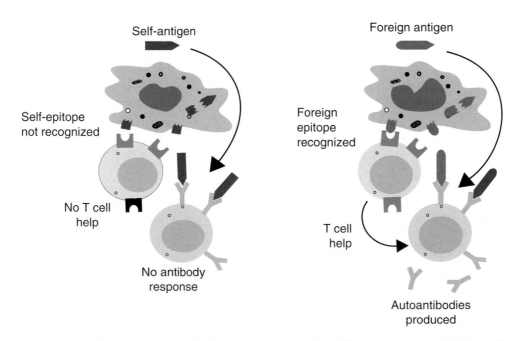

Figure 32-2.   Cross-reactions with foreign antigens may be sufficient to trigger a T helper cell population that will promote an autoimmune response by B cells. Thus a helper effect triggered by a foreign antigen may inadvertently permit an autoimmune response to occur.

infected with this organism mount an initial immune response to the bacterium, which may then become an autoimmune response. In about 10% of patients with Lyme arthritis, antibiotics fail to resolve the disease suggesting that, once triggered, the autoimmune process can proceed in the absence of the bacterium.

Antibodies against microbial heat-shock proteins are found in the serum of humans and rats with rheumatoid arthritis, ankylosing spondylitis, and SLE. Injection of killed *Mycobacterium tuberculosis* in Freund's complete adjuvant can cause arthritis in rats, and T cells from these animals can transfer arthritis to normal syngeneic recipients. These T cells are responding to HSP 60, a mycobacterial heat-shock protein (Chapter 23). Because heat shock proteins are highly conserved and T cells from rheumatoid arthritis patients are also directed against HSP 60 it has been suggested that molecular mimicry between microbial and mammalian HSP 60 may be important in rheumatoid arthritis.

Ankylosing spondylitis is an autoimmune arthritis of humans that affects the sacroiliac joints, spine, and peripheral joints. Patients also develop acute anterior uveitis (inflammation of the iris and neighboring structures in the eye). More than 95% of whites with ankylosing spondylitis possess the MHC class I allele HLA-B27, whereas in the normal population the prevalence of this allele is less than 8%. It is believed that the disease results from molecular mimicry between the hypervariable region of HLA-B27 and antigens found in *Klebsiella pneumoniae* and related bacteria. *Klebsiella pneumoniae* is found more frequently than normal in the intestine of patients with active ankylosing spondylitis and uveitis, and patients with active disease have elevated levels of IgA against *Klebsiella* in their sera. Cloning of B27 into mice and subsequent infection of these animals with *K. pneumoniae* causes an acute spondylitis.

HLA-B27-like alleles have been cloned from bonobos, gorillas, rhesus, and cynomolgus monkeys, and HLA-B27-associated ankylosing spondylitis has been described in gorillas. In fact up to 20% of wild gorillas may have spondylitis, and the disease has also been described in a gibbon, in baboons, and in rhesus macaques.

In porcine enzootic pneumonia caused by *Mycoplasma hyopneumoniae*, antibodies to the mycoplasma cross-react with pig lungs, and in contagious bovine pleuropneumonia there is cross-reactivity between *Mycoplasma mycoides* antigens and normal bovine lung. It is not known to what extent these autoantibodies contribute to the pathogenesis of these diseases. There is a clearer relationship between *Leptospira interrogans* and the development of periodic ophthalmia, the leading cause of blindness in horses (Chapter 33).

Some microbial superantigens may also trigger autoimmunity. Thus the superantigen staphylococcal enterotoxin B activates the same T cells that react with myelin and induces an autoimmune encephalitis. It has been suggested that a bacterial superantigen may trigger rheumatoid arthritis since the T cells in affected joints are enriched in cells bearing certain T-cell receptor V domains. The only known agents that can alter V gene expression in this way are superantigens.

Alterations in Antigen Processing

In some cases autoimmunity seems to result from a normal immune response against an exogenous antigen that subsequently "spreads" to recognize self-antigens. Thus when an autoimmune response is initiated, the immune response is first directed against a single epitope on the inciting antigen. However, as the process continues, the T- and B-cell responses diversify and responses begin to be directed against additional epitopes. At first they will be other epitopes on the same protein. Eventually responses may spread to epitopes on other autoantigens. Epitope spreading has been demonstrated in many autoimmune diseases such as thyrotoxicosis and diabetes and may account for the difficulties encountered in controlling these diseases.

ABNORMAL IMMUNE RESPONSES

Failure of Regulatory Control

Although autoimmunity may be triggered by responses to hidden epitopes, a sustained response is necessary for disease to develop. This may result from a failure of the normal control mechanisms of the immune system and can be demonstrated simply by injecting mice with rat red blood cells. Following such an injection, mice not only make antibodies to the rat cells but also develop a self-limiting and transient autoimmune response to their own red blood cells. This autoimmune response is rapidly controlled by regulatory cells and lasts for only a few days. If, however, regulatory cell activity in these mice is impaired, as occurs in New Zealand Black (NZB) mice, for example, then these autoantibodies will persist to cause red blood cell destruction and anemia.

It is common to find autoimmune diseases associated with lymphoid tumors. For example, myasthenia gravis, an autoimmune disease involving the neuromuscular junction, is commonly associated with the presence of a thymic carcinoma. In humans, there is a fourfold increase in the incidence of rheumatoid arthritis in patients with malignant lymphoid tumors, and there is evidence for a similar association in other mammals. Since many lymphoid tumors result from a failure in immunological control mechanisms, a simultaneous failure in self-tolerance may also occur. Alternatively, some tumors may represent the development of a forbidden clone of cells producing autoantibodies. It is also possible that some lymphoid tumors may result from long-term stimulation of the immune system by autoantigens.

Potentially harmful, self-reactive lymphocytes are normally destroyed in the thymus by apoptosis triggered through the death receptor CD95 (fas) (Chapter 17). Defects in CD95 or its ligand, CD154 (fas-L) cause autoimmunity by permitting abnormal T cells to survive and cause disease. This is well demonstrated in the *lpr* strain of mice. These animals have a mutation in their CD95 gene that alters the structure of its intracellular domain. A mutation (called *gld*) in fas ligand has a similar effect. Both *lpr* and *gld* mice develop multiple auto-immune lesions accompanied by lymphoproliferation. Some investigators have suggested that mutations in CD95 may contribute to the pathogenesis of lupus in other mammals.

Virus-Induced Autoimmunity

Many autoimmune diseases appear to be triggered by virus infections. For example, mice infected with certain reoviruses develop an autoimmune polyendocrine disease characterized by diabetes mellitus and retarded growth. These reovirus-infected mice make autoantibodies against normal pituitary, pancreas, gastric mucosa, nuclei, glucagon, growth hormone, and insulin. Likewise, in NZB mice, persistent infection with a type C retrovirus leads to the production of autoantibodies against nucleic acids and red blood cells.

The situation with spontaneous disease is less clear. Many attempts have been made to isolate viruses from patients with autoimmune disease but with mixed results. For example, SLE of dogs and humans has been associated with either a type C retrovirus or paramyxovirus infection. Small quantities of the Epstein-Barr virus genome can be found in the salivary glands of humans with Sjögren's syndrome. Moreover, epidemiological evidence points to some form of a viral trigger for diseases such as multiple sclerosis, rheumatoid arthritis, and insulin-dependent diabetes mellitus in children.

Just how viruses can induce autoimmunity is unclear. One possible mechanism described above is molecular mimicry. An equally plausible mechanism is called bystander activation. Thus viruses may induce an inflammatory response that results in the release of multiple cytokines. These cytokines may activate previously dormant T cells. As a result the T cells may attack auto-antigens that they previously ignored. Evidence suggests that Coxsackie-virus-induced diabetes is mediated in large part through bystander activation (Figure 32-3).

AUTOIMMUNE DISEASE AND VACCINATION

It is widely believed that the prevalence of autoimmune disease in domestic pets, especially dogs, has risen in recent years. Some investigators have attributed this rise to excessive use of potent vaccines. This link is by no means proven; nevertheless, there is some evidence that supports a causal association between vaccination and autoimmunity.

First, it is well recognized that Guillain-Barré syndrome, an autoimmune neurological disease of humans, can be triggered by administration of some vaccines such as

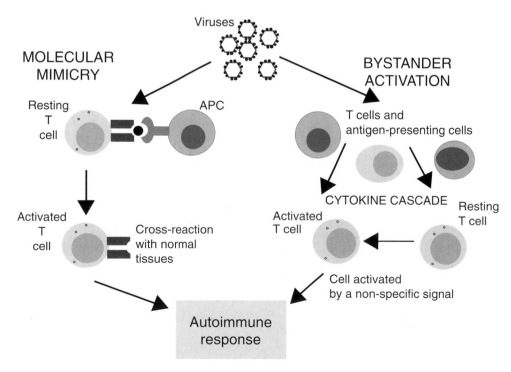

Figure 32-3. Viruses may trigger autoimmune responses either by molecular mimicry or by bystander activation.

influenza vaccine. Likewise, in animals, the administration of potent, adjuvanted vaccines stimulates the transient production of a variety of autoantibodies. For example, immunization of beagle puppies with a rabies vaccine triggers a significant increase in antithyroglobulin antibodies about 6 months later. Whether these antibodies can cause autoimmune disease is unknown. More significantly, a case-control study has identified a link between vaccination and the development of autoimmune hemolytic anemia in dogs a few weeks later. Vaccines containing potent adjuvants may trigger the development of low levels of autoantibodies to connective tissue components such as fibronectin and laminin. Thus there is growing evidence that vaccination may trigger some forms of autoimmunity; however, it remains unclear just how significant this might be, and in all likelihood such an event would occur only rarely.

Microchimerism

During pregnancy mothers and their fetuses may exchange cells. As a result, fetal cells can persist in a mother's body for many years after pregnancy, whereas, conversely, the mother's cells may survive for many years in her offspring. These cells are accepted by a tolerant immune system. A growing amount of evidence suggests that these persistent cells may be the cause of some autoimmune diseases. This is especially true in humans where autoimmune diseases are much more common in women than in men. The process is called fetal microchimerism. Thus in many women with the autoimmune disease scleroderma, it is possible to find fetal T, B, and NK cells as well as fetal monocytes in their blood. It is suggested that this autoimmune disease is a form of graft-versus-host disease in these patients. Increased numbers of fetal cells have also been identified in humans with autoimmune thyroiditis. Transfer of cells from mother to fetus may also cause autoimmunity. Thus small numbers of maternal cells can be detected in the blood of almost all boys with the autoimmune disease dermatomyositis. In all of these cases the number of foreign cells in an individual is clearly insufficient to be the sole cause of the autoimmune disease, so that additional, poorly understood factors must also be involved.

PREDISPOSING FACTORS

Genetic Predisposition

Although viruses or other infectious agents may trigger autoimmune responses, it is clear that not all infected individuals develop autoimmune disease. This is because genetic factors are key determinants of disease susceptibility. Genetic analysis of mice has led to the identification of at least 25 genes that contribute to autoimmunity if deleted or overexpressed. These include genes that

code for cytokines, cytokine receptors, costimulators, molecules that regulate apoptosis, molecules that regulate antigen clearance, and members of cytokine or antigen-signaling cascades. Some diseases result from a defect in a single gene such as the *lpr* or *gld* mutations. Others result from inherited complement deficiencies. More commonly, the role of genes is complex. Thus genes influence the severity of disease and no specific gene is necessary or sufficient for disease expression. Even if an animal has a complete set of susceptibility alleles at multiple loci, presence of overt disease may be contingent on the genetic background of the animal. (This is called incomplete penetrance.) This genetic complexity probably also contributes to differences in disease presentation since these may be determined by different sets of contributing genes. Genetic analysis is also complicated because different susceptibility genes may or may not interact with each other. The vulnerability of a target organ to autoimmune damage may also be inherited.

The most important genes that influence naturally occurring autoimmune diseases are those in the MHC. MHC molecules regulate the presentation of processed epitopes. In theory, therefore, they determine resistance or susceptibility to many diseases. In practice, there is strong selection against genes that predispose to susceptibility to infectious agents, so that MHC genes have been selected for a strong response to most common infectious pathogens. In contrast, autoimmune diseases in old, post-reproductive animals do not offer a selective disadvantage and MHC-linked predispositions can be found. Studies of human populations have shown that almost all autoimmune diseases are linked to certain MHC alleles. Presumably an essential prerequisite for any autoimmune disease is that the autoantigen is appropriately processed and presented on an MHC molecule. Thus the structure of the MHC antigen–binding groove determines if a specific autoantigen will trigger an immune response. Some MHC alleles protect against autoimmunity, and any predisposition to autoimmunity may be the result of the net effect of both enhancing and protective genes.

Instead of being closely linked to a single MHC gene, some autoimmune diseases are associated with combinations of MHC molecules. For example, in humans the combination of HLA-A1, B8, and DR3 is associated with increased risk of diabetes, myasthenia gravis, and SLE.

Many domestic dogs, especially those from rare breeds, are significantly inbred and show restricted MHC polymorphism. This can increase autoimmune disease susceptibility. In the dog there are a number of recognized associations between autoimmunity and MHC alleles. Thus diabetes mellitus is associated with DLA-A3, A7, and A10 and DLA-B4; antinuclear antibodies are associated with DLA-12; SLE is associated with DLA-A7; and autoimmune polyarthritis is associated with the class III gene for C4.

Breed Predispositions

The three major classes of immunologically mediated disease (autoimmunity, immunodeficiency, and atopy) tend to be encountered in some dog breeds more commonly than in others. Thus, Old English sheepdogs are unusually prone to develop autoimmune blood diseases. Certain autoimmune diseases, such as polyarteritis nodosa and hypothyroidism, have familial associations (Table 33-1).

Breeds are, of course, an artificial phenomenon. They have been developed as a result of aggressive phenotypic selection, in many cases resulting in inbreeding and a lack of genetic diversity. This has had two effects. First, it has permitted deleterious autosomal recessive genes to be expressed, as is seen in the increased incidence of immunodeficiency syndromes and other immunological disorders. Second, it has resulted in a loss of MHC polymorphism. For example, DRB1*04 is found in a majority of boxers, DRB1*2401 may be restricted to akitas, DRB1*01 predominates in West Highland white terriers, DQA*0203 is restricted to Dobermans, there is a high incidence of DQA*0102 in Irish wolfhounds and chows, and DRB1*0101 is common in Irish setters. These limited haplotypes ensure that the dogs in these breeds will respond to an unusually narrow range of antigens, thus reducing their resistance to infectious agents. Such dogs will also be more susceptible to autoimmune diseases because they are restricted in the range of immune responses they may mount. The increasing incidence of immunological diseases seen in dogs is largely attributable to careless breeding practices.

Inbred lines of other species have been produced that are associated with spontaneous development of autoimmune disease. For example, chickens of the OS strain develop an autoimmune thyroiditis. An inbred line of dogs has been used for studies of SLE. Inbred NZB mice spontaneously develop a syndrome that bears a striking resemblance to SLE (Chapter 34). NZB mice develop immune complex glomerulonephritis. They become hypergammaglobulinemic and hypocomplementemic, and they develop an autoimmune hemolytic anemia. Some also develop lymphoid tumors. These mice produce autoantibodies against nuclear antigens, red blood cells, and T cells, and their B cells are polyclonally activated. New Zealand White (NZW) mice are phenotypically normal, but the F1 cross between NZW and NZB mice has an even more severe lupus-like syndrome. In these animals, kidney disease is severe and is associated with high titers of antibodies to nucleic acids. Studies on the inheritance of these traits in mice suggest that they are controlled by a small number of unlinked major genes and a large number of minor genes. In diabetic mice it has been determined that from three to six unlinked genes determine susceptibility.

MECHANISMS OF TISSUE DAMAGE IN AUTOIMMUNITY

Autoimmune disease results when tissues are damaged by autoreactive T cells or antibodies. The mechanisms by which the damage is caused are examples of hypersensitivity. However, it should be pointed out that many of these diseases are due to multiple mechanisms and that these may vary with time. For example, autoimmune responses may be initiated by Th1 cells and subsequently involve Th2 responses.

Type I Hypersensitivity

Milk allergy in cattle is an autoimmune disease in which milk (α casein), normally found only in the udder, gains access to the general circulation and so stimulates an immune response. This happens when milking is delayed and intramammary pressure forces milk proteins into the circulation. For some reason the immune response stimulated by α casein is mediated through Th2 cells and IgE autoantibodies are produced. As a result, affected cows may develop acute anaphylaxis (Chapter 26). A similar condition is seen occasionally in other domestic mammals such as the mare. Although antibodies in milk proteins are commonly found in human serum after rapid weaning, type I hypersensitivity is not a usual sequel.

Type II Hypersensitivity

Autoantibodies against cell surface antigens may cause cell lysis with the assistance of complement or cytotoxic cells. If autoantibodies are directed against red blood cells, then autoimmune hemolytic anemia may result; if directed against platelets, thrombocytopenia will occur; and if against thyroid cells, thyroiditis will result. In one form of this process in humans, autoantibodies against thyroid-stimulating hormone (TSH) receptors on thyroid cells stimulate thyroid activity rather than its destruction. Cell surface receptors are common targets of autoimmune attack. In addition to the TSH receptor, autoantibodies attack the acetylcholine receptor in myasthenia gravis, and the insulin receptor in some forms of diabetes. Autoantibodies to β-adrenoceptors (Chapter 26) have been detected in some patients with asthma. By blocking β-receptors, these antibodies make the airways highly irritable and affected individuals are prone to severe asthma.

Type III Hypersensitivity

Autoantibodies form immune complexes with autoantigens, and these complexes may cause inflammation. This is most significant in SLE, a disease in which many different autoantibodies are produced. Immune complexes deposited in glomeruli provoke a membranoproliferative glomerulopathy (Chapter 28). Similarly, in rheumatoid arthritis, immune complexes are deposited in joints and contribute to the local inflammatory response.

Type IV Hypersensitivity

Many autoimmune disease lesions are infiltrated with mononuclear cells, and Th1 responses probably contribute to the pathogenesis of disease of this type. Cytotoxic T cells cause demyelination in experimental allergic encephalitis and human multiple sclerosis. Insulin-dependent diabetes mellitus may be due to a cell-mediated response because the diseased pancreatic islets may be infiltrated by lymphocytes and lymphocytes from diabetics may be cytotoxic for pancreatic islet cells in vitro.

Although cytotoxic T cells can kill cells directly, cytokines from these cells can also cause tissue damage. Examples of this include interleukin-1, which stimulates nitric oxide production; the nitric oxide in turn kills cells. Likewise, tumor necrosis factor-α released by these cells is pro-inflammatory and up-regulates cell adhesion molecules, including selectins, and so facilitates immigration of neutrophils into the lesions.

SOURCES OF ADDITIONAL INFORMATION

Bach JF: The effect of infections on susceptibility to autoimmune and allergic diseases, *N Engl J Med* 347:911-918 2002.

Barinaga M: Cells exchanged during pregnancy live on, *Science* 296:2169-2172, 2002.

Benoist C, Mathis D: The pathogen connection, *Nature* 394:227-228, 1998.

Charron D: Molecular basis of human leukocyte antigen class II disease associations, *Adv Immunol* 48:107-159, 1990.

Davidson A, Diamond B: Autoimmune diseases, *N Engl J Med* 345:340-348, 2001.

Hang L, Aguado MT, Dixon FJ, Theofilopoulous AN: Induction of severe autoimmune disease in normal mice by simultaneous action of multiple immunostimulators, *J Exp Med* 161:423-428, 1985.

Janeway C: Beneficial autoimmunity, *Nature* 299:396-397, 1982.

Kantor FS: Autoimmunities: diseases of dysregulation, *Hosp Pract* 23:75-84, 1988.

Khansari N, Fudenberg MH: Immune elimination of autologous senescent red cells by Kupffer cells in vivo, *Cell Immunol* 80:426-430, 1983.

Kotzin BL: Superantigens and their role in disease, *Hosp Pract* 28:11, 59-70, 1994.

Lahita RG: Sex steroids and autoimmunity, *Adv Inflamm Res* 8:143-164, 1984.

Morahan G, Morel L: Genetics of autoimmune diseases in humans and in animal models, *Curr Opin Immunol* 14:803-811, 2002.

Oldstone MBA: Molecular mimicry and immune-mediated diseases, *FASEB J* 12:1255-1265, 1998.

Shoenfeld Y, Schwartz RS: Immunologic and genetic factors in autoimmune diseases, *N Engl J Med* 311:1019-1029, 1984.

Sinha AA, Lopez MT, McDevitt HO: Autoimmune diseases: the failure of self tolerance, *Science* 248:1380-1388, 1990.

Steinman L: Escape from "Horror autotoxicus," *Cell* 80:7-10, 1995.

Zinkernagel RM: Maternal antibodies, childhood infections, and autoimmune diseases, *N Engl J Med* 345:1331-1335, 2001.

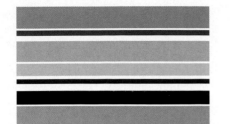

Organ-Specific Autoimmune Diseases

CHAPTER 33

T his chapter considers those autoimmune diseases that mainly affect a single organ or tissue. These diseases presumably result from an abnormal response to a small number of self- or foreign antigens and do not necessarily reflect significant loss of control of the immune system as a whole. It is likely that all organs of the body are potentially susceptible to this form of immunological attack.

AUTOIMMUNE ENDOCRINE DISEASE

Although domestic animals develop autoimmune endocrine diseases, such diseases differ from those in humans insofar as they tend to present as single disorders, rather than involving multiple endocrine glands. Occasionally a dog may experience two or more autoimmune endocrine disorders simultaneously (autoimmune polyglandular syndrome), but this is very uncommon.

Lymphocytic Thyroiditis

Dogs, humans, and chickens suffer from a naturally occurring autoimmune thyroiditis. In dogs the disease is asymptomatic until about 75% of the thyroid is destroyed when clinical signs appear. It results from the production of autoantibodies against thyroglobulin. These antibodies may also react with triiodothyronine (T_3) or thyroxine (T_4). Affected dogs may also show a delayed skin reaction to intradermally injected thyroid extract, suggesting that cell-mediated mechanisms also participate in the disease. Several dog breeds are predisposed to the disease (Table 33-1), and relatives of affected animals may have antithyroid antibodies although clinically normal. A familial form of hypothyroidism has been demonstrated in beagles and Great Danes. Dogs from high-risk breeds such as Dobermans tend to develop the disease when young whereas dogs from low-risk breeds tend to develop it when older. Unfortunately, by the time the disease is diagnosed the dog may already have been

TABLE   33-1
Breed Susceptibility to Major Autoimmune Diseases

	Thyroiditis	IDDM	Pancreatitis	Meningitis	VKH	AIHA	AITP	MG
Great Danes	+							
Borzois	+							
Doberman pinschers	+							
Golden retrievers	+				+			+
Dachshunds	+							+
Cocker spaniels	+					+	+	
Miniature schnauzers	+							
Irish setters	+				+	+		
Beagles	+							
Old English Sheepdogs	+					+	+	
Samoyeds		+			+	+		
German shepherds			+	+				+
Rough-coated collies			+					
Boxers				+				
Bernese mountain dogs				+				
Siberian huskies					+			
Saint Bernards					+			
Australian Sheepdogs					+			
Shetland Sheepdogs					+			
Akitas					+		+	
Miniature dachshunds						+		
Scottish terriers						+	+	
Vizslas						+		
Poodles							+	
Short-haired pointers							+	
Chihuahuas							+	

bred several times. Affected thyroids are infiltrated with plasma cells and lymphocytes, and germinal center formation may occur (Figure 33-1). The infiltrating cells probably cause epithelial cell destruction through antibody-dependent cell-mediated cytotoxicity (ADCC) and T-cell cytotoxicity.

The clinical signs of autoimmune thyroiditis are those of hypothyroidism; that is, the animals are fat and inactive and show patchy hair loss. The most common problems are a dry, dull, coarse coat; scaling; hypotrichosis; slow hair regrowth; hyperpigmentation; myxedema; and pyoderma. Other signs include myopathy, hyperlipidemia, hypothermia, anestrus, galactorrhea, diarrhea or constipation, and polyneuropathy. Tests of thyroid function such as a radioimmunoassay for plasma T_4 or T_3 only confirm the existence of hypothyroidism. A thyroid-stimulating hormone (TSH) response test is more useful because it can confirm the inability of the affected thyroid to respond to TSH. (Plasma T_4 levels are measured before and after injection of TSH.) In order to confirm autoimmune thyroiditis, a biopsy must show the characteristic lymphocytic infiltration. Antithyroid antibodies must be detected in serum using enzyme-linked immunosorbent assay (ELISA) or an indirect fluorescent

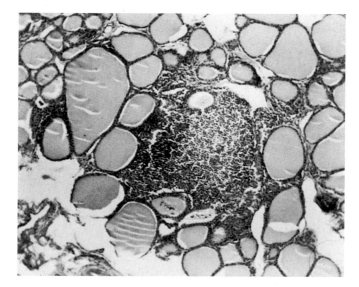

Figure 33-1. A lymphocytic nodule in the thyroid of a dog suffering from autoimmune thyroiditis. Original magnification ×100. (From a specimen provided by Dr. BN Wilkie.)

antibody test. There is little correlation between antithyroid antibody titers and disease severity. Management of autoimmune thyroiditis involves replacement therapy with sodium levothyroxine (synthetic T_4). Improvement should be seen within 4 to 6 weeks. There is no cure for this disease and the success of treatment depends on effective replacement therapy.

An autoimmune thyroiditis also occurs in the OS (obese) strain of white Leghorn chickens. The thyroid tissue of these birds is heavily infiltrated by lymphocytes and plasma cells. Autoantibodies are directed against thyroglobulin, and affected birds are hypothyroid. These birds also make antibodies against their adrenal gland, exocrine pancreas, and proventricular cells. Neonatal thymectomy prevents the development of lesions.

Hyperthyroidism

Hyperthyroidism is a disease of old cats. Autoantibodies to thyroid peroxidase have been demonstrated in almost one third of cases of feline hyperthyroidism whereas about 10% of these animals may also have antinuclear antibodies. Lymphocytic infiltration is also observed in about one third of cases, and it is possible that these cases may be immunologically mediated.

Lymphocytic Parathyroiditis

Dogs and cats develop autoimmune hypoparathyroidism. Affected animals usually have a history of neurological or neuromuscular disease, especially seizures. On investigation affected animals are profoundly hypocalcemic, and serum parathormone levels are severely reduced. On histology normal parathyroid tissue is replaced by a massive infiltration of lymphocytes and a few plasma cells. Once hypocalcemic tetany is controlled, these animals may be managed by oral vitamin D and calcium administration. It would be logical to administer immunosuppressive therapy.

Insulin-Dependent Diabetes Mellitus

In humans, insulin-dependent diabetes mellitus (IDDM) is an autoimmune disease mediated by autoantibodies against an islet cell enzyme called glutamic acid decarboxylase. At least some cases of spontaneous IDDM in dogs may also be immunologically mediated. The canine disease is associated with pancreatic islet atrophy and a loss of β cells. In some cases, the islets are infiltrated by lymphocytes. Experimentally, circulating mononuclear cells from diabetic dogs have caused cultured mouse islet cells to release insulin. If the islet cells were stimulated to release insulin by exposure to glucose, then the mononuclear cells suppressed insulin release. Serum from IDDM dogs lysed these islet cells in the presence of complement. (Figure 33-2). When dog serum was tested for antibodies against cultured β cells by immunofluorescence, 9 of 23 diabetic dogs showed strongly positive reactions and an additional 3 showed a weak reaction. Only 1 of 15 normal dogs gave a positive response. Thus cytotoxic cells or antibodies or both may be responsible for β-cell destruction in dogs. Therefore if autoimmune diabetes is diagnosed, treatment should include immunosuppressive therapy including prednisolone, cyclophosphamide, or azathioprine. A familial predisposition to IDDM has been observed in Samoyeds.

Diabetes mellitus is rare in cattle. Affected animals have atrophy and reduced numbers of pancreatic islets with partial or complete loss of β cells. Lymphocytes commonly infiltrate the remaining islets.

Atrophic Lymphocytic Pancreatitis

The commonest cause of an exocrine pancreatic deficiency in dogs is an atrophic condition associated with lymphocyte infiltration. It is seen predominantly in German shepherds and rough-coated collies. The infiltrating lymphocytes are primarily CD4+ and CD8+ T cells. The CD8+ cells are associated with areas of

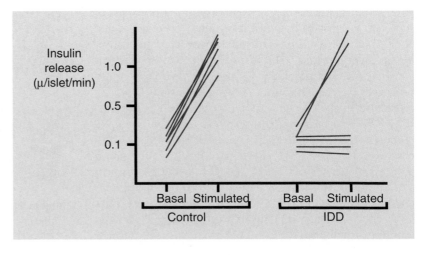

Figure 33-2. Insulin release from islets incubated in vitro in the presence of six individual control or insulin-dependent diabetic dog sera, plus complement. Four of the six diabetic dog sera inhibited insulin release from cultured islets. (From Sai P, Debray-Sachs M, Jondet A, et al: *Diabetes* 33: 135-140, 1984.)

pancreatic necrosis. Some of these dogs have low levels of antibodies against pancreatic acinar cells so this may be an autoimmune disease.

Autoimmune Adrenalitis

Dogs may suffer from lymphocyte-mediated destruction of the adrenal cortex. Affected animals present with depression, weak pulse, bradycardia, abdominal pain, vomiting, diarrhea, dehydration, and hypothermia. As a result of excessive sodium and chloride loss, animals develop hypovolemia and acidosis leading to circulatory shock, hyperkalemia, and cardiac dysrhythmias. Blood corticosteroid levels are low in these animals. This disease has been observed in association with hypothyroidism.

AUTOIMMUNE NEUROLOGICAL DISEASE

An autoimmune brain disease known as experimental allergic encephalomyelitis may be produced by injecting animals with brain tissue emulsified in Freund's complete adjuvant. After a few weeks, dogs or cats develop erratic focal encephalitis and myelitis, possibly with paralysis. The brain lesions consist of focal vasculitis, mononuclear cell infiltration, perivascular demyelination, and axon damage. Antibodies to brain tissue can be detected in the serum of these animals, although the lesion itself is a result of a cell-mediated response.

Similar encephalitis used to occur following administration of rabies vaccines containing brain tissue to humans. For this reason, the use of adult brain tissue was stopped and suckling mouse brain tissue taken before myelination is used in the production of rabies vaccines. Postdistemper demyelinating leukoencephalopathy may also be of autoimmune origin, although the production of antimyelin antibodies appears to be common response to central nervous tissue damage, regardless of its cause.

Equine Polyneuritis

Equine polyneuritis (neuritis of the cauda equina) is an uncommon disease of horses affecting the sacral and coccygeal nerves. Affected horses show hyperesthesia followed by progressive paralysis of the tail, rectum, and bladder and localized anesthesia in the same region. The disease may also be associated with facial and trigeminal paralysis. Although sacral and lumbar involvement is usually bilateral, the cranial nerve involvement is often unilateral. A chronic granulomatous inflammation develops in the region of the extradural nerve roots. Affected nerves are thickened and discolored. They show a loss of myelinated axons, infiltration by macrophages, lymphocytes, giant cells, and plasma cells and deposition of fibrous material in the perineurium. In severe cases the nerve trunks may be almost totally destroyed. Affected horses have circulating antibodies to a peripheral myelin protein called P2. P2 can induce experimental allergic neuritis in rodents (see below). Although equine polyneuritis may be an autoimmune disease, equine adenovirus 1 has been isolated from its lesions, so that the cause is complex. Because of the extensive nerve damage, immunosuppressive or anti-inflammatory therapy is rarely successful.

Canine Polyneuritis

Canine polyneuritis or coonhound paralysis affects dogs following a bite or scratch from a raccoon. It presents as an ascending symmetrical flaccid paralysis with mild sensory impairment. The bitten limb is usually affected first but the disease is progressive and will worsen for 10 to 12 days following the bite. In severe cases the dog may develop flaccid quadriplegia and lose the ability to swallow, bark, or breathe. The disease is, however, self-limiting, and if respiration is not impaired the prognosis is good. Dogs usually recover completely. Affected nerves show demyelination and axonal degeneration with macrophage infiltration. An acute polyneuritis similar to coonhound paralysis has also been described following vaccination of dogs with rabies or other vaccines.

Coonhound paralysis and postvaccinal polyneuritis both closely resemble Guillain-Barré syndrome in humans. This syndrome may follow upper respiratory tract infection, gastrointestinal disease, or even vaccination. It is mediated by autoantibodies against peripheral nerve gangliosides. Management of Guillain-Barré syndrome and canine polyneuritis involves the administration of corticosteroids and the use of a respirator if required.

If sciatic nerve tissue is used to immunize experimental dogs, it provokes experimental allergic neuritis. After a latent period of 6 to 14 days, ascending polyneuritis and gradual paralysis develop (Figure 33-3). The disease is a result of peripheral nerve demyelination as a result of autoimmune attack. Therefore experimental allergic encephalomyelitis is an excellent model of all the diseases described above.

Steroid-Responsive Meningitis-Arteritis

Corticosteroid-responsive meningitis is characterized by sterile inflammation of the meningeal arteries and meningitis. Affected dogs show anorexia, fever, lameness, and listlessness followed by progressive spinal rigidity; hyperesthesia; generalized, cervical, or spinal pain; ataxia; seizures; and behavioral changes. These dogs may have concurrent immune-mediated polyarthritis. Administration of prednisolone leads to rapid clinical improvement. Once the disease is in remission, the dose should be gradually reduced to the minimum necessary to prevent

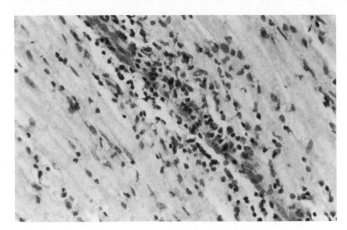

Figure 33-3. A section of rat sciatic nerve showing a mononuclear cell infiltration. This is the lesion of experimental allergic neuritis produced by inoculation of rat sciatic nerve in Freund's complete adjuvant. Original magnification ×400. (Courtesy of Dr. BN Wilkie.)

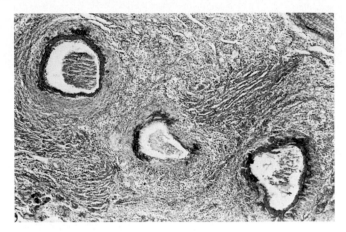

Figure 33-4. Meningeal arteries from a dog with meningeal arteritis. Note the periarteritis with fibrinoid necrosis. Original magnification ×125. (From Harcourt RA: *Vet Rec* 102: 519-522, 1978.)

relapses. It may not be possible to discontinue treatment completely. Large dogs, such as boxers, German shepherds, or Bernese mountain dogs, are commonly affected although the disease has also been reported in beagles.

The cerebrospinal fluid of these animals contains high IgA and CXCL8 levels and mature neutrophils. Serum IgA is also elevated. About 30% of these dogs have a positive LE cell test but no detectable antinuclear antibody activity (Chapter 34). On necropsy, the spinal meningeal arteries show fibrinoid degeneration, intimal or medial necrosis, and hyalinization, and are infiltrated with lymphocytes, plasma cells, and macrophages, and a few neutrophils (Figure 33-4). Complete obliteration of the blood vessel lumina may occur while rupture and thrombosis of inflamed vessels may lead to hemorrhage, compression, and infarction.

Immune-mediated vasculitis is usually associated with immune complex deposition and neutrophil infiltration in blood vessel walls. However, in the meningitis described above, the cellular infiltration may not contain neutrophils. In the beagle cases, no immunoglobulin deposits were detected in the lesions although numerous IgG-containing plasma cells were present in the leptomeninges and in the walls of affected vessels. This may be an autoimmune disease involving local production of IgA or IgG.

Degenerative Myelopathy

In this neurological disease, affected dogs show progressive ataxia affecting the hindlimbs until they can no longer walk. Forelimb problems eventually develop, and dogs die in 6 to 12 months after disease onset. Affected dogs have a degenerative myelopathy with widespread demyelination and loss of axons in the

thoracolumbar region. The cause of the disease is unknown but some investigators believe it to be immune mediated. Affected dogs have circulating immune complexes, depressed lymphocyte mitogenic responses, and deposits of IgG and C3 in the lesions and nearby normal tissues.

Cerebellar Degeneration

A cerebellar degeneration has been observed in Coton de Tulear puppies. It is associated with a depleted granular cell layer and microglial cell activation caused by T-cell destruction of granular cells.

AUTOIMMUNE EYE DISEASE

Equine Recurrent Uveitis

The most common cause of blindness in horses is equine recurrent uveitis (or periodic ophthalmia). Horses have recurrent attacks of uveitis, retinitis, and vasculitis. In acute cases they have blepharospasm, lacrimation, and photophobia. Each attack gets progressively more severe and gradually spreads to involve other eye tissues until complete blindness results. The eye lesions are infiltrated with Th1 cells and neutrophils with extensive fibrin and C3 deposition. The major autoantigen implicated is the interphotoreceptor retinoid-binding protein with subsequent epitope spreading to the S protein. Affected horses also have circulating antibodies to *Leptospira interrogans*. The titer of these antibodies tends to rise during a flare-up of the lesion and drop while in remission. If horses are immunized with either equine cornea or killed *L. interrogans* of certain serovars, they develop corneal opacity 10 days later when antibodies appear in the bloodstream. It has been possible to show partial antigenic identity between equine corneas and these *L. interrogans* serovars. Thus some cases may be due to an autoimmune attack on ocular tissues as a result of molecular mimicry with *L. interrogans*. Other cases may be due to infection with *Borrelia burgdorferi* or with the nematode *Onchocerca cervicalis*.

Systemic and topical corticosteroid therapy is required to bring the inflammation under control although the disease usually recurs.

Uveodermatological Syndrome

Uveodermatological syndrome is a sporadic disease of dogs. A similar disease, Vogt-Koyanagi-Harada syndrome, occurs in humans. Affected dogs exhibit severe eye disease (uveitis) and skin depigmentation with whitening of the hair (poliosis) and skin (vitiligo). The eye lesions develop first. Thus most animals present with sudden blindness or chronic uveitis. The early lesions vary from a severe panuveitis to a bilateral anterior uveitis. Some dogs may have retinal detachment and there may be progressive depigmentation of the retina and iris. Depigmentation of the hair and skin gradually follows the onset of the eye lesions. It may be generalized and commonly involves the eyelids, nasal planum, lips, scrotum, and foot pads (Figure 33-5). These depigmented areas may become ulcerated and crusted.

Histologic examination shows a diffuse infiltration of the uveal tract with lymphocytes, plasma cells and macrophages. Many of the macrophages contain ingested melanin. The skin lesions consist of a mononuclear (macrophages, giant cells, lymphocytes, plasma cells) infiltration of the dermal–epidermal junction (Figure 33-6). The amount of melanin in the epidermis and hair follicles is greatly reduced.

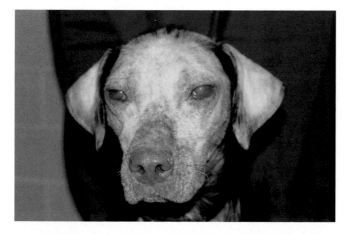

Figure 33-5. A case of uveodermatological syndrome. Note ocular clouding, alopecia, and depigmentation of the nasal planum. (Courtesy of Drs. Robert Kennis, Joan Dziezc, and Larry Wadsworth.)

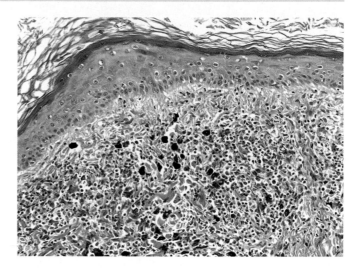

Figure 33-6. Histological section of skin from a case of uveodermatological syndrome. Note the major lymphocyte infiltration associated with the skin melanocytes. It is the destruction of these melanocytes that leads to depigmentation. (Courtesy of Dr. Joanne Mansell.)

In humans, Vogt-Koyanagi-Harada syndrome is believed to be a result of an autoimmune response against melanocytes. In dogs no consistent immunological abnormalities have been observed.

Management of the eye lesions with ocular glucocorticoids and of the skin lesions with systemic corticosteroids has been beneficial although the disease may recur when therapy is terminated. Azathioprine may also be given if glucocorticoids are insufficient to stop disease progression.

AUTOIMMUNE REPRODUCTIVE DISEASES

If the testes are damaged so that hidden antigens are released, then an autoimmune response may exacerbate the orchitis. Experimentally, autoimmune orchitis may be produced in male animals by injection of testicular extracts emulsified in Freund's complete adjuvant. Autoantibodies to sperm may also be detected in the serum of some animals following injury to the testes or long-standing obstruction of the seminiferous ducts. For example, dogs infected with *Brucella canis* have chronic epididymitis and become sensitized by sperm antigens carried to the circulation after phagocytosis by macrophages. These sperm antigens stimulate the production of IgG or IgA autoantibodies. The autoantibodies can agglutinate and immobilize sperm, causing infertility.

In stallions antisperm autoantibodies may be associated with reduced fertility or infertility. In cows, antibodies to sperm can reach high levels and cause infertility. In certain lines of black mink, 20% to 30% of the older males are infertile as a result of high levels of antisperm antibodies. The animals have a monocytic orchitis and immune complexes are deposited along the basal lamina of the seminiferous tubules.

Dermatologists recognize an autoimmune dermatitis in which intact female dogs develop a hypersensitivity to endogenous progesterone or estrogen. The disease presents as a bilaterally symmetrical and intense pruritus, erythema, and papular eruption. Its development usually coincides with estrus or pseudopregnancy. Corticosteroid treatment may have little effect, but testosterone may help.

Recently there has been an increased interest in production-enhancing vaccines. These vaccines commonly interfere with normal hormone production or reproductive behavior by inducing an autoimmune response. Thus a vaccine designed to neutralize production of gonadotropin-releasing hormone effectively castrates male animals. Its use results in improved meat quality, faster growth, and reduced aggressive behavior. This vaccine is also used to castrate male pigs and block the production of steroids associated with boar taint, the offensive odor associated with boar meat. Similar vaccines may be used as contraceptives. Thus if dogs are immunized with bovine or ovine luteinizing hormone (LH), the autoantibodies produced may neutralize their own LH. Similarly, it is possible to produce autoantibodies that neutralize LH-releasing hormone. As a result, the reproductive cycle is abolished in females and testicular, epididymal, and prostatic atrophy occurs in male dogs, leading to sterility. Other experimental immunocontraceptive vaccines have been directed against prostaglandin $F_{2\alpha}$, reproductive steroids, the LH receptor, and zona pellucida protein.

Sheep immunized with polyandroalbumin (androstenedione-7-carboxyethyl thioester linked to human serum albumin) have about 23% more lambs than untreated sheep. The ewes are given two doses of this vaccine before lambing. It is believed that the vaccine induces autoantibodies that reduce serum androstenedione levels.

Turkeys immunized against vasoactive intestinal peptide show reduced broodiness and a significant increase in egg production.

AUTOIMMUNE SKIN DISEASES

Many different autoimmune skin diseases have been identified. They are characterized by local destruction or cell separation within the skin and the consequent development of bullae (blisters or vesicles) (Figure 33-7). As a result, dermatologists use the terms *pemphigus* or *pemphigoid* to describe them, after the Greek word *pemphix* meaning "blister."

The Pemphigus Complex

The pemphigus complex consists of four skin diseases that have been described in humans, dogs, horses, and

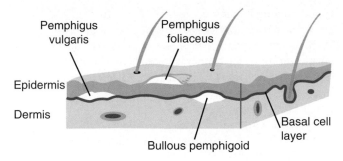

Figure 33-7. The differential histology of the autoimmune skin diseases. Note the location of the vesicle in relation to the epidermis.

cats. The most severe is pemphigus vulgaris. In this disease, bullae develop in the skin around the mucocutaneous junctions, especially the nose, lips, eyes, prepuce, and anus, and on the tongue and the inner surface of the ear. These bullae rupture readily, leaving weeping, denuded areas that may become secondarily infected. Histological examination of intact bullae shows a separation of the skin cells (acantholysis) in the suprabasal region of the lower epidermis (Figure 33-8). The acantholysis results from an autoantibody attack on a cell adhesion protein called desmoglein-3. The combination of antibodies with desmoglein-3 triggers keratinocytes to secrete proteases. These digest the adhesion proteins and so allow the keratinocytes to separate from each other. Eventually this leads to acantholysis and bulla formation. Pemphigus vegetans is a rare and mild variant of pemphigus vulgaris in which either bullae or pustules form and papillomatous proliferation of the base of these occurs on healing.

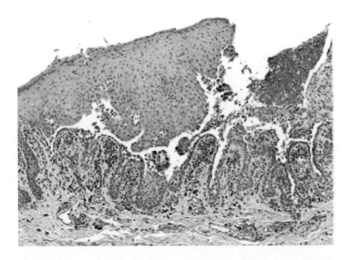

Figure 33-8. A section of an oral lesion of pemphigus vulgaris in a dog. Note the cleft formation at the base of the epidermis accompanied by extensive cellular infiltration. (Courtesy of Dr. Joanne Mansell.)

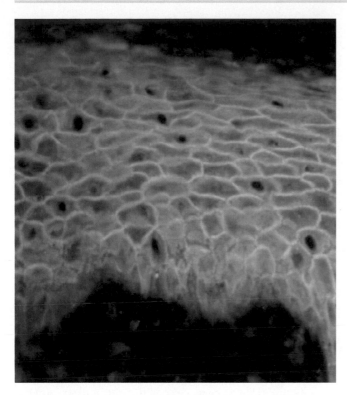

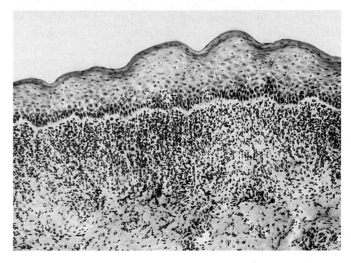

Figure 33-10. Section from an oral lesion of bullous pemphigoid in a dog. Note that the cleft is formed below the epidermis. Inflammatory cells are present in the superficial dermis and, to a lesser extent, in the epithelium. (From Bennett D, Lauder IM, Kirkham D, McQueen A: *Vet Rec* 106:497, 1980.)

Figure 33-9. Direct immunofluorescent micrograph of a section of normal dog skin that has been incubated in serum from a dog with pemphigus vulgaris. The intercellular cement is stained. (Courtesy of Dr. K Credille.)

Pemphigus foliaceus is a milder and more common disease than pemphigus vulgaris. It has been described in humans, dogs, cats, goats, and horses. It too is a vesicular disease, but the bullae are not confined to mucocutaneous junctions or muzzle. Histology of the skin reveals that the vesicle formation occurs superficially in the subcorneal region. The bullae are very fragile and therefore rarely persist. The autoantigen in humans has been identified as desmoglein-1, a cell adhesion protein found in the squamous cell desmosomes. Some cases of canine pemphigus foliaceus appear be a result of thiol groups from drugs binding to cell membranes. The disease has developed following the use of antibiotics such as trimethoprim-sulfadiazine, oxacillin, cephalexin, and ampicillin.

A mild variant of pemphigus foliaceus is pemphigus erythematosus. The lesions in pemphigus erythematosus tend to be confined to the face and ears and are very similar to those of systemic lupus erythematosus. Indeed, some dogs with pemphigus erythematosus may have antinuclear antibodies in their serum.

Direct immunofluorescent examination of skin lesions reveals immunoglobulins deposited on the intercellular cement in a typical "chicken-wire" pattern (Figure 33-9).

It is important to differentiate between the two major forms of pemphigus for prognostic reasons. Pemphigus vulgaris has a relatively poor prognosis; treatment tends to be unsatisfactory and the lesions are persistent. In contrast, pemphigus foliaceus is milder and the results of treatment may be more satisfactory. Treatment of either disease involves the use of large doses of corticosteroids. In refractory cases, azathioprine, cyclophosphamide, cyclosporine, or gold salts such as aurothioglucose may be of assistance. As with other autoimmune diseases, the disease often recurs when treatment is stopped.

A third form of pemphigus, called paraneoplastic pemphigus, is seen in humans and has been recorded in a dog. It develops in association with lymphoid or solid tumors. It resembles pemphigus vulgaris but multiple autoantibodies against skin antigens are present.

Skin Basement Membrane Diseases

A second set of blistering diseases is associated with the development of autoantibodies against components of the skin basement membrane. Several of these have been identified in dogs and other domestic animals. They include bullous pemphigoid, linear IgA dermatosis, and epidermolysis bullosa acquisita.

Bullous Pemphigoid
Bullous pemphigoid is a rare skin disease that resembles pemphigus vulgaris. Collies, Shetland sheepdogs, and Dobermans appear to be predisposed to this disease. It has also been described in humans, pigs, horses, and cats. Multiple bullae develop around mucocutaneous junctions and in the groin and axillae. However, the disease differs from pemphigus vulgaris in that the bullae develop in the subepidermis (and are therefore less likely

to rupture). They tend to be filled with fibrin as well as mononuclear cells or eosinophils, and they heal spontaneously (Figure 33-10). Bullous pemphigoid results from the development of autoantibodies against type XVII collagen. This molecule is located in the hemidesmosomes, the structures that attach basal keratinocytes to the basement membrane (Figure 33-11). The deposition of IgG on the basement membrane may be demonstrated by immunofluorescence that reveals intense linear staining. The prognosis of bullous pemphigoid is usually poor, but mild cases may recover after treatment with corticosteroids. More commonly aggressive treatment, such as high doses of prednisolone supplemented if necessary with cyclophosphamide, azathioprine, and chlorambucil, may be required. Some dogs may develop a bullous pemphigoid-like disease in response to autoantibodies against the basement membrane protein laminin-5.

Linear IgA Dermatosis

Another group of skin diseases is characterized by the deposition of IgA in the lamina lucida of the skin basement membrane. One such disease, called dermatitis herpetiformis, has been recorded in a beagle, whereas a linear IgA dermatosis has been recorded in dachshunds. Both diseases present with pruritic pustular and papular lesions, resembling pyoderma, with eosinophil-filled subepidermal vesicles. The autoantigen has been identified as a processed extracellular form of collagen XVII. The drug dapsone has been recommended as the specific treatment for these diseases.

Epidermolysis Bullosa Acquisita

A generalized skin disease characterized by severe blistering and ulcerative lesions has been identified in a Great Dane. The vesicles originate from erythematous areas on the skin and rapidly progress to ulcers. There is generalized urticaria, oral ulceration, and eventually cutaneous sloughing. A localized variant of the disease has been observed in a German short-haired pointer. The dermis and epidermis separate and neutrophils accumulate within the superficial dermis. The neutrophil infiltration may eventually result in microabcess formation. Secondary changes include ulceration, necrosis, and bacterial infection. Affected animals develop IgA and IgG autoantibodies against the anchoring fibrils of the lower basement membrane (lamina densa). These autoantibodies are specific for type VII collagen and distinctly different from those responsible for bullous pemphigoid. Immunosuppressive therapy may be of benefit although secondary bacterial infection can cause difficulties.

Alopecia Areata

Alopecia areata is an autoimmune disease directed against cells in hair follicles. It is characterized by the development of multiple round spots of hair loss in the absence of obvious inflammation. It has been reported in humans and other primates, dogs, cats, horses, and cattle. In dogs, the lesions are infiltrated with CD4+ and CD8+ T cells and Langerhans cells. IgG antibodies directed against the lower hair follicles can also be detected. C3 or IgM may also be present. The targets of this immunological attack are unclear but may be bulbar keratinocytes, hair follicle keratins, or bulbar melanocytes. (The disease sometimes spares unpigmented hairs.) Alopecia areata responds to corticosteroid treatment.

Relapsing Polychondritis

A disease involving autoimmunity against type II cartilage has been described in humans and in cats. The animals present with bilateral curling of the ears and ocular changes. The cartilage is infiltrated with plasma cells and lymphocytes.

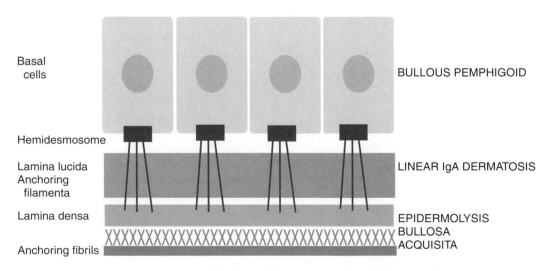

Figure 33-11.   Structures on the dermal basement membrane that act as autoantigens.

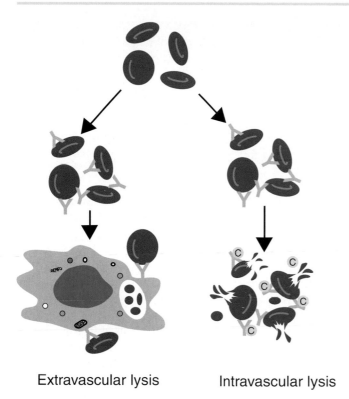

Extravascular lysis   Intravascular lysis

Figure 33-12. Differences between intravascular and extravascular hemolysis.

AUTOIMMUNE NEPHRITIS

Horses may develop autoantibodies to glomerular basement membranes, which may provoke glomerulonephritis and renal failure. Immunofluorescence studies of affected kidneys show that the basement membrane is evenly coated with a smooth, linear deposit of immunoglobulin. The autoantibodies may provoke proliferation of the glomerular epithelial cells and epithelial crescent formation.

AUTOIMMUNE HEMOLYTIC ANEMIA

Autoantibodies to red blood cell antigens provoke their destruction and cause autoimmune hemolytic anemia (AIHA). These hemolytic anemias are well recognized in humans and dogs and have been recorded in cattle, horses, cats, mice, rabbits, and raccoons.

Affected dogs are anemic. Thus pallor, weakness, and lethargy are accompanied by fever, icterus, and hepatosplenomegaly. The anemia may be associated with tachycardia, anorexia, vomiting, or diarrhea. Clinical signs are contingent on the speed of development of the disease, its severity, and the mechanism of red cell destruction. This destruction may result from intravascular hemolysis (destruction within the bloodstream) mediated by complement or, much more commonly, by removal of antibody-coated red cells by the macrophages of the

spleen and liver (extravascular hemolysis) (Figure 33-12). In dogs the disease occurs more often in females (2:1 ratio) and with an average age of onset around 4 to 5 years. There is evidence for a genetic predisposition to AIHA in some animals (Table 33-1). The causes of AIHA are unknown although some cases may be attributable to alterations in red surface antigens induced by drugs or viruses. In dogs the autoantibodies are primarily directed against red cell glycophorins, the cytoskeletal protein spectrin, and the membrane anion exchange protein (CD233 or band 3). About one third of cases of AIHA are associated with other immunological abnormalities such as systemic lupus (Chapter 34) or autoimmune thrombocytopenia and with lymphoid tumors such as feline leukemia. Its onset may be associated with obvious stress such as vaccination (Chapter 22), viral disease, or hormonal imbalances as in pregnancy or pyometra.

AIHAs in dogs are classified according to the antibody class involved, the optimal temperature at which the autoantibodies react, and the nature of the hemolytic process (Table 33-2).

Class I: This form of AIHA is caused by autoantibodies that agglutinate red cells at body temperature. The agglutination may be seen when a drop of blood is placed on a glass slide. Both IgG and IgM antibodies are involved. Since IgG does not activate complement efficiently, the red cells are mainly destroyed by phagocytosis in the spleen. In very severe cases, a blood smear may show erythrophagocytosis by neutrophils and monocytes.

Class II: IgM antibodies activate complement and destroy red cells by intravascular hemolysis. This results in hemoglobinemia, hemoglobinuria, icterus, and very severe anemia. Affected dogs are anemic, weak, possibly jaundiced, and hemoglobin may appear in the urine. Kupffer cells in the liver or in lymph nodes preferentially remove red cells with complement on their surface, so these animals develop hepatomegaly and lymphadenopathy.

Class III: Most cases of AIHA in dogs and cats are mediated by IgG1 and IgG4 antibodies, which bind to red cells at 37° C but do not activate complement or agglutinate the red cells. IgG antibodies can only form short bridges (15 to 25 nm) between cells. As a result, they cannot counteract the zeta potential of the red cells and will not cause direct agglutination. [In contrast, IgM antibodies form long bridges (30 to 50 nm) and so can agglutinate cells despite their zeta potential.] Affected red cells are opsonized and removed by splenic macrophages. Splenomegaly is a consistent feature of class III disease.

Class IV: Some IgM antibodies cannot agglutinate red cells at body temperature but only do so when the blood is chilled. These antibodies are called "cold-agglutinins." They can be detected by cooling blood to between 10° C and 4° C, at which point clumping occurs. The agglutination is reversed on rewarming. As blood circulates through the extremities (tail, toes, ears, and so forth) of affected animals it may be sufficiently

TABLE   33-2
Classification of Autoimmune Hemolytic Anemias

Class	Predominant Antibody	Activity	Optimal Temp. (°C)	Site of Red Cell Removal	Clinical Effect
I	G >> M	Agglutinin	37	Spleen	Intravascular agglutination
II	M	Hemolysin	37	Liver	Intravascular hemolysin
III	G	Incomplete	37	Spleen	Anemia
IV	M	Agglutinin	4	Liver	Cyanosis of extremities
V	M	Incomplete	4	Liver	Anemia

cooled to permit hemagglutination within capillaries. This can lead to vascular stasis, blockage, tissue ischemia, and, eventually, necrosis. Affected animals may therefore present with necrotic lesions at the extremities and anemia may not be a significant feature. As might be anticipated, this form of AIHA is severest in the winter.

Class V: This is mediated by IgM antibodies that will bind red cells when chilled to 4° C but will not agglutinate them. These antibodies can only be identified by an antiglobulin test conducted in the cold. They do not induce necrosis of extremities but can activate complement leading to intravascular hemolysis.

Diagnosis

The hematology of affected animals reflects the severe anemia and a regenerative response by the bone marrow. Blood smears commonly show spherocytes, which are small round red cells that lack a central pale area. These spherocytes result from the partial phagocytosis of antibody-coated red cells. The number of spherocytes in blood is a measure of the intensity of red cell destruction.

To diagnose AIHA associated with the presence of nonagglutinating or incomplete antibodies (classes II, III, V), it is necessary to use a direct antiglobulin test (Chapter 16). The red cells of the affected animal are collected in anticoagulant, washed free of serum, and incubated in an antiglobulin serum. The best antiglobulin for these purposes is one with activity against IgM, IgG, and complement. Red cells coated with autoantibody or complement will be cross-linked and agglutinated by the antiglobulin. Occasionally IgM may have a low affinity for the red cells, so it elutes, leaving only complement on their surface. It is important to emphasize that samples for immunological testing should be collected before immunosuppressive therapy begins. It is also important to note that in the cat, most cases of antiglobulin-positive hemolytic anemia are secondary to feline leukemia virus or *Mycoplasma haemofelis (Haemobartonella felis)* infections. Treatment for AIHA involves management of the anemia and administration of corticosteroids to reduce phagocytosis of red cells. As a result, the most effective treatment is that for disease mediated by IgG. Corticosteroids are of much less benefit in the management of intravascular hemolysis mediated by IgM and complement and do not induce significant immunosuppression in animals so

affected. Treated animals may respond within 24 to 48 hours. Corticosteroid treatment may be supplemented with cyclophosphamide and/or azathioprine in acute cases. Splenectomy should only be considered when more conservative therapy has failed. Although splenectomy may be of assistance in cases of refractory class III disease, no controlled trials have confirmed this.

Acute immunologically mediated anemias have been observed in horses following infection with *Streptococcus fecalis*, in sheep following leptospirosis, in cats with mycoplasmosis (hemobartonellosis), and in pigs with eperythrozoonosis. In these cases IgM cold agglutinins are produced that can clump red cells from normal animals of the same species when chilled. Hemoglobin itself may act as an autoantigen, and antibodies to hemoglobin are detectable in the serum of cattle severely infected with *Arcanobacterium pyogenes*, perhaps as a result of bacterial hemolysis.

AIHA occurs in horses with lymphosarcomas and melanomas. The animals are depressed and pyrexic, and exhibit splenomegaly, jaundice, and hemoglobinuria. Some show red cell autoagglutination. On antiglobulin testing the horses are positive for IgG on their red cells. Dexamethasone treatment induces remission.

Immune Suppression of Hematopoiesis

It has been demonstrated in humans, and surmised in dogs, that autoimmune responses may be directed against hematopoietic stem cells. Thus autoantibodies to erythroid precursors may cause red cell aplasia, and autoantibodies to myeloid precursors may provoke an immune neutropenia. In dogs, red cell aplasia has been associated with the presence of IgG that inhibits erythroid stem cell differentiation. These diseases can only be diagnosed by careful hematological analysis and by demonstration of autoantibodies by immunofluorescence on bone marrow smears. Affected animals may benefit from high doses of corticosteroids or immunosuppressive therapy.

AUTOIMMUNE THROMBOCYTOPENIA

Autoimmune thrombocytopenia (AITP) due to production of autoantibodies to platelets has been reported in horses, dogs, and, rarely, cats. The clinical sign is excessive bleeding. Thus affected animals usually present with multiple petechiae in the skin, gingiva, other mucous membranes, and conjunctiva. Epistaxis may occur and dogs may show melena and hematuria. The predominant cause of death in these dogs is severe gastrointestinal hemorrhage. Antibodies against platelet surface antigens lead to extravascular destruction of opsonized platelets in the spleen. These antibodies may also interfere with normal platelet function. Affected animals have unusually low platelet counts and a prolonged bleeding time. The condition is commonly observed in association with AIHA and SLE. The thrombocytopenia seen in animals with multiple myeloma or other lymphoid tumors, in ehrlichiosis, or following certain drug treatments may be due to the nonspecific binding of IgG to platelets. In dogs, the average age of onset is 6 years. Predisposed breeds include Old English sheepdogs, cocker spaniels, and poodles. Antibodies to platelets may be measured by direct immunofluorescence on bone marrow aspirates looking for positive reactions on megakaryocytes. However, the best test for this purpose is one that measures the release of factor 3 from platelets following exposure to autoantibodies. This may be performed by incubating platelet-rich plasma with a globulin fraction of the serum under test and estimating the amount of procoagulant activity released. In about 75% of cases the antibodies are of the IgG class. In cats most cases of AITP are probably secondary to feline leukemia virus infection.

Corticosteroids are used in the management of AITP. Additional immunosuppression with azathioprine or cyclophosphamide may be required for patients who do not respond to corticosteroid therapy. Vincristine may also produce a good clinical response. This drug binds to platelets and so kills macrophages when they phagocytose the antibody-coated platelets. Splenectomy may be of value when other forms of therapy have failed.

AUTOIMMUNE MUSCLE DISEASE

Myasthenia Gravis

Myasthenia gravis in humans, dogs, and cats is a disease of skeletal muscle characterized by abnormal fatigue and weakness after relatively mild exercise. It results from a failure of transmission of nerve impulses across the motor endplate of striated muscle as a result of a deficiency of acetylcholine receptors (Figure 33-13). In Jack Russell terriers, Springer spaniels, and fox terriers, a congenital form of the disease occurs as a result of an inherited deficiency of the acetylcholine receptors. This congenital form is therefore a disease of young dogs.

In adult dogs, however, the acetylcholine receptor deficiency is due to IgG autoantibodies. These antibodies accelerate degradation of the receptors, block the acetylcholine-binding sites, and trigger complement-mediated damage. As a result, the number of available, functional

acetylcholine receptors is significantly reduced. Dogs may also make autoantibodies against titin, an intracellular muscle protein and the ryanodine receptor—a Ca^{2+} release channel in striated muscle.

In normal muscles, the binding of acetylcholine to its receptor opens a sodium channel to produce a localized endplate potential. If the amplitude of the endplate potential is sufficient, this will generate an action potential and trigger muscle contraction. The endplate potential from a normal neuromuscular junction is more than sufficient to generate a muscle action potential. In myasthenic junctions, however, the endplate potentials fail to trigger action potentials in many muscle fibers. This is manifested as muscle weakness. Repeating the stimulus leads to a progressive increase in weakness as transmission failure occurs at more and more neuromuscular junctions since the amount of acetylcholine released from a nerve terminal usually declines after the first few impulses.

The disease may develop in any breed of dog but certain breeds appear to be predisposed to the disease (Table 33-1). Large dogs such as German shepherds, golden retrievers, and Labradors, appear to develop more severe disease. Rottweilers appear to be at low risk. In cats there appears to be a breed predisposition for Abyssinians and related Somalis.

Clinically different disease forms may be recognized. Thus almost 60% of cases are generalized and the rest are focal. In some animals the thymus may show medullary hyperplasia, germinal center formation, or even a thymic carcinoma, and surgical thymectomy may result in clinical improvement. About 3% of dog cases and 20% of cat cases are associated with the presence of a thymic tumor.

Animals may present with a history of swallowing difficulty, regurgitation, labored breathing, and generalized muscle weakness. Megaesophagus is common. The disease can be classified as focal myasthenia gravis when an animal presents with megaesophagus and various degrees of facial paralysis without limb muscle weakness; generalized myasthenia gravis where limb muscle weakness is associated with facial paralysis and megaesophagus; and acute fulminating myasthenia gravis when the disease rapidly leads to quadriplegia and respiratory difficulty. Without treatment about half of affected animals will die whereas the others may show spontaneous remissions. Aspiration pneumonia is the main cause of death in myasthenic dogs.

Administration of a short-acting anticholinesterase drug such as edrophonium chloride (tensilon) leads to a rapid gain in muscle strength. The anticholinesterase, by permitting the acetylcholine to accumulate at the neuromuscular junction, enables the remaining receptors to be stimulated more effectively. Myasthenia gravis is managed with long-acting anticholinesterase drugs such as pyridostigmine bromide or neostigmine methyl sulfate. Dogs may also be immunosuppressed with prednisone or

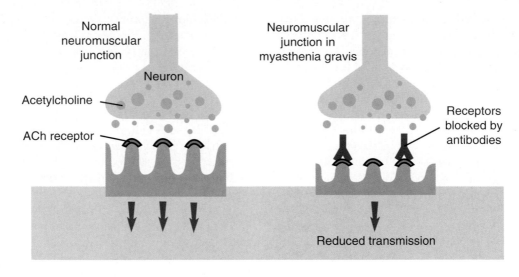

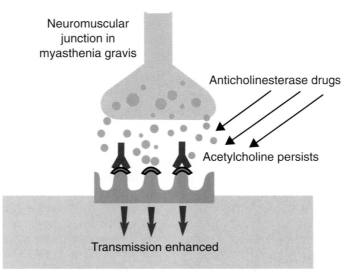

Figure 33-13. The pathogenesis of myasthenia gravis. Destruction of acetylcholine receptors prevents effective neuromuscular transmission. Blockage of cholinesterase activity by anticholinesterase drugs permits acetylcholine to accumulate and so enhances neuromuscular transmission.

azathioprine or both. However, corticosteroid treatment may result in transient exacerbation of symptoms. Plasmapheresis has been used for short-term therapy to stabilize patients prior to thymectomy.

Polymyositis

A generalized autoimmune myositis occurs in large dogs such as German shepherds. The disease may be acute or gradual in onset. The animals show progressive muscle weakness not associated with exercise. Changes in laryngeal muscle function lead to a change in the voice. Megaesophagus may lead to dysphagia and if severe can result in aspiration pneumonia. Affected animals may develop a shifting lameness. Animals may be febrile and develop leukocytosis and eosinophilia. Biopsies show muscle fiber degeneration, necrosis, and vacuolation, and affected muscles may be infiltrated by lymphocytes

and plasma cells. About 50% of affected dogs have antinuclear antibodies or antibodies to sarcolemma or both. Corticosteroids are the treatment of choice.

Autoimmune Masticatory Myopathy

Dogs can develop a myopathy confined to the muscles of mastication. They present with pain and atrophy or swelling of the masticatory muscles manifested by difficulty in opening (trismus) or closing the jaw. Affected animals may also have ocular lesions such as conjunctivitis or exophthalmos. Histology of affected muscles shows inflammatory or degenerative lesions with atrophy and fibrosis. Myositis with lymphocytes and plasma cells predominates, and some lesions may contain many eosinophils. Myofiber atrophy, perimysial or endomysial fibrosis, and muscle fiber necrosis are consistent features. Immunoglobulins can be detected in biopsies of affected muscles, and circulating antibodies to the masticatory muscle fibers have been demonstrated. The masticatory muscles contain an isoform of myosin that is different from that found in the limb muscles, leading to selective attack on these muscles. Corticosteroids such as long-term prednisone are used for treatment, but the prognosis is guarded.

Canine Cardiomyopathy

English cocker spaniel dogs can develop a cardiomyopathy with antinuclear and antimitochondrial autoantibodies, and reduced serum IgA levels associated with a specific C4 allotype (C4:4). The autoantigen has not been identified, but in humans some forms of cardiomyopathy have been associated with autoantibodies against the adenine nucleotide translocator of mitochondria.

CHRONIC ACTIVE HEPATITIS

Doberman pinschers may develop an autoimmune hepatitis. The symptoms are typical of liver disease with anorexia, depression, weight loss, diarrhea, polydipsia, polyuria, icterus, and eventually ascites. The disease commonly presents between 3 and 6 years of age but may have been present subclinically for many years. On histology, the liver shows intense inflammation and scar tissue formation around small hepatic vein branches. The lesions contain lymphocytes, plasma cells, and macrophages. The disease eventually causes progressive fibrosis and destruction of hepatocytes. About half of affected dogs develop antibodies to hepatocyte cell membranes. These antibody-positive dogs have more severe disease than dogs lacking such antibodies. In addition, lymphocytes from about 75% of affected dogs respond to liver membrane protein in vitro. Hepatocytes from affected dogs, but not from normal Dobermans, express MHC class II antigens. This MHC expression correlated with the severity of the disease. Corticosteroid treatment reduced both MHC expression and disease severity. It has been suggested therefore that the disease results from a cell-mediated attack on abnormally expressed MHC molecules or an antigen associated with them.

SOURCES OF ADDITIONAL INFORMATION

Day MJ: Detection of equine antisperm antibodies by indirect immunofluorescence and the tube-slide agglutination test, *Equine Vet J* 28:494-496, 1996.

Day MJ: Inheritance of autoantibody, reduced serum IgA and autoimmune disease in a canine breeding colony, *Vet Immunol Immunopathol* 53:207-219, 1996.

Dewey CW: Acquired myasthenia gravis in dogs, *Compend Contin Educ Pract Vet* 19:1340-1354, 1997.

Fenger CK, Hoffsis GF, Kociba GJ: Idiopathic immune-mediated anemia in a calf, *J Am Vet Med Assoc* 201:97-99, 1992.

Gilmour MA, Morgan RV, Moore FM: Masticatory myopathy in the dog: a retrospective study of 18 cases, *J Am Anim Hosp Assoc* 28:300-306, 1992.

Happ GM. Thyroiditis: model canine autoimmune disease, *Adv Vet Sci Comp Med* 39:97-129, 1995.

Hoenig M, Dawe DL: A qualitative assay for beta cell antibodies. Preliminary results in dogs with diabetes mellitus, *Vet Immunol Immunopathol* 32: 195-203, 1992.

Kennedy RL, Thoday KL: Autoantibodies in feline hyperthyroidism, *Res Vet Sci* 45: 300-306, 1988.

Mackin A: Canine immune-mediated thrombocytopenia, *Compend Contin Educ Pract Vet* 17:353-362, 515-533, 1995.

Meric SM, Perman V, Hardy RM: Corticosteroid-responsive meningitis in ten dogs, *J Am Anim Hosp Assoc* 21:677-684, 1985.

Morgan RV: Vogt-Koyanagi-Harada syndrome in humans and dogs, *Compend Contin Educ Pract Vet* 11:1211-1218, 1989.

Olivry T, Fine J-D, Dunston SM, et al: Canine epidermolysis bullosa acquisita: circulating autoantibodies target the amino terminal noncollagenous (NC1) domain of collagen VII in anchoring fibrils, *Vet Dermatol* 9:19-31, 1998.

Olivry T, Moore PF, Naydan DK, et al: Antifollicular cell-mediated and humoral immunity in canine alopecia areata, *Vet Dermatol* 7:67-79, 1996.

Parma AF, Santisteban CG, Villalba JS, Bowden RA: Experimental demonstration of an antigenic relationship between *Leptospira* and equine cornea, *Vet Immunol Immunopathol* 10: 215-224, 1985.

Poitout F, Weiss DJ, Armstrong PJ: Cell-mediated immune responses to liver membrane protein of canine chronic hepatitis, *Vet Immunol Immunopathol* 57:169-178, 1997.

Romeike A, Brügmann M, Drommer W: Immunohistochemical studies in equine recurrent uveitis (ERU), *Vet Pathol* 35: 515-526, 1998.

Scott-Moncrieff JC, Azcona-Olivera J, Glickman NW, et al: Evaluation of antithyroglobulin antibodies after routine vaccinations in pet and research dogs, *J Am Vet Med Assoc* 221:515-521, 2002.

Stanley JR: Autoantibodies against adhesion molecules and structures in blistering skin disease, *J Exp Med* 181: 1-4, 1995.

Taniyama H, Shirakawa T, Furuoka H, et al: Spontaneous diabetes mellitus in young cattle: histologic, immunohistochemical and electron microscopic studies of the islets of Langerhans, *Vet Pathol* 30:46-54, 1993.

Tipold A, Vandevelde M, Zurbriggen A: Neuroimmunological studies in steroid-responsive meningitis-arteritis in dogs, *Res Vet Sci* 58:103-108, 1995.

White SD, Carlotti DN, Pin D, et al: Putative drug-related pemphigus foliaceus in four dogs, *Vet Dermatol* 13:195-202, 2002.

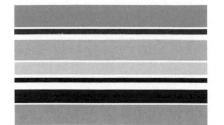

The Systemic Immunological Diseases

CHAPTER 34

Animals may suffer from autoimmune diseases that involve multiple organ systems. In human medicine these have been called "rheumatic" diseases, "connective tissue" diseases, or "collagen" diseases based on outdated views on their pathogenesis. These systemic diseases or syndromes are interrelated and have many overlapping clinical features (Figure 34-1). Because they share many features, it is sometimes difficult to come to a definitive diagnosis of the precise syndrome involved. These diseases include systemic lupus erythematosus, rheumatoid arthritis, nonerosive arthritides, various vasculitides, dermatomyositis, and Sjögren's syndrome.

All these diseases have some form of autoimmune component. Unlike the diseases described in Chapter 33, however, they are not simply diseases in which a local autoimmune response leads to tissue destruction. Most are associated with the presence of circulating immune-complexes or the long-term deposition of immune-complexes and complement in tissues. This immune-complex deposition leads to chronic inflammation. The initiating antigens are unknown but may well be infectious agents. All exhibit a significant genetic predisposition, commonly with linkage to the MHC.

SYSTEMIC LUPUS ERYTHEMATOSUS

Systemic lupus erythematosus (SLE) is a complex disease syndrome that has been described in humans, other primates, mice, horses, dogs, and cats. It is characterized by a broad and bewildering diversity of different symptoms and a wide variety of disease courses as symptoms flare and recede over time.

Pathogenesis

The factors that lead to the development of lupus are complex, multifactorial, and poorly defined. Its development is affected by environmental factors, including infectious agents, drugs, and food, in association with many different genes. Patients develop a variety of autoantibodies, changes in T cell function, defective phagocytosis and oncogene expression. One key defect in lupus patients appears to be the impaired clearance of apoptotic cells. Normally, apoptotic cells are removed by phagocytosis by macrophages without causing inflammation. Macrophages from SLE patients, however, show defective phagocytosis of apoptotic cells, which as a result accumulate in tissues. Nuclear fragments from these cells may be trapped and processed by dendritic cells, thereby triggering autoantibody formation. The defect is most obvious in the skin of affected animals where UV radiation may lead to accumulation of apoptotic cells. Antigens, especially nucleic acids, from these cells then act as autoantigens and trigger autoantibody formation. These autoantibodies in turn lead to immune complex deposition and tissue damage. Other processes may induce lupus. For example, some inherited complement deficiencies impair phagocytosis of immune complexes so that these are deposited in excessive amounts in tissues (Figure 34-2).

One consistent feature of lupus is the development of autoantibodies against antigens located within the cell nucleus. These antinuclear antibodies (ANAs) are found in 97% to 100% of dogs with lupus as compared with 16% to 20% of normal control animals. About 16 different nuclear antigens have been described in humans. Dogs differ from humans in that they develop

400

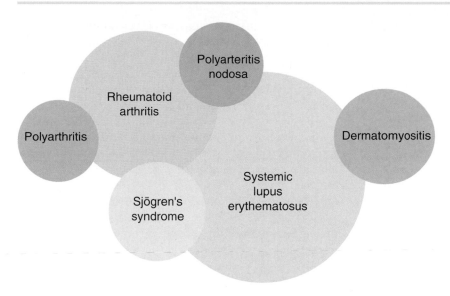

Figure 34-1. The interrelationships among the diseases discussed in this chapter. The diagram is somewhat simplified, since polyarthritis may be associated with polymyositis.

autoantibodies not against native, double-stranded DNA, but against nuclear proteins such as histones and ribonucleoproteins. Antinuclear antibodies can cause tissue damage by several mechanisms. They can combine with free antigens to form immune-complexes that are deposited in glomeruli causing a membranous glomerulonephropathy (Chapter 28). They may be deposited in arteriolar walls, where they cause fibrinoid necrosis and

fibrosis, or in synovia, where they provoke arthritis. Antinuclear antibodies also bind to the nuclei of degenerating cells to produce round or oval structures called hematoxylin bodies in the skin, kidney, lung, lymph nodes, spleen, and heart. Within the bone marrow, opsonized nuclei may be phagocytosed, giving rise to lupus erythematosus (LE) cells (Figure 34-3).

Lupus patients apparently make antibodies to nucleic acids because of a defect in the mechanisms by which apoptotic cells are removed. Bacterial DNA is a potent antigen and immune stimulant. Since mammalian DNA and bacterial DNA have a conserved backbone structure, it is possible that patients with lupus may respond to bacterial infection by producing cross-reactive antibodies that react with mammalian DNA. For example, the NZB/NZW mouse strain spontaneously develops a lupus-like syndrome when immunized with bacterial DNA by producing cross-reactive antibodies to mammalian dsDNA. These anti-DNA antibodies may form immune complexes and cause arthritis, skin rashes, and

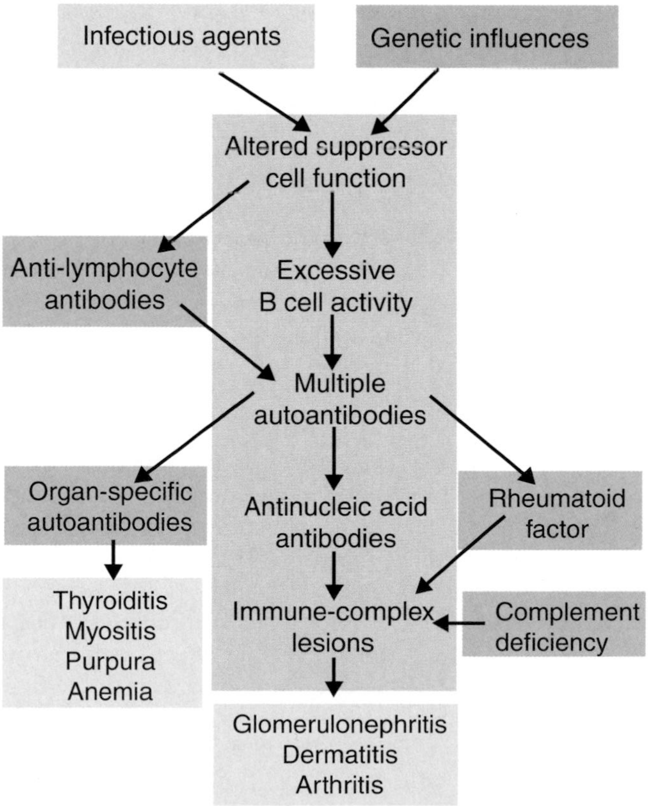

Figure 34-2. A diagram showing a possible pathogenesis of systemic lupus erythematosus.

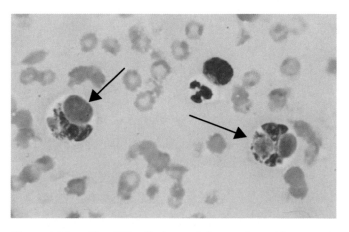

Figure 34-3. Two LE cells (*arrows*) from a dog with systemic lupus erythematosus (×1300).

vascular disease. Antibody-DNA immune complexes may bind to TLR9 and activate autoreactive B cells by triggering both the TLR and antigen-receptors.

Although ANAs are characteristic of lupus, many other autoantibodies are produced, suggesting that affected animals may also have abnormal B cells. Affected animals show abnormalities in B cell signaling and migration, overexpression of CD154 (CD40L), and enhanced production of IL-6 and IL-10. Some experimental mouse models show overexpression of B cell stimulatory molecules by T cells and dendritic cells. It is therefore possible that the production of multiple autoantibodies in lupus is a combined result of defective apoptosis, overstimulation of B cells, and a failure to eliminate self-reactive B cells.

Autoantibodies to red cells induce a hemolytic anemia. Antibodies to platelets induce a thrombocytopenia. Antilymphocyte antibodies may interfere with immune regulation. About 20% of dogs with lupus produce antibodies to IgG (rheumatoid factors). Antimuscle antibodies may cause myositis, and antimyocardial antibodies may provoke myocarditis or endocarditis. Antibodies to skin basement membrane cause a dermatitis characterized by changes in the thickness of the epidermis, focal mononuclear cell infiltration, collagen degeneration, and immunoglobulin deposits at the dermo-epidermal junction. These deposits form a "lupus band," seen in many other autoimmune skin diseases in addition to lupus (Figure 34-4). In humans especially, lupus skin lesions are commonly restricted to the bridge of the nose and the area around the eyes since apoptosis is exacerbated by UV radiation in sunlight. The results of this excessive immune reactivity are also reflected in a polyclonal gammopathy, enlargement of lymph nodes and spleen, and thymic enlargement with germinal center formation.

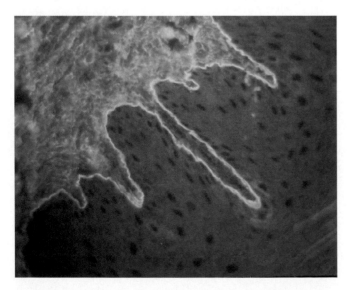

Figure 34-4. A lupus band in a section of monkey esophagus. The indirect immunofluorescence assay shows IgG deposition on the skin basement membrane. (Courtesy of Dr. F Heck.)

The great variety of autoantibodies produced in lupus can cause an equally great variety of clinical symptoms. Polyarthritis, fever, proteinuria, anemia, and skin diseases are the most common abnormalities but pericarditis, myocarditis, myositis, lymphadenopathy, and pneumonia have also been reported.

Although lupus likely involves a failure of apoptosis, leading to activation of autoimmune B cells and multiple autoimmune disorders, its initiating cause remains obscure. There is good evidence for a genetic predisposition in humans, dogs, and mice. It is also associated with an inherited deficiency of certain complement components and certain Fcγ receptors. Hormones clearly influence the development of the disease as shown by the fact that women develop lupus about 8 times as often as men and because it is much more severe during pregnancy. Estrogens affect apoptosis through fas, fas-L, IFN-γ and nitric oxide and interfere with B cell tolerance. Virus infections may initiate the syndrome. Thus individuals with lupus commonly have high levels of antibodies to parainfluenza 1 and measles. Myxovirus-like structures have been seen in renal endothelial cells from lupus patients, and type C retroviruses have been isolated from patients and associated with the disease.

As described in Chapter 15, some lupus patients have a deficiency of the complement receptor CD35. As a result, immune-complexes are not bound to red cells or platelets and therefore are not effectively removed from the circulation. These immune-complexes may then be deposited in the glomeruli or in joints. Lupus is also associated with defects in apoptosis. Thus the mouse *lpr* mutation in CD95 (fas) leads not only to a failure of apoptosis but specifically, a failure of negative selection within the thymus (Chapter 17). In addition, the failure of apoptosis and of the removal of dying cells may result in the body being flooded with nucleic acid fragments that may trigger antinuclear antibody formation.

Equine lupus. Equine lupus presents as a generalized skin disease (alopecia, dermal ulceration, and crusting), accompanied by an antiglobulin-positive anemia. The disease is remarkable insofar as affected horses may be almost totally hairless (Figure 34-5). Affected horses are ANA-positive, although LE cell tests are equivocal in this species. Skin biopsies show basement membrane degeneration and immunoglobulin deposition typical of lupus. Affected horses may also have glomerulonephritis, synovitis, and lymphadenopathy. Treatment of reported cases has been unsuccessful.

Canine lupus. Lupus affects middle-aged dogs (between 2 and 12 years of age) and affects males more than females. The disease is commonly seen in collies, German shepherds, and Shetland sheepdogs, but beagles, Irish setters, poodles and Afghan hounds are also affected. Lupus (or positive lupus serology) may occur in related animals, supporting the importance of genetic factors. For example, dogs possessing the MHC class I antigen DLA-A7 are at increased risk and those possessing -A1

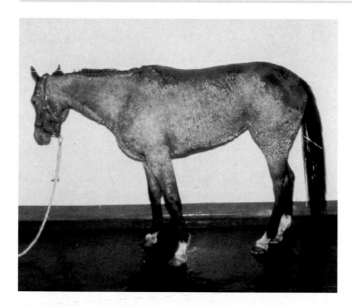

Figure 34-5. A filly with systemic lupus erythematosus. Note the generalized alopecia and crusting. (From Geor RJ, Clark EG, Haines DM, Napier PG: *J Am Vet Med Assoc* 197:1489, 1990.)

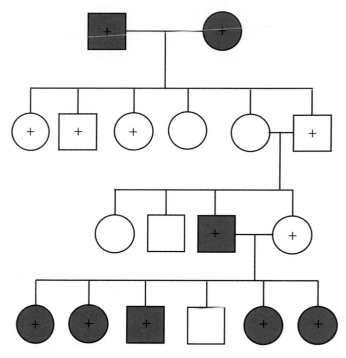

Figure 34-6. The inheritance of canine systemic lupus erythematosus. This diagram shows four generations of a single family of dogs. Colored squares or circles denote those animals exhibiting clinical signs of systemic lupus; a "+" denotes animals positive for antinuclear antibodies. (From Teichner M, Krumbacher K, Doxiadis I, et al: *Clin Immunol Immunopathol* 55:225, 1990.)

and -B5 are at decreased risk for developing disease (Figure 34-6) When dogs affected by lupus are bred, the number of affected offspring is higher than can be accounted for genetically, suggesting that the disease may be vertically transmitted. Cell-free filtrates from asymptomatic but LE cell–positive dogs, when administered to newborn mice, have been reported to provoke the appearance of ANA and the development of some lymphoid tumors. Type C retroviruses have been isolated from these tumors, and antisera to these viruses may be used to demonstrate viral antigens on the lymphocytes and in the glomeruli of humans with lupus. Cell-free filtrates of these mouse tumors have also been reported to induce the formation of ANA and the production of LE cells in newborn puppies.

Dogs may present with one or more signs of disease. However, the disease is progressive so that the severity of the lesions and the number of organ systems involved gradually increases in untreated cases. The most characteristic presentation is a fever accompanied by a symmetrical, nonerosive polyarthritis. Indeed, as many as 90% of dogs with lupus may develop arthritis at some stage. Other common presenting signs include renal failure (65%), skin disease (60%), lymphadenopathy and/or splenomegaly (50%), leukopenia (20%), hemolytic anemia (13%), and thrombocytopenia (4%). Dogs may also show myositis (8%) or pericarditis (8%) and neurological abnormalities (1.6%). The leukopenia involves a major loss of CD8+ T cells with a somewhat smaller loss of CD4+ T cells so that the CD4/CD8 ratio may climb as high as 6, compared with a normal value of about 1.7. The skin lesions are highly variable but are commonly localized in areas exposed to sunlight. With this great

variety of clinical presentations to choose from, it is not surprising that lupus is so difficult to diagnose.

Bullous systemic lupus is a very rare variant characterized by lupus plus vesicular erosive and ulcerative skin lesions, subepidermal vesicles, and circulating antibodies against type VII collagen. It may be treated with prednisolone and dapsone.

Feline lupus. Lupus is uncommon in cats, in which it usually presents as an antiglobulin-positive anemia. Other clinical manifestations include fever, skin disease, thrombocytopenia, polyarthritis, and renal failure. The ANA test must be interpreted with care in cats since many normal cats are ANA-positive.

Diagnosis

A simple diagnostic rule for lupus could be stated as follows: Suspect lupus in an animal with multiple disorders such as those described above and either a positive test for ANA or a positive test for LE cells (Table 34-1).

Antinuclear antibodies are normally demonstrated by immunofluorescence. Cultured cells or frozen sections of mouse or rat liver on a microscope slide are used as a source of antigen. Dilutions of a patient's serum are applied to this, and the material is incubated and then washed off. The binding of ANA to the cell nuclei is

TABLE 34-1
Diagnostic Criteria for Systemic Lupus Erythematosus

Any two of the following must be present:
Characteristic skin lesions
Polyarthritis
Antiglobulin-positive hemolytic anemia
Thrombocytopenia
Proteinuria
And either
A positive ANA test
Or
A positive LE cell test

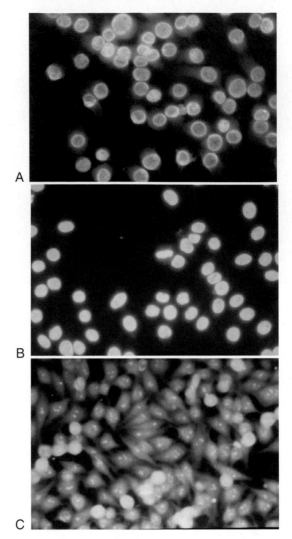

Figure 34-7. Three positive ANA reactions. These are indirect fluorescent antibody reactions, in which dog serum under test is layered onto a cell culture. After washing, the bound antibody is detected using a fluorescent antiglobulin. Although "rim" fluorescence **(A)** has traditionally been considered a positive reaction, the staining pattern obtained appears to depend in large part on the way the cells are fixed. These can therefore show diffuse staining **(B)** or nucleolar fluorescence **(C)**. (Courtesy of Dr. FC Heck.)

revealed by incubating the tissue in a fluorescein-labeled antiserum to canine or feline immunoglobulins and then rewashing. A variety of different nuclear staining patterns have been described for humans, and their clinical correlations have been analyzed. In animals, staining patterns have been less thoroughly investigated, and their significance is currently unclear. Some investigators believe that the staining pattern depends greatly on the way the cells are first fixed. Evidence suggests, however, that a homogeneous staining pattern or staining of the nuclear rim is of greatest diagnostic significance but that nucleolar fluorescence is not (Figure 34-7). Dogs whose serum shows a speckled fluorescence pattern tend to have autoimmune diseases other than lupus. Some normal dogs, dogs undergoing treatment with certain drugs (griseofulvin, penicillin, sulfonamides, tetracyclines, phenytoin, procainamide), and some dogs with liver disease or lymphosarcoma may have detectable ANAs. Thus nonspecific ANAs may be a result of many different neoplastic, inflammatory, and autoimmune diseases. Consequently, this test must not be used as the only diagnostic test for lupus. Administration of propylthiouracil to cats with hyperthyroidism may result in the development of a syndrome resembling lupus. This may include the development of an antiglobulin-positive anemia, as well as positive ANA reactions.

LE cells, as previously mentioned, are neutrophils (PMNs) that have phagocytosed nuclei from dead and dying cells (see Figure 34-3). Their presence may be detected in the bone marrow and occasionally in buffy coat preparations from animals with lupus. It is usually necessary, however, to produce them in vitro. This can be accomplished by allowing the blood of an affected animal to clot and then incubating it at 37° C for 2 hours. During this time, normal PMNs will phagocytose the nuclei of any dying or damaged cells. Pressing it through a fine mesh then disrupts the clot, the resulting cell suspension is centrifuged, and the buffy coat is smeared, stained, and examined. LE cells are not a reliable diagnostic feature of systemic lupus in domestic animals since

there is a high incidence of both false-positive and false-negative results.

Treatment

Lupus in animals usually responds well to high doses of corticosteroids (prednisolone or prednisone) accompanied, if necessary, by cyclophosphamide, azathioprine, or chlorambucil. Levamisole (Chapter 37) has also been used with success. However, more drastic measures, such as plasmapheresis, may be needed in refractory cases.

DISCOID LUPUS ERYTHEMATOSUS

Discoid lupus erythematosus is a mild, uncommon variant of SLE characterized by the occurrence of facial skin lesions alone. There are no other pathological lesions, and ANA and LE tests are negative. It occurs in dogs, cats, horses, and humans. Discoid lupus has been described in collies and collie crosses, German shepherds, Siberian huskies, and Shetland sheepdogs. They commonly present with nasal dermatitis with depigmentation, erythema, erosion, ulceration, scaling, and crusting. Occasionally the feet may be affected, and some dogs may have oral ulcers. C3, IgA, IgG, or IgM may be detected in the skin basement membrane in a typical lupus band. The skin lesions may be infiltrated with mononuclear and plasma cells. It is treated with corticosteroids, and the prognosis is good. Since the lesions are exacerbated by sunlight, it is appropriate to use sunscreens and encourage the owner to keep the animal out of intense sunlight.

Discoid lupus in cats is characterized by a nonpruritic scaling and crusting dermatitis almost totally confined to the pinnae of the ear. There may be some ulceration and papule or pustule formation. Skin biopsy shows mononuclear infiltration of the basal cell layer with degeneration of basal cells. Direct immunofluorescence of skin sections shows a lupus band. Affected cats have negative or low ANA titers and negative LE cell tests. Treatment with corticosteroids is effective.

SJÖGREN'S SYNDROME

The triad of keratoconjunctivitis sicca, xerostomia, and rheumatoid factor (RF) constitute an autoimmune syndrome called Sjögren's syndrome. In this syndrome, autoimmune attack on salivary and lacrimal glands leads to conjunctival dryness (keratoconjunctivitis sicca) and mouth dryness (xerostomia). Affected animals subsequently develop gingivitis, dental caries, and excessive thirst. Sjögren's syndrome is often associated with rheumatoid arthritis, systemic lupus, polymyositis, and autoimmune thyroiditis. The first two cases described in dogs were found in a colony maintained for investigations into canine lupus. Affected dogs develop antibodies to nictitating membrane epithelial cells and, less consistently, to lacrimal and salivary glands or to the pancreas, and these organs may be extensively infiltrated with lymphocytes and other mononuclear cells. Most affected animals (90%) are hypergammaglobulinemic and have ANAs (40%) and RFs (34%). Many have other autoimmune diseases such as polyarthritis, hypothyroidism, or glomerulonephritis.

Keratoconjunctivitis Sicca

In keratoconjunctivitis sicca, one of the most common ophthalmic diseases of dogs, lacrimal gland secretion is greatly reduced and animals experience corneal dryness. The resulting abrasion leads to inflammation of the cornea and conjunctiva. There is a mucoid or mucopurulent ocular discharge, as well as blepharitis, conjunctivitis, and secondary bacterial infections. Corneal ulceration may occur; this can progress to perforation if untreated.

The disease is diagnosed by use of the Schirmer tear test. A 5 × 30 mm strip of filter paper is placed in the medioventral cul-de-sac for 1 minute. Normal dog tears wet between 14 and 24 mm of paper/minute, but in keratoconjunctivitis sicca cases the tears usually wet less than 10 mm and many wet less than 5 mm. The breeds at highest relative risk include English bulldogs, West Highland white terriers, Lhasa apsos, pugs, cocker spaniels, and Pekinese. The disease may be treated by use of artificial tears. It is also logical to use immunosuppressive agents in refractory cases. For example, cyclosporine ophthalmic drops appear to be effective, although it takes 2 to 3 weeks before improved lacrimation is seen.

Keratoconjunctivitis sicca has been reported in a horse. The 3-year-old animal presented with bilateral ulcerative keratoconjunctivitis sicca and improved clinically with ophthalmic cyclosporine therapy. Histological examination of the lacrimal glands showed an eosinophil infiltration with lesser numbers of lymphocytes, plasma cells, and macrophages. Although this suggests an immunological origin for the disease, it must be pointed out that nonimmunological mechanisms such as facial nerve damage can also result in corneal dryness.

Chronic Superficial Keratitis

Chronic superficial keratitis is a common ocular disease of dogs in which blood vessels, lymphocytes, plasma cells, and melanocytes invade the superficial corneal stroma. Immunoglobulin deposits may be present. Eventually the pigmented granulation tissue causes corneal opacity. The disease is believed to be immune-mediated, although its cause is unknown. It is more prevalent in dogs living at high altitudes, where UV exposure is great.

AUTOIMMUNE POLYARTHRITIS

Animals can develop immunologically mediated joint diseases. Most are associated with the deposition of immunoglobulins or immune-complexes within joints. They may be classified into two groups based on the presence or absence of joint erosion.

Erosive Polyarthritis

Rheumatoid Arthritis

The most important immune-mediated erosive polyarthritis in humans is rheumatoid arthritis. Rheumatoid arthritis is a common, crippling disease affecting about 1% of the human population. A very similar disease is seen in domestic animals, especially dogs, in which there is no obvious breed or sex predilection. Dogs with rheumatoid arthritis may present with chronic depression, anorexia, and pyrexia in addition to lameness, which tends to be most severe after rest (for example, immediately after waking in the morning). The disease mainly affects peripheral joints, which show symmetrical swelling and stiffness. Rheumatoid arthritis tends to be progressive and eventually leads to severe joint erosion and deformities. In advanced cases affected joints may fuse as a result of the formation of bony ankyloses. Radiological findings are variable, but the swelling usually involves soft tissues only, and there may be subchondral rarefaction, cartilage erosion and narrowing of the joint space.

Pathogenesis. Rheumatoid arthritis is a chronic inflammatory disease. It commences as a synovitis with lymphocytes in the synovia and neutrophils in the joint fluid. As the inflammation continues, the synovia swell and proliferate. Outgrowths of the proliferating synovia eventually extend into the joint cavities, where they are called pannus. Pannus consists of fibrous vascular tissue that, as it invades the joint cavity, releases proteases that erode the articular cartilage and, ultimately, the neighboring bony structures. As the arthritis progresses, the infiltrating lymphocytes can form lymphoid nodules and germinal centers within the synovia. Amyloidosis, arteritis, glomerulonephritis, and lymphatic hyperplasia are occasional complications of rheumatoid arthritis (Figure 34-8).

It is probable that many different stimuli, especially infectious agents, trigger the disease in susceptible animals. Infectious agents implicated in the human disease include Epstein-Barr virus (a herpesvirus), parvoviruses, and mycobacteria. Lyme disease arthritis has many similarities to rheumatoid arthritis. In domestic mammals, *Mycoplasma hyorhinis*, *Erysipelothrix rhusiopathiae*, and *Borrelia burgdorferi* produce a chronic arthritis that resembles rheumatoid arthritis. Dogs with rheumatoid arthritis have antibodies to canine distemper in their synovial fluids, antibodies that are not present in dogs

with osteoarthritis. Immune-complexes can be precipitated out of the synovial fluid of dogs with rheumatoid arthritis, and analysis of these complexes by Western blotting showed the presence of canine distemper virus antigens. Thus canine distemper virus may be present in canine rheumatoid joints and may play a role in the pathogenesis of the disease.

Rheumatoid arthritis is also a genetic disorder. Susceptibility and severity of rheumatoid arthritis in humans are mainly associated with possession of certain MHC class II molecules (HLA-DR). This susceptibility is associated with the presence of a conserved amino acid sequence located in the HLA-DRB1 antigen-binding groove and known as the "RA shared epitope." Presumably these molecules can bind and present self-peptides. It is interesting to note that this same conserved RA shared epitope is found on canine DLA-DRB1 and is also associated with susceptibility to RA in some dog breeds. Some MHC class III genes also affect susceptibility to canine RA. For example, there is an association between possession of the C4 allotype C4-4, low serum C4 levels, and the development of autoimmune polyarthritis. Despite these examples, it has been estimated that non-MHC genes contribute as much as 75% of the genetic susceptibility to rheumatoid arthritis.

Although rheumatoid arthritis is generally regarded as an autoimmune disease, the identity of the autoantigens involved is unclear. Three major autoantigens that have been implicated are IgG, collagen, and glycosaminoglycans (Figure 34-9). The development of autoantibodies to IgG is characteristic of rheumatoid arthritis. These autoantibodies, called rheumatoid factors, are directed against epitopes on the C_H2 domains of antigen-bound IgG. They can belong to any immunoglobulin class, including IgE, although IgG RFs are by far the most common. The IgG in rheumatoid arthritis patients is less glycosylated than normal IgG, and it may be that this abnormal IgG can act as an immunogen in a susceptible animal. RFs are found not only in rheumatoid arthritis but also in lupus and other diseases in which extensive

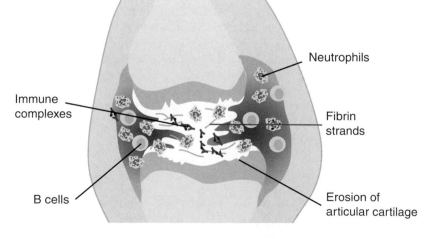

Figure 34-8. A schematic diagram showing how joints are damaged in rheumatoid arthritis.

Neutrophils

Immune complexes

Fibrin strands

B cells

Erosion of articular cartilage

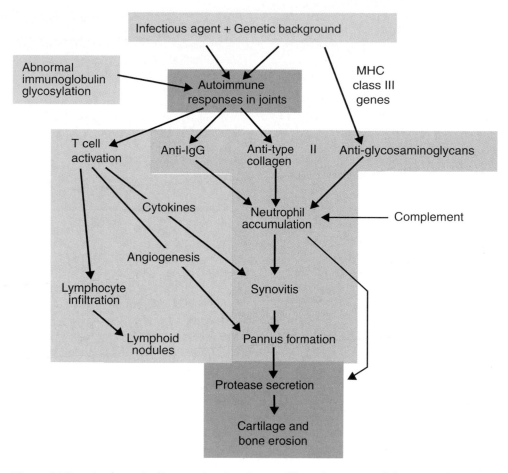

Figure 34-9. A schematic diagram showing the possible pathogenesis of rheumatoid arthritis.

immune-complex formation occurs. RFs are also found in the serum and synovial fluid of some dogs with osteoarthritis (including cruciate disease) or infective arthritis.

RFs can be detected by allowing them to agglutinate antibody-coated particles. In humans, latex beads coated with IgG are used for this purpose. In dogs, it is easier to make a canine antisheep erythrocyte serum and coat sheep erythrocytes with this in a subagglutinating dose. After washing, these erythrocytes agglutinate when mixed with RF-positive dog serum.

Although RFs are of diagnostic importance, their clinical significance is unclear. RFs are found in joint fluid, where their titer tends to correlate with the severity of the lesions, and the lesions themselves may be exacerbated by intra-articular inoculation of autologous immunoglobulins. Nevertheless, some individuals with rheumatoid arthritis may not have detectable RFs, and it is not uncommon to find others who have no arthritis despite the presence of RF in their serum. Thus the measurement of RF in dogs is of doubtful specificity.

Other evidence suggests that autoantibodies to collagen may be important. Type II collagen is the predominant form of collagen in articular cartilage and so may serve as an autoantigen. Autoantibodies to type II collagen can be detected in the serum and synovial fluid of dogs with rheumatoid arthritis, infective arthritis, and osteoarthritis. Autoantibodies to both type I and type II collagen are found in synovial fluid following cruciate ligament rupture (secondary to osteoarthritis). These antibodies are largely bound in immune-complexes. Although collagen-anticollagen complexes may contribute to the pathology of these diseases, they are very unlikely to be of major significance and probably represent a secondary response to local tissue damage. Affected humans develop a cell-mediated response to denatured collagens II and III, and horses with chronic, nonsuppurative arthritis, osteoarthritis, or traumatic arthritis develop antibodies to horse collagens I and II. These antibodies, as well as immune-complexes, can therefore be found in the synovial fluid of horses with many different joint diseases. An experimental autoimmune disease that closely resembles rheumatoid arthritis develops in rats immunized with type II collagen.

Evidence from experimental mice and some humans suggests that T cells directed against such glycosaminoglycans as hyaluronic acid, heparin, and chondroitin sulfates may induce an arthritis resembling rheumatoid arthritis.

Whatever the precise initiating factors, the first stage in the development of rheumatoid arthritis involves activation of macrophages within the synovial membrane. As inflammation develops within the synovia, many macrophage cytokines are produced. These include IL-1, IL-6, GM-CSF and TNF-α. There are much lower levels of the T cell–derived cytokines IFN-γ and IL-2. In addition, inflammatory chemokines such as CCL2 (MCP-1), CCL3 (MIP-1α) and CXCL8 (IL-8) accumulate. The presence of these chemokines, as well as C5a, leukotriene B$_4$, and platelet-activating factor results in the accumulation of large numbers of neutrophils within the synovial fluid. Activation by phagocytosis of immune-complexes and tissue debris leads to protease escape and the release of oxidants. IL-1 and TNF-α stimulate cartilage degradation by activating chondrocytes and stimulating the release of metalloproteases. Thus metalloproteases-2 and -9 from chondrocytes and macrophages are raised in canine RA joint fluid. This, together with activation of kinins and plasmin, leads to intense inflammation. The metalloproteases degrade the articular cartilage and ligaments, leading to the characteristic joint pathology.

Macrophage cytokines also trigger formation of new blood vessels within synovia. Circulating lymphocytes home to these newly formed capillaries, emigrate into the tissues, and aggregate around the blood vessels. These infiltrating lymphocytes are primarily activated CD4$^+$ T cells. B cell emigration into the tissues eventually leads to local RF production. The RFs form large immune-complexes and activate the complement system. Some of the immune-complexes may precipitate out within the superficial layers of the articular cartilage.

The progressive development of inflammation within the joint leads first to morning stiffness. The joints become warm as the blood flow increases, but because the inflammation is restricted to the synovia, the skin rarely becomes red. The animal may show depression and fatigue as a result of the systemic effects of IL-1 and TNF-α. If the joints develop effusions, they will be obviously swollen. As the disease progresses, the grossly inflamed synovia invades the cartilage, ligaments, and bone and results in the destruction of articular cartilage. Synovial lining cells, small blood vessels and fibroblasts proliferate. Large numbers of macrophages are found in the pannus, as well as MHC class II–positive nonphagocytic cells—probably B cells and dendritic cells.

Diagnosis. Diagnosis of rheumatoid arthritis in animals is generally based on the criteria established for human rheumatoid arthritis. At least five of the major clinical features should be present, and any one of the first five shown in Table 34-2 should have been present for at least 6 weeks. In addition, steps should be taken to exclude systemic lupus (by testing for ANA) and to exclude an infectious cause for the arthritis.

Treatment. Treatment of canine rheumatoid arthritis with drugs tends to be unsatisfactory, and the long-term

---

TABLE **34-2**
Diagnostic Criteria for Canine Rheumatoid Arthritis

Any four of the following signs must be present:
Morning stiffness lasting at least 1 hour for at least 6 weeks
Arthritis affecting three joints or joint swelling or exudation lasting at least 6 weeks
Arthritis affecting the hand joints for longer than 6 weeks
Symmetrical arthritis lasting at least 6 weeks
Rheumatoid nodules
Presence of serum rheumatoid factor measured by a reliable test
Characteristic radiographic changes in the wrists or hands

---

prognosis of the disease is poor. Nonsteroidal antiinflammatory drugs, such as aspirin, carprofen, or etodolac, have been the first choice in treating early, uncomplicated cases of rheumatoid arthritis, although their efficacy is unclear. Corticosteroids such as prednisolone should be reserved for late, severe cases in which salicylates have proved inadequate. Local steroid injections into affected joints will produce rapid relief and clinical remission. However, the joints are still subjected to stress, disease progression is not slowed, and the corticosteroids delay healing and promote articular degeneration. Their use may therefore permit articular damage to proceed unabated. Recently, good success has been achieved in humans by the aggressive use of the immunosuppressive agent, methotrexate. Monoclonal antibodies to TNF-α (infliximab), to CD4, to thymocytes, or to IL-2R have also had significant success in preventing bone erosions in humans as has administration of recombinant TNF-α receptors (etanercept). The immunosuppressive drug, leflunomide, appears to be as effective as methotrexate. Slow-acting immunosuppressive agents, such as sodium aurothiomalate and aurothioglucose, and anti-malarials, such as chloroquine, are also used in humans, but they are expensive, results have been erratic, and experience with these in animals is limited. Surgical procedures may improve joint stability and reduce pain.

Nonerosive Polyarthritis

The second major group of immune-mediated arthritides are those in which the joint cartilage is not eroded and the inflammatory lesion is largely confined to the joint capsule and synovia. Many of these clinically resemble rheumatoid arthritis but may be differentiated by their nonerosive character.

Equine Polyarthritis

Polyarthritis has been reported in the horse in association with a lupus-like syndrome. In these cases affected foals (up to 3 months of age) present with multiple swollen joints involving all four limbs and a persistent fever. In some cases other synovial sheaths, including tendon sheaths and bursae, are affected. The synovial effusions are sterile, but synovial biopsies show lymphocyte and plasma cell infiltration with some immunoglobulin deposits. The cells in the joint fluid are mainly neutrophils. These animals are negative for RF, ANA, and LE cells. Many of these animals have a lesion within the thorax, especially pneumonia, due to *Rhodococcus equi*. It is possible that immune-complexes originating in the lungs may lodge in the synovia to trigger the synovitis.

Canine Polyarthritis

Dogs may develop several distinct nonerosive polyarthritides, which can be divided into at least three major categories: arthritis associated with systemic lupus, arthritis associated with a myositis, and an idiopathic polyarthritis. Breeds that are predisposed to polyarthritis include German shepherds, Irish setters, Shetland sheepdogs, cocker spaniels, and Springer spaniels. The main clinical features of polyarthritis are stiffness, pyrexia, anorexia, and lethargy.

Lupus polyarthritis. Polyarthritis is a common feature of systemic lupus. Diagnosis is contingent on making a firm diagnosis of lupus. Thus it is necessary to show multiple system involvement, a significant titer of serum ANAs, and immunopathological features consistent with lupus.

Polyarthritis with polymyositis. A disease characterized by both nonerosive polyarthritis and polymyositis is recognized in young dogs. Most recorded cases have been seen in spaniels. The animals are stiff and have painful joints, fever, lethargy, weakness, muscle atrophy, and muscle pain. They are negative for ANA, thus excluding a diagnosis of systemic lupus, and negative for RF. The arthritis is nonerosive and symmetrical, involving multiple joints. The animals have a symmetrical inflammatory myopathy with myalgia, atrophy, and muscle contracture. The synovial fluid shows high white cell counts, especially neutrophils. Muscle biopsies show a neutrophil or mononuclear cell infiltrate, or both, with muscle fiber atrophy and degeneration. Synovial biopsies show a neutrophil and mononuclear cell infiltration with a fibrinous exudate. IgG, IgM, and complement are deposited in the walls of the synovial vessels. Treatment is with corticosteroids and immunosuppressive agents such as cyclophosphamide.

Idiopathic polyarthritis. Most cases of canine polyarthritis fit none of the categories described above. Although these cases are nonerosive and possess the characteristics of type III hypersensitivity, their precise etiology is unknown. Four types of idiopathic polyarthritis have been identified according to their disease associations (Table 34-3): type I is uncomplicated; type II cases are characterized by an infection elsewhere in the body; type III cases are associated with gastrointestinal disease; and type IV cases are associated with the presence of a tumor elsewhere in the body.

TABLE 34-3
Classification of Nonerosive Polyarthritis in Dogs

Type	Disease Associations
I	Uncomplicated polyarthritis without other disease associations
II	Polyarthritis associated with infectious lesions remote from the joints (e.g., respiratory or urinary infections)
III	Polyarthritis associated with gastrointestinal disease
IV	Polyarthritis associated with neoplastic disease remote from the joints

From Bennett DJ: *Small Anim Pract* 28:909-928, 1987.

An example of type I polyarthritis is the juvenile-onset polyarthritis syndrome seen in Akitas between the ages of 9 weeks and 8 months. These dogs have a cyclical high fever lasting 24 to 48 hours before resolving and evidence of severe, incapacitating joint pain with soft tissue swelling. Radiology shows hepatosplenomegaly and lymphadenopathy. Some animals may have meningitis or meningoencephalitis. Their erythrocytes may be antiglobulin-positive. Synovial fluid shows no evidence of infection, although large numbers of neutrophils are present. The dogs are usually negative for RF and ANA. Pedigree analysis suggests that the disease is inherited. Some dogs respond positively to corticosteroid treatment. In refractory cases azathioprine may also be required.

Type II disease is a reactive arthritis associated with infections in the respiratory or urinary tract, tooth infections, or cellulitis. This association between arthritis and respiratory disease is also seen in foals, as described above. Type III disease is associated with the presence of gastroenteritis, diarrhea, or ulcerative colitis. It is not clear whether this type of disease is truly distinguishable from type II disease. Type IV disease is associated with the presence of tumors, including seminomas, and carcinomas of several types.

Idiopathic polyarthritis tends to be most common in male dogs, and about half of the cases are seen in young dogs between 1 and 3.5 years. Most of the animals show systemic signs such as fever, anorexia, and lethargy. The animals are lame and have a history of stiffness after rest. The most commonly affected joints include the stifle, elbow, and carpus. The onset of lameness is sudden in most cases and is associated with obvious muscle atrophy. There is no significant joint erosion although periarticular soft tissue swelling and synovial effusion are common. Some cases may have proliferative periosteal changes. All cases are negative for RF and ANA. The joint fluid is sterile. Synovial biopsies show hypertrophy with a neutrophil and/or a mononuclear cell infiltration. Fibrin deposits are seen in most cases, as is fibrosis. Most lesions contain IgM, IgG, and complement deposits and some contain IgA-producing plasma cells. Some affected dogs may show evidence of glomerulonephritis.

Treatment is with corticosteroids. The prognosis for idiopathic polyarthropathy is generally better than that for the other forms of immune-mediated arthritis.

Feline Polyarthritis

Chronic progressive polyarthritis of male cats is characterized by polyarthritis with either osteopenia or periosteal new bone formation. Periarticular erosions and eventual collapse or subchondral erosions, joint instabilities and deformities closely resembling those of rheumatoid arthritis are also seen. Affected cats are commonly infected with feline syncytia-forming virus (FSV) or feline leukemia virus (FeLV), or both. (The incidence of FSV in these cats is two to four times higher, and the incidence of FeLV is six to ten times higher than in normal cats.) It is described here because of suggestions that it is of immunological origin. These suggestions are based on the massive lymphocyte and plasma cell infiltration of affected joints and the presence of an immune-complex type of glomerulonephritis. However, affected cats are RF- and ANA-negative, and their serum immunoglobulin levels tend to be close to normal. Corticosteroids lessen the severity of clinical signs. Combination therapy with corticosteroids and azathioprine or cyclophosphamide can induce temporary remissions.

DERMATOMYOSITIS

A familial disease of dogs that resembles dermatomyositis in humans has been described in collies and Shetland sheepdogs. It is a clinical syndrome of dermatitis with a less obvious myositis. Puppies appear normal at birth, but skin lesions develop between 7 and 11 weeks of age and myositis develops between 12 and 23 weeks. In other studies, the dermatitis developed at 3 to 6 months of age, and myositis was detected after the dermatitis was diagnosed. The onset and progression of the disease are correlated with a rise in circulating immune-complexes and serum IgG, but the reason for these increases is unclear. Circulating immune-complexes and IgG levels return to normal as the disease resolves, suggesting a causative association. Many dogs outgrow the disease and are left with moderate hyperpigmentation, some hypopigmentation and alopecia, and some atrophy of the muscles of mastication. Other dogs develop a progressive disease with severe dermatitis and myositis. Dogs with progressive disease may also develop signs of immunosuppression especially pyoderma and septicemia, as well as demodicosis. If the muscles of the esophagus are affected, megaesophagus may develop and secondary aspiration pneumonia results. Generalized lymphoid hyperplasia may also develop in these dogs. On necropsy myositis may be seen in the esophagus and arteritis in the skin, muscle, and bladder. Crystalline virus-like structures have been seen in endothelial cells within muscle tissues.

The skin lesions first develop on the face; subsequently, lesions may spread to the limbs and trunk, especially over bony prominences. These early lesions are erythematous and eventually lead to vesicle and pustule formation. Once the vesicles rupture, they ulcerate and crust. Older lesions are found on the bridge of the nose and around the eyes and show hair loss and changes in pigmentation. There may be enlargement of the lymph nodes, draining the affected areas. The development of the skin lesions is cyclical so that the clinical course and severity are variable. The skin lesions usually resolve by 1 year of age. Muscle disease follows the onset of skin disease, but there is no correlation between the severity of the two lesions. The most common sign of myositis is masseter and temporal muscle atrophy. Some severely affected puppies may have difficulty eating as a result of the myositis. Consequently, they also grow poorly.

Skin histology shows a nonspecific inflammatory dermatitis. Muscle biopsy, especially of the temporal muscle, shows multifocal accumulations of lymphocytes, plasma cells, and macrophages, as well as a few neutrophils and eosinophils. The myofibers are atrophied and may show fragmentation and vacuolation (Figure 34-10). Hematology and serum biochemistry are usually normal. The disease is inherited as an autosomal dominant condition, although expression is highly variable. Symptomatic and corticosteroid treatment may be of benefit in severely affected cases.

IMMUNE VASCULITIS

Several forms of immune vasculitis have been described in domestic animals. Their precise relationships are unclear, and as a result, they have been given several

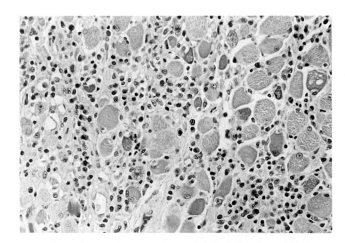

Figure 34-10.   A section of esophagus from a dog with dermatomyositis. Note the fragmented myofibers, as well as the infiltration by lymphocytes, plasma cells, and macrophages (H&E stain, ×200). (From Hargis AM, Prieur DJ, Haupt KH, et al: *Am J Pathol* 123:480-496, 1986.)

different names, including canine juvenile polyarteritis, polyarteritis nodosa, and leukocytoclastic vasculitis.

Canine juvenile polyarteritis primarily affects beagles less than 2 years of age. The animals show episodes of anorexia, persistent fever of greater than 40° C, and a hunched stance with lowered head and a stiff gait, indicating severe neck pain. The clinical signs may show cyclical remissions and relapses. The animals have a neutrophilia and elevated acute-phase proteins. These dogs have elevated serum IgM and IgA but normal IgG. The proportion of B cells in the blood is increased, but their T cells are decreased, as is their response to mitogens.

On necropsy there are few gross lesions. There may be some hemorrhage in lymph nodes. Histologically there is a systemic vasculitis and perivasculitis. In the acute disease there is necrotizing vasculitis with fibrinoid necrosis and a massive inflammatory cell infiltration involving the small and medium-sized arteries of the heart, mediastinum, and cervical spinal cord (Figure 34-11). Immunoglobulins are deposited in the walls of small- and medium-sized arteries. During remissions the vascular lesions consist of intimal and medial fibrosis and a mild perivasculitis, the residue of previous acute vasculitis. Chronically affected dogs may develop generalized amyloidosis. In many ways, this disease resembles Kawasaki disease of children, the leading cause of acquired heart disease in the United States.

Polyarteritis nodosa is seen in humans, pigs, dogs, and cats. It is characterized by a widespread, focal necrosis of the media of small- and medium-sized muscular arteries. The lesions are found in many organs, especially in the kidney. Vessels in the skin are rarely involved.

On occasion, focal vascular lesions characterized by neutrophil infiltration may develop in small blood vessels throughout the body, but especially in skin. Affected dogs have mucocutaneous ulcers, bullae, edema, polyarthropathy, myopathy, anorexia, intermittent fever, and lethargy. Although called hypersensitivity vasculitis, a foreign antigen can be found in only a small proportion of cases. For this reason, a better name for this condition may be leukocytoclastic vasculitis. The cause or causes of polyarteritis nodosa and hypersensitivity vasculitis are unknown. The histology of both diseases suggests that they are a form of type III hypersensitivity reaction, perhaps due to the presence of an infectious agent. Immunosuppression with corticosteroids, together with cyclophosphamide, has given good results in treating hypersensitivity vasculitis in dogs. Polyarteritis nodosa is usually detected as an incidental finding on necropsy, although ocular defects may present clinically if the arteries of the eye are involved.

SOURCES OF ADDITIONAL INFORMATION

Bell SC, Carter SD, Bennett D: Canine distemper viral antigens and antibodies in dogs with rheumatoid arthritis, *Res Vet Sci* 50:64-68, 1991.

Coughlan AR, Robertson DHL, Bennett D, et al: Matrix metalloproteinases 2 and 9 in canine rheumatoid arthritis, *Vet Rec* 143:219-223, 1998.

Dougherty SA, Center SA, Shaw EE, Erb HA: Juvenile-onset polyarthritis syndrome in Akitas, *J Am Vet Med Assoc* 198: 849-856, 1991.

Feldmann M: Development of anti-TNF therapy for rheumatoid arthritis, *Nature* 2:364-370, 2002.

Felsburg PJ, HogenEsch H, Somberg PW, et al: Immunologic abnormalities in canine juvenile polyarteritis syndrome: a naturally occurring animal model of Kawasaki disease, *Clin Immunol Immunopathol* 65:110-118, 1992.

Geor RJ, Clark EG, Haines DM, Napier PG: Systemic lupus erythematosus in a filly, *J Am Vet Med Assoc* 197:1498-1492, 1990.

Graninger W, Smolen J: Treatment of rheumatoid arthritis by TNF-blocking agents, *Int Arch Allergy Appl Immunol* 127: 10-14, 2002.

Halliwell REW, Werner LL, Baum DE, et al: Incidence and characterization of canine rheumatoid factor, *Vet Immunol Immunopathol* 21:161-176, 1989.

Harris ED: Rheumatoid arthritis: pathophysiology and implications for therapy, *N Engl J Med* 322:1277-1289, 1990.

Hermann M, Voll RE, Kalden JR: Etiopathogenesis of systemic lupus erythematosus, *Immunol Today* 21:424, 2000.

Kaswan RL, Salisbury MA: Canine keratoconjunctivitis sicca: etiology, clinical signs, diagnosis and treatment. Part II. Diagnosis and treatment with cyclosporine, *J Vet Allerg Clin Immunol* 2:8-12, 1993.

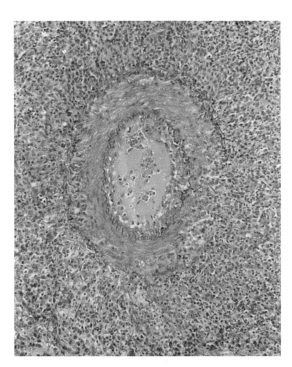

Figure 34-11. An extramural coronary artery from a beagle suffering from juvenile polyarteritis. This medium-sized muscular artery is characterized by medial necrosis, ruptured elastic laminae, and severe perivascular accumulations of neutrophils, lymphocytes, and macrophages. (H&E stain.) (From Snyder PW, Kazacos EA, Scott-Moncrieff JC, et al: *Vet Pathol* 32:337-345, 1995.)

Lipsky PE: Systemic lupus erythematosus: an autoimmune disease of B cell hyperactivity, *Nature Immunol* 2:764-766, 2001.

Marshall E: Lupus: Mysterious disease holds it secrets tight, *Science* 296:689-691, 2002.

May C, Hughes DE, Carter SD, Bennett D: Lymphocyte populations in the synovial membranes in dogs with rheumatoid arthritis, *Vet Immunol Immunopathol* 31:289-300, 1992.

Monestier M, Novick KE, Karam ET, et al: Autoantibodies to histone, DNA, and nucleosome antigens in canine systemic lupus erythematosus, *Clin Exp Immunol* 99:37-41, 1995.

Olivry T, Savary KCM, Murphy M, Dunston SM, et al: Bullous systemic lupus erythematosus (type I) in a dog, *Vet Rec* 145:165-169, 1999.

Osborne AC, Carter SD, May SA, Bennett D: Anti-collagen antibodies and immune complexes in equine joint diseases, *Vet Immunol Immunopathol* 45:19-30, 1995.

Teichner M, Krumbacher K, Doxiadis I, et al: Systemic lupus erythematosus in dogs: association to the major histocompatibility complex class I antigen DLA-A7, *Clin Immunol Immunopathol* 55:255-262, 1990.

Vinuesa CG, Goodnow CC: DNA drives autoimmunity, *Nature* 416:595-598, 2002.

Vyse TJ, Kotzin BL: Genetic susceptibility to systemic lupus erythematosus, *Annu Rev Immunol* 16:261-292, 1998.

Wang JY, Roehrl MH: Glycosaminoglycans are a potential cause of rheumatoid arthritis, *Proc Natl Acad Sci* 99: 14362-14367, 2002.

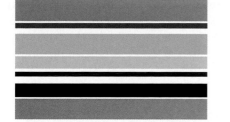

Primary Immunodeficiencies

CHAPTER 35

Any defect in either the innate or acquired immune systems usually becomes apparent when affected animals show unusual susceptibility to infectious or parasitic diseases. These diseases may be due to pathogenic organisms or, if the defect is very severe, opportunistic infections by organisms that are not normally able to cause disease. Deficiencies in the immune systems may be a result of inherited defects—primary immunodeficiencies, or alternatively, the deficiencies may be a direct result of some other cause—secondary or acquired immunodeficiencies. This chapter describes some of the primary immunodeficiencies recorded in domestic animals.

One feature of primary immunodeficiencies in domestic animals is breed susceptibility. Thus there may be significant differences in disease susceptibility among animal breeds, especially in those breeds with reduced genetic diversity. Examples of breed-associated immunodeficiencies include the increased risk for canine parvoviral enteritis in Doberman pinschers and Rottweilers. German shepherd dogs may have increased susceptibility to canine distemper. Mexican hairless dogs may have defective cell-mediated immune responses. It must also be recognized that the genetic composition of many breeds varies geographically, and problems with a specific breed in one country may not occur in others.

INHERITED DEFECTS IN INNATE IMMUNITY

Inherited deficiencies in innate immunity include defects in the various stages of phagocytosis, as well as the

413

complement deficiencies described previously (Chapter 15). Phagocytic defects are well recognized in domestic animals.

Chédiak-Higashi Syndrome

Chédiak-Higashi syndrome is an inherited disease of cattle, Aleutian mink, blue smoke Persian cats, white tigers, Hereford, Japanese black, and Brangus cattle, beige (*bg/bg*) mice, orcas, and humans. It is an autosomal recessive disease resulting from a mutation in a gene (*LYST*) that regulates lysosomal trafficking within cells. The *LYST* gene is found on bovine chromosome 28. It encodes a protein that controls membrane fusion. In Chédiak-Higashi cattle there is a missense A:T → G:C mutation that results in replacement of a histidine with an arginine residue. The defect produces abnormally large granules in neutrophils, monocytes, and eosinophils and enlarged melanin granules in pigment cells (Figure 35-1). The enlarged neutrophil granules result from the fusion of primary and secondary granules. In other cells the lysosomes are abnormal. The leukocyte granules of affected animals are more fragile than those of normal animals, rupturing spontaneously and causing tissue damage, such as cataracts in the eye. These leukocytes have defective chemotactic responsiveness, reduced motility, and reduced intracellular killing as a result of defective granule fusion and a deficiency of elastase.

Clinically, the syndrome is associated with multiple abnormalities, including dilution of hair pigmentation

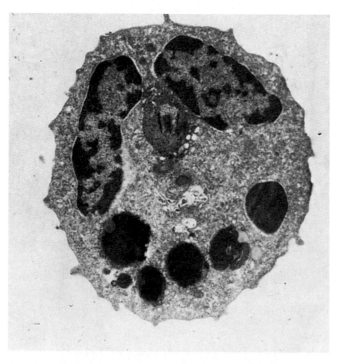

Figure 35-1. A neutrophil from a Chédiak-Higashi syndrome calf with enlarged cytoplasmic granules. (Courtesy of Dr. HW Leopold.)

(sometimes only obvious in the newborn), eye abnormalities, increased susceptibility to infection, and a bleeding tendency. In hair, the melanin granules fuse together. As a result, the abnormal melanin granules cause the dilution of coat color and light-colored irises (pseudoalbinism). Eye abnormalities include photophobia, and animals may develop cataracts. Their eyes have a red fundic light reflection rather than the normal yellow-green.

Because of the neutrophil defects, affected animals may be more susceptible to respiratory infections and neonatal septicemia. Some affected breeds of cattle, such as Herefords, tend to be more susceptible to infection than others, such as Japanese black cattle. The Chédiak-Higashi gene also impairs the function of natural killer (NK) cells. As a result, affected animals may show increased susceptibility to tumors and to viruses such as the Aleutian disease virus in mink.

Platelets from affected animals also contain enlarged granules, and their function is abnormal. Affected animals tend to bleed abnormally after surgery and develop hematomas at injection sites. Death from acute hemorrhage is common.

Chédiak-Higashi syndrome may be diagnosed by examining either a stained blood smear for the presence of grossly enlarged granules within leukocytes or by examining hair shafts for enlarged melanin granules. Treatment is symptomatic.

Pelger-Huët Anomaly

Pelger-Huët anomaly is an inherited disorder characterized by a failure of granulocyte nuclei to segment into lobes. As a result, their nuclei remain round in shape. The neutrophils therefore appear on first sight to be very immature (a left shift). The anomaly is usually detected when an animal is observed to have a persistent left shift that cannot be reconciled with its good health. Although Pelger-Huët neutrophils closely resemble band forms, their nuclear chromatin is condensed, reflecting their maturity. The disorder in humans is due to a mutation in the gene coding for lamin B, a nuclear membrane receptor that interacts with chromatin to determine the shape of the nucleus. Pelger-Huët anomaly has been observed in humans, domestic shorthair cats, and various dog breeds such as cocker spaniels, basenjis, Boston terriers, foxhounds, and coonhounds. In foxhounds and Australian shepherds the disorder is inherited as an autosomal dominant trait.

Pelger-Huët anomaly has a minimal effect on the health of animals. Nevertheless, fewer pups are weaned from affected dogs than from unaffected ones. In addition, Pelger-Huët neutrophils are less able to emigrate from blood vessels in vivo. It has been suggested that this reduced mobility is due to inflexible nuclei. B cell responses may also be impaired in these dogs since normal canine B cells exposed to serum from affected dogs show depressed responses to antigens.

Canine Leukocyte Adhesion Deficiency

In order for neutrophils to leave inflamed blood vessels and enter tissues, they must first bind to the vascular endothelial cells. This adherence is mediated by integrins on the neutrophil surface that bind ligands on vascular endothelial cells. In the absence of integrins, neutrophils cannot bind firmly to blood vessel walls and cannot emigrate from the vessels into tissues (Figure 35-2). Thus bacteria within tissues can grow freely without fear of attack by neutrophils. Canine leukocyte adhesion deficiency (CLAD) results from a defect in the integrin CD11b/CD18 (Mac-1). In CD11b/CD18–deficient dogs, neutrophils cannot respond to chemotaxins, bind to particles coated with iC3b (Mac-1 is a complement receptor), or bind to endothelial cells. Affected dogs have recurrent infections, while at the same time, they have large numbers of neutrophils in their blood.

CLAD has been described in Irish red setters (as well as in the related red and white setter breed), in which it is an autosomal recessive disease. Affected animals die early in life as a result of recurrent severe bacterial infections (osteomyelitis, omphalophlebitis, gingivitis), lymphadenopathy, impaired pus formation, delayed wound healing, weight loss, and fever.

Animals have a marked leukocytosis (>200,000/μl), primarily a neutrophilia and eosinophilia. Although these granulocytes look normal, functional tests reveal defects in adherence-dependent activities, including impaired adhesion to glass or plastic surfaces or to nylon wool fibers. They cannot ingest C3b-opsonized particles. Normal canine granulocytes aggregate after activation with phorbol myristate acetate, but those of CLAD animals do not. Migration in response to chemotactic stimuli is poor. Neither CD11b nor CD18 can be detected by immunofluorescence.

The lesion results from a single missense mutation at position 107 in the β chain of the CD18 gene, which results in the replacement of a highly conserved cysteine residue (Cys36) by a serine. As a result, the mutation disrupts a disulfide bond in CD18, altering its structure and function. CD11b (the α chain) is not expressed because it must be associated with the β chain before the dimer can be expressed on the cell surface.

A diagnostic test for the CLAD mutation has been developed. Thus genomic DNA is amplified by PCR using primers for the mutated region. The products of this reaction may then be sequenced and the presence of the mutation determined.

Canine granulocytopathy syndrome was an autosomal recessive disease observed in Irish setters. Some investigators have suggested that the disease is identical to CLAD, but because it was described before integrins were discovered, this cannot be confirmed. These animals had suppurative skin lesions, gingivitis, osteomyelitis, pododermatitis, and lymphadenopathy. Affected dogs had a pronounced leukocytosis, and their neutrophils were morphologically normal, although there was a persistent left shift. The affected animals were hypergammaglobulinemic and anemic as a result of the persistent infections. Their lymph nodes showed diffuse, suppurative, nongranulomatous lymphadenitis, which is inconsistent with a diagnosis of CLAD. Examination of the neutrophils of these dogs showed that their respiratory burst was depressed, as reflected by a decrease in glucose oxidation. Nevertheless, they were more effective than normal cells at reducing nitro-blue tetrazolium, implying that O_2^- was produced in greater quantities than normal or, perhaps, that it was not effectively removed. In spite of this, these cells were unable to kill opsonized *Escherichia coli* or *Staphylococcus aureus*, suggesting that they had a killing defect rather than an adhesion defect.

Bovine Leukocyte Adhesion Deficiency

An integrin deficiency occurs in Holstein calves. It is an autosomal recessive trait characterized clinically by recurrent bacterial infections, anorexia, oral ulceration, gingivitis, periodontitis, chronic pneumonia, stunted growth, delayed wound healing, peripheral lymphadenopathy, and a persistent extreme neutrophilia. Affected calves usually die between 2 and 7 months of age. The survivors grow slowly and may develop amyloidosis. These calves have large numbers of intravascular neutrophils but very few extravascular neutrophils, even in the presence of invading bacteria.

The disease results from a point mutation in the gene coding for CD18 (Figure 35-3). As a result, an aspartic acid residue is replaced by glycine, and functional CD18 is not produced. In the absence of this integrin, neutrophils fail to attach firmly to vascular endothelial cells and cannot emigrate from blood vessels. Healthy carriers have a single copy of the mutated gene and so have

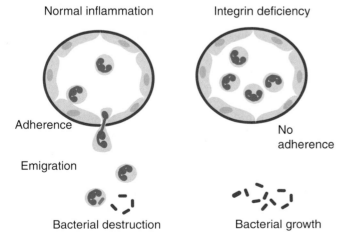

Figure 35-2. Integrins are required to bind neutrophils firmly to blood vessel walls. This permits the neutrophils to emigrate to sites of bacterial invasion. In the absence of integrins, neutrophil emigration fails to occur. As a result, invading bacteria can grow unmolested in the tissues.

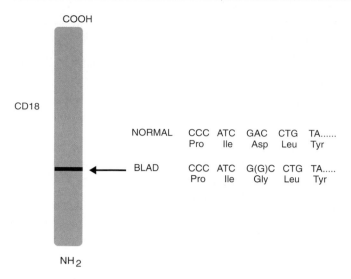

Figure 35-3. The BLAD mutation. The mutation involves replacement of a cytosine by a guanosine in the CD18 gene. As a result, an aspartic acid residue is replaced by a glycine residue. The mutation occurs in a highly conserved region of the CD18 molecule and prevents formation of a biologically active molecule.

abnormally low levels of CD18 (Figure 35-4). Through the use of a test based on the DNA polymerase chain reaction, the presence of the altered gene can be demonstrated. In this way it has been shown that one bull, Osborndale Ivanhoe, with thousands of registered sons

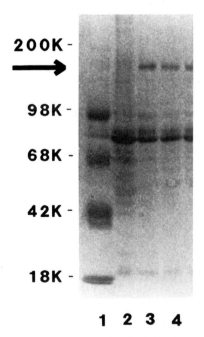

Figure 35-4. A Western blot of bovine Mac-1. An extract has been made from the neutrophils of a BLAD calf (*lane 2*) or from clinically normal calves (*lanes 3 and 4*). The extracts have been electrophoresed and blotted onto nitrocellulose. The bands are stained to show the presence of glycoproteins. Note that CD18 (*arrow*) is absent from the lysate of neutrophils from a BLAD calf. Lane 1 shows molecular weight standards (kD). (From Kehrili ME et al: *Am J Vet Res* 51:1826-1836, 1990.)

and daughters, was a carrier of this gene. As a result, the defective gene was widespread and common among Holstein cattle in the United States (14% of bulls, 5.8% of cows). Fortunately, carrier animals can now be rapidly detected and removed from breeding programs.

Because CD18 is also employed by T cells moving to sites of antigen invasion, BLAD calves show delayed or poor type IV responses to intradermal skin testing. In addition, their neutrophils show reduced responsiveness to chemotactic stimuli, and diminished superoxide production and myeloperoxidase activity. They have increased expression of Fc receptors but decreased binding and expression of C3b and IgM on neutrophil surfaces, implying an alteration in receptor function. This is reflected by greatly reduced endocytosis and killing of *Staphylococcus aureus*.

Canine Cyclical Neutropenia

Canine cyclical neutropenia (gray collie syndrome) is an autosomal recessive disease of collies. Affected dogs have dilution of skin pigmentation, eye lesions, and regular cyclic fluctuations in leukocyte numbers. Their hair is characteristically a silver gray color. The loss of neutrophils occurs about every 11 to 12 days and lasts for about 3 days. It is followed by normal or elevated neutrophil counts for about 7 days. Severe neutropenia suppresses inflammation and increases susceptibility to bacterial and fungal infections. (Their neutrophils also have reduced myeloperoxidase activity, so the disease is not entirely due to a neutrophil deficiency). The nature of the defect is not clear but is probably a result of fluctuations in myeloid stem cell numbers due to abnormalities in growth factor production. Some ultrastructural changes have been observed in neutrophil precursors. The animals have severe enteric disease, respiratory infections, mouth infections (gingivitis), bone disease (arthralgia), and lymphadenitis and rarely live beyond 3 years. Because platelet numbers also cycle, affected dogs may also have bleeding problems, including gingival hemorrhage and epistaxis. Immunoglobulin levels rise as a result of the recurrent antigenic stimulation, but complement levels cycle in conjunction with the neutropenia. The disease begins to express itself as maternal immunity wanes. Affected puppies are weak, grow poorly, have wounds that fail to heal, and have a high mortality. If they are kept alive by aggressive antibiotic therapy, the chronic inflammation may lead to amyloidosis.

Treatment involves the repeated use of antibiotics to control the recurrent infections. If endotoxin is administered repeatedly, it can stimulate the bone marrow and stabilize neutrophil, reticulocyte, and platelet numbers. Lithium carbonate has a similar effect. Unfortunately, both endotoxin and lithium carbonate are toxic, and the disease recurs when the treatment is discontinued.

Other Examples of Defective Neutrophil Function

An inherited defect in neutrophil bactericidal activity has been reported in Dobermans. Dogs had bronchopneumonia and chronic rhinitis that developed soon after birth and persisted despite antimicrobial therapy. Although their chemotaxis and ingestion were apparently normal, their neutrophils were unable to kill *S. aureus*. Since these cells showed reduced reduction of nitroblue tetrazolium and superoxide production, it was suggested that there was a defect in the respiratory burst pathway.

Young Weimaraner dogs have been described with recurrent fevers, diarrhea, pneumonia, pyoderma, osteomyelitis, stomatitis, and osteomyelitis. They had defective neutrophil function, as shown by a depressed chemiluminescent response to phorbol ester, implying a defect in the respiratory burst mechanism. Although their IgG and IgM levels were somewhat low, all the other immunological parameters of these animals were within normal ranges.

A persistent neutropenia attributable to a deficiency of granulocyte colony-stimulating factor (G-CSF) has been reported in a 3-year-old male Rottweiler. The animal had a fever due to multiple recurrent infections, especially a chronic bacterial arthritis in the presence of a persistent neutropenia. A bioassay showed that the animal was not making any G-CSF. Its myeloid stem cells responded readily to additional G-CSF, suggesting that they were functionally normal. Bone marrow examination suggested that its neutrophil precursors had failed to mature.

A possible autosomal recessive neutropenia has been described in border collies. This resulted in recurrent bacterial osteomyelitis and gastroenteritis. Animals presented with persistent fever and lameness due to lytic bone lesions. They had myeloid hyperplasia and dense accumulations of neutrophils in the marrow but few in the blood. The neutropenia apparently resulted from an inability of the neutrophils to escape from the bone marrow into the bloodstream, perhaps as a result of a deficiency of GM-CSF. In humans this disease has been called myelokathexis.

INHERITED DEFECTS IN THE ACQUIRED IMMUNE SYSTEM

The inherited immunological defects have served to confirm the overall arrangement of the immune system, as outlined in Figure 35-5. For example, if both the cell- and antibody-mediated immune responses are defective, it may be assumed that the genetic lesion operates at a point before thymic and bursal cell processing—that is, a stem-cell lesion. A defect that occurs only in thymic development is reflected in an inability to mount cell-mediated immune responses, although antibody production may be normal. Similarly, a lesion restricted to B cells is reflected by impaired antibody responses.

IMMUNODEFICIENCIES OF HORSES

Horses are among the few domestic animals whose economic worth has permitted a thorough analysis of neonatal mortality. As a result, a significant number of primary immunodeficiency syndromes have been identified in this species (Figure 35-6).

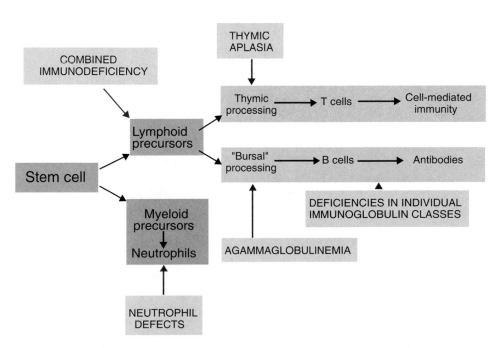

Figure 35-5. The points in the immune system where development blocks may lead to immunodeficiencies.

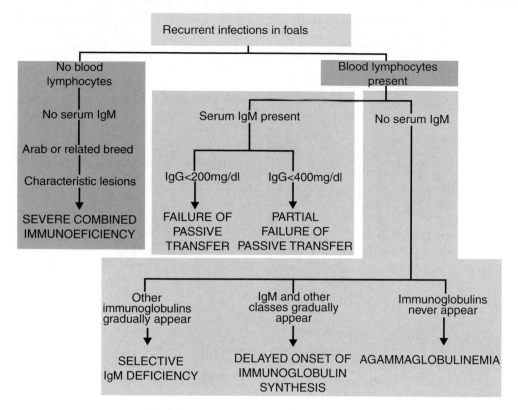

Figure 35-6.   The differential diagnosis of the equine immune deficiencies.

Severe Combined Immunodeficiency

The most important congenital equine immunodeficiency is the severe combined immunodeficiency syndrome (SCID). Affected foals fail to produce functional T or B cells and have very few circulating lymphocytes. If they suckle successfully, they will acquire maternal immunoglobulins. Once these have been catabolized, however, these foals cannot produce their own antibodies and eventually become agammaglobulinemic. Affected foals are therefore born healthy but begin to sicken by 2 months of age. The precise time of onset depends on the quantity of colostral antibodies absorbed. All die by 4 to 6 months as a result of overwhelming infection by a variety of low-grade pathogens. Severe bronchopneumonia is the predominant presenting sign. Organisms that have been implicated in this bronchopneumonia include equine adenovirus, *Rhodococcus equi*, and *Pneumocystis carinii* (an opportunistic fungal pathogen). The disease is manifested by a nasal discharge, coughing, dyspnea, weight loss, and fevers. Affected foals may also develop enteritis, omphalophlebitis, and many other infections. *Cryptosporidium parvum* and many different bacteria have been implicated in the enteritis.

On necropsy, the spleens of these foals lack germinal centers and periarteriolar lymphoid sheaths. Their lymph nodes lack lymphoid follicles and germinal centers, and there is cellular depletion in the paracortex. The thymus in these animals may be difficult to find.

By using large quantities of blood, it is possible to demonstrate the presence of functional NK cells. Neutrophil and monocyte functions are also normal in these foals.

SCID is an autosomal recessive disease, and its occurrence therefore indicates that both parents carry the mutation. Accurate diagnosis is of great importance, since the presence of the mutation significantly reduces the value of the parent animals. Thus all suspected cases must be confirmed by postmortem examination. The clinical diagnosis of SCID requires that at least two of the following three criteria be established: (1) very low (consistently below 1000/ mm^3) circulating lymphocytes; (2) histology typical of SCID—that is, gross hypoplasia of the primary and secondary lymphoid organs; and (3) an absence of IgM from presuckle serum. (The normal equine fetus synthesizes IgM. As a result, IgM in normal newborn foals is about 160 µg/ml. If the foal successfully suckles, it will obtain immunoglobulins of all isotypes from the mare's colostrum. However, the half-life of IgM is only about 6 days, so maternal IgM will disappear within a few days of birth. Thus a normal foal will always have some IgM in its serum, but a SCID foal will have none.)

The presence of the mutant SCID gene in horses can be detected by means of a polymerase chain reaction (PCR) procedure. A sample of DNA is obtained from horse skin cells. A set of primers designed to amplify only DNA containing the 5-base pair deletion and another set designed to amplify only the normal allele are used to determine whether the mutant gene is present. This test has demonstrated that the frequency of the SCID gene in Arabian horses is 8.4%. Based on this, it would be expected that 0.18% of Arabian foals would be homozygous for the trait and hence clinically affected. Pedigree analysis suggests that the SCID trait was introduced to the United States by a single stallion in the 1920s.

Molecular Basis of Equine SCID

When the antigen receptors (BCRs and TCRs) are synthesized, large segments of DNA are excised so that V, D, and J gene segments can be rejoined (Chapter 14). Several enzymes are involved in this recombination process. Some cut the DNA strands, and others rejoin them. Studies on the cells of SCID foals show that although the enzymes that cut the DNA are normal, there is a defect in the large multicomponent enzyme that rejoins the cut ends. The specific defect lies in the gene coding for the catalytic subunit of an enzyme called DNA-dependent protein kinase (DNA-PK$_{CS}$) (Figure 35-7). In the mutant DNA-PK$_{CS}$ gene, a loss of five nucleotides results in a frameshift, premature termination of the peptide chain, and a deletion of 967 amino acids from the C-terminus of the molecule, including its entire kinase domain (Figure 35-8). Functional DNA-PK$_{CS}$ is totally absent from affected foals. Because of this deficiency, broken DNA strands cannot be rejoined, and neither T cells nor B cells can form functional V regions. In the absence of both TCRs and BCRs, affected foals cannot respond to antigens.

Since DNA-PK$_{CS}$ is needed to rejoin broken strands of DNA, it also plays a key role in other DNA repair processes. Thus when normal foal cells are irradiated, they can repair the damage to DNA caused by the ionizing radiation. The cells from SCID foals, in contrast, are unable to repair their DNA. These cells are much more susceptible to radiation-induced damage (Figure 35-9).

Immunoglobulin Deficiencies

Primary agammaglobulinemia is a rare disease of foals. Affected animals have no identifiable B cells (cells with surface immunoglobulins) and have very low immunoglobulin levels. Their lymphoid tissues contain no primary follicles, germinal centers, or plasma cells. Nevertheless, their blood lymphocytes can respond to mitogens and produce the cytokine, migration inhibitory factor (MIF). Intradermal inoculation of phytohemagglutinin induces a typical type IV delayed hypersensitivity reaction. Affected foals experience recurrent bacterial infections but can survive for 17 to 18 months. The disease should be suspected in a foal having a normal lymphocyte count but lacking both IgM and IgG. It may be confirmed by showing normal T cell responses to mitogens and an absence of B cells.

Selective IgM deficiencies have been described in foals. Serum IgM levels in these animals are at least two standard deviations below normal, but IgG and IgA levels and B cell numbers are normal. In most cases, foals have septicemia or recurrent respiratory tract infections, often involving *Klebsiella pneumoniae* or *R. equi*, and die by 10 months of age. Some affected foals live longer and respond to therapy but fail to grow, have recurrent respiratory infections, and die by 24 months of age.

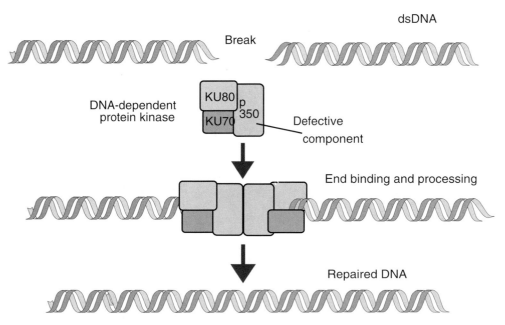

Figure 35-7. The defect in DNA dependent protein kinase that prevents DNA repair in SCID foals.

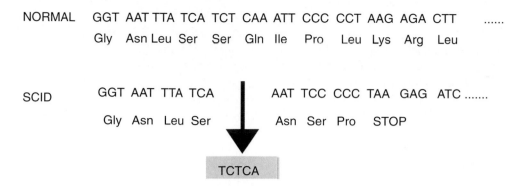

NORMAL	GGT	AAT	TTA	TCA	TCT	CAA	ATT	CCC	CCT	AAG	AGA	CTT	......
	Gly	Asn	Leu	Ser	Ser	Gln	Ile	Pro	Leu	Lys	Arg	Leu	

SCID	GGT	AAT	TTA	TCA		AAT	TCC	CCC	TAA	GAG	ATC	....
	Gly	Asn	Leu	Ser		Asn	Ser	Pro	STOP			

TCTCA

Figure 35-8. The gene deletion in the equine DNA-PK gene that leads to premature termination of the molecule.

Most affected foals have been Arabians or quarter horses, suggesting that the disease may have a genetic basis.

A single case of IgG deficiency has been described in a 3-month-old foal with salmonellosis. The animal had normal IgA and IgM but no germinal centers, lymphoid follicles, splenic follicles, or periarteriolar lymphoid sheaths. Serum IgG was extremely low.

Between 2 and 3 months of age, some foals experience a transient hypogammaglobulinemia as a result of a delayed onset of immunoglobulin synthesis. These animals may have recurrent infections during the period when their immunoglobulin levels are low. Lymphocyte numbers and responsiveness remain normal at this time.

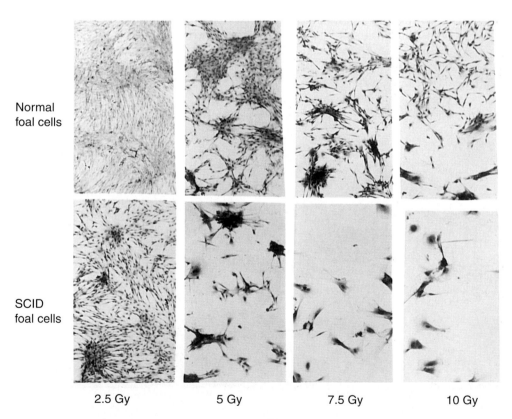

Normal foal cells

SCID foal cells

2.5 Gy   5 Gy   7.5 Gy   10 Gy

Figure 35-9. The effect of radiation on normal foal fibroblasts and on fibroblasts from a SCID foal. Equivalent numbers of cells were exposed to varying amounts of ionizing radiation as indicated and cultured in chamber slides. Five days later the slides were fixed, stained, and photographed. Note that there are many fewer SCID cells surviving this treatment since they are unable to repair their DNA. (From Wiles R, Leber R, Moore BB, et al: *Proc Natl Acad Sci USA* 93:11485-11489, 1995. Courtesy of Dr. K Meek.)

Common Variable Immunodeficiency

Common variable immunodeficiency (CVID) is the most prevalent primary immunodeficiency disease in humans. It is a heterogeneous group of sporadic diseases all characterized by a failure of B cells to make antibodies. In most cases, the B cell defect is secondary to a defect in helper T cell signaling. Unlike the other primary immunodeficiencies, most cases are diagnosed in adults. Cases of common variable immunodeficiency have been recorded in horses. Although they resemble primary immunodeficiencies in their sporadic nature and severity, they occur in animals older than 3 years of age. Typically, the horses present with recurrent infections that are not responsive to medical treatment. Their serum contains only trace levels of IgG and IgM, no detectable IgG3, and very low IgA levels. T cell numbers are normal, but B cells are undetectable and there is no response to the B cell mitogen LPS. On necropsy, there are no B cells in lymphoid organs, blood, or bone marrow. Some horses may have severe liver disease, a feature also seen in humans. It is suspected that these individuals have an underlying defect that is only expressed when the immune system is stressed by infection. Other cases have included horses between 2 and 5 years old with a selective IgM deficiency. Many develop a concurrent lymphosarcoma, and limited evidence suggests that they have excessive suppressor T cell function.

Fell Pony Immunodeficiency Syndrome

An autosomal recessive disease consisting of anemia, peripheral, ganglionopathy, and immunodeficiency has been reported in Fell pony foals in the UK. Affected foals appear normal at birth but fail to thrive. The disease develops at 4 to 12 weeks of age as maternal immunity wanes. The foals become extremely anemic, and opportunistic infections, expressed as diarrhea or respiratory disease, occur. The foals usually die or are euthanized by 3 months of age as a result of infections with Cryptosporidium or adenoviruses. Affected animals have an absence of germinal centers and a lack of plasma cells, suggesting some form of B cell deficiency. Indeed, B cell numbers in affected foals are less than 10% of normal levels, although CD4 and CD8 T cell numbers are within the normal range. Immunoglobulin levels are relatively normal, but an immunoglobulin deficiency may be masked by maternal antibodies. Neutrophil counts are normal.

Incidence

The most important immunodeficiency in foals is not inherited but results from a failure to absorb sufficient colostral antibodies from the mare (see Chapter 19). This failure of passive transfer may affect up to 10% of all foals. Severe combined immunodeficiency occurs in 2% to 3% of Arab foals and is 10 times more common than selective IgM deficiency. Selective IgM deficiency is, in turn, 10 times more common than agammaglobulinemia.

IMMUNODEFICIENCIES OF CATTLE

Severe Combined Immunodeficiency

A combined immunodeficiency has been recorded in an Angus calf. The animal was apparently normal when born and suckled normally. It became ill, however, at 6 weeks of age when it developed pneumonia and diarrhea. The animal was lymphopenic and severely hypogammaglobulinemic. It had undetectable IgM and IgA and a low level of IgG, which was believed to be the residue of passively acquired maternal antibodies. The animal died within a week with systemic candidiasis. It had a hypoplastic thymus consisting of epithelial cells but no thymocytes. It had no detectable lymph nodes and a hypoplastic spleen that had no lymphocytes within its periarteriolar lymphoid sheaths. The syndrome thus closely resembled equine SCID.

Selective IgG2 Deficiency

IgG2 deficiency has been reported in red Danish cattle. About 1% to 2% of this breed is completely deficient in this immunoglobulin subclass and as a result have increased susceptibility to pneumonias and gangrenous mastitis. Up to 15% may also have low IgG2 levels, although they do not appear to have any ill effects in consequence.

Hereditary Parakeratosis

Certain Black Pied Danish and Friesian cattle carry an autosomal recessive trait of thymic and lymphocytic hypoplasia (Trait A-46). Affected calves are born healthy, but by 4 to 8 weeks they begin to experience severe skin infections. If untreated, they die within a few weeks, and none survive for longer than four months. Affected calves have exanthema, hair loss on the legs, and parakeratosis around the mouth and eyes. There is depletion of lymphocytes in the GALT and atrophy of the thymus, spleen, and lymph nodes. These animals are T cell–deficient and have depressed cell-mediated immunity but normal antibody responses. Thus they have a normal antibody response to tetanus toxoid but respond poorly to dinitrochlorobenzene or tuberculin, both of which induce cell-mediated reactions. If these calves are treated by oral zinc oxide or zinc sulfate, they recover the ability to mount normal cell-mediated responses. If however the zinc supplementation is stopped, the animals will relapse within a few weeks. It is probable that these animals have a reduced ability to absorb zinc from the intestine.

Zinc is an essential component of the thymic hormone thymulin (Chapter 36) and is therefore required for a normal T cell response.

Transient Hypogammaglobulinemia

A transient hypogammaglobulinemia associated with a delayed onset of immunoglobulin synthesis has been recorded in a Simmental heifer.

Hypotrichosis With Thymic Aplasia

A case of thymic aplasia with absence of hair has been described in calves. It is probably similar to the "nude" mutation seen in mice and cats (p. 426).

IMMUNODEFICIENCIES OF DOGS

Combined Immunodeficiencies

A severe combined immunodeficiency resulting from a defect in the catalytic subunit of the DNA-dependent protein kinase (DNA-PK$_{cs}$) has been identified in Jack Russell terriers. From a single breeding pair of terriers, 12 of 32 siblings died from opportunistic infections between 8 and 14 weeks of age. These animals showed a SCID phenotype with lymphopenia, agammaglobulinemia, and thymic and lymphoid aplasia. The disease appeared to be inherited as an autosomal recessive condition. It results from a point mutation, leading to stop codon formation and premature termination of the peptide chain 517 amino acids before the normal C-terminus. Affected dogs show severely diminished expression of DNA-PK$_{cs}$. As in equine SCID, the defect blocks gene splicing during V(D)J recombination in TCR and immunoglobulin variable regions. The carrier frequency of this gene is 1.1%.

An X-linked severe combined immunodeficiency has been recorded in Basset hounds and Cardigan Welsh corgis. The disease is characterized by stunted growth, increased susceptibility to infections, and absence of lymph nodes. Clinically, animals are healthy during the immediate neonatal period as a result of maternal antibodies. However by 6 to 8 weeks, as the levels of maternal antibodies decline, the animals begin to develop infections. At first these are relatively mild infections, such as superficial pyoderma and otitis media. Eventually, they become more severe, and untreated animals die of severe pneumonia, enteritis, or sepsis by 4 months of age. Common infections include canine distemper, generalized staphylococcal infections, adenoviral and parvoviral infections, and cryptosporidiosis. It is interesting to note that *P. carinii* pneumonia has not been recorded in these dogs. This immunodeficiency is an X-linked disorder since breeding of a carrier female to a normal sire results in approximately half the males in each litter being affected and all the females being phenotypically normal.

On examination these dogs usually have reduced blood lymphocyte numbers ~1000/μl but are not profoundly lymphopenic. Their CD4/CD8 ratio is, however, approximately 15:1 as compared with normal dogs that have a CD4/CD8 ratio of 1.7:1. This indicates a major drop in CD8$^+$ cell numbers. The absolute number of T cells persists at less than 20% of normal. The dogs have normal numbers of B cells. The few lymphocytes in the blood are unresponsive to mitogens. The puppies have normal IgM levels but very low, or no, IgG and IgA. The dogs do not make antibodies against antigens such as tetanus toxoid.

On necropsy the thymus of affected dogs is approximately 10% of the normal weight and lacks a defined cortex (Figure 35-10). The total number of thymocytes is approximately 0.3% of normal. Their lymph nodes and tonsils are very small and dysplastic and may be very difficult to find. When present, the nodes are disorganized and contain very few small lymphocytes. Their spleens contain large periarteriolar lymphoid nodules with occasional small lymphocytes and few plasma cells. The bone marrow in these dogs appears normal. Approximately 40% of the thymocytes of these dogs are CD4$^-$/CD8$^-$ compared with 16% of the thymocytes of normal dogs.

The disease results from a mutation in the gene coding for the γ chain of the IL-2R (IL-2Rγ). The same chain is

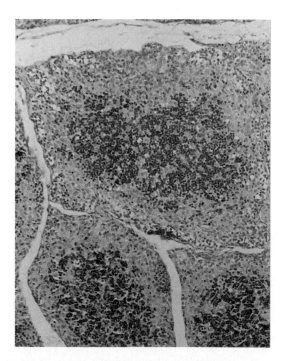

Figure 35-10. Photomicrograph of the thymus of a Basset hound with X-linked immunodeficiency. Note the lack of a defined cortex and the scattered foci of dark-staining lymphocytes. (H&E stain.) (From Snyder PW, Kazacos EA, Felsburg PJ: *Clin Immunol Immunopathol* 67:55-67, 1993.)

also a component of the IL-4, IL-7, IL-9, and IL-15 receptors and has been designated the common γ-chain, γc. In affected Basset hounds, a loss of four bases in the γc gene causes a frameshift. As a result, of this frameshift a stop codon is generated. Thus, instead of the complete protein, only a small peptide is produced and no functional protein is made. A second SCID mutation has been described in Cardigan Welsh corgis. In these animals a single cytosine residue is inserted into the γc gene so that a stop codon is generated before the transmembrane domain resulting in a failure to synthesize the complete chain (Figure 35-11). As a result this peptide is not expressed on the cell surface. In both cases, the mutation does not interfere with IL-2 production, but the lymphocytes of these animals are unresponsive to IL-2. In the absence of a γc chain mature T cells will not develop.

Experimentally, affected dogs may be "cured" by bone marrow allografts. Reconstitution with normal bone marrow results in the presence of normal donor T cells and a mixed chimerism ranging from 30% to 50% donor B cells.

Immunoglobulin Deficiencies

A selective IgM deficiency has been reported in two related Doberman pinschers. One animal was asymptomatic, whereas the other had a chronic mucopurulent nasal discharge and bronchopneumonia. Both these animals had raised IgA, low IgG, and very low IgM. They experienced only a chronic nasal discharge, so the clinical significance of this deficiency is in doubt.

Selective deficiencies of IgA have been observed in several breeds of dogs. German shepherds are predisposed to a range of infectious disorders, including mycoses, anal furunculosis, deep pyoderma, and small intestinal bacterial overgrowth. This suggests that they may have deficiencies in mucosal immunity. Consistent with this is the observation that normal German shepherds in the United Kingdom have normal IgM and IgG levels but significantly reduced levels of IgA (~80 mg/dl as opposed to 170 mg/dl in the control group.) Likewise, dogs of this breed have significantly lower concentrations of IgA in their tears as compared with other breeds. They have normal numbers of IgA-producing plasma cells, implying that the deficiency may be due to defective synthesis or secretion of IgA.

Shar-pei puppies with recurrent cough, nasal discharge, conjunctivitis, and pneumonia, as well as demodicosis and *Microsporum canis* infections, have been identified as having a selective IgA deficiency (<15 mg/dl). Likewise, abnormally low IgA concentrations have been found in a high percentage of clinically normal shar-pei dogs. A high incidence of atopic disease is observed in these dogs, a feature also seen in IgA-deficient humans.

A primary selective IgA deficiency has been described in an inbred beagle colony. The colony had a history of parainfluenza and endemic kennel cough due to *Bordetella bronchiseptica*. Despite extensive vaccinations, these animals continued to experience recurrent respiratory tract infections and otitis. Immunoelectrophoresis and radial immunodiffusion showed that the affected dogs had normal serum IgG and IgM levels but very

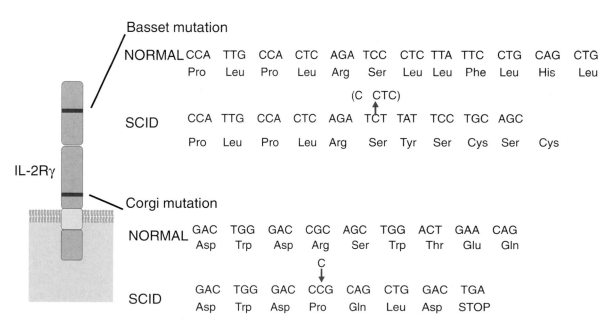

Figure 35-11. The two defined canine X-linked SCIF mutations in the IL-2Rγ gene. In the corgi mutation, the insertion of a single cytosine residue into the gene leads to the generation of a stop codon and premature termination of peptide synthesis. In the basset mutation, deletion of four bases causes a frameshift mutation and also leads to the generation of a stop codon (not shown). (Data from Henthorn PS, Somberg RL, Fimiani VM, et al: *Genomics* 23:69-74, 1994; and from Somberg RL, Pullen RP, Casal ML, et al: *Vet Immunol Immunopathol* 47:203-214, 1995.)

little IgA (<5mg/dl). Phenotypically normal parent dogs had very low IgA levels. Four affected dogs had circulating anti-IgA antibodies. Their T and B lymphocyte numbers and lymphocyte responses to mitogens were normal, as was their response to tetanus toxoid. They had a normal number of plasma cells secreting IgG and IgM but no plasma cells secreting IgA. When two affected animals were mated, four out of five pups in a litter were IgA-deficient. The disease was not sex-linked.

A transient hypogammaglobulinemia has been seen in two animals from a litter of Spitz puppies that experienced recurrent upper respiratory tract infections between 8 and 16 weeks of age. These dogs had normal T cell numbers and mitogen responses. They had low immunoglobulin levels and low antibody titers to vaccine antigens at 16 weeks. These puppies responded very weakly to tetanus toxoid when it was administered at 4 months. By 6 months, however, immunoglobulins had risen to normal levels and the puppies regained their health. It is believed that these puppies experienced a delayed onset of immunoglobulin synthesis. Symptomatic treatment is sufficient to carry these animals until their immune system becomes functional.

T Cell Deficiencies

A family of inbred Weimaraner dogs has been reported as having immunodeficiency and dwarfism. The animals appeared normal at birth, but at 6 to 7 weeks of age they developed a wasting syndrome characterized by emaciation and lethargy. The dogs began to experience recurrent infections that eventually killed them. On necropsy their thymuses were atrophied and lacked a cortex. These animals had normal immunoglobulin levels, their helper cell activity was unimpaired, and their secondary lymphoid organs appeared normal. The lymphocytes of these dogs were unresponsive to mitogens.

Growth hormone treatment caused thymic cortical regeneration and a dramatic clinical improvement. However, growth hormone did not restore lymphocyte responsiveness to mitogens. The disease is almost certainly due to a deficiency of growth hormone as a result of a lesion in the hypothalamus and confirms that the thymus requires growth hormone to function.

Bull terriers suffer from lethal acrodermatitis. This is a complex immunodeficiency syndrome associated with growth retardation, skin lesions (acrodermatitis, chronic pyoderma, paronychia), diarrhea, recurrent pneumonia, and abnormal behavior. The puppies were weak at birth and did not nurse well. Some showed a lighter pigmentation than their littermates. When weaned, they had difficulty in eating and failed to grow. Small, crusted lesions developed between the digits, and a pustular dermatitis developed around the eyes and mouth at 6 to 10 weeks. The lesions developed into a severe pyoderma. Fungi such as *Malassezia* and *Candida* were readily isolated from the lesions. Diarrhea developed early in the disease, and respiratory tract infections were common. The puppies became depressed and sluggish and died by 15 months of age, with a median survival of 7 months. They had a neutrophilia, normal IgG and IgM levels but significantly lower IgA levels, and hypercholesterolemia. Plasma zinc levels were unusually low. They showed depressed lymphocyte mitogen responses.

On necropsy there was a severe loss of T cells and the puppies lacked a thymus, and the lymph nodes and spleen were very small. The disease is inherited as an autosomal recessive disease, and the parents of affected puppies could be traced to one common ancestor. Because of its similarities to trait A-46 of cattle, these dogs were treated with oral zinc (p. 421). Very high doses resulted in some clinical improvement, but this could not be sustained.

Pneumocystis carinii pneumonia has been observed repeatedly in young miniature dachshunds. The affected animals are usually less than 1 year old and appear to be immunodeficient. Serum electrophoresis shows a marked reduction in IgM, IgG, and IgA. In addition, lymphocyte responses to both phytohemagglutinin and pokeweed mitogens are severely depressed. There is a reduction in B cell numbers. Although the *Pneumocystis* pneumonia responds to aggressive therapy, these animals rarely do well and die young. *P. carinii* pneumonia has also been described in Cavalier King Charles spaniels. Some of these dogs were hypogammaglobulinemic with low levels of IgG.

Uncharacterized Immunodeficiencies

German shepherd dog pyoderma is, as its name implies, a chronic skin disease that occurs in middle-aged German shepherd dogs associated with infection with coagulase-positive staphylococci. These cases do not respond well to antibiotic therapy, and it is believed to reflect some form of underlying genetic or immunological defect. Although affected dogs appear to mount normal humoral responses, limited studies have shown reduced lymphocyte responses to mitogens, an imbalance of lymphocyte subsets (CD4 cells are depressed, CD8 cells are increased), and a decline in the level of CD21$^+$ B cells. (CD21 plays a role in B cell activation). Unfortunately, it is unclear whether these alterations represent primary defects or whether they are a result of the chronic bacterial infection.

The veterinary literature contains several reports of dogs with severe recurrent infections caused by organisms that are not normally considered to be highly pathogenic Protothecosis has been recorded in dogs. One third of the cases have been in collies suggesting an inherited predisposition. Weimaraners are unusually susceptible to some systemic bacterial infections; German shepherds are susceptible to generalized systemic *Aspergillus* infections, whereas some Rottweiler and Doberman families are unusually susceptible to parvovirus infection. None of these have been shown to be due to primary immunodeficiencies, and all require further investigation.

It has been suggested that some cases of deep pyoderma in dogs may result from immunological defects. Some breeds, especially German shepherds, appear to be unusually susceptible to the disease. As pointed out above, this breed appears to be unusually susceptible to small intestinal bacterial overgrowth as a result of an IgA deficiency. When the number of CD3+ T cells and B cells were examined in normal dog skin and in the skin of dogs with deep pyoderma, it was found that the B cell numbers were similar but that the number of T cells infiltrating the lesions in German shepherds was significantly reduced. Studies on T cell function in these animals have also demonstrated a functional defect. This suggests that T cell dysfunction may play a role in the pathogenesis of deep pyoderma in this breed.

IMMUNODEFICIENCIES OF CATS

Hypotrichosis with Thymic Aplasia

The nude mouse has long been accepted as an important mouse model of immunodeficiency. Nude mice are a strain of hairless mice that fail to develop a functional thymus. This disease has been described in rats, guinea pigs, and calves. A similar mutation has been described in Birman kittens. These kittens were born without any body hair (Figure 35-12). On necropsy they also had no thymus and had depletion of lymphocytes in the paracortex of lymph nodes, spleen, and Peyer's patches. Thus they were essentially T cell–deficient. Analysis of the pedigree suggested that the disease was inherited as an autosomal recessive disease.

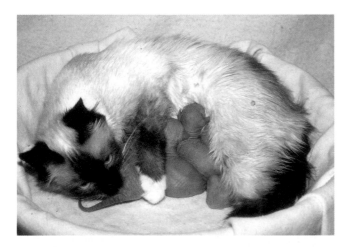

Figure 35-12. Kittens born with an autosomal recessive form of congenital hypotrichosis with thymic aplasia—nude kittens. (From *J Am Anim Hosp Assoc* 30:601, 1994. Courtesy of Dr. MJ Casal.)

IMMUNODEFICIENCIES OF CHICKENS

Birds of the hypothyroid OS strain have a selective IgA deficiency. Birds of the UCD 140 line have a selective IgG deficiency called hereditary dysgammaglobulinemia. These birds have normal immunoglobulin levels for about 50 days after hatching; then their IgG drops and their IgM and IgA rise. In addition to hypogammaglobulinemia, UCD 140 strain birds develop immune-complex lesions, and it has been suggested that a vertically transmitted virus mediates this disease.

IMMUNODEFICIENCIES OF HUMANS

A large number of well-characterized immunodeficiency syndromes have been reported in humans. It is anticipated that investigators will succeed eventually in identifying most of these syndromes in domestic animals as well.

The most important phagocytic deficiency syndrome of humans is chronic granulomatous disease. This has not yet been reported as occurring in domestic animals, although it undoubtedly does. Children affected with chronic granulomatous disease have recurrent infections characterized by the development of septic granulomata in lymph nodes, lungs, bones, and skin. The neutrophils of these children are less capable than normal cells of destroying organisms such as staphylococci and coliforms. Their specific lesion is a defect in one of the subcomponents of the NADPH oxidase (NOX) complex.

Infants suffer from several different forms of combined immunodeficiency. The most severe is reticular dysgenesis, which results from a defect in the development of both myeloid and lymphoid stem cells. Other combined immunodeficiencies result from blocks in the development of both T and B lymphoid stem cells. Some of these CID cases are due to a deficiency of the enzyme adenosine deaminase. In other cases there is a defect in the genes coding for IL-2 or IL-7 receptors, for recombinase-activating gene proteins, for CD25, for CD3γ chain, or for MHC class I or class II molecules. The standard treatment for all these diseases is a bone marrow allograft.

T Cell Deficiencies

The DiGeorge anomaly results from a failure of the third and fourth thymic pouches to develop. In consequence, no thymic epithelial tissue develops and few cells populate the T-dependent areas of the secondary lymphoid tissues. Since these individuals have no functional T cells, they can neither mount a delayed hypersensitivity reaction nor reject allografts. The importance of T cells in protection against viruses is emphasized by the observation that individuals with the DiGeorge anomaly generally die of virus infections but remain resistant to bacteria.

B Cell Deficiencies

The most severe of the B cell deficiencies, called Bruton-type agammaglobulinemia, is an X-linked recessive disease; affected infants are devoid of all immunoglobulin classes. They experience recurrent infections due to bacteria such as pneumococci, staphylococci, and streptococci but are usually resistant to viral, fungal, and protozoan infections. The disease results from a mutation in a receptor tyrosine kinase. Inherited deficiencies of individual immunoglobulin classes have also been recorded in humans. As might be anticipated, there are many possible combinations of deficiencies in IgG, IgM, IgA, and IgE, and a tendency to give each a specific name leads to confusion. One of the most important of these is the Wiscott-Aldrich syndrome. In this disease, a selective IgM deficiency is associated with multiple infections, eczema, and thrombocytopenia. Another such syndrome is ataxia-telangiectasia, in which serum IgA and IgE levels are extremely low or absent and cerebellar and cutaneous abnormalities exist. Affected children, lacking an effective surface immune system, have recurrent bacterial respiratory tract infections. Ataxia-telangiectasia results from a defect in DNA repair mechanisms. In another disease called hyper-IgM syndrome, a defect in the CD40-ligand leads to a failure in the IgM switch so that affected individuals have high levels of IgM but no other antibody classes.

IMMUNODEFICIENCIES OF MICE

Nude Mice (Nu)

The best-known mouse model of immunodeficiency is the nude mouse. Nude mice are a strain of hairless mice that fail to develop a functional thymus. (Similar mutations have been observed in rats, guinea pigs, calves, and cats.) Because the T cells fail to develop with the thymus, nude mice are deficient in mature T cells but possess a limited number of immature T cells and B cells so that occasional lymphocytes may be found in peripheral blood. Normal thymus grafts, by restoring epithelial-cell function, permit the T cells of nude mice to mature and develop immune competence. Nude mice are deficient in conventional cell-mediated immune responses, as reflected by prolonged allograft survival and lack of responses to T-cell mitogens. Their IgG and IgA levels also are depressed, presumably as a result of a loss of helper T cells.

Although nude mice show enhanced susceptibility to virus-induced tumors, they fail to develop more than the normal level of spontaneous tumors. This observation was, for many years, a major objection to the immunological surveillance theory, because if T cells destroy tumors, T cell-deficient animals should have an increased incidence of neoplasia. However, nude mice do possess normal numbers of NK cells, which may protect them in the absence of T cells.

Severe Combined Immunodeficiency Mice (SCID)

SCID mice have very low numbers of B cells and T cells. Development of B cells is halted before expression of cytoplasmic or cell-membrane immunoglobulins. T cell development is also arrested at a very early stage, and those lymphocytes that do reach the bloodstream are CD4$^-$/CD8$^-$. They have no immunoglobulins and are unable to mount cell-mediated immune responses. *Scid* mice survive relatively well for about a year in specific-pathogen-free facilities but eventually die of *P. carinii* pneumonia. The defects in *scid* mice result from an inability to rearrange their BCR or TCR V region genes correctly. Several different mutations in the DNA joining enzymes have been identified. As a result the cells cannot produce functional receptors, and no functional T or B cells are produced. As in SCID horses, the mouse *scid* mutations also increase sensitivity to ionizing radiation since these animals are unable to repair DNA damage. About 15% of *scid* mice are "leaky" so that they have low levels of immunoglobulins of limited heterogeneity and can reject allografts. Antigen-presenting cells, myeloid and erythroid cells, and NK cells are normal in *scid* mice.

Moth-Eaten Mice (ME)

Moth-eaten mice have a defective T cell system but produce excessive quantities of immunoglobulins and develop autoimmune disease. Their name comes from their appearance. Within a few days of birth, neutrophils invade their hair follicles and cause patchy loss of pigment. These animals lack cytotoxic T cells and NK cells. Mice that are *me/me* have a short life span and usually die as a result of lung damage. The thymus of these animals involutes unusually early, and the emigration of prethymocytes into the thymus is impaired. The B cell hyperactivity may be due to excessive production of some B cell–stimulating cytokines.

X-Linked Immunodeficiency (XID)

Mice that are *xid* have a recessive, X-linked B cell defect so that they are unable to respond to certain T-independent carbohydrate antigens. They lack certain B cell subsets. Mice that are *bg/nu/xid* are severely immunosuppressed since they lack T, B, and NK cells. Lightly irradiated *bg/nu/xid* mice can accept human bone marrow grafts.

SOURCES OF ADDITIONAL INFORMATION

Allan FJ, Thompson KG, Jones BR, et al: Neutropenia with a probable hereditary basis in border collies, *NZ Vet J* 44: 67-72,1996.

Bernoco D, Bailey E: Frequency of the SCID gene among Arabian horses in the USA, *Anim Genet* 29:41-42, 1998.

Buckley RH: Primary immunodeficiency diseases due to defects in lymphocytes, *N Engl J Med* 343:1313-1325, 2000.

Casal ML, Straumann U, Sigg C, et al: Congenital hypotrichosis with thymic aplasia in nine Birman kittens, *J Am Anim Hosp Assoc* 30:600-602, 1994.

Day MJ: An immunopathological study of deep pyoderma in the dog, *Res Vet Sci* 56:18-23, 1994.

Debenham SL, Millington A, Kijas J, et al: Canine leucocyte adhesion of deficiency in Irish red and white setters, *J Small Anim Pract* 43:74-75, 2002.

Ding Q, Bramble L, Yuzbasiyan-Gurkan V, et al: DNA-PKcs mutations in dogs and horses: allele frequency and association with neoplasia, *Gene* 283:263-269, 2002.

Flaminio MJB, LaCombe V, Kohn CW, Antczak DF: Common variable immunodeficiency in a horse, *J Am Vet Med Assoc* 221:1296-1302, 2002.

Hagiwara Y, Fujiwara S, Takai H, et al: *Pneumocystis carinii* pneumonia in a cavalier King Charles spaniel, *J Vet Med Sci* 63:349-351, 2001.

Henthorn PS, Somberg RL, Fimani VM, et al: IL-2Rγ gene microdeletion demonstrates that canine X-linked severe combined immunodeficiency is a homologue of the human disease, *Genomics* 23:69-74, 1994.

Jensen AL, Thomsen MA, Aaes H, et al: Polymorphonuclear neutrophil granulocyte chemotactic hyperresponsiveness in a case of canine acromegaly, *Vet Immunol Immunopathol* 37:329-336, 1993.

Kehrli ME, Schmalstieg FC, Anderson DC, et al: Molecular definition of the bovine granulocytopathy syndrome: identification of the deficiency of the Mac-1 (CD11b/CD18) glycoprotein, *Am J Vet Res* 51:1826-1836, 1990.

Kijas JMH, Bauer Jr TR, Gäfvert S, et al: A missense mutation in the β-2 integrin gene *(ITGB2)* causes canine leukocyte adhesion deficiency, *Genomics* 61:101-107, 1999.

Lanevschi A, Daminet S, Niemeyer GP, Lothrop CD: Granulocyte colony-stimulating factor deficiency in a Rottweiler with chronic idiopathic neutropenia, *J Vet Intern Med* 13:72-75, 1999.

Latimer KS, Campagnoli RP, Danilenko DM: Pelger-Huet anomaly in Australian shepherds: 87 cases (1991-1997), *Comp Haematol Internat* 10:9-13, 2000.

Lobetti RG, Leisewitz AL, Spencer JA: *Pneumocystis carinii* in the miniature dachshund: case report and literature review, *J Small Anim Pract* 37:280-285, 1996.

Lunn DP, McClure JT, Schobert CS, Holmes MA: Abnormal patterns of equine leukocyte differentiation antigen expression in severe combined immunodeficiency foals suggests the phenotype of normal equine natural killer cells, *Immunology* 84:495-499, 1995.

Mackay ER, Rosen FS: Immunodeficiency diseases caused by defects in phagocytes, *N Engl J Med* 343:1703-1713, 2000.

McEwan NA: Malassezia and Candida infections in bull terriers with lethal acrodermatitis, *J Small Anim Pract* 42:291-297, 2001.

Meek K, Kienker L, Dallas C, et al: SCID in Jack Russell terriers: a new animal model of DNA-PKcs deficiency, *J Immunol* 167:2142-2150, 2001.

Nachreiner RF, Refsal KR, Graham PA, Bowman MM: Prevalence of serum thyroid hormone autoantibodies in dogs with clinical signs of hypothyroidism, *J Am Vet Med Assoc* 220:466-471, 2002.

Rosen FS, Cooper MD, Wedgewood RJP: The primary immunodeficiencies, *N Engl J Med* 333:431-439, 1995.

Scholes SFE, Holliman A, May PDF, Holmes MA: A syndrome of anaemia, immunodeficiency and peripheral ganglionopathy in Fell pony foals, *Vet Rec* 142:128-134, 1998.

Shiflett SL, Kaplan J, Ward DM: Chédiak-Higashi syndrome: a rare disorder of lysosomes and lysosome related organelles, *Pigment Cell Res* 15:251-257, 2002.

Shin EK, Perryman LE, Meek K: A kinase-negative mutation of DNA-PKcs in equine SCID results in defective coding and signal joint formation, *J Immunol* 158:3565-3569, 1997.

Shiraishi M, Kawashima S, Moroi M, et al: A defect in collagen receptor-Ca2$^+$ signaling system in platelets from cattle with Chediak-Higashi syndrome, *Thromb Haemost* 87:334-341, 2002.

Shuster DE, Kehrli ME, Ackermann MR, Gilbert RO: Identification and prevalence of a genetic defect that causes leukocyte adhesion deficiency in Holstein cattle, *Proc Natl Acad Sci USA* 89:9225-9229, 1992.

Somberg RL, Pullen RP, Casal ML, et al: A single nucleotide insertion in the canine interleukin-2 receptor gamma chain results in X-linked severe combined immunodeficiency disease, *Vet Immunol Immunopathol* 47:203-213, 1995.

Somberg RL, Robinson JP, Felsburg PJ: T lymphocyte development and function in dogs with X-linked combined immunodeficiency, *J Immunol* 153:4006-4016, 1994.

Thomas GW, Bell SC, Phythian C, et al: Aid to the antemortem diagnosis of Fell pony foal syndrome by the analysis of B lymphocytes, *Vet Rec* 152:618-621, 2003.

Ward DM, Shiflett SL, Kaplan J: Chediak-Higashi syndrome: a clinical and molecular view of a rare lysosomal storage disorder, *Curr Mol Med* 2:469-477, 2002.

Wiler R, Leber R, Moore BB, et al: Equine severe combined immunodeficiency: a defect in V(D)J recombination and DNA-dependent protein kinase activity, *Proc Natl Acad Sci USA* 92:11485-11489, 1995.

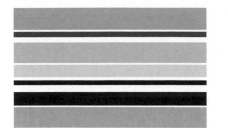

Secondary Immunological Defects

CHAPTER 36

The immune system, like any body system, is subject to destruction and dysfunction as a result of attacks by a variety of pathogenic agents or mechanisms. Among the most important of these agents are microorganisms, especially viruses, toxins, stress of various types, and malnutrition.

VIRUS-INDUCED IMMUNOSUPPRESSION

Viruses that affect the immune system may be divided into those that affect primary lymphoid tissues and those that affect secondary lymphoid tissues. For example, in chickens, the virus of infectious bursal disease (IBDV) destroys lymphocytes in the bursa of Fabricius. IBDV is not completely specific for bursal cells; it also destroys cells in the spleen and thymus. These tissues usually recover, however, whereas the bursa atrophies. The results of this disease, as might be predicted, are most evident in young birds infected soon after hatching, when the bursa is actively engaged in generating B cells.

The most important virus-induced immunodeficiency disease is acquired immune deficiency syndrome (AIDS), a disease of humans resulting from infection with one of the human immunodeficiency viruses (HIV-1 or HIV-2). Many viruses cause similar diseases in animals. Two that closely resemble human AIDS are simian AIDS and feline AIDS (Figure 36-1). Another animal virus that infects and destroys secondary lymphoid organs is canine distemper. Canine distemper virus, although it can multiply in many different cell types, has a predilection for lymphocytes, for epithelia, and for nervous tissue. The distemper virus spreads from the tonsils and bronchial lymph nodes to the spleen, lymph nodes, and bone marrow, where it replicates. The shedding of infected cells from these organs enables the virus to reach epithelial tissues and the brain. Canine distemper virus destroys lymphocytes and so produces a lymphopenia. It also depresses the activities of macrophages. Thus canine distemper virus suppresses production of IL-1 and IL-2 while stimulating prostaglandin release by macrophages. As a result, lymphocyte responses to mitogens are depressed, immunoglobulin levels fall, and immediate hypersensitivity and skin graft rejection are suppressed. This immunosuppression accounts, in large part, for the clinical signs of canine distemper, and a significant proportion of dogs with distemper develop *Pneumocystis carinii* pneumonia. (*P. carinii* is a fungus that occurs in the lungs. It never causes disease in immunocompetent animals but produces a severe pneumonia in animals with suppressed immune function. Indeed, the development of *Pneumocystis* pneumonia is clear evidence of a significant immunodeficiency.) If germfree dogs are infected by virulent distemper virus, they develop a mild disease, presumably because secondary infection cannot occur (Figure 36-2).

Loss of lymphocytes is common in virus infections, since viral survival and persistence may require immune

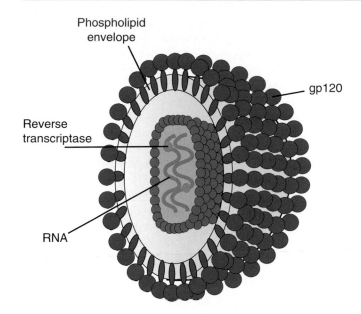

Figure 36-1. The structure of a typical retrovirus such as feline leukemia virus or feline lentivirus.

suppression. Thus a lymphopenia occurs in feline panleukopenia, canine parvovirus-2 infection, feline leukemia, and African swine fever. Bovine virus diarrhea virus (BVDV) causes a lymphopenia and destruction of both B and T cells in the lymph nodes, spleen, thymus, and Peyer's patches. As in canine distemper, surviving B cells fail to make immunoglobulins and respond poorly to mitogens. Viral destruction of the Peyer's patches causes intestinal ulceration and leads to secondary bacterial

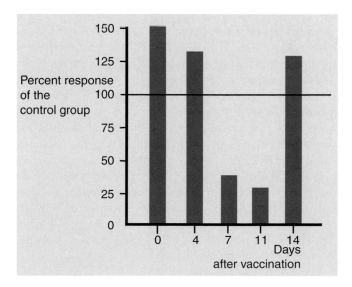

Figure 36-2. The immunosuppressive effect of viruses. The effect of administering a mixed vaccine (containing canine distemper, canine adenovirus, canine parainfluenza, canine parvovirus-2, and leptospira) on the response of a puppy's lymphocytes to the mitogen phytohemagglutinin. Control levels were 100%. (From Phillips TR, Jensen JL, Rubino MJ, et al: *Can J Vet Res* 53:154-160, 1989.)

invasion. Both persistently infected cattle and normal cattle infected with cytotoxic BVDV show depressed neutrophil functions such as degranulation and antibody-dependent cellular cytotoxicity. Bacterial clearance from blood is also impaired. A related virus, border disease virus, preferentially infects CD8+ T cells and interferes with their cytotoxic and immunoregulatory functions.

Herpesviruses are also immunosuppressive. For example, equine herpesvirus-1 causes a drop in T cell numbers and depresses cell-mediated responses in foals. Bovine herpesvirus-1 (BHV-1) also causes a drop in T cells and in the responses to T cell mitogens. Although BHV-1 stimulates bovine alveolar macrophages to express increased amounts of MHC class II molecules and promotes antibody-mediated phagocytosis, it also depresses macrophage-mediated cytotoxicity and IL-1 synthesis. Parainfluenza 3 and infectious bovine rhinotracheitis viruses have long been known to interfere with alveolar macrophage function. They inhibit phagosome-lysosome fusion, thus paving the way for secondary infections with *Mannheimia hemolytica* in stressed calves.

The effect of some viruses on the immune system may be relatively complex or anomalous (Box 36-1). In canine distemper, for instance, lymphocyte responses to phytohemagglutinin are depressed, but allograft rejection may

---

BOX 36–1

Viruses That Affect Lymphoid Tissues of Animals

VIRUSES THAT DESTROY LYMPHOID TISSUES
Human immunodeficiency virus
Measles virus
Simian immunodeficiency virus
Simian retrovirus, type D
Feline immunodeficiency virus
Feline leukemia virus
Feline panleukopenia virus
Equine herpesvirus 1
Canine distemper virus
African swine fever virus
Bovine virus diarrhea virus
Mouse thymus herpesvirus
Infectious bursal disease virus
Newcastle disease virus

VIRUSES THAT STIMULATE LYMPHOID TISSUE ACTIVITY
TO AN UNUSUAL EXTENT
Maedi-visna virus
Aleutian disease virus
Malignant catarrhal fever virus

VIRUSES THAT CAUSE LYMPHOID NEOPLASIA
Marek's disease virus
Feline leukemia virus
Bovine leukemia virus
Mouse leukemia virus
Human T cell leukemia virus 1

be normal. In visna, a neurological disease of sheep caused by a retrovirus, cell-mediated immune responses such as graft rejection are suppressed, whereas B cell responses are enhanced. Some leukemia viruses can exert selective depressive effects, so that depression of the IgG response is greater than that of the IgM response. In equine infectious anemia, the IgG3 response is variably depressed, whereas synthesis of the other immunoglobulin classes remains unaffected. It has been claimed that chickens infected with Marek's disease virus show both enhanced graft-versus-host disease and depressed graft rejection!

The results of virus-induced lymphoid tissue destruction are readily seen. Animals are lymphopenic and have reduced lymphocyte responses to mitogens. For example, the responses to phytohemagglutinin are depressed in influenza, measles, canine distemper, Marek's disease, Newcastle disease, feline leukemia, bovine virus diarrhea, and lymphocytic choriomeningitis. Destruction of lymphoid tissue may also result in hypogammaglobulinemia or a reduced response to antigens. Thymic atrophy and lymphopenia are common manifestations of many virus infections, and before a primary immunodeficiency syndrome is diagnosed, rigorous steps must be taken to exclude the possibility that it is, in fact, secondary to a virus infection.

RETROVIRUS INFECTIONS IN PRIMATES

Human immunodeficiency virus (HIV-1) almost certainly originated from a strain of simian immunodeficiency virus (SIV_{cpz}), which normally infects chimpanzees (*Pan troglodytes*) in parts of central Africa. SIV_{cpz} probably jumped to humans and mutated slightly to become HIV-1. It can infect but very rarely causes disease in chimpanzees. Other primates such as pig-tailed macaques (*Macaca nemestrina*) can only be transiently infected with HIV-1 but are not immunosuppressed and remain healthy. A distantly related virus, HIV-2, can cause disease in baboons (*Papio cyanocephalus*) and pig-tailed macaques, but its natural reservoir is the sooty mangabey (*Cercocebus atys*). Rhesus (*Macaca mulatta*) and cynomolgus (*M. fascicularis*) macaques may be persistently infected with HIV-2 but do not develop disease. There are several interesting nonprimate models of HIV infection. Rabbits are susceptible to persistent HIV infection but, like macaques, do not develop disease. When reconstituted with human lymphocytes, *scid* mice can harbor HIV, but the virus destroys their T cells very rapidly in a manner unlike the natural disease.

Many different lentiviruses have been isolated from primates, especially African species. These simian immunodeficiency viruses include SIV_{mac} isolated from a rhesus macaque in a laboratory; SIV_{agm} from an African green monkey; SIV_{sm} from a sooty mangabey; SIV_{mnd} from a mandrill; and most important, SIV_{cpz} from a chimpanzee. As pointed out previously, SIV_{cpz} is probably the ancestor of HIV-1, whereas SIV_{sm} is the ancestor of HIV-2. All these isolates selectively invade CD4+ T cells. When SIV_{mac} infects rhesus macaques and other Asian species, it causes an immunodeficiency syndrome similar to human AIDS. Sexual transmission is suspected. The animals develop lymphadenopathy, severe weight loss, chronic diarrhea, lymphomas, neurological lesions and opportunistic infections by organisms such as *P. carinii*, *Mycobacterium avium-intracellulare*, *Candida albicans*, and *Cryptosporidium parvum*. The macaques are immunosuppressed as a result of depletion of CD4+ T cells and macrophages. About 25% of infected animals do not mount a significant response to SIV and die within 3 to 5 months, with the remainder usually dying 1 to 3 years after infection. Spontaneous recovery does not occur. The other SIVs cause persistent viremia but rarely result in disease in African primates.

Type D Simian Retroviruses

An acquired immunodeficiency syndrome develops in primates infected with one of several endogenous type D simian retroviruses (SRVs). These viruses, much more common than the lentiviruses, are transmitted by biting, with inoculation of saliva or blood; vertical transmission rarely occurs. SRVs have a much broader tissue tropism than the SIVs and, in addition to lymphocytes and macrophages, can also infect fibroblasts, epithelial cells, and the central nervous system. The SRVs destroy both B and T cells leading to death from opportunistic infections. The syndrome is associated with a profound drop in serum IgG and IgM levels and a severe lymphopenia. Monocyte function is unimpaired, but surviving lymphocytes do not respond to mitogens. Affected monkeys are also profoundly neutropenic. On necropsy, the monkeys have a generalized lymphadenopathy, hepatomegaly, and splenomegaly. There is a loss of lymphocytes from the T-dependent areas of the secondary lymphoid organs. B cell areas show an initial hyperplasia of the secondary follicles followed by the loss of these follicles and an absence of plasma cells. These histological changes are very similar to those seen in AIDS in humans. In many cases, normally innocuous agents such as *P. carinii*, cytomegalovirus, *C. parvum*, and *C. albicans* cause infection. Some affected monkeys develop tumors such as fibrosarcomas. About one half of the infected animals develop neutralizing antibodies and survive the disease. The others die from septicemia or diarrhea with wasting.

RETROVIRUS INFECTIONS IN CATS

Feline Leukemia

Feline leukemia virus (FeLV) is an oncogenic retrovirus that can cause both proliferative and degenerative diseases in cats. Three naturally occurring viral subgroups are recognized based on the structure of their gp70 protein. FeLV-A is the predominant, naturally transmitted subgroup. It is present in all FeLV-infected cats. The viruses of the other subgroups are only found in association with FeLV-A. When FeLV-A combines with endogenous retroviral sequences (sequences that are stably integrated into the cat genome and are normally never expressed but are genetically transmitted), FeLV-B is formed. FeLV-B is found in about 50% of viremic cats and has a greater propensity than FeLV-A to cause tumors. FeLV-C is found in about 1% to 2% of infected cats and arises from FeLV-A through a mutation in the envelope gene. It is much more suppressive for bone marrow than FeLV-A.

FOCMA. In many cases of feline lymphosarcoma, a unique surface protein is expressed on infected cells. This protein is called feline oncornavirus cell membrane antigen (FOCMA). Endogenous retroviral genes within the cat genome code for FOCMA. It is not expressed on normal cells but on cells infected with FeLV or FeSV. It was originally believed that the presence of FOCMA on a cell membrane identified the cell as an FeLV-induced tumor cell. Of those cats that fail to make neutralizing antibodies to FeLV and so remain viremic, about 80% develop antitumor activity by making antibodies against FOCMA. A cat that makes antibodies to FOCMA can usually destroy virus-induced tumor cells. Unfortunately, antibodies to FOCMA do not confer protection against the FeLV-induced degenerative diseases, and viremic cats that fail to produce anti-FOCMA antibodies are fully susceptible to all the FeLV syndromes, including lymphosarcoma. Some feline lymphosarcoma cells may express FOCMA in the absence of any evidence of FeLV infection.

Transmission. FeLV is shed in body secretions, especially saliva and nasal secretions and is thus transmitted between cats as a result of grooming. On natural exposure to FeLV, about 70% of cats become infected, but the remaining 30% do not. Of the infected cats, about 60% become immune and 40% become viremic. Of viremic cats, 10% cure spontaneously, whereas the remaining 90% remain infected for life. Of these persistently viremic animals, about 15% live normal healthy lives, but the remaining animals die within 3 to 5 years from FeLV disease. Lymphoid tumors develop in 15% to 20% of FeLV-infected cats. Persistently viremic cats have a half-life of 1 year.

Pathogenesis. Once FeLV infects a cat, the virus first grows in the lymphoid tissues of the pharynx and tonsils. This is followed by a transient viremia as it spreads throughout the body and infects all the other lymphoid organs. A mild lymphopenia occurs 1 to 2 weeks after infection. This is of variable duration but lasts longer in young cats than in adults. There is also a variable

neutropenia. Antibodies develop between 7 and 42 days after the onset of infection and the virus is cleared between 28 and 42 days. Virus can be found in the thymus at day 1, in blood between 2 and 145 days, and in lymphoid organs between 3 and 28 days. The presence of both antibodies and virus results in the formation of large amounts of immune-complexes and the development of a glomerulopathy. Some cats may lose their viremia but remain latently infected. In latently infected animals, the virus persists in the bone marrow, but there is no virus in the blood and virus-neutralizing antibodies are present. Treatment with steroids or culturing bone marrow cells in vitro allows productive reexpression of the virus. Stress (for example, steroid treatment, crowding, or shipping) may cause a recurrence of viremia in 5% to 10% of cats. The presence of neutralizing antibodies does not correlate well with the disease state, and challenging recovered cats may not provoke a secondary antibody response. Prenatal or early infection of kittens with FeLV can also result in a persistent viremia.

Tumors. Cats probably have the highest prevalence of lymphoid tumors of any domestic mammal. Most of these lymphoid tumors are caused by FeLV. They include lymphosarcoma, reticulum cell sarcoma, erythroleukemia, and granulocytic leukemias. The lymphosarcoma caused by FeLV is usually a T cell neoplasm, although FeLV grows in cells of many types and is not restricted to lymphoid tissues. Some FeLV lymphomas in the intestine may be of B cell origin. When tumors develop in FeLV-infected cats, not all can be shown to contain the virus. The proportion of positive cases range from 100% of myeloid leukemias to 30% of alimentary lymphomas. In young cats FeLV-induced tumors are mainly of T cell origin. In older cats they tend to be both T and B cell in origin.

Immunosuppression. Feline leukemia virus destroys lymphocytes and suppresses their function.

T cell defects. Cats infected with FeLV develop T cell tropic variants as a result of the development of mutations in their envelope. These immunodeficiency-inducing variants can replicate to high numbers in T cells. They enter T cells by binding to two receptors. One receptor is a phosphate transporter protein (Pit1). The second is a novel cell surface protein called FeLIX ("FeLV infectivity X-essory protein"). The lymphopenia in FeLV-infected cats is due to a loss of CD4+ T cells. CD8+ T cells may also drop in the early stages of the disease so that the CD4:CD8 ratio can remain within normal limits. (The CD4:CD8 ratio in normal cats ranges from about 0.4 to 3.5, with a median value of about 1.9.) CD8+ T cell numbers eventually recover so that the CD4:CD8 ratio may then drop. B cell numbers may also be depressed, but this depends on the severity of secondary infections. Kittens infected with FeLV develop a wasting syndrome associated with thymic atrophy and recurrent infections. Depending on the severity of the secondary infections, this may be associated with either lymphoid atrophy or lymphoid hyperplasia. In cats without secondary infection, lymphoid atrophy is associated with loss of cells from the paracortical areas of lymph nodes. The changes in the spleens of these animals are less marked but may result in a reduction in the entire white pulp. As a result of T cell loss, FeLV infected cats have depressed cell-mediated immunity. The surviving T cells show depressed responses to mitogens. This depression is probably due to the effects of p15e, the immunosuppressive envelope protein of the FeLV virus, which is produced in very large quantities by dying cells. p15e suppresses the responses of cats to FOCMA, suppresses lymphocyte mitogen responses, and blocks the responses of T cells to IL-1 and IL-2. As a result, FeLV-infected cats may carry skin allografts for about twice as long as normal cats (24 days as compared with 12). The leukocytes of cats infected with FeLV produce significantly less IL-2 than leukocytes from normal cats. This decline in IL-2 production is especially marked in cats with leukemia or lymphosarcoma arising in the thymus. This immunosuppression also predisposes viremic cats to secondary diseases such as feline infectious peritonitis, hemobartonellosis, toxoplasmosis, septicemia, and fungal infections. Bone marrow stem cells are also inhibited by p15e, preventing production of erythroid cells and causing a nonregenerative anemia.

B cell defects. In contrast to the severe T cell dysfunction, B cell activities in FeLV infected cats are only mildly impaired. There may be poor responses to low doses of antigen, as well as reduced IgM production, but serum IgG levels remain normal. Because B cell function and antibody production are relatively normal in chronically infected cats, antibodies to the virus are produced in large quantities. These antibodies combine with circulating virions or soluble proteins to form immune-complexes. The immune-complexes are deposited in the renal glomeruli and cause severe MPGN, leading to hypoproteinemia, edema, uremia, and death. Viral antigens binding to erythrocytes can also cause an antiglobulin-positive hemolytic anemia. Immune-complexes also activate the classical complement pathway. As a result, complement will be consumed and FeLV cats may have very low levels of complement. This loss may reduce resistance to tumors since normal cat serum infused into leukemic cats can cause tumor regression.

FeLV-AIDS. During natural FeLV infection a form of the virus may develop that is profoundly immunosuppressive. Called FeLV-AIDS, this causes fatal immunodeficiency in nearly 100% of infected cats. The isolate consists of two virus populations. One, designated 61E, is replication-competent but does not induce immunodeficiency disease by itself. The other, 61C, is replication-defective, but when inoculated together with 61E, it induces a fatal immunodeficiency syndrome. A viral chimera has been constructed that has properties intermediate between those of the two originating strains.

The immunodeficiency syndrome is characterized by progressive weight loss and lymphoid hyperplasia followed by severe lymphoid depletion, chronic diarrhea, and opportunistic infections. The onset of clinical disease is preceded by the accumulation of unintegrated viral DNA in the bone marrow and by an early and drastic drop in CD4+ T cells, whereas CD8+ T cell and B cell numbers remain normal. Genetic analysis has shown that the immunodeficiency is associated with mutations in a 34 amino acid sequence at the C-terminus of viral gp70. The mutation changes the conformation of the surface glycoprotein, which affects the ability of the virus to bind to cell receptors and block infection by additional virions leading to subsequent cell killing. The defect in FeLV-AIDS is an inability to mount antibody responses, although in vitro B cell function appears to be normal. An inability to respond to T-independent antigens precedes the loss of CD4+ T cells. Thus, as early as 9 weeks after infection, the CD4+ T cells produce lower levels of B cell stimulatory cytokines.

Immunity. About 40% of cats infected with FeLV do not mount an adequate immune response against the virus and become persistently infected. Persistently infected cats remain viremic. About 60% of infected cats mount a strong immune response. These cats develop virus-neutralizing antibodies to the major envelope glycoprotein, gp70. Immune cats also develop virus-specific cytotoxic T cells to viral gag/pro antigens. These prevent the virus from invading cells, and these cats become strongly immune. Antibodies against antigens other than gp70 may also play a role in immunity.

Three types of effective vaccines have been developed against FeLV. One type contains supernatant fluid from a cell line persistently infected with FeLV. This fluid contains several of the major protein antigens of FeLV. The second and most common type of FeLV vaccine consists of inactivated whole virions, which are usually administered with a powerful adjuvant. The third type of FeLV vaccine contains pure gp70 obtained from recombinant *Escherichia coli*. Resistance to FeLV is associated with a response to gp70, but other virion antigens are required for maximal protection. Widespread vaccination has significantly reduced the prevalence of this disease in the United States.

Diagnosis. FeLV viremia may be detected by an ELISA, by the membrane filter technique, or by rapid immunochromatography on a blood or serum sample. A direct immunofluorescent test on a buffy coat smear using antibodies to group-specific antigen can detect cell-associated antigen (Figure 36-3). Some of these tests may detect infection before the development of viremia, since soluble virus antigens are shed into the bloodstream. Alternative testing methods include testing saliva

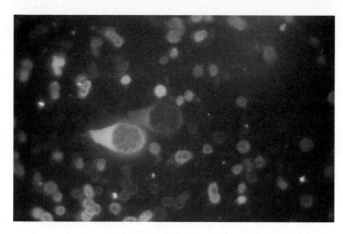

Figure 36-3. A positive indirect immunofluorescence assay for FeLV in a peripheral blood smear. (Courtesy of Dr. FC Heck.)

or tears using material collected on a swab or filter paper strips. Polymerase chain reaction (PCR)–based assays may be used to detect viral nucleic acid.

Feline Immunodeficiency Virus

Feline immunodeficiency virus (FIV) was originally isolated from cats with clinical immunodeficiency. The virus is an enveloped, single-stranded RNA virus belonging to the lentivirus subgroup of retroviruses. It is differentiated from FeLV (a gammaretrovirus) by the biochemical requirements of its reverse transcriptase. (FIV reverse transcriptase requires magnesium, whereas FeLV requires manganese). FIV is related to HIV, the cause of AIDS (Figure 36-4). FeLV and FIV are distinctly different viruses, and antibodies made against one do not react with the other. Nevertheless, approximately 12% to 33% of FIV-infected cats may also be infected with FeLV, an especially potent immunosuppressive mixture. At least five different genetic subtypes of FIV have been identified.

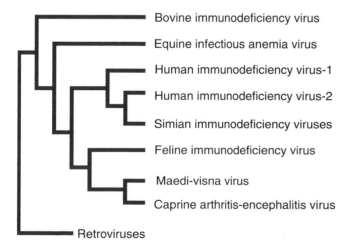

Figure 36-4. A dendrogram showing the relationships of the major lentiviruses.

Subtype variations may account for differences in pathogenicity, tissue tropism, and clinical disease.

Transmission. FIV is spread by territorial free-roaming male cats through aggressive biting. As a result, it occurs predominantly in old male cats that spend a lot of time outdoors. Oral exposure is a potential route of infection in suckling kittens, and chronically infected queens transmit viruses to more than half their kittens in utero. Noninfected kittens from chronically infected queens show reduced neonatal viability. FIV can also be sexually transmitted. In households where cats live together nonaggressively, sharing food or water bowls and undergoing mutual grooming, the infection is poorly spread. In the United States, 1% to 3% of normal healthy cats and 10% to 15% of chronically ill cats are infected with FIV. In some countries, such as Japan, the infection rate may be as high as 44%.

Pathogenesis. Experimental infection of cats with FIV is characterized by four distinct clinical stages. The acute stage lasts for several weeks. Infected cats develop a fever about 3 to 10 weeks after exposure to FIV. The virus is carried to local lymph nodes, where it replicates in T cells. It then spreads to other lymph nodes throughout the body. FIV can be isolated from infected cats as early as 10 to 14 days after infection. Viremia increases until day 21, peaks again at 7 to 8 weeks and then declines. Disease severity varies from no clinical signs to generalized lymphadenopathy and lymphoid hyperplasia. Cats can develop fever, anorexia, dehydration, and diarrhea with mild pneumonitis, conjunctivitis, and nephritis. They may develop a mild lymphopenia and a severe neutropenia at this time. The lymphopenia is due to a loss of CD4+ T cells. Cats rarely die at this stage unless they are also infected with FeLV, in which case they die of a panleukopenia. Antibodies to FIV develop 2 to 6 weeks after infection and persist throughout infection. Most cats recover from this stage and appear normal.

The asymptomatic, or latent, stage may last as long as 10 years and is longer in young than in older cats. Cats are clinically healthy during this stage, but there is a progressive drop in their CD4+ T cell numbers. Their lymph nodes show gradual hypoplasia, leading to aplasia. Cats may also develop signs of bone marrow suppression, including leukopenia and anemia. Thus this stage is marked by progressive impairment of immune function, but it may be many years before severe immunodeficiency and AIDS-like signs develop.

The gradual onset of progressive generalized lymphadenopathy marks the third stage of the disease. This lasts for months to years and is associated with vague signs of ill health, such as recurrent fever, inappetence, weight loss, chronic stomatitis, arthritis, and behavioral abnormalities. Lymph nodes develop follicular hyperplasia. As a result of the growing immunodeficiency, cats may develop secondary but not opportunistic infections. These are mainly bacterial infections affecting the oral cavity, skin, and digestive tract. Cats will show some weight loss (less than 20%), anemia, lymphopenia, and neutropenia.

The final stage is a severe AIDS-like disease that lasts for a few months until the cat dies. Lymphoid tissue shows follicular involution. Cats show a weight loss of greater than 20%. Because of their severe immunodeficiency, opportunistic infections develop. These can include feline herpesvirus type 1, rodent poxviruses, vaccine-induced rabies, FeLV, staphylococcal infections, anaerobic infections, tuberculosis (*M. avium/intracellulare*), *Cryptococcus*, toxoplasmosis, mange, lungworms, and heartworms. The animals have anemia, lymphopenia, and neutropenia. Malignancies and ocular and neurological disease also occur. In naturally infected cats, clinical findings are highly variable because of the great variety of potential secondary infections. They can include chronic fever, oral cavity disease (periodontitis/gingivitis/stomatitis) leading to inappetence or pain on eating, chronic upper respiratory tract disease, chronic enteritis leading to persistent diarrhea, and conjunctivitis. Some cats may experience cystitis, chronic skin disease, fever, anorexia, lethargy, abortion or reproductive problems, vomiting, anemia, leukopenia, lymphosarcoma, and myeloproliferative disorders. Neurological signs have been described in FIV-infected cats, and the virus has been shown to infect the central nervous system. Half of FIV-infected cats have neurological dysfunction, as demonstrated by abnormal behavior, convulsions, ataxia, paralysis, and nystagmus. FIV is associated with demyelination in the dorsal columns of the spinal cord, vacuolization of the myelin sheaths in the spinal nerve roots, and perivascular and perineuronal mononuclear cell infiltration. Ocular lesions, especially anterior uveitis, conjunctivitis, and glaucoma have also been noted.

Immunosuppression. FIV can replicate in CD4+ and CD8+ T cells, B cells, megakaryocytes, neuronal cells, and in macrophages. Some strains only replicate well in lymphocytes, whereas other strains replicate well in both lymphocytes and macrophages. Some FIV strains can also grow in fibroblasts in vitro. Primary targets of FIV infection are the lymphocytes. However, as infection persists, the virus increasingly affects macrophages. In clinically ill cats with a high viral load, macrophages are the major sites of viral replication. FIV-infected cats have fewer neutrophils, a lower proportion of T cells, and a higher proportion of B cells compared with uninfected animals.

FIV does not bind to T cells through CD4 but through the feline homolog of CD134, as well as the α-chemokine receptor CXCR4 (CD184) in a manner similar to HIV. Most naturally infected cats have a critical loss of CD4+ T cells (Figure 36-5). This loss is a result of destruction of infected cells, decreased production, and premature apoptosis. The surviving CD4 cells may show reduced responses to mitogens. FIV cats may show a shift away from a Th1 cytokine production pattern. They may also show an increase in CD8+ T cells. As a result, the CD4:CD8 ratio of FIV-infected cats may drop from a normal value of about two to less than one.

The lymphopenia that develops in both FeLV and FIV infections is due to a loss of T cells. CD4+ T cells are depressed in both, but the depression is much greater in FIV-infected animals than in FeLV-infected animals. FIV infected cats show a rapid drop in T cell numbers, whereas B cells are unaffected. Their CD8+ T cells recover, but their CD4+ T cells fail to do so. Within 6 months of FIV infection, there is a measurable drop in CD4+ T cells and in the lymphocyte response to pokeweed mitogen (PWM), a B cell mitogen. (The B cell response to PWM requires functional CD4+ T cells). The response

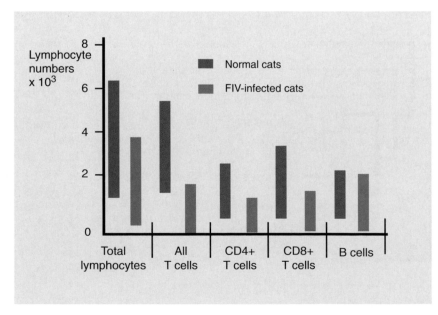

Figure 36-5. The numbers of cells in different lymphocyte populations (pan T, CD4, CD8, B cells) for 11 normal cats and 11 cats infected with feline immunodeficiency virus. (From Novotney C, English RV, Housman J, et al: *AIDS* 4:1213-1218, 1990.)

to thymus-dependent and -independent antigens remains unchanged. By 2 to 3 years after the onset of infection, however, the drop in CD4+ T cells continues, and the response to the T cell mitogen, Con A, becomes depressed. The response to thymus-dependent antigens is profoundly depressed by this stage, but the response to thymus-independent antigens is normal. Other changes that occur in FIV-infected cats include depressed responses to phytohemagglutinin and lipopolysaccharide, reduced production of IL-2, and depressed responses to IL-2. Affected cats may upregulate IL-10 transcription, which may contribute to their immunodeficiency. FIV-infected cats may have normal numbers of CD8+ T cells and B cells and normal levels of IgM and IgA. More than 25% of FIV-infected cats may be hypergammaglobulinemic as a result of polyclonal B cell activation 6 to 8 weeks after infection. Despite this, the response of FIV-infected cats to antigens such as diphtheria toxoid may be depressed. Affected cats may have high levels of immune complexes in their serum and deposited in renal glomeruli.

Immunity and diagnosis. Clinical symptoms are not sufficient to reliably diagnose FIV infection. The infection is therefore diagnosed by testing for antibodies in serum by ELISA or immunochromatography and should be confirmed by Western blotting or PCR. Antibodies appear as early as 2 weeks after infection, and most cats are positive by 60 days. These antibodies persist for the life of the animal. In the terminal stages antibodies may fall to undetectable levels. Maternal antibodies persist in most kittens born to FIV-positive queens for the first 8 to 12 weeks of life regardless of whether the kitten is infected. Some may remain seropositive up to 16 weeks. These antibodies afford protection since passive immunization is effective, and kittens that receive high levels of antibodies from vaccinated or infected queens are protected.

Once infected with FIV, a cat will remain infected for life. However, viral regression may occur in kittens vertically infected by their mothers. At 3 to 4 months of age, these kittens may lose detectable antibody and virus in their blood, although the virus persists at low levels in bone marrow and lymph nodes. The presence of very low levels of viruses in an animal can be detected by PCR.

Envelope glycoproteins do stimulate strong cell-mediated and humoral immunity in cats. Good results have been obtained using inactivated whole FIV and certain DNA vaccines; a killed vaccine against FIV has recently been licensed. Like HIV, the antigenic diversity of FIV subtypes complicates vaccine development, and it is likely that a multisubtype vaccine will be required to provide optimal immunity.

Treatment. Treatment of FIV infection is symptomatic and can involve the use of antibiotics to control bacterial infections, fluid therapy, and possibly dietary supplements. AZT (zidovudine, azidothymidine) is the only drug known to have an antiviral effect in clinically affected cats. It appears to improve the health of affected cats and increases both their quality of life and survival. Unfortunately, AZT-resistant strains of FIV may develop, and the drug seems to be of limited benefit in clinically ill cats. Encouraging results have also been obtained by the use of bone marrow allografts in association with antiviral therapy.

RETROVIRUS INFECTIONS IN CATTLE

Bovine Immunodeficiency Virus

Bovine immunodeficiency virus (BIV) is a lentivirus originally isolated from a cow with lymphosarcoma. The BIV-infected animal showed lymph node hyperplasia, lymphocytosis, central nervous system lesions, loss of weight, and weakness. When used to infect calves, BIV shows limited pathogenicity. The animals develop transient lymphocytosis, lymphadenopathy, and a non-suppurative meningoencephalitis. BIV infection may also cause minor changes in the response of bovine lymphocytes to mitogens and may suppress some neutrophil functions such as ADCC several months after infection. BIV can also infect sheep. In this species, infection is associated with an increase in CD2+ and CD4+ T cells, as well as in the CD4:CD8 ratio between 6 and 8 months after inoculation. The sheep showed no signs of illness by 1 year after inoculation and appeared to have normal immune function. BIV can also cause a chronic infection of rabbits, which leads to splenomegaly and lymphadenopathy.

Jembrana disease is a lentivirus infection that occurs in Balinese cattle (*Bos javaensis*). It causes intense lymphoproliferation in the lymph nodes and spleen in these cattle. Animals that recover are completely immune.

RETROVIRUS INFECTIONS IN DOGS

A lentivirus has been isolated from the mononuclear cells of a leukemic German shepherd dog in Israel. It has been called canine immunodeficiency virus (CIV). This virus does not appear to be closely related to the other major lentiviruses. On inoculation into newborn beagles, it caused pronounced lymphadenopathy. It is anticipated, however, that several years would pass before major disease symptoms presented themselves.

Another retrovirus has been isolated from a dog with a severe acquired immunodeficiency syndrome in the United States. This animal had anemia, neutropenia, lymphopenia, and thrombocytopenia, as well as depressed humoral and T cell–mediated immune responses. On necropsy the dog showed depletion of lymphoid organs and bone marrow hypoplasia. Yet it also had plasma cell infiltrates in many organs, as well as multiple secondary infections. The retrovirus isolated from this animal was of the C-type, and it possessed a gene that cross-reacted with the polymerase gene of bovine leukemia virus. It is also interesting to note that this animal had received multiple blood transfusions, a route of infection well recognized for HIV.

A lentivirus has been isolated from a dog with hemorrhagic gastroenteritis. This animal showed a lymphopenia and agammaglobulinemia with lymphoid and bone marrow hypoplasia. A retrovirus was isolated that could grow in canine lymphocytes and thymocytes; it had a magnesium-dependent reverse transcriptase. The virus was present in bone marrow, intestine, and lymph nodes. It caused reduced synthesis of IL-2 by canine cells, reduced their responsiveness to IL-2, and was cytotoxic for lymphocytes.

CIRCOVIRUS INFECTIONS

Circoviruses are small, nonenveloped DNA viruses that have a propensity to damage lymphoid tissues. They include the chicken anemia agent, which infects hemocytoblasts in the bone marrow and precursor T cells in the thymus, beak-and-feather disease virus, which can cause lymphoid atrophy in psittacine birds, and porcine circovirus-2 (PCV2), which may cause postweaning multisystemic wasting syndrome (PMWS). PMWS is an acquired immunodeficiency syndrome of piglets characterized by postweaning wasting, lymphadenopathy, and respiratory disease with occasional pallor, jaundice, and diarrhea. Some affected piglets have a profound lymphopenia, initially involving CD4, CD8, and double-positive T cells. T cell areas in tonsils and lymph nodes are depleted, and there is an absence of follicles. IgM$^+$ B cells are also reduced in more chronic cases. Lymphoid depletion is directly related to viral load in lymphoid organs. Piglets suffer from a variety of secondary and opportunistic infections. While PCV2 is the most likely causative agent, it has proved difficult to reproduce the disease consistently, and other factors are clearly required. These include environmental factors, other infectious agents, and possibly immune stimulation.

JUVENILE LLAMA IMMUNODEFICIENCY SYNDROME

A severe immunodeficiency syndrome affecting young llamas has been recognized. It has not been reported in other South American camelids. The disease is not due to failure of passive transfer, since the median age of onset is approximately 1 year (range 2 to 30 months). Most affected animals are clinically normal and grow well until weaning. Initial signs include failure to grow, weight loss,

and repeated multiple opportunistic infections with a variety of bacteria, fungal, and protozoan organisms. Respiratory tract infections are common. *P. carinii* infection has been recorded in some animals. The animals have low to low-normal lymphocyte numbers. They have depressed lymphocyte responses to mitogens such as phytohemagglutinin, concanavalin A, and streptococcal protein A. Lymph node biopsies show marked depletion of T cells in the paracortical areas, and the primary follicles in the B cell areas appear small and lack germinal centers. The animals also have low serum IgG levels and respond very poorly to *Clostridium perfringens* vaccines. Thus both T and B cell responses are depressed. The cause of this syndrome is unknown. Some investigators have detected reverse transcriptase activity in tissues and seen particles on electron microscopy that are compatible with a retrovirus infection. Nevertheless, the consistent occurrence of this disease in young llamas suggests that it may be inherited. Although treatment is supportive, the long-term prognosis for these animals is poor.

OTHER CAUSES OF SECONDARY IMMUNODEFICIENCY

Microbial and Parasite Infections

Immunosuppression generally accompanies infestation with *Toxoplasma* or trypanosomes, helminths such as *Trichinella spiralis*, arthropods such as *Demodex*, and bacteria such as *Mannheimia haemolytica*, the actinobacilli, and some streptococci.

Toxin-Induced Immunosuppression

Many environmental toxins such as polychlorinated biphenyls, polybrominated biphenyls, dieldrin, iodine, lead, cadmium, methyl mercury, and DDT are immunosuppressive. $CdCl_2$ and $HgCl_2$ both inhibit phagocytosis by bovine leukocytes at very low concentrations. Higher concentrations are required to inhibit NK cell function and cell proliferation. Mycotoxins may be important immunosuppressants in cases where cattle or poultry are given feed containing moldy grain. These include T-2 toxin from *Fusarium*, which depresses the response of calf lymphocytes to mitogens and decreases the chemotactic migration of neutrophils. T-2 toxin also reduces IgM, IgA, and C3 levels in cattle. Aflatoxins increase the susceptibility of chickens to *Salmonella* as a result of depressed phagocytic activity. They depress piglet growth and reduced immune responses to *Mycoplasma*. Fumonisin B1 inhibits division of both T and B cells in piglets, increases IFN-γ production while suppressing IL-4 production, and increases susceptibility to *E. coli* infections. Ochratoxins and trichothecenes are also immunosuppressive in pigs and birds. Toxin-induced immunosuppression may be especially important in wild carnivores situated at the top of the food chain. A good example of this is seen in seals feeding on environmentally contaminated fish. These animals show depressed responses to vaccines, impaired mitogenic responses, lowered delayed hypersensitivity responses, and reduced NK cell numbers. This immunosuppression may decrease their resistance to phocine morbillivirus.

Malnutrition and the Immune Response

It has long been recognized that famine and disease are closely associated, and we tend to assume that malnutrition leads to increased susceptibility to infection. This is not necessarily true, however, because the effects of malnutrition on immune functions are complex. For example, malnutrition can include not only deficiencies but also excesses or imbalances of individual nutrients.

In general, severe nutritional deficiencies reduce T-cell function and therefore impair cell-mediated responses, at the same time sparing B cell function and humoral immunity. Thus starvation rapidly induces thymic atrophy and a reduction in the level of thymic hormones. The number of circulating T cells drops, and cells are lost from the T-cell areas of secondary lymphoid tissue. Delayed hypersensitivity reactions are reduced, allograft rejection is delayed, and interferon production is impaired. Some studies have suggested that protein starvation selectively suppresses Th2 responses such as IL-4 and IgE production, leading to increased susceptibility to parasite invasion. This starvation-induced immunosuppression is likely mediated through the hormone leptin. The levels of leptin found in blood are proportional to body fat mass since leptin is primarily secreted by adipocytes. Starvation thus lowers blood leptin levels. Leptin acts on Th1 cells to enhance cytokine levels and on macrophages to promote phagocytosis. Starved animals with reduced blood leptin are therefore immunosuppressed and have reduced resistance to some infections. This immunosuppression can be reversed by administration of leptin to starved animals.

Severe starvation has little effect on B cell functions. The B cell areas in lymphoid tissues and the number of circulating B cells remain unchanged. Serum immunoglobulins of all classes may remain normal or even rise. Secretory IgA levels commonly drop, but secretory IgE may rise, suggesting abnormal immunoregulation. Starvation will, however, result in depressed complement levels and impairment of neutrophil and macrophage chemotaxis, the respiratory burst, release of lysosomal enzymes, and microbicidal activity.

Several trace elements and vitamins are required for optimal functioning of the immune system. The most important trace elements are zinc, copper, selenium, and iron. Deficiencies of any of these are immunosuppressive. Zinc is especially critical for the proper functioning of the immune system. Zinc deficiency is associated with lymphoid atrophy and delayed cell-mediated responses such as allograft rejection. Zinc-deficient pigs have reduced thymus weight, depressed cytotoxic T cell activity, depressed B cell activity and depressed NK cell activity. They show decreased antibody production to T-dependent antigens. If pregnant animals are deprived of zinc, their offspring are immunosuppressed. Phagocytic cells from zinc-deficient animals show reduced chemotaxis and microbial ingestion. Mild zinc supplementation may promote immune responses. Copper deficiencies are also immunosuppressive. Thus a copper deficiency reduces neutrophil numbers and function by depressing superoxide production. It also reduces lymphocyte responsiveness to mitogens, reduces T, B, and NK cell numbers, and enhances mast cell histamine release. Selenium deficiency depresses the function of most immune cells, reducing neutrophil activity, T and NK cell responses, and IgM production. Supplementation with selenium upregulates the expression of the IL-2R and prevents oxidative damage to immune cells. Iron deficiency is immunosuppressive for cell-mediated responses. However, the effects of this on resistance to infection may be complex, since many pathogens require iron to replicate. Other important minerals include magnesium, where a deficiency suppresses immunoglobulin levels.

In general, the antioxidant vitamins A and E are most important for proper immune function. Thus deficiencies of vitamin A reduce lymphocyte proliferation, NK cell activity, and cytokine and immunoglobulin production. Vitamin E is a major antioxidant in cell membranes and is important therefore in regulating the oxidants produced by phagocytic cells. Vitamin E deficiency depresses immunoglobulin levels through its effects on regulatory T cells and results in decreased lymphocyte responses to mitogens. Animals deficient in vitamin E also show reduced IL-2 and transferrin receptor expression and depressed phagocytic function. Vitamin E is one of the few vitamins where supplementation has been shown to enhance immune responses and disease resistance. Other vitamins essential for proper immune function include vitamin B12 and folic acid required for cell-mediated immune responses. Some B vitamins are required to maintain immunoglobulin levels, while vitamin D is required for proper macrophage development.

Taurine deficiencies in cats can result in a neutropenia, although mononuclear cell numbers may rise. The neutrophils of taurine-deficient cats show decreased respiratory burst activity and phagocytosis. Although these cats may show a hypergammaglobulinemia, there is regression of follicular centers, suggesting a loss of B cell activity.

The effects of malnutrition may be reflected in altered resistance to infectious diseases. Because bacteria can readily survive and multiply in body tissues despite malnutrition of the host, starvation commonly increases the severity of bacterial infections such as pneumonia.

Viruses, in contrast, usually require healthy host cells in which to grow. Malnutrition, by rendering host cells unhealthy, can therefore increase resistance to viruses. Overnutrition can also influence susceptibility to viruses. For example, overfed dogs show an increased susceptibility to canine distemper and canine adenovirus 1. Since obesity and overeating are functionally immunosuppressive, it follows that animals in high-yielding production systems may also be immunosuppressed.

Exercise and the Immune Response

Regular moderate exercise boosts immune function. Increased antibody responses are seen in mice that get moderate exercise as compared with unexercised control mice. Exercise raises blood neutrophil levels, enhances NK cell activity, promotes lymphocyte responses to mitogens, and increases blood levels of IL-1, IL-6, and TNF-α. As a result, regularly exercised mice show a delay in tumor growth after administration of syngeneic tumor cells. On the other hand, strenuous exercise is stressful and enhances susceptibility to infectious disease. Thus, although mild exercise is good for immune function, high-intensity exercise, prolonged exhaustive exercise, or overtraining may induce a functional immunodeficiency. A decreased proliferative response of blood lymphocytes can be found in horses for up to 16 hours after a race. It is also clear that acute exercise in the unfit animal can be especially stressful. Unfit horses subjected to acute exercise showed significantly raised steroid levels, which corresponded to reduced proliferation of their lymphocytes to mitogens and influenza

virus antigens and reduced neutrophil chemotactic responsiveness and chemiluminescence (a measure of respiratory burst activity) (Figure 36-6). These animals show a decline in the CD4:CD8 ratio, as well as a decline in both the number and activity of NK cells. The age of an animal can moderate the effect of exercise on immune responses. Thus strenuous exercise significantly reduces lymphocyte proliferative responses in young horses yet has much less effect on older animals. This resistance of older horses to exercise-induced immunosuppression is probably a result of a reduced steroid production in the older animals. Bulls subjected to stressful exercise become more susceptible to experimental *Mannheimia* pneumonia.

Posttraumatic Immune Deficiency

Severely traumatized or burnt animals commonly die of sepsis as a result of an immunodeficiency. This is largely due to the production of large amounts of IL-10 and other immunosuppressive cytokines by macrophages. Corticosteroids, prostaglandins from damaged tissues, and a small protein called suppressive active peptide, which appears in serum following a burn, all have immunosuppressive properties. The deficiency occurs within minutes or hours and recovers as wounds heal. It affects T cell, macrophage, and neutrophil function, but B cell function appears to be normal. As a result, delayed hypersensitivity reactions, allograft rejection, and T-dependent antibody responses are all impaired. IL-2 and IL-2R production are reduced. CD8$^+$ cells are increased in injured individuals, suggesting that regulatory cell function may be enhanced. Macrophages lose antigen-presenting ability as

Figure 36-6. Although a moderate amount of exercise is good for the immune system, excessive exercise causes severe stress that can be immunosuppressive. In this example, six thoroughbred horses were subjected to a treadmill-based exercise challenge of various intensities (speed and incline). Blood samples were assayed for plasma cortisol levels by radioimmunoassay and influenza virus-specific lymphocyte proliferation was assayed by thymidine incorporation. A clear relationship exists between exercise intensity, the stress response, and immune responsiveness. (From data kindly provided by Drs. SG Kamerling, PA Melrose, DD French, and DW Horohov.)

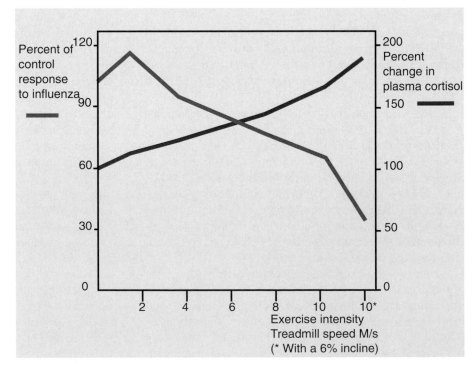

they express decreased levels of MHC class II molecules. Neutrophil and macrophage phagocytosis and respiratory burst activities are both impaired. Although surgery can result in some suppression of lymphocyte responses to mitogens, evidence suggests that routine surgery has no significant effect on the response of healthy animals to vaccination.

Age and the Immune Response

Innate, cell-mediated, and humoral immune responses all decline with advancing age. For example, as dogs age lymphocyte numbers, T cells, CD4+ cells, and CD8+ cells all decline. B cells tend to decline faster than T cells. Not only do macrophage numbers decline in aged animals, but they also express significantly lower levels of all TLRs. As a result, when stimulated with known TLR ligands, they secrete significantly lower amounts of IL-6 and TNF-α. Aged macrophages show reduced responses to activating agents such as IFN-γ.

As animals age, there is significant thymic involution, leading to a decline in the numbers of CD4+ T cells and in the export of cells from the thymus. In addition, these animals' peripheral lymphocyte population changes from a naive population to a memory cell population. T cells from aged animals lose their ability to progress through the cell cycle. As a result, early events in the T-cell response to antigens, such as activation of protein kinase C and the rise in intracellular calcium, are impaired. Even after expressing IL-2 receptors and being exposed to IL-2, aged T cells may not be able to respond effectively to antigens. T cells from old dogs and horses show a decline in proliferative responses to mitogens. Analysis shows that some aged T cells continue to produce normal amounts of IL-2, but many do not. Thus aged T cell populations are mixtures of fully functional and impaired cells. In old horses (older than 20 years), there is a significant decrease in the proportion of CD8+ T cells and a rise in the CD4:CD8 ratio compared with young animals.

The bone marrow is relatively unaffected by old age, and an aged bone marrow can reconstitute the body as well as a young one. If aged B cells are mixed with young T cells, the response is relatively normal. If the reverse is attempted (i.e., mixing young B cells with aged T cells), the B cells respond poorly. Somatic mutation in immunoglobulin V region genes ceases in old animals so that antibody affinity tends to be lower than in young animals. Nevertheless, immunoglobulin concentrations do not decline in old-age. The aging process does not affect antigen processing and presentation. Old dogs show little decline in antibody responses, although old horses have reduced antibody responses to influenza vaccination. Horses over 20 years of age have reduced lymphocyte responses to mitogens, and this deficiency cannot be overcome by exposure to additional IL-2.

Despite the previous comments, young animals may show poorer resistance to some invaders than mature animals. This seems to be especially important in sheep. Thus lambs are more susceptible than mature sheep to parasitic and infectious diseases during the first year of life. Older sheep tend to show greater resistance to internal parasites such as *Haemonchus*, *Trichostrongylus*, and *Ostertagia*. Sheep younger than 1 year of age are more susceptible than mature sheep to virus diseases such as bluetongue and contagious ecthyma. Young sheep, 4 to 8 months of age, have a lower proportion of CD4+ T cells in their blood than mature sheep. Lymphocytes from these young sheep produced less IFN-γ than those from adult sheep. Older sheep produced more antibodies to *Brucella abortus* lipopolysaccharide and responded more intensely to the contact sensitizer dinitrochlorobenzene. However, the two age groups did not differ in B cell or WC1+ T cell numbers and mounted comparable responses to diphtheria toxoid and tetanus. This mild immunodeficiency in lambs presumably reflects the immaturity of the immune system during the first year of life.

Other Secondary Immunodeficiencies

Immunodeficiencies may result from a wide variety of insults to the body. For example, immunoglobulin synthesis is generally reduced in individuals with absolute protein loss (patients with the nephrotic syndrome, heavily parasitized or tumor-bearing individuals, and patients who have experienced severe burns or trauma). Stress may result in immunodeficiencies. For example, it is possible to provoke a combined immunodeficiency

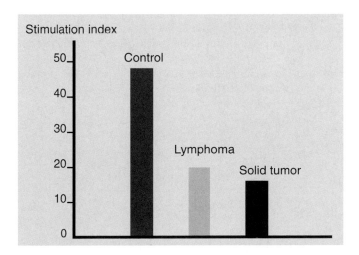

Figure 36-7.   Immunosuppression in dogs with lymphomas or solid tumors as compared to normal control dogs. The stimulation index is a measure of the response of lymphocytes to the mitogenic lectin phytohemagglutinin. (Data taken from Weiden PL, Storb R, Kolb HJ, et al: *J Natl Cancer Inst* 53: 1049-1056, 1974.)

syndrome by chilling newborn puppies for 5 to 10 days. Stresses such as rapid weaning, sleep deprivation, general anesthesia, prolonged transportation, and overcrowding are all effective immunosuppressants in animals. Physical destruction of lymphoid tissues can result in immunodeficiencies. For example, loss of lymphoid tissue leading to immunosuppression may occur in tumor-bearing animals, especially if the tumors themselves are lymphoid in origin (Figure 36-7). Adult horses with chronic diarrhea are immunosuppressed, as reflected by reduced IgA and reduced lymphocyte responses to mitogens. Some endocrine diseases such as thyrotoxicosis and diabetes mellitus may also result in immunosuppression.

SOURCES OF ADDITIONAL INFORMATION

Anderson NV, Houanes YD, Vestweber JG, et al: The effects of stressful exercise on leukocytes in cattle with experimental pneumonic pasteurellosis, *Vet Res Commun* 15:189-204, 1991.

Burkhard MJ, Hoover EA: Feline immunodeficiency virus (FIV): clinical manifestations and management, *Feline Pract* 27:10-13, 1999.

Diehl LJ, Hoover EA: Early and progressive helper T-cell dysfunction in feline leukemia virus-induced immunodeficiency, *J AIDS* 5:1188-1194, 1992.

Dua N, Reubel G, Moore PF, et al: An experimental study of primary feline immunodeficiency virus infection in cats and a historical comparison to acute simian and human immunodeficiency virus diseases, *Vet Immunol Immunopathol* 43: 337-355, 1994.

Flynn, JN, Cannon CA, Lawrence, CE, Jarrett O Polyclonal B-cell activation in cats infected with feline immunodeficiency virus, *Immunology* 81:626-630, 1994.

Greeley EH, Ballam JM, Harrison JM, et al. The influence of age and gender on the immune system: a longitudinal study in Labrador retriever dogs, *Vet Immunol Immunopathol* 82: 57-71, 2001.

Greeley EH, Kealy RD, Ballam JM, et al: The influence of age on the canine immune system, *Vet Immunol Immunopathol* 55:1-10, 1996.

Hoffman-Goetz L, Pedersen BK: Exercise and the immune system: a model of the stress response? *Immunol Today* 15: 382-387, 1994.

Horohov DW, Kydd JH, Hannant D: The effect of aging on T cell responses in the horse, *Dev Comp Immunol* 26:121-128, 2002.

Hutchison JM, Garry FB, Johnson LW, et al: Immunodeficiency syndrome associated with wasting and opportunistic infection in juvenile llamas: 12 cases (1988-1990), *J Am Vet Med Assoc* 201:1070-1076, 1992.

Ing R, Su Z, Scott ME, Koski KG: Suppressed T helper 2 immunity and prolonged survival of a nematode parasite in protein malnourished mice, *Proc Natl Acad Sci USA* 97: 7078-7083, 2000.

Keadle TL, Pourciau SS, Melrose PA, et al. Acute exercise stress modulates immune function in unfit horses, *J Eq Vet Sci* 13:228-231, 1993.

Levy JK, Ritchey JW, Rottman JB, et al: Elevated interleukin-10-to-interleukin-12 ratio in feline virus-infected cats predicts loss of type 1 immunity to *Toxoplasma gondii*, *J Infect Dis* 178:503-511, 1998.

Mancuso P, Gottschalk A, Phare SM, et al: Leptin-deficient mice exhibit impaired host defense in gram-negative pneumonia, *J Immunol* 168:4018-4024, 2002.

McEwan NA: *Malassezia* and *Candida* infections in bull terriers with lethal acrodermatitis, *J Small Anim Pract* 42:291-297, 2001.

McKenzie RC, Rafferty TS, Beckett GJ: Selenium: an essential element for immune function, *Immunol Today* 19:342-345, 1998.

Modiano JF, Getzy DM, Akol KG, et al: Retrovirus-like activity in an immunosuppressed dog: pathological and immunological findings, *J Comp Pathol* 112:165-183, 1995.

Pardi D, Hoover EA, Quackenbush SL, et al: Selective impairment of humoral immunity in feline leukemia virus-induced immunodeficiency, *Vet Immunol Immunopath* 28:183-200, 1991.

Pollock JM, Rowan TG, Dixon JB, et al: Alterations of cellular immune responses by nutrition and weaning in calves, *Res Vet Sci* 55:298-306, 1993.

Torres B, Elyar JS, Okada S, Yamamoto JK: Fundamentals of FIV infection: is a vaccine possible? *Feline Pract* 25:6-11, 1997.

Trogdon Hines M, Schott HC, Bayly WM, Leroux AJ: Exercise and immunity: a review with emphasis on the horse, *J Vet Intern Med* 10:280-289, 1996.

Renshaw M, Rockwell J, Engleman C, et al: Cutting edge: impaired toll-like receptor expression and function in aging, *J Immunol* 169:4697-4701, 2002.

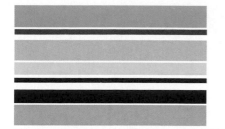

Drugs and Other Agents That Affect the Immune System

CHAPTER 37

Many situations exist in which it is desirable to stimulate or suppress the immune system, and many different drugs and techniques are available to do this. Indeed, this area of immunology is a discipline in its own right—immunopharmacology.

SUPPRESSION OF THE IMMUNE SYSTEM

The methods available for inhibiting immune responses may be classified into two main groups. The most widely employed techniques involve administering treatment that, by inhibiting all cell division, reduces the response of T and B cells to antigens. This approach is crude and dangerous, since other rapidly proliferating cell populations, such as intestinal epithelium and bone marrow cells, may also be severely damaged with potentially disastrous consequences. Alternatively, it is possible to use techniques that selectively eliminate T or B cells. This can be done using specific antisera or monoclonal antibodies or by the use of highly selective immunosuppressive drugs.

NONSPECIFIC IMMUNOSUPPRESSION

Radiation

X-radiation can be immunosuppressive. It affects cells by several different mechanisms. The simplest of these is through ionizing rays hitting an essential, unique molecule, such as DNA, within the cell. A loss of even one nucleotide results in a permanent mutation of a gene, with potentially lethal effects on the progeny of the affected cell. Radiation also causes ionization of water and the formation of highly reactive free oxygen and hydroxyl radicals in the environment of the cell. The hydroxyl radicals can react with dissolved oxygen to form peroxides that have toxic effects on many cell processes, especially cell division. Although X-radiation is of some use in prolonging graft survival in experimental animals, especially laboratory rodents, the amount of radiation required for effective prolongation of graft survival in the dog is so high that it is lethal to the animal.

Corticosteroids

Corticosteroids are among the most commonly used immunosuppressive and antiinflammatory agents. Their potency, however, differs significantly among species. Mammals may be classified as corticosteroid-sensitive or corticosteroid-resistant on the basis of the ease by which they can be depleted of lymphocytes. Laboratory rodents and humans are much more sensitive to the immunosuppressive effects of corticosteroids than the major domestic mammals, and care should therefore be taken not to extrapolate laboratory animal results directly to other animals.

The effects of glucocorticosteroids on cell function have a common pathway (Figure 37-1). Corticosteroids are absorbed directly into cells, where they bind to cytoplasmic receptors. The corticosteroid-receptor complexes are then transported to the nucleus, where they stimulate the synthesis of a protein called IκB-α. IκB-α is a inhibitor of the transcription factor NF-κB. In a resting cell, NF-κB is bound to IκB-α. When a lymphocyte is

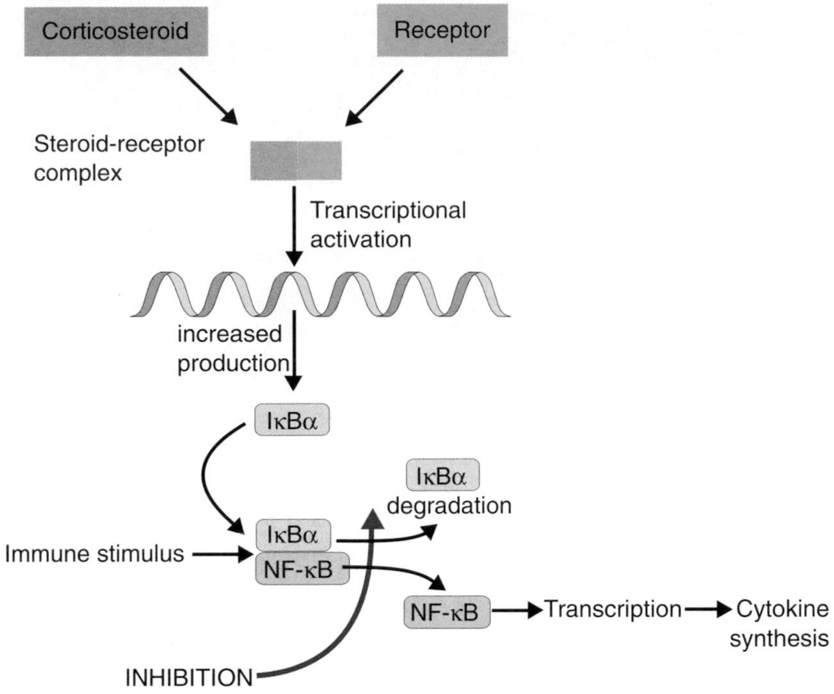

Figure 35-5. A schematic diagram showing the mode of action of corticosteroids. Normally, signal transduction and cytokine synthesis occur when the transcription factor NF-κB dissociates from its inhibitor IκB-α. The released IκB-α is rapidly degraded. Glucocorticosteroids stimulate the synthesis of excessive amounts of IκB-α, which binds to NF-κB and so inhibits its actions.

stimulated, the two molecules dissociate, the IκB-α is degraded, and the released NF-κB moves to the nucleus and activates many genes involved in inflammation and immunity. Corticosteroids, however, stimulate the production of excess IκB-α. This excess is not degraded but rebinds to NF-κB and continues to block all NF-κB–mediated processes, including cytokine synthesis. As a result, corticosteroids suppress both immunological and inflammatory processes.

Corticosteroids influence immunity in four areas (Box 37-1): they have effects on leukocyte circulation; they influence the effector mechanisms of lymphocytes; they modulate the activities of inflammatory mediators; and they modify protein, carbohydrate, and fat metabolism.

The effects of corticosteroids on leukocyte circulation vary among species. In horses and cattle, the number of circulating eosinophils, basophils, and lymphocytes declines abruptly when corticosteroids are administered. The numbers of neutrophils, on the other hand, increase as a result of decreased adherence to vascular endothelium and reduced emigration into inflamed tissues. Neutrophil, monocyte, and eosinophil chemotaxis is suppressed by corticosteroids, but neutrophil random migration is enhanced. Corticosteroids suppress the cytotoxic and phagocytic abilities of neutrophils in some species, but in others, such as the horse and goat, they have no effect on phagocytosis. Macrophage production of prostaglandins and interleukin 1 is reduced in some species.

Corticosteroids may kill thymocytes and suppress the ability of T cells to produce cytokines. The most important exception to this is IL-2, which is not controlled by NF-κB. Lymphocyte proliferation in the mixed

---

BOX 37–1

The Effects of Corticosteroids on the Immune System

NEUTROPHILS
Neutrophilia
Depressed chemotaxis
Depressed margination
Depressed phagocytosis
Depressed ADCC
Depressed bactericidal activity

MACROPHAGES
Depressed chemotaxis
Depressed phagocytosis
Depressed bactericidal activity
Depressed IL-1 production
Depressed antigen processing

LYMPHOCYTES
Depressed proliferation
Depressed T cell responses
Impaired T cell–mediated cytotoxicity
Depressed IL-2 production
Depressed lymphokine production

IMMUNOGLOBULINS
Minimal decrease

COMPLEMENT
No effect

lymphocyte reaction is suppressed, suggesting that there is interference with the recognition of MHC class II molecules. Corticosteroids also block production of lymphotoxin and monocyte chemotactic molecules. NK and some antibody-dependent cellular cytotoxicity (ADCC) reactions may be refractory to corticosteroid treatment and in cattle corticosteroids may increase serum interferon levels. The effects of corticosteroid therapy on antibody responses are variable and depend on the timing of administration and on the dose given. In general, B cells tend to be corticosteroid-resistant, and enormous doses are usually required to depress antibody synthesis. It is interesting to note, however, that in horses, moderate doses of dexamethasone suppresses IgG1 and IgG4 responses while having no apparent effect on IgG3 responses. Glucocorticosteroids characteristically cause apoptosis of thymocytes, especially those with the double positive phenotype (CD4+, CD8+). Corticosteroids also upregulate the expression of CD121b. This is a decoy receptor that can bind active IL-1 but will not transduce a signal, effectively suppressing the activity of IL-1.

The synthetic glucocorticoids are able to suppress acute inflammation. They inhibit the increase in vascular permeability and vasodilatation. As a result they prevent edema formation and fibrin deposition. At the same time, corticosteroids block the emigration of leukocytes from capillaries. They inhibit the release of lysosomal enzymes and impair antigen processing by macrophages. Corticosteroids can also inhibit the effects of phospholipases and so prevent the production of leukotrienes and prostaglandins. These effects of corticosteroids may mask the signs of tissue damage. In the later stages of inflammation, they inhibit capillary and fibroblast proliferation (perhaps by blocking IL-1 production) and enhance collagen breakdown. As a result, corticosteroids delay wound and fracture healing.

When corticosteroid therapy is initiated, prednisolone is usually the agent selected for small animal treatment, and betamethasone and dexamethasone are commonly employed in large animal practice. Cats may require significantly higher doses than dogs to achieve a significant clinical response. Once a response has been induced, the dose of corticosteroids can be gradually reduced by lengthening the dose interval and then decreasing the amount given. This treatment is not without risks since it has the potential to suppress the pituitary-adrenal axis and induce Cushing's syndrome. Also, by suppressing inflammation and phagocytosis, corticosteroids may render an animal highly susceptible to infection.

Cytotoxic Drugs

The major immunosuppressive cytotoxic drugs, having been designed to inhibit cell division, act on nucleic acid synthesis and activity. The three major drugs currently used are cyclophosphamide, azathioprine, and methotrexate.

The alkylating agents cross-link DNA helices, preventing their separation and thus inhibiting template formation. The most important of these is cyclophosphamide (Figure 37-2). Cyclophosphamide is toxic for resting and dividing cells, especially for dividing immunocompetent cells. It impairs both B and T cell responses, especially the primary immune response. It blocks mitogen and antigen-induced cell division and the production of cytokines such as IFN-γ. It prevents the B cell from renewing its antigen receptors. Early in therapy, cyclophosphamide tends to destroy more B cells than T cells. In long-term therapy it affects both cell populations. It also suppresses macrophage function and therefore has an anti-inflammatory effect. Cyclophosphamide may be administered parenterally or orally and is inactive until biotransformed in the liver. It has a half-life of about 6 hours and is largely excreted through the kidney. It is of interest to note that corticosteroids enhance the metabolism of cyclophosphamide and so reduce its potency. The main toxic effect of cyclophosphamide is bone marrow suppression, leading to leukopenia with a predisposition to infection. Other effects may include thrombocytopenia, anemia, and bladder damage. Cyclophosphamide is of benefit in the treatment of lymphoid neoplasia and in the treatment of immune-mediated skin diseases.

Purine analogs are also used as immunosuppressive agents since they compete with purines in the synthesis of nucleic acids. The most widely employed of these is azathioprine. Unlike cyclophosphamide, azathioprine affects only proliferating, not resting, lymphocytes; it is therefore a less potent immunosuppressor. It can suppress both primary and secondary antibody responses if given after antigen exposure. Azathioprine has a significant antiinflammatory action as a result of its ability to inhibit the production of macrophages. It has no effect on the production of cytokines by lymphocytes and affects both T and B responses equally. Like cyclophosphamide, its major toxic effect is bone marrow depression that tends to affect leukocytes rather than platelets or red cells. Azathioprine is useful in the control of allograft rejection but is ineffective in preventing xenograft rejection. It is favored by many clinicians for the treatment of immune-mediated skin diseases because of its combination of antiinflammatory and immunosuppressive activity. It is commonly used in association with corticosteroid therapy. If azathioprine is used in dogs, marrow function should be carefully monitored and the dose reduced if adverse effects occur.

Methotrexate is a folic acid antagonist that binds to dihydrofolate reductase and so blocks the synthesis of tetrahydrofolate, leading to failure to synthesize thymidine and purine nucleotides. It can suppress antibody formation, and its side effects are similar to those seen with cyclophosphamide and azathioprine.

Some drugs used in the therapy of autoimmune disorders are also immunosuppressive. These include the gold

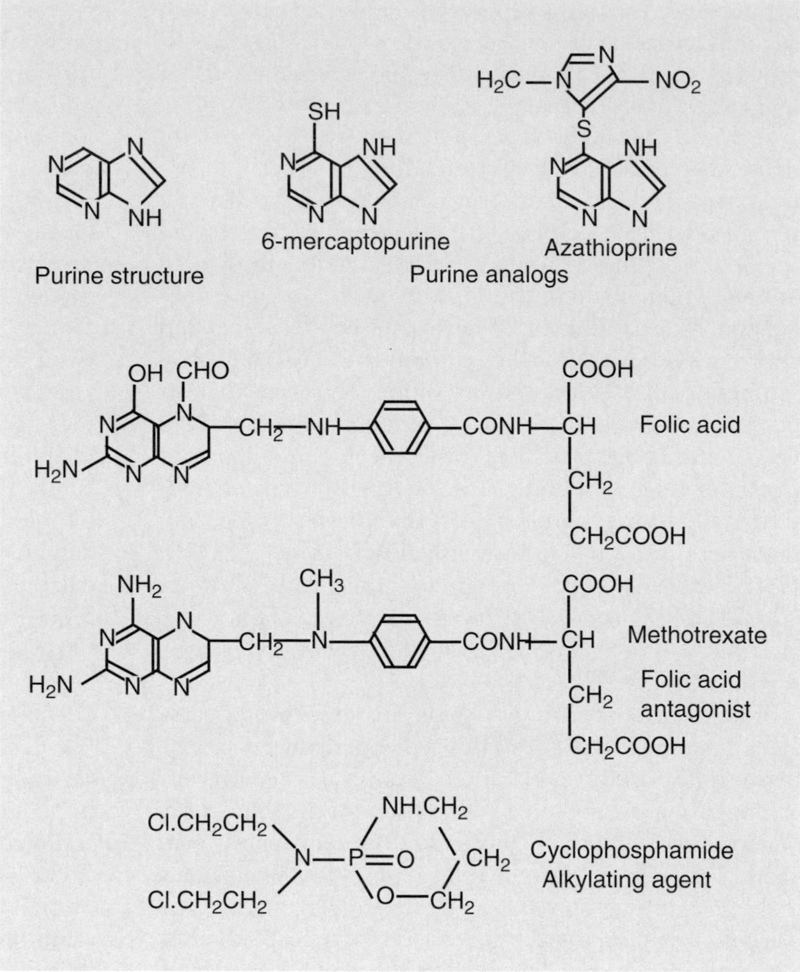

Figure 37-2. The structure of some commonly employed immunosuppressive drugs and the normal compounds with which they compete. Cyclophosphamide acts by cross-linking DNA chains.

salts, sodium aurothiomalate, and aurothioglucose, which act on protein kinase C to depress antigen-induced cell division. Gold therapy can reduce the levels of autoantibodies and has an antiinflammatory effect. Although gold therapy is effective in treating some autoimmune disease cases, it is associated with significant adverse side effects, including allergic reactions, thrombocytopenia, dermatitis, and renal failure.

SELECTIVE IMMUNOSUPPRESSION

Immunosuppressive Drugs

Perhaps the single most important step in the development of routine, successful organ allografting has been the development of very potent but selective immunosuppressive agents. Of these, cyclosporine (Sandimmune) has been by far the most successful. Cyclosporine is an immunosuppressive polypeptide derived from certain fungi. These fungi yield several natural forms of cyclosporin, of which the most important is cyclosporin A, a peptide consisting of 11 amino acids arranged in a circle (Figure 37-3). Because of this structure, cyclosporine has

two distinct surfaces, or faces, that allow it to bind two proteins simultaneously. Thus, when it enters the cytoplasm, one face binds to an intracellular receptor called cytophilin, while the other face binds and blocks the intracellular transmitter calcineurin, a serine/threonine phosphatase. As a result, cyclosporine inhibits signal transduction and prevents production of IL-2 and IFN-γ by T cells. The net effect of cyclosporine treatment is therefore the blocking of the Th1 response.

Because cyclosporine inhibits the production of IFN-γ by activated T cells, it will block IFN-γ induction of MHC class I expression in grafts. Since corticosteroids have a similar effect, the combination of corticosteroids and cyclosporine is especially potent and can enhance survival of allografts while at the same time leaving other immune functions intact. It therefore has a significant advantage over other older immunosuppressants. The use of cyclosporine has made tissue transplantation a routinely successful and safe procedure. In cats that have received renal allografts from unrelated blood-group–compatible donors and that were treated with cyclosporine and prednisolone, mean survival is greater than 12 months. Paradoxically, cyclosporine does enhance production of TGF-β and so may promote tumor growth.

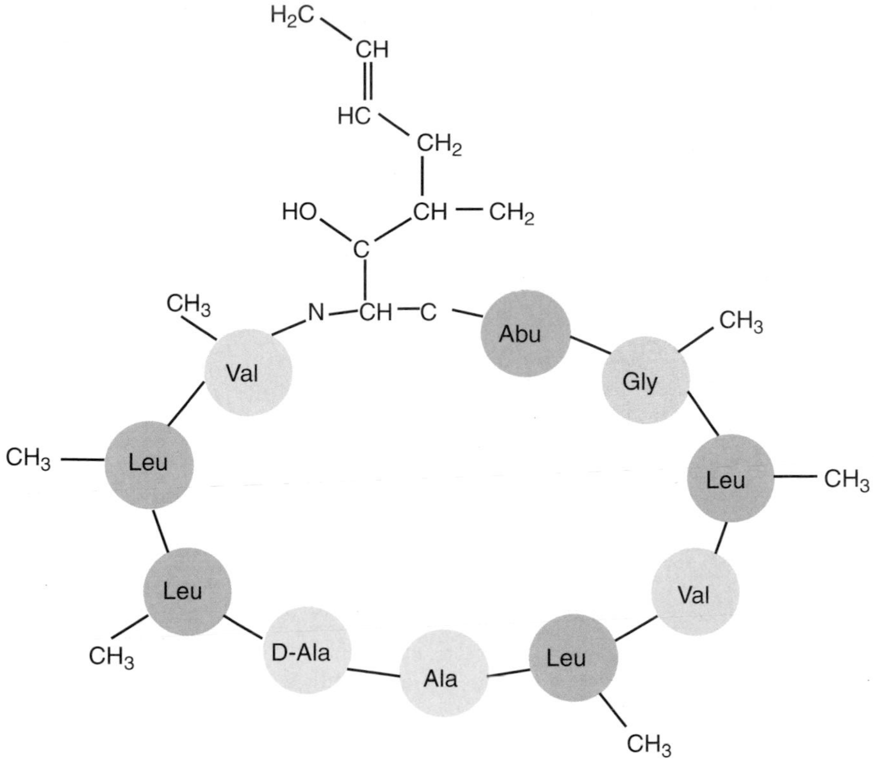

Figure 37-3. The structure of cyclosporine.

Tacrolimus and sirolimus (rapamycin) are macrolide antibiotics with similar biochemical and clinical effects to cyclosporine. They inhibit the production of several key cytokines, including IL-2, IL-3, IL-4, IL-5, IFN-γ, and TNF-α. Tacrolimus and sirolimus are much more potent than cyclosporine in inhibiting T and B cell responses. They are also superior to cyclosporine in preventing or reversing allograft and xenograft rejection in humans and can prevent graft vascular disease (Chapter 30). Unfortunately, they both have severe intestinal toxicity in dogs, causing ulceration, vasculitis, anorexia, and vomiting, although they can completely block renal allograft rejection. Sirolimus also inhibits wound healing.

Newly developed immunosuppressive drugs that may be useful in veterinary medicine include 15-deoxyspergualin, a spermidine polyamine that binds to HSP 70 and interferes with antigen processing; mycophenolate mofetil, a synthetic compound that inhibits purine synthesis; and brequinar sodium and leflunomide, which are inhibitors of pyrimidine synthesis.

Mycophenolate mofetil, like many of the others, significantly prolongs canine allograft survival but is severely toxic to the canine gastrointestinal tract. Leflunomide is a malononitriloamide that is very effective in suppressing both T and B cell proliferation. It is metabolized in the intestine to trimethyl fluoroanaline, which inhibits pyrimidine synthesis. When given along with cyclosporine to dogs, mycophenolate mofetil completely prevents renal allograft rejection between unrelated mongrel dogs. It is very effective in controlling canine autoimmune diseases such as immune-mediated thrombocytopenia, autoimmune hemolytic anemia, nonsuppurative meningoencephalitis, polymyositis, and pemphigus foliaceus, as well as systemic histiocytosis (Chapter 6).

Depletion of Lymphocytes

Because of the many adverse side effects of the nonspecific immunosuppressive drugs (not the least important of which is an increased predisposition to infection), a considerable effort has been made to find more specific alternative immunosuppressive procedures. One relatively simple technique that largely depletes T cells is to administer an antiserum specific for T lymphocytes. Antilymphocytic serum (ALS) suppresses the cell-mediated immune response and leaves the humoral immune response relatively intact. In practice, ALS has proved to be of variable efficiency and causes severe side effects. ALS-treated mice have been shown to accept rat xenografts, whereas clinical use of ALS in humans has not been universally accepted as useful. A much more specific antiserum with precise targeting is monoclonal anti-CD3. Anti-CD3 is directed only against T cells and appears to be very effective in reversing graft rejection in humans. An even more specific monoclonal antibody is anti-IL-2R, which attacks only activated lymphocytes. Anti-IL-2R helps prevent renal graft rejection and has fewer side effects than traditional antilymphocyte globulin.

Monoclonal antibodies against canine CD4 and CD8 have been used to control rejection of renal allografts. They are very effective, even with highly mismatched mongrel dogs. Both anti-CD4 and anti-CD8 must be used together, and their immunosuppressive effect lasts for about 10 days. (The dogs develop neutralizing antibodies against these monoclonal antibodies.) These monoclonal antibodies are very effective in combination with cyclosporine.

STIMULATION OF THE IMMUNE SYSTEM

There are many situations in veterinary medicine in which it is desirable to enhance either innate or acquired immunity; for example, the enhancement of resistance to infection and the treatment of immunosuppressive conditions. Immunostimulants vary according to their origin, their mode of action, and the way in which they are used. In contrast to adjuvants, immunostimulants need not be administered together with an antigen to enhance an immune response.

Bacteria and Bacterial Products

A wide variety of bacteria have been employed as immunostimulants. These most probably bind and stimulate one or more toll-like receptors. As a result, they activate macrophages and dendritic cells and stimulate cytokine synthesis. Their immunostimulating effects are probably due to the release of a mixture of cytokines. The most potent of these cytokine synthesis enhancers is BCG, the live, attenuated vaccine strain of *Mycobacterium bovis*. BCG generally enhances B and T cell–mediated responses, phagocytosis, graft rejection, and resistance to infection. Unfortunately, whole BCG induces tuberculin hypersensitivity in treated animals and is therefore unacceptable for use in farm animals. In order to prevent sensitization, purified cell wall fractions of BCG have been employed. These have been used to treat equine sarcoids and ocular squamous cell carcinoma. They are also of benefit in the treatment of upper respiratory tract infections in horses. Fractionation of BCG has resulted in the isolation of several active constituents. One of these is trehalose dimycolate. It promotes nonspecific immunity against several bacterial infections and may provoke regression of some experimental tumors. Muramyl dipeptide (MDP), a simple glycopeptide also purified from *Mycobacteria*, enhances antibody production, stimulates polyclonal activation of lymphocytes, and activates macrophages. Because MDP is rapidly excreted in the urine, its biological activity is greatly enhanced by incorporation into liposomes. Polymerization and conjugation with glycopeptides or synthetic antigens can also enhance the immunostimulating effects of MDP. MDP has been shown to be of benefit in prolonging survival time and decreasing metastases in dogs with osteosarcoma.

Killed anaerobic corynebacteria, such as *Propionibacterium acnes*, promote antibody formation. These bacteria are phagocytosed by macrophages and presumably stimulate cytokine synthesis through TLRs. *P. acnes* has a complex activity since it stimulates macrophages and the antibody response to thymus-dependent antigens, but it has a variable effect on the response to thymus-independent antigens. (It may selectively promote a Th2 response). These organisms have a general immunostimulating action, leading to enhanced antibacterial and antitumor activity. Killed *P. acnes* has been of benefit in the treatment of staphylococcal pyoderma, malignant oral melanoma in dogs, feline leukemia in cats, and respiratory disease in horses.

Staphylococcal cell walls (especially staphylococcal phage lysate), some streptococcal components, and products from *Bordetella pertussis*, *Brucella abortus*, *Bacillus subtilis*, and *Klebsiella pneumoniae* all have immunostimulating activity.

Unmethylated CpG nucleotides can bind to the dendritic cell/macrophage receptor TLR9, activate antigen-presenting cells, and trigger a potent Th1 cytokine response. When administered with antigens, these nucleotides act as potent adjuvants. When administered alone, they can act as potent immunostimulants and greatly enhance innate immunity.

Complex Carbohydrates

Certain complex carbohydrates derived from yeasts—namely, zymosan, glucans, aminated polyglucose, and lentinans—can also activate macrophages. These may function as adjuvants and potentiate resistance to infectious agents. Acemannan, a complex carbohydrate derived from the *Aloe vera* plant, is a cytokine synthesis enhancer with antitumor and antiviral activities. It has been used to treat feline leukemia and fibrosarcomas in cats and dogs. Fish such as trout, salmon, and catfish appear to respond well to these immunostimulants when incorporated in the diet. As a result, immunostimulation by carbohydrates, especially glucans, is becoming routine in many aquaculture operations.

Immunoenhancing Drugs

A broad-spectrum anthelmintic, levamisole, functions in a manner similar to the thymic hormone thymopoietin (Chapter 8); that is, it stimulates T cell differentiation and T cell response to antigens. Levamisole enhances bovine lymphocyte blastogenesis at suboptimal mitogen concentrations, enhances interferon production, and increases FcR activity in bovine macrophages. It probably also enhances cell-mediated cytotoxicity, lymphokine production, and suppressor cell function. Levamisole stimulates the phagocytic activities of macrophages and neutrophils. Its effects are greatest in animals with depressed T cell function; it has little or no effect on the immune system of healthy animals. Levamisole may therefore be of assistance in the treatment of chronic infections and neoplastic diseases, but it may exacerbate disease caused by excessive T cell function.

Vitamins

Vitamin E and selenium affect immune responses and disease resistance in poultry, pigs, and laboratory animals. A deficiency of vitamin E ([*dl*]-α-tocopheryl-acetate) results in immunosuppression and reduced resistance to disease. On the other hand, supplementation of diets with vitamin E can enhance certain immune responses and lead to increased resistance to disease. Lymphocyte responses to pokeweed mitogen are higher in pigs with high vitamin E levels. Vitamin E supplementation given to cows for several weeks before calving prevents the decline in neutrophil function (superoxide production) and macrophage function (IL-1 production and MHC class II expression) that normally occurs in the immediate postparturient period. Vitamin E promotes B cell prolif eration; the effect is most marked in the primary immune response. It can act as an adjuvant when administered with *Brucella ovis* vaccine, clostridial toxoid, and *E. coli* J5 vaccine. In some cases this increased antibody production may lead to increased disease resistance. The mode of action of vitamin E in enhancing immunity is unclear, but certainly supplemental vitamin E may act as a significant stimulus of immunity in some animals.

Cytokines

Since purified cytokines produced by recombinant DNA techniques are now available, many investigators have investigated whether they can be used to treat disease. By administering additional cytokines, one assumes that the amount of these molecules in the normal animal is rate-limiting and that administering additional material in pure form will somehow promote disease resistance or healing. This also assumes that by administering a single new cytokine, one will not trigger mechanisms that will regulate its activity and perhaps neutralize its effects. None of these assumptions may be valid. The major cytokines (IL-1, IL-2, IL-12, colony-stimulating factors, and the interferons) have all been tested on animals in vivo. Unfortunately, the administration of purified cytokines has usually had minimal effects on disease processes and has been accompanied by significant adverse effects.

Interferons

It was predicted for many years that the interferons would prove to be effective antiviral agents if they were made available in large quantities for animal treatment. Theoretically, administration of interferons should inhibit virus replication as well as stimulate some cellular functions such as neutrophil activity, thereby promoting disease resistance. This has proved to be an oversimplification. High doses of interferons are very toxic and cause severe fever, malaise, and appetite loss. They inhibit hematopoiesis and so cause thrombocytopenia and granulocytopenia. They can also cause liver, kidney, and neural toxicity. In addition, interferons seem to be relatively poor antiviral agents.

Recombinant human interferon-α (rHuIFN-α) has been administered to calves to treat rhinopneumonitis caused by bovine herpesvirus 1 (BHV-1). Although treated calves were less severely affected than controls, toxic effects such as fever and depression were seen. Multiple doses were required, and some calves developed antibodies against the interferon. rHuIFN-α has also been used to treat rotavirus-induced diarrhea in calves. It caused some clinical improvement but had no effect on virus shedding. Recombinant bovine interferon (rBoIFN-α or rBoIFN-γ) has also been administered to calves. rBoIFN-α significantly reduced disease symptoms in calves experimentally inoculated with BHV-1 and *Mannheimia hemolytica*. It was ineffective when given orally for the treatment of experimental transmissible gastroenteritis in piglets. Prophylactic treatment of healthy calves with rBoIFN-α1 significantly reduced the incidence of respiratory disease in these animals. rBoIFN-γ increased the secondary antibody response to vesicular stomatitis virus. It also enhanced neutrophil-mediated killing of *B. abortus*, but it had a mixed effect on the ability of calves to survive challenge with virulent *Salmonella enterica typhimurium*, since some treatment regimens reduced calf survival. Recombinant porcine interferon decreased the mortality of pigs challenged with *Actinobacillus pleuropneumoniae*. Dairy cattle that received intramammary rBoIFN-γ 24 hours before challenge with *E. coli* had considerably less mastitis than untreated controls. There was no mortality in the treated group, but the control group had 42% mortality within 3 days.

It is possible that interferons may have a more consistent positive therapeutic effect if, instead of being used on healthy animals, they are used on immunosuppressed, stressed animals. Glucocorticosteroids decrease the ability of animals to produce interferon, and rBoIFN-γ does reduce the severity of *Histophilus somni*–induced pneumonia in dexamethasone-treated calves.

Human and bovine interferon-α have been used for the treatment of feline leukemia.. The most impressive results were obtained with low-dose oral IFN-α in experimentally infected cats, in which significant protection was observed. Interferon-γ has been used to treat canine parvoviral enteritis

In conclusion, the use of high doses of interferons for the treatment of infectious diseases of cattle and swine has produced some positive responses. These are, however, not particularly impressive, and the interferon induces major toxic side effects such as fever, inappetence, and malaise. Low doses of interferon administered orally may produce more consistent positive results without these adverse side effects.

Interleukins

Recombinant interleukin 2 was administered to animals at the same time that they were vaccinated against a variety of organisms. In general this resulted in a somewhat increased level of protection. For example, rHuIL-2 administered to pigs at the same time that they received an *A. pleuropneumoniae* bacterin induced a considerably greater protection on challenge. A similar result was obtained using pigs immunized with a pseudorabies subunit vaccine. Calves that were vaccinated against BHV-1 and injected with rBoIL-2 showed enhanced responses to the virus and showed less severe signs of infection after challenge. Unfortunately, IL-2 is very toxic. It causes severe side effects, including a capillary leak syndrome, diarrhea, and fever (Chapter 31). Intramammary infusions of rBoIL-2 do induce local macrophage and neutrophil infiltration and increase mastitis cure rates. It is also interesting to note that relatively low doses of rHuIL-2, when injected locally into papillomas or carcinomas of the vulva in cattle, induced a response in over 80% of cases and some complete regressions were observed.

Other Cytokines

In addition to the trials described above, studies have been conducted using interleukin-1 and GM-CSF. rBoIL-1β treatment of calves simultaneously vaccinated against BHV-1 resulted in no change in disease severity, although it is an effective adjuvant in BHV-1 immunization. OvIL-1β has been used to enhance the response of sheep to purified, adjuvanted blowfly antigens. Although this treatment did not increase antibody levels, the animals showed enhanced delayed hypersensitivity and protection. It also appeared to have a protective effect against *Streptococcus suis* challenge in pigs. rBoGM-CSF increased neutrophil functions in corticosteroid-treated calves, enhancing their ability to phagocytose *Staphylococcus aureus* and suggesting that it might be useful in disease treatment. Encouraging results have, however, been obtained by the administration of IL-12, which promotes Th1 cell function. Administration of IL-12 to pigs receiving an inactivated pseudorabies vaccine effectively enhances their cell-mediated responses. BoIL-12 has helped to promote a Th1 response to *Salmonella enterica typhimurium* in calves. Despite this, the clinical trials of purified cytokines have generally produced disappointing results. The main reason for this may be that in vivo the immune system is regulated not by a single cytokine but by a complex mixture of cytokines. It is therefore likely that the best clinical responses will be obtained by using nonspecific cytokine synthesis enhancers.

SOURCES OF ADDITIONAL INFORMATION

Akiyama K, Sugii S, Hirota Y: A clinical trial of recombinant bovine interferon α1 for the control of bovine respiratory disease in calves, *J Vet Med Sci* 53:449-452, 1993.

Brassard DL, Grace MJ, Bordens RW: Interferon-α as an immunotherapeutic protein, *J Leukoc Biol* 71:565-577, 2002.

Calne RY: Immunosuppression in liver transplantation, *Lancet* 343:1154-1155, 1994.

Campos M, Godson D, Hughes H, Babiuk L: The role of biological response modifiers in disease control, *J Dairy Sci* 76:2407-2417, 1993.

Chapes SK, Chitko CG, Thaler RC, et al. Activated porcine alveolar macrophages: are biological response modifiers the answer? *Vet Immunol Immunopathol* 22:91-99, 1989.

Finch JM, Turner RJ: Effects of selenium and vitamin E on the immune responses of domestic animals, *Res Vet Sci* 60:97-106, 1996.

Fruman DA, Burakoff SJ, Bierer BE: Immunophilins in protein folding and immunosuppression, *FASEB J* 8:391-400, 1994.

Guelfi JF, Courdouhji MK, Alvinene M, Toutain PL: *In vivo* and *in vitro* effects of three glucocorticoids on blood leukocyte chemotaxis in the dog, *Vet Immunol Immunopathol* 10:245-252, 1985.

Hughes HPA, Babiuk LA: Potentiation of the immune response by cytokines. In Myers MJ, Murtaugh MP, editors: *Cytokines in animal health and disease*, New York, 1994, Marcel Dekker.

Jarosinski KW, Wei J, Sekellick MJ, et al: Cellular responses in chickens treated with IFN-α orally or inoculated with recombinant Marek's disease virus expressing IFN-α, *J Interferon Cytokine Res* 21:287-296, 2001.

Jenkins WL: Concurrent use of corticosteroids and antimicrobial drugs in the treatment of infectious diseases in large animals, *J Am Vet Med Assoc* 185:1145-1149, 1984.

Kawashima K, Platt KB: The effect of human recombinant interleukin-2 on the porcine immune response to a pseudorabies virus subunit vaccine, *Vet Immunol Immunopathol* 22: 345-353, 1989.

McCaw DL, Boon GD, Jergens AE, et al. Immunomodulation therapy for feline leukemia virus infection, *J Am Anim Hosp Assoc* 37:356-363, 2001.

Murray FA, Chenault JR: Effects of steroids on bovine T-lymphocyte blastogenesis in vitro, *J Anim Sci* 55: 1132-1138, 1982.

Reddy DN, Reddy PG, Xue W, et al: Immunopotentiation of bovine respiratory disease virus vaccines by interleukin-1α and interleukin-2, *Vet Immunol Immunopathol* 37:25-38, 1993.

Reddy PG, Blecha F, Minocha HC, et al: Bovine recombinant interleukin-2 augments immunity and resistance to bovine herpesvirus infection, *Vet Immunol Immunopathol* 23:61-74, 1989.

Roth JA, Kaeberle ML: Effect of glucocorticoids on the bovine immune system, *J Am Vet Med Assoc* 180:894-901, 1982.

Secombes CJ: Enhancement of fish phagocyte activity, *Fish Shellfish Immunol* 4:421-436, 1994.

Slack J, Risdahl JM, Valberg SJ, et al: Effects of dexamethasone on development of immunoglobulin G subclass responses following vaccination of horses, *Am J Vet Res* 61:1530-1531, 2000.

Takehara K, Kikuma R, Ishikawa S, et al: Production and in vivo testing of a recombinant bovine IL-12 as an adjuvant for *Salmonella typhimurium* vaccination in calves, *Vet Immunol Immunopathol* 86:23-30, 2002.

Thompson AW: FK-506 enters the clinic, *Immunol Today* 11:35-36, 1990

Thompson AW, Forrester JV: Therapeutic advances in immunosuppression, *Clin Exp Immunol* 98:351-357, 1994.

Weiss RC, Oostrom-Ram T: Effect of recombinant human interferon-alpha in vitro and in vivo on mitogen-induced lymphocyte blastogenesis in cats, *Vet Immunol Immunopathol* 24:147-158, 1990.

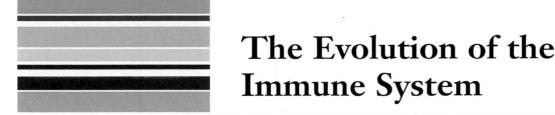

The Evolution of the Immune System

CHAPTER
38

All animals (and plants!), regardless of their complexity or evolutionary history, must be able to defend themselves against invading organisms that might cause disease or death. Both invertebrates and vertebrates possess innate immune defenses triggered by "danger signals" such as tissue damage or microbial invasion. The acquired immune system, however, evolved only after the emergence of the jawless fishes or cyclostomes. Thus, acquired immune mechanisms such as antibody production or antigen-sensitive lymphocytes are found only in the advanced vertebrates.

IMMUNITY IN INVERTEBRATES

Invertebrates are classified based on the presence of a body cavity or coelom (Figure 38-1). The acoelomates include the sponges and coelenterates (jellyfish and sea anemones). The coelomates evolved further into two major lines. One line includes the annelids, mollusks, and arthropods, collectively called the protostomes. The other line, including the echinoderms, protochordates, and chordates, is called the deuterostomes. It is from deuterostome-like ancestors that the vertebrates evolved. Invertebrates rely exclusively on physical barriers and innate immune defenses to exclude microbial invaders.

Physical Barriers

Physical barriers are most obvious in the arthropods. Tough chitinous exoskeletons can protect arthropods against all types of attackers. The horseshoe crab (*Limulus polyphemus*) not only has a hard exoskeleton but also can protect itself against bacterial endotoxins in polluted water by secreting a specialized glycoprotein through pores in the carapace. On contact with endotoxins, this glycoprotein coagulates, sealing the pores and immobilizing any invading bacteria. Likewise, if gram-negative bacteria enter horseshoe crab hemolymph, clotting factors are activated by lipopolysaccharides and result in local clot formation that traps invaders. Other invertebrates such as the coelenterates, annelids, molluska, and echinoderms secrete masses of sticky mucus when attacked, thus immobilizing potential invaders. This mucus may contain antimicrobial peptides such as defensins.

Innate Immunity

Invertebrates use three major innate defense mechanisms: phagocytosis by blood or body cavity cells; protease cascades that lead to fluid clotting, melanin formation, and opsonization; and the production of a wide variety of antimicrobial peptides.

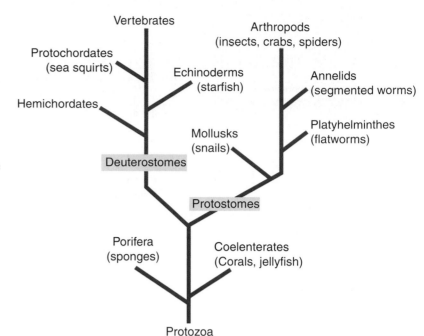

Figure 38-1. A phylogenetic tree showing the major divisions of the invertebrates.

Phagocytosis

In 1884 Elie Metchnikoff discovered the process of phagocytosis when examining starfish larvae. He showed that mobile cells attacked rose thorns introduced into the coelom of these larvae. Since then, phagocytosis has been shown to be a universal defense mechanism within the animal kingdom. Many different types of phagocytic cells are recognized in coelomate invertebrates. They occur in blood (hemocytes) and in the body cavity (coelomocytes). These cells behave in a manner similar to mammalian phagocytes and undertake chemotaxis, adherence, ingestion, and digestion. They contain proteases and in some invertebrates, such as mollusks, they produce potent oxidants. Some phagocytic cells can aggregate and plug wounds to prevent bleeding. In some cases in which phagocytic cells are unable to control invaders, they may be walled off in cellular nodules somewhat similar to vertebrate granulomas.

Invertebrates can produce cytokine-like molecules. One of these, an IL-1–like molecule, may activate phagocytic cells and stimulate phagocytosis. Lipopolysaccharide stimulation of mollusk hemocytes may stimulate the release of TNF-like, IL-6–like, or IL-1–like proteins. Cell surface adhesive proteins such as integrins are found in arthropods such as *Drosophila* or freshwater crayfish. These may promote hemocyte degranulation and activation of the prophenoloxidase system.

The Prophenoloxidase (proPO)-Activating System

This system, found in arthropod hemolymph, consists of multiple enzymes that, when activated, generate a cascade of proteases leading to the production of the pigment melanin (Figure 38-2). The system is activated by the interaction of bacterial and fungal lipopolysaccharides,

peptidoglycans, and glucans with hemocytes. Activation also occurs through cuticular and hemolymph proteases. The proPO system generates phenoloxidase, a sticky enzyme that binds to foreign surfaces. This enzyme acts on tyrosine and dopamine to generate melanin and deposit it around inflammatory sites. Melanin enhances phagocytosis, plasma coagulation, and killing of bacteria and fungi.

Antimicrobial Peptides

When insects are injected with bacteria, their PAMPs are recognized by toll-like receptors. In contrast to

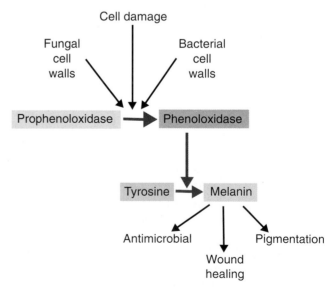

Figure 38-2. The prophenoloxidase pathway is an enzyme cascade system found in many invertebrates, where it serves a key defensive role.

mammals, where TLRs directly recognize pathogens, Drosophila Toll is activated by a protein ligand (called spätzle) that is generated after pathogen recognition. As a result, their cells produce antimicrobial peptides. These peptides are mainly produced in the fat body (the functional equivalent of the mammalian liver), although some may be produced locally on body surfaces. The peptides appear about 2 hours after exposure to the bacteria and reach peak levels at 24 hours. In some insects, the activity is short-lived and disappears in a few days; in others, it may last for several months. About 400 different antimicrobial peptides have been identified in invertebrates. One important group includes the defensins, small peptides that disrupt the cell walls of pathogens. Defensins are found not only in insects but also in mammals (Chapter 2) and plants.

A second important group of antimicrobial peptides is the lectins, proteins that can bind microbial carbohydrates such as lipopolysaccharides, glucans, mannans, and sialic acid. They include C-type lectins and pentraxins and are thus analogous to mammalian acute-phase proteins. These lectins act as opsonins and enhance activation of the prophenoloxidase system. Insects also produce the antibacterial enzyme lysozyme.

The complement system is very ancient, probably originating 600 to 700 million years ago, long before the emergence of vertebrates. Complement-like proteins have been traced back as far as the echinoderms, because both C3 and C2/factor B have been identified in sea urchins. Lectins homologous to mammalian MBL and ficolins, two MASPs, C3, C2/factor B, and a C3 receptor have been identified in ascidians (sea squirts). Thus invertebrates have both alternative and lectin pathways. Once activated through these pathways, invertebrate complement can opsonize microbial invaders.

Invertebrates do not make antibodies. The ability to mount adaptive immune responses arose with the jawed vertebrates. Nevertheless, proteins belonging to the immunoglobulin superfamily have been detected in arthropods, echinoderms and mollusks, as well as in protochordates.

Graft Rejection

Acquired immune responses do not occur in invertebrates since they are unable to generate diverse antigen-binding receptors. Nevertheless, invertebrates can reject allografts and xenografts. For example, cell-mediated allograft rejection occurs in sponges, coelenterates, annelids, and echinoderms. Thus when two identical sponge colonies are placed side by side and made to grow in contact with each other, no reaction occurs. If, however, sponges from two different colonies are made to grow in contact, local destruction of tissue occurs along the area of contact as each sponge attempts to destroy the other.

Annelids such as earthworms can reject both allografts and xenografts. The rejection of xenografts (from other species of earthworms) takes about 20 days. Cells invade the graft. The grafted tissue turns white, swells, becomes edematous, and eventually dies. If the recipient worms are grafted with a second piece of skin from the same donor, the second graft is rejected faster than the first. This ability to rapidly reject second grafts may be adoptively transferred by coelomocytes from sensitized animals.

IMMUNITY IN VERTEBRATES

There are seven classes of living vertebrates: the jawless fish, the cartilaginous fish, the bony fish, the amphibians, the reptiles, the birds, and the mammals (Figure 38-3).

The fish emerged 350 to 500 million years ago, long before the appearance of the mammals. The least complex living fish belong to the class Agnatha, the jawless fish, or cyclostomes such as the lampreys and the hagfish. Considerably more complex than the cyclostomes are the Chondrichthyes. These are the fish with cartilaginous skeletons and include the rays and sharks (the elasmobranchs). The most complex fish are the bony fish of the class Osteicthyes, which include the overwhelming majority of modern fish, the teleosts. Because they evolved so long ago, fish are much more heterogeneous than mammals, and major differences exist between the immune systems of each class.

There are two major orders of amphibians: the less evolved Urodela, which includes long bodied, tailed amphibians such as the salamanders and newts; and the Anura, an advanced, tailless order that includes the frogs and toads. These too differ significantly in their immune capabilities.

Three subclasses of reptiles currently exist: the Anapsida, which includes the turtles; the Lepidosaura, which consists of the lizards and snakes; and the Archosauria, which includes the crocodiles and alligators.

The dinosaurs, although related to the reptile Archosauria, were sufficiently different from true reptiles to be classified in a class of their own, the Dinosaura. Although the great majority of dinosaurs disappeared 65 million years ago at the end of the cretaceous period, their modern descendants are probably the birds, the members of the class Aves. Unlike the reptiles, birds are (and dinosaurs probably were) endothermic, or warm blooded. As a result of this, birds share with mammals all the benefits that come from greatly increased physiological and biochemical efficiency.

The mammals consist of three orders: the monotremes, or egg-laying mammals, such as the platypus and the echidna; the marsupials, or pouched mammals, such as the opossum and the kangaroos; and the eutherians, or placental mammals. The bulk of this book is devoted to the immunology of this final order.

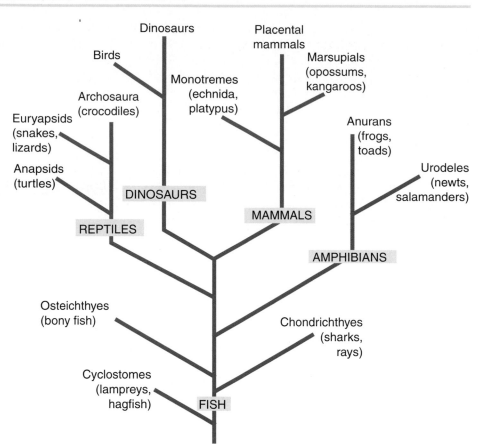

Figure 38-3. A simplified phylogenic tree showing the major relationships among the vertebrates.

IMMUNITY IN CYCLOSTOMES

The most primitive of living vertebrates are the cyclostomes, the fish without jaws, including the lampreys and the hagfish. These fish make proteins that can bind to bacteria and enhance phagocytosis by leukocytes. However, these proteins are not antibodies but are complement-like. Their amino acid sequences resemble C3, C4, and C5, and they contain a hidden thioester bond. Cyclostomes do not make immunoglobulins.

Cyclostomes possess both the alternate and lectin pathways but lack the later lytic components of complement. The lamprey complement system thus promotes phagocytosis rather than lysis. Because cyclostomes do not have antibodies, complement-mediated innate reactions play an essential role in their defense. Lamprey C3 has features of the common ancestor of mammalian C3 and C4 and lamprey factor B resembles the common ancestor of factor B and C2.

Cyclostomes have two types of blood leukocytes. One population is monocyte-like; members of the other population look like lymphocytes but do not respond to foreign antigens. Hagfish kept under good conditions in a warm environment can reject skin allografts. First grafts take about 72 days at 18° C to be rejected; second grafts are rejected in about 28 days. This rejection is presumably due to innate mechanisms.

The Immunological "Big-Bang"

The acquired immune system depends on possession of two key antigen receptor systems, the TCR and the BCR. Both of these require the rearrangement of V, D, and J gene segments to form functional, antigen-binding receptors. Invertebrates and cyclostomes cannot rearrange these genes, but cartilaginous and bony fish can. Sometime during the 100 million years between the divergence of jawless and jawed vertebrates and the emergence of cartilaginous and bony fish, about 450 million years ago, the enzymic machinery needed for the recombination of V gene segments emerged. The mechanism of this sudden appearance is unknown. It has been suggested, however, that a transposon carrying the precursors of the recombinase-activating genes (RAG1 and RAG2); most likely a bacterial integrase was successfully inserted into an immunoglobulin superfamily V-like gene within the germ line of the early jawed vertebrates (Figure 38-4). As a result, the immunoglobulin gene could be expressed only after rejoining mediated by the RAG enzymes. Thus emerged, in a major evolutionary leap, the ability to generate antigen-binding sites and functional immunoglobulins. This, for the first time, permitted animals to respond specifically to previously encountered antigens. The advantages of this new "improved" system were such that it is now a feature of all jawed vertebrates. This did not, of course, result in

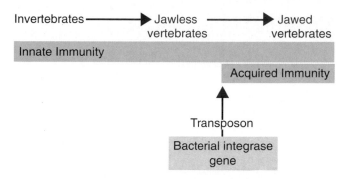

Figure 38-4.   Innate immunity is a feature of all animals, both vertebrates and invertebrates. Acquired immunity, in contrast, is found only in the jawed vertebrates, that is, animals more evolved than the jawless fish. It has been suggested that the ability to mount an acquired immune response depended on the transfer of a bacterial integrase gene to a vertebrate germ cell through a transposon.

discarding of the innate immune defenses. Thus lectins, the complement system, and the NK cell system remain essential components of vertebrate immunity.

IMMUNITY IN JAWED FISH

Innate Immunity

Phagocytosis in fish is similar to that described for mammals. For example, fish granulocytes enter inflammatory sites first and their numbers peak around 12-24 hours. This is followed by a later wave of macrophages and possibly lymphocytes. The granulocytes are attracted by microbial products and soluble tissue mediators. The response tends to be prolonged, and macrophage numbers peak at 2 to 7 days. In fish, granulocytes originate from the anterior kidney, whereas the macrophages develop from blood monocytes. Fish macrophages are found in many sites, especially the mesentery, splenic ellipsoids, kidney, and atrium of the heart.

Teleost neutrophils are similar in morphology and probably function to mammalian neutrophils and are frequently seen in inflammatory lesions. These neutrophils are phagocytic, and their numbers increase in response to infections. They possess most of the enzymes of mammalian neutrophils. It has been suggested that in some species neutrophils may carry out their bactericidal function extracellularly rather than intracellularly. The release of oxidants from neutrophils at inflammatory sites may cause severe tissue damage. The fat of fish is highly polyunsaturated as an adaptation to low temperatures. Polyunsaturated fats are prone to oxidation, and free radicals may therefore oxidize tissue lipids. Fish, therefore, require a powerful means of modulating this response. The brown pigment melanin can quench free radicals, and melanin-containing cells are common in the

lymphoid tissues of most bony fish, as well as in inflammatory lesions. It probably protects tissues against oxidants produced by phagocytic cells.

Both bony and cartilaginous fish can produce lysozyme, lectins, defensins, complement, and acute-phase proteins. Lysozyme is present in fish eggs and may protect the developing embryo. This fish lysozyme is much more broadly reactive than the mammalian enzyme and is active against both gram-positive and -negative bacteria. Fish acute-phase proteins include C-reactive protein, serum amyloid A, and serum amyloid P. However, their rise is much less pronounced than in mammals. A mannose binding lectin has been identified in species such as the Atlantic salmon. Natural cytotoxic cells similar to mammalian natural killer (NK) cells have been described in bony fish. They are produced in the anterior kidney.

Cartilaginous and bony fish possess all three complement pathways: namely, the classical, alternate, and lectin activator pathways. The fish lytic pathway generates a membrane attack complex similar to that formed in mammals, although it works at a lower optimum temperature (~25° C). Unlike other vertebrates, in which C3 is coded for by a single copy gene, in bony fish, C3 is produced in multiple functional isoforms. Thus rainbow trout have four C3 isoforms, carp have eight, and sea bream have five. They differ in their structure and in their ability to bind to different activating surfaces. It has been suggested that this complement polymorphism permits the most effective destruction of different invading microorganisms. As in mammals, C3 is the complement component at highest concentration in fish serum. Regulatory proteins similar to C4-binding protein and factor H have been identified in sand bass.

Acquired Immunity

Both cartilaginous and bony fish can mount acquired immune responses and have a complete set of lymphoid organs except for a bone marrow (Figure 38-5). Thus they have a thymus located just above the pharynx. It

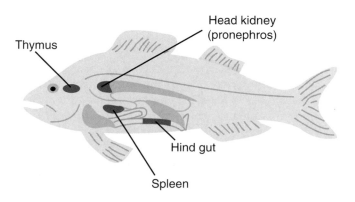

Figure 38-5.   The lymphoid organs of a bony fish.

arises from the first gill arches. In immature fish small pores lead from the pharynx to the thymus, suggesting that it may be stimulated directly by antigens in the surrounding water. Thymectomy in fish can lead to prolongation of allograft survival and reduced antibody responses. Antibodies or antigen-binding cells may be detected in the thymus during an immune response, suggesting that it contains both T-like and B-like cells. Although the thymus may involute in response to hormones or season, age involution is inconsistent and the thymus may be found in many older fish.

The kidney of fish differentiate into two sections. The opisthonephros or posterior kidney is an excretory organ that serves the same function as the mammalian kidney. In contrast, the pronephros or anterior kidney is a lymphoid organ containing antibody-forming cells and phagocytes. It thus performs a function analogous to mammalian bone marrow and lymph nodes. Fish have a spleen whose structure and location are similar to those in mammals.

Aggregates of lymphocytes are prominent in the fish intestinal tract. In addition, lymphomyeloid structures that appear to produce granulocytes are found in the submucosa of the esophagus (Leydig organ) and in the gonads (epigonal organ) of sharks. Some species possess both, but others may have only one of these organs. The epigonal organ and the Leydig organ in cartilaginous fish express RAG proteins, as well as TdT (Chapter 14) and other B cell–specific transcription factors and appear to be primary lymphoid organs. The epigonal organ appears to function like mammalian bone marrow as a source of B cells throughout life.

Fish possess aggregations of macrophages that contain pigments such as melanin and hemosiderin. These melanomacrophage centers are found in the spleen, liver, and kidney. Antigens may persist in these centers for long periods, and they may have a function similar to germinal centers in more evolved vertebrates.

Fish possess true lymphocytes that resemble those described in mammals. Thus B cells can be found in the thymus, anterior kidney, spleen, Leydig organ, and blood, and their surface membrane immunoglobulin acts as an antigen receptor. These B cells can mature into plasma cells. Both helper and cytotoxic T cells can be detected in fish.

Immunoglobulins

Immunoglobulins are seen for the first time in cartilaginous fish because they possess the recombinant activator genes RAG 1 and RAG 2. The manner in which these immunoglobulin molecules are coded for by light and heavy chain genes and the structures of the V, J, and C gene segments are similar to those seen in mammals. Nevertheless, they differ from mammals in the organization of immunoglobulin gene segments within the genome. For example, sharks and other elasmobranch fish have clustered immunoglobulin genes, where V, D, J,

and C segments form clusters that are duplicated many times; thus:

-VDJC—VDJC—VDJC—VDJC—VDJC—

There are 200 to 500 of these VDJC clusters in sharks; each cluster is about 16 kilobases in size. About half of these clusters appear to be functional. (This arrangement is somewhat similar to that seen in the TCR-γ, and TCR-β genes in mammals). Teleost fish, in contrast, have an immunoglobulin heavy chain gene arrangement similar to that of mammals, with multiple Vh genes arranged thus (called the translocon pattern):

-V-V-V-V-V-V-V-V-D-D-J-J-J-J-C—

Teleost light chain genes, however, are found in the clustered pattern. Thus, for example, in catfish, heavy chains are constructed in the translocon pattern, and light chain genes are in the clustered pattern. Shark immunoglobulins show evidence of somatic hypermutation.

IgM is the most ancient of the immunoglobulin classes and is found in both bony and cartilaginous fish (Figure 38-6). Cartilaginous fish usually have both pentameric and monomeric serum IgM. Bony fish have tetrameric and monomeric IgM. These different forms may compensate for a lack of IgG. Recently, several additional isotypes have been identified in elasmobranchs. These include IgNAR (new antigen receptor) in the nurse shark, IgW in the sandbar shark, and IgR in the skate. IgNAR consists only of heavy chains with no associated light chains. IgNAR sequences in young sharks are infrequently mutated, but mutation increases significantly as the fish mature. The heavy chain of IgW contains six C_H domains, two more than IgM. Sequence

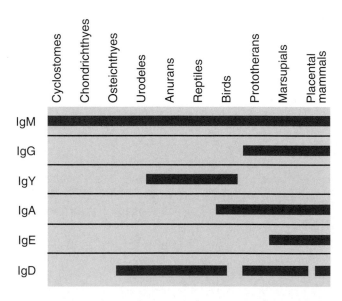

Figure 38-6. The evolution of the major immunoglobulin classes.

analysis raises the possibility that it may be an evolutionary forerunner of IgD or IgA. The IgW isotype occurs in two forms: a conventional form and a short, truncated form similar to the truncated form of IgY. IgR, on the other hand, has only two C_H domains. Peptides homologous to the J chain have been described in some fish but not in others. In the absence of J chains, the IgM monomers are held together by noncovalent bonds. IgD genes and products have been identified in catfish, halibut, salmon, and cod. They have some similarities to mammalian IgD, including coexpression with IgM on the B cell surface as a result of alternative splicing. The function of teleost IgD is unknown. Light chain isotypes have been described in catfish, salmon, and trout. Their number varies from 1 to 3. None is closely homologous to mammalian κ and λ chains. Fish antibody responses are characterized by the predominance of IgM and by their relatively poor secondary responses.

An unusual feature of elasmobranch immunity is the existence of immunoglobulin genes rearranged in the germ line. These appear to play a role early in development but tend to be silenced in later life when their function is replaced by rearranging genes. Thus in the nurse shark, the predominant immunoglobulin in neonates is coded for by a germ line–rearranged gene. This might be a transitional stage between innate and acquired immunity.

Fish antibodies in the presence of normal serum as a source of complement can lyse target cells. Likewise, fish antibodies are effective at agglutination. There is no evidence that fish antibodies can function as opsonins, nor have Fc receptors been detected on fish phagocytic cells. The blood vessel walls of fish are permeable to IgM. As a result, antibodies are found in most tissue fluids (plasma, lymph, skin mucus). Transfer of antibodies from immunized females to their eggs has been described in the plaice.

Not all antigens are effective immunogens in fish. Soluble protein antigens are poorly immunogenic, but particulate antigens such as bacteria or foreign erythrocytes are highly immunogenic. Many cartilaginous fish show seasonal effects on antibody production; that is, under constant conditions of light and temperature, immune responses are poorer in winter than in summer. Social interactions can also influence their immune response; fish kept at high population density are immunosuppressed.

Cell-Mediated Immunity

The acquisition of recombinase activity enabled fish to generate rearranged TCRs, and TCR homologs have been identified in both elasmobranchs and teleosts. Their overall structure is similar to that in mammals. The germ line TCR genes are not rearranged and are organized in the cluster pattern. Fish have both MHC class I and II genes. The basic structure of each MHC molecule has been conserved, as has the organization of

the class I and class II genes. In teleost fish, however, class I and II loci are on different chromosomes.

Cartilaginous fish reject scale allografts slowly, whereas bony fish reject them much more rapidly. Repeated grafting leads to accelerated rejection. The rejected allografts are infiltrated by lymphocytes and show destruction of blood vessels and pigment cells. As in all ectotherms, graft rejection is slower at lower temperatures. Many different cytokines have been identified in fish, including IL-1, IL-2, IL-3, IL-6, TNF-α, TGF-β, IFN-β, and IFN-γ.

IMMUNITY IN AMPHIBIANS

As vertebrates have evolved, they have shown a progressive increase in the complexity of their immune systems (Figure 38-7). This is well seen in amphibians, in which there are marked differences between the less complex urodeles (tailed amphibians such as the newts and salamanders) and the much more evolved anurans such as the frogs and toads. In addition, amphibians go through a complex metamorphosis as they change from the tadpole into an adult form. This has significant effects on the development of the immune system.

An interesting feature of the amphibians is the presence of very potent antimicrobial peptides in their skin. Amphibians also possess a complement system that, although similar to that of mammals, is more effective at 16° C.

Urodele Amphibians

Urodeles generally lack a bone marrow, although some salamanders may have a small amount of lymphoid tissue within their long bones. They have a thymus that

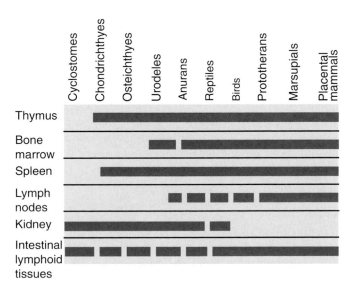

Figure 38-7. The evolution of the major lymphoid organs in vertebrates.

develops slowly, only appearing at the seventh week of life. Thymectomy delays or blocks rejection of skin allografts. The thymus of urodeles is not divided into cortex and medulla. The kidney retains its lymphoid function, as in fish. Stem cells arise from the intertubular areas of the kidney in both urodeles and anurans. In the spleen the red and white pulps are not separate.

Urodeles produce a monomeric IgM and can mount a good but slow antibody response against bacterial antigens. They do not respond to soluble protein antigens such as serum albumin or ferritin.

It takes about 28 to 42 days for a skin allograft to be rejected in urodele amphibians. The allograft looks healthy for about 3 weeks, and it is then slowly rejected. Destruction of the pigment cells makes rejection of the graft readily visible because it turns white. Second-set rejection takes about 8 to 20 days in the newt, and the alloimmune memory lasts at least 90 days.

Anuran Amphibians

In contrast to urodeles, a fully functional bone marrow is present in anurans (frogs and toads). Their thymus arises from the second pharyngeal pouches and involutes by about 1 year of age. It also involutes during metamorphosis from the tadpole to the adult stage and then rapidly regenerates. The thymus lies just below the skin posterior to the middle ear. In contrast to the thymus of the fish, it shows a distinct separation between the outer cortex and central medulla. The thymic cortex is full of proliferating lymphocytes. The medulla contains fewer lymphocytes, but thymic corpuscles are present. Immunoglobulins can be found on about 80% of these thymocytes. Larval thymectomy in the toad reduces the response to foreign red blood cells, but the response to bacterial lipopolysaccharide is unaffected, suggesting this is a T-independent response. Thymectomy also slows but does not completely prevent allograft rejection in toads. Some residual T cell function redevelops several months after larval thymectomy, suggesting that extrathymic T cell development may occur in these animals. In frogs and toads, for the first time, boundary layer cells separate the red pulp and the periarteriolar white pulp of the spleen. Structures that resemble lymph nodes are seen in some anuran amphibians. These protolymph nodes consist of a mass of lymphocytes surrounding blood sinusoids. As a result, they filter blood rather than lymph. Nodular lymphoid aggregates do not seem to be present in the intestine of urodeles but are seen in anurans.

Larval anurans such as the bullfrog tadpole have lymphomyeloid organs in their branchial region called ventral cavity bodies. Sinusoids in these organs are lined with macrophages that effectively remove injected particulate antigens from the blood. Removal of these organs renders tadpoles incapable of making antibodies to soluble antigens. They disappear at metamorphosis. Lymphocytes are found in large numbers in the subcapsular region of the liver in fish, amphibians, and reptiles. These lymphocyte accumulations occur close to blood sinuses and may have a stem cell function.

Both adult and larval amphibians have circulating B and T cells. They probably originate in the ventral cavity bodies or the liver. The thymic lymphocytes and about 80% of circulating lymphocytes carry surface IgM. Frogs possess NK-like and T cytotoxic–like killer cells.

Anuran amphibians have two or three immunoglobulin classes and are the least evolved vertebrates to show isotype switching. Their IgM consists of either pentamers or hexamers (in *Xenopus*) and one or two low-molecular–weight molecules. IgY with a 66 kDa υ heavy chain and IgX with a 64 kDa χ heavy chain. (IgX is a distinctly different immunoglobulin class not found in other vertebrates [Figure 38-8].) *Xenopus* immunoglobulins also contain two types of light chain (perhaps homologous to mammalian κ and λ chains). Anuran amphibians possess secretory immunoglobulins in bile and the intestine (but not in skin mucus). These consist of IgM and IgY but not IgA. In the axolotl (*Ambystoma mexicanum*) IgY is a secretory immunoglobulin found in close association with secretory component-like molecules. This is different from *Xenopus*, in which IgY behaves like avian IgY or mammalian IgG. Amphibian antibody diversity is generated in a fashion similar to that in mammals.

Frogs given bacteria or foreign erythrocytes will produce only IgM. Bacteriophages or soluble foreign proteins induce both IgM and IgY. Soluble antigens and bacteriophage can induce the production of both IgY and IgM in adult toads. The IgY takes up to a month to appear, and its level is very low. Anuran larvae will make only IgM antibodies unless immunized several times when low levels of IgY are produced. Amphibians do not mount a secondary immune response to erythrocytes and bacteria, but memory develops in response to the antigens that stimulate an IgY response. Studies on immunological memory are complicated by the fact that antigens may persist in the circulation for several months following injection. Anaphylactic (or anaphylactoid) reactions have been described in amphibians and reptiles.

Amphibians have T cells with functional TCRs, and anurans such as bullfrogs and toads show a fairly rapid allograft rejection. A first-set reaction takes about 14 days at 25° C. The graft shows capillary dilation, lymphocyte infiltration, and disintegration of pigment cells. Second allografts do not even become vascularized and are destroyed within a few days. If these amphibians are kept in the cold, a skin allograft may take as long as 200 days to be rejected. Delayed hypersensitivity reactions have been described in the axolotl (*Ambystoma*) and *Xenopus* in response to mycobacterial sensitization.

During amphibian metamorphosis from larval stage to adult, there is a temporary immunosuppression as shown by slowing of allograft rejection. Some allografts may even be tolerated at this time. As tadpoles change into

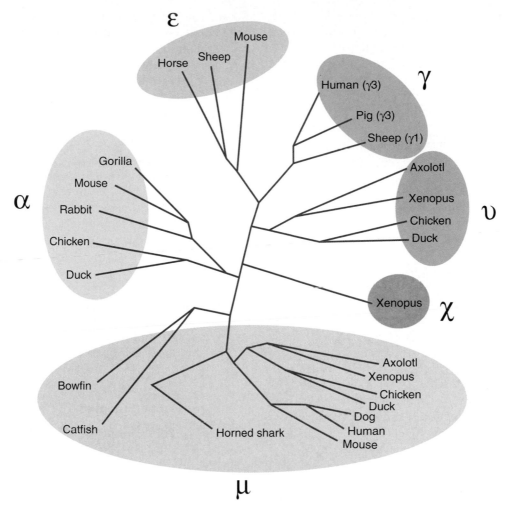

Figure 38-8. The evolutionary relationships among the major vertebrate immunoglobulin heavy chains. This is a distance tree constructed by aligning the amino acid sequences of representative vertebrate Ig H-chain constant regions. (From Warr GW, Magor KE, Higgins DA: *Immunology Today* 16:392-398, 1995.)

frogs or toads, the thymus shrinks and there is a drop in the numbers of B cells and antibody levels.

Cytokines identified in amphibians include IL-1, IL-2, and the interferons. *Xenopus* lymphocytes possess a receptor resembling IL-2R and can be stimulated by human IL-2 in vivo. *Xenopus* peritoneal cells generate IL-1–like activity.

Xenopus has a well-characterized MHC with class I, II, and III regions called XLA. The class II region contains genes for both α and β chains. These are 30 to 35 kDa transmembrane glycoproteins. About 20 class I and 30 class II alleles are believed to exist. The class III region contains a gene for C4. It is interesting to note that although MHC class II molecules are expressed early in larval development on B cells and tadpole epithelia, MHC class I molecules are not expressed before larval metamorphosis.

IMMUNITY IN REPTILES

The reptilian thymus develops from the pharyngeal pouches and is structurally similar to that seen in other classes of vertebrates. Both age and seasonal involution of the reptile thymus have been reported. The thymus shrinks in winter and enlarges in summer. The reptilian spleen usually shows a clear separation between red and white pulps.

Lymphomyeloid nodes that resemble lymph nodes are seen in reptiles. They have a simple structure consisting of a lymphoid parenchyma with phagocytes and intervening sinusoids. Primitive lymph nodules surrounding the aorta, vena cava, and jugular veins are also found. Lymphocytes and plasma cells are found in nodules in the intestinal wall of all the more evolved vertebrates. Some turtles and snakes (but not alligators) have lymphoid aggregations that project into the cloacal lumen, called the cloacal complex. These aggregates are larger in adults than in young turtles and are therefore not primary lymphoid organs and cannot be regarded as a primitive bursa. A few lymphocytes are found in the kidney of reptiles.

The reptiles that have been studied possess both IgM and IgY. The IgM of turtles is comparable to mammalian IgM in size, chain structure, and carbohydrate content. The IgY is found in both the full-sized and truncated isoforms (although some turtles may have only the truncated isoform). Alligators possess two different forms of immunoglobulin light chain, perhaps homologs of mammalian κ and λ.

Three C3 genes are present in the cobra. One codes for functional C3 in serum. The other two are expressed only in the venom gland and encode a C3c-like molecule present in venom that forms a stable C3-convertase in the presence of factor B.

Turtles and lizards immunized with bovine serum albumin, pig serum, or red blood cells can mount both primary and secondary antibody responses. The antibody produced in the primary response is IgM; the antibody produced in the secondary response is IgY. All reptile antibody responses appear to be T-dependent. Secondary responses and IgY antibody production do not occur in response to certain bacterial antigens such as *Salmonella enterica adelaide*, *Brucella abortus*, or *S. enterica typhimurium*. The reader may recollect that a similar situation occurs in mammals, in that thymus-independent antigens such as *E. coli* lipopolysaccharide induce a prolonged IgM response that is distinctly different from that induced by soluble protein antigens (Chapter 18).

As in other ectotherms, the rate of allograft rejection is temperature-dependent. Turtles, snakes, and lizards reject allogeneic skin grafts in about 40 days at 25° C. Graft-versus-host disease can be induced by injection of cells from their parents into newborn turtles and can lead to death. The severity of the disease depends on the genetic disparity between the turtles. Mortality, however, is greater at 30° C than at 20° C. Other evidence of cell-mediated immune responses such as mixed lymphocyte reactions and delayed hypersensitivity reactions have been demonstrated in reptiles.

IMMUNITY IN BIRDS

It must be recognized that the vast majority of studies on the avian immune system have focused on chickens. Thus the statements below, while generally true of chickens, may not necessarily apply to many of the other approximately 9000 bird species. The thymus in birds and in primitive mammals is similar to that seen in eutherian mammals. Germinal centers are not seen in fish, amphibian, or reptile spleens. In contrast, the germinal centers of bird lymphoid organs are large and well-defined. Although birds are commonly considered not to possess lymph nodes, they do possess structures that can be considered to be their functional equivalent. These avian

lymph nodes consist of a central sinus that is the main lumen of a lymphatic vessel. It is surrounded by a sheath of lymphoid tissue that contains germinal centers (Figure 38-9). Avian lymph nodes have no external capsule.

The bursa of Fabricius has been described in Chapter 8. Bursectomy results in a loss of antibody production, although bursectomized birds can still reject skin allografts. These results have been interpreted to suggest that the bursa is a primary lymphoid organ whose function is to serve as a maturation and differentiation site for the cells of the antibody-forming system. The bursa, however, contains some T cells; it can trap antigens and undertake some antibody synthesis. Birds also have large numbers of lymphocytes in the cecal tonsils and in the skin.

Bird lymphocytes originate in the yolk sac and migrate either to the bursa or to the thymus. Immature lymphocytes that enter the thymus mature under the influence of factors derived from thymic epithelial cells, and cells with recognizable T-cell markers emigrate from the thymus. In avian blood, T cells constitute between 60% and 70% of the total lymphocyte population. Immature lymphocytes that enter the bursa emigrate as immunoglobulin positive B cells.

Immunoglobulin Classes

There are three principal immunoglobulin classes in birds (chickens): IgY, IgM, and IgA. No avian IgD gene has yet been identified.

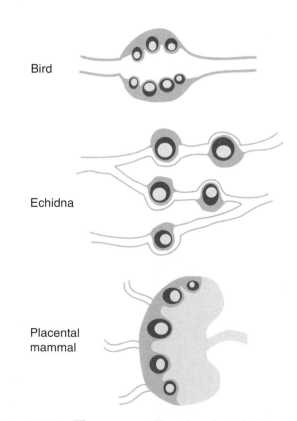

Figure 38-9. The structure of lymph nodes in birds, echidna, and placental mammals.

Immunoglobulin Y

The principal immunoglobulin in chicken serum is called IgY. Although somewhat similar to mammalian IgG, it has sufficient molecular differences to warrant a different designation. Some investigators have reported the existence of three immunoglobulin subclasses—termed IgY1, IgY2, and IgY3—although this has not been completely substantiated.

Like the immunoglobulins of mammals, IgY consists of two heavy and two light chains (Figure 38-10). The heavy chains, called upsilon (υ) chains, usually consist of one variable and four constant domains, and the complete molecule has a molecular weight of about 180 kDa (7.8 S). However, some birds have a truncated isoform that has only two constant domains (it lacks the third and fourth constant domains). This isoform has a molecular weight of about 120 kDa (5.7 S). Some birds such as ducks and geese have both full-sized and truncated IgY. Others, such as chickens, have only full-sized molecules.

The truncated isoform of IgY is produced as a result of alternative splicing of heavy chain mRNA. Its correct name is therefore IgY(ΔFc). Because the molecule lacks an Fc region, it cannot activate complement or bind to Fc receptors. Its function is unclear. There has, however, been a tendency during evolution to make low-molecular–weight immunoglobulins. Thus similar truncated immunoglobulins have also been described in some fish (IgM[ΔFc]), some turtles, and in the quokka (*Setonix brachyurus*), a marsupial. These low-molecular–weight molecules may offer some selective advantage. For example, it has been suggested that they will not trigger potentially lethal hypersensitivity reactions.

Both isoforms of IgY lack a hinge region. Thus, although bivalent, these molecules are somewhat inflexible and can cause precipitation or agglutination only in the presence of high-salt concentrations. They tend to show somewhat restricted diversity and limited affinity

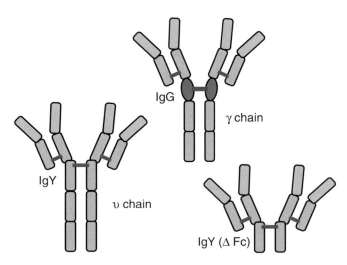

Figure 38-10. The structure of IgY and IgY(ΔFc) compared with mammalian IgG.

maturation. Studies on the interrelationships of the vertebrate immunoglobulins clearly show that IgY is related to both IgG and IgE in mammals (see Figure 38-8). In fact, it may have arisen from an evolutionary precursor of these two classes.

It is of interest to note that chickens can develop anaphylaxis. The signs of acute anaphylaxis in chickens and other birds are similar to those in mammals, although it is likely mediated by IgY. They show increased salivation, defecation, ruffling of feathers, dyspnea, convulsions, cyanosis, collapse, and death. The major target organ is probably the lung, and death is due to pulmonary arterial hypotension, right-sided heart dilation, and cardiac arrest. The pharmacological agents involved include histamine, serotonin, the kinins, and leukotrienes.

Immunoglobulin M

Birds produce primary and secondary responses in a manner similar to mammals. The predominance of IgM production in the primary immune response and of IgY in the secondary response is less marked than in mammals. A monomeric IgM can be detected in chicken eggs and in 1-day-old chicks. It is thought to be derived from oviduct secretions in the hen.

Immunoglobulin A

The structure of chicken IgA is similar to IgA in mammals. The only significant difference is that chicken IgA has four heavy chain C domains, whereas mammalian IgA has only three. Chicken serum IgA exists in both dimeric (340 kDa) and monomeric (170 kDa) forms. Intestinal IgA is associated with secretory component (SC).

Generation of Antibody Diversity

Chickens generate antibody diversity in a manner that is quite unlike that seen in mammals. In most mammals, the primary antibody repertoire is created through the recombination of immunoglobulin variable (V), diversity (D), and joining (J) genes. They thus have a large number of V, D, and J genes that are selected randomly and combine to form many different variable regions. Chickens, on the other hand, have only one functional V gene and one J gene for both light and heavy chains, although they do have 16 different D genes. Chicken immunoglobulin diversity is therefore generated by gene conversion. Although they have only one functional V gene, chickens have a large number of V pseudogenes that serve as sequence donors to diversify the functional light chain V gene by gene conversion. During recombination of the V and J genes, single bases are also added to each gene (N-region addition), and joining occurs at random. Chicken immunoglobulins are further diversified by somatic hypermutation and imprecise V-J joining.

A second major difference involves the timing of the process. In mammals, rearrangement of immunoglobulin genes is an ongoing process. Chickens, in contrast, rearrange their immunoglobulin genes as a single wave between 10 and 15 days of embryogenesis, at a period when there is clonal expansion of B cells in the bursa of Fabricius. During that 5-day period, birds generate all the antibody specificities they will need for the rest of their lives. The chicken can generate about 10^6 different immunoglobulin molecules. This is approximately one order of magnitude less than the mouse.

Chicken T cells can respond to phytohemagglutinin and concanavalin A. Avian T cells can participate in delayed hypersensitivity reactions, graft-versus-host disease, and allograft rejection. Avian homologs of mammalian γ/δ TCR (TCR-1) and α/β TCR (TCR-2 and TCR-3) have been identified. TCR-2 and TCR-3 are subsets of α/β TCRs that use distinctly different V_β gene segments. TCR-2 cells undergo V-DJ joining by gene deletion, whereas TCR-3 cells undergo V-DJ joining by chromosome inversion. The structure of the avian CD3 signaling complex is different from that in mammals insofar as it contains only two dimers, δ/γ-ϵ and ζ-ζ, rather than three. There is evidence that chickens possess both Th1 and Th2 cells. For example, chicken IL-18 stimulates IFN-γ release from CD4+ T cells.

Birds reject skin allografts in about 7 to 14 days. Histological examination shows massive infiltration of the grafted tissue with lymphocytes. These cells are believed to be T cells, since neonatal thymectomy results in a failure to reject grafts. If chicken T cells are dropped onto the chorioallantoic membrane of 13- to 14-day-old chick embryos, the cells will attack the chick tissues. This will result in pock formation on the membrane and splenic enlargement. The grafted cells attack the hematopoietic cells of the recipient. A few days after hatching, chicks become resistant to this form of graft-versus-host attack.

IMMUNITY IN MONOTREMES AND MARSUPIALS

The least evolved mammals, the monotremes, such as the duck-billed platypus (*Ornithorynchus anatinus*) and the echidna (*Tachyglossus aculeatus*), have a spleen, thymus, and gut-associated lymphoid tissues that are as well developed as those in marsupials and eutherian mammals. However, instead of typical mammalian lymph nodes, they have lymphoid nodules that consist of several lymphoid nodules, each containing a germinal center, suspended by its blood vessels within the lumen of a lymphatic plexus. Thus, each nodule is bathed in lymph. There is usually just one germinal center per nodule. The evolution of the predominant blood immunoglobulin from IgY to IgG probably occurred very early in mammalian evolution since monotremes possess not IgY but IgG. They have two IgG subclasses, IgG1 and IgG2,

as well as IgE and IgM. Although distinctly different from marsupial and eutherian IgG and IgE, these show overall structural similarity to other mammalian immunoglobulins. Thus all the major structural changes that gave rise to the immunoglobulin classes expressed in modern mammals evolved before the separation of the monotremes from the marsupials and placental mammals and probably soon after the split from reptile lineages 300 mya. Monotremes, like other mammals, produce predominantly IgM in the primary immune response and IgG in secondary immune responses.

Marsupials produce immunoglobulins in a manner similar to eutherian mammals. They possess four immunoglobulin isotypes: IgM, IgG, IgE, and IgA. The marsupial opossum (*Didelphis*) resembles more primitive vertebrates in that it responds well to particulate antigens, such as bacteria, but responds poorly to soluble antigens. When opossums were inoculated with sheep red blood cells, the primary immune response was long-lived and reasonably strong. The secondary response was weaker than the first and lasted for a much shorter period.

Mammals possess a very large number of V gene segments. When the sequences of these are analyzed, they can be shown to form different Vh gene families. Thus 7 gene families have been identified in humans and 15 in mice. Further analysis of these families shows that they form three major "clans" (clans I, II, and III). Comparative studies have shown that these three clans have probably existed for more than 400 million years. Fish Vh sequences are most closely related to mammalian clan III. However, fish possess two additional clans not found in mammals. The monotremes and marsupials have Vh genes that also belong to clan III. Likewise, although chickens, rabbits, and pigs have relatively few Vh genes, the V genes of these three species belong to clan III. This has led to the assumption that clan III is the most ancient of the mammalian clans. However, cattle and sheep also express only a single Vh gene family, and this belongs to clan II. This may be due to inactivation and loss of clan III in these species.

MAMMALIAN PHYLOGENY

This book has focused on immunity in a small group of domestic mammals. These mammals have been selected not as representatives of mammalian diversity but for the behavioral traits that lend them to domestication or for the ease with which they are maintained in captivity. If we examine their place in mammalian phylogeny (Figure 38-11), we can see that most domestic animal species are relatively closely related. Even domestic pets such as dogs and cats are closer to farm animal species than to primates. Likewise, laboratory animals tend to cluster in a separate group. It is unsurprising, therefore, that significant differences exist among the immune

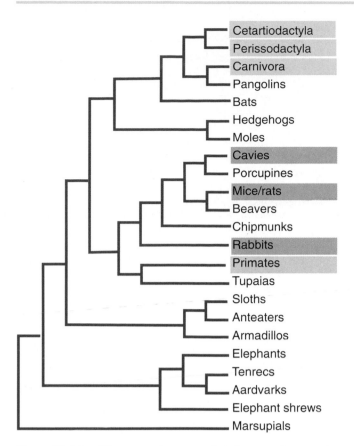

Figure 38-11. The currently accepted phylogeny of mammals. Note that none of the domestic animal species can be considered representative of mammals as a whole.

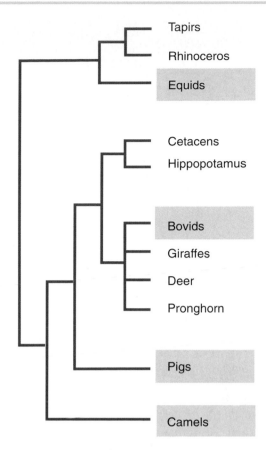

Figure 38-12. The phylogeny of the domestic herbivores. Many gaps remain in our knowledge of the immunology of these species.

systems of species of interest to veterinarians. It is also clear that if we are to understand the significance of these differences and how they evolved, we must examine the immune systems of other, unrelated mammals. Even within the major domestic herbivores (Figure 38-12), their phylogeny demonstrates why there are significant variations in their immune systems and hints at other, unsuspected but possibly important differences.

FEVER

Vertebrates generally respond to antigens faster and more intensely at higher temperatures. Conversely, low temperatures in ectotherms may be significantly immunosuppressive. Thus in chilled fish, the lag period may be long or there may be a complete absence of an antibody response. Only certain phases of the antibody response are temperature-dependent. For example, secondary immune responses can be elicited at low temperatures provided primary immunization is carried out at a high temperature. The cells that are sensitive to low temperature in fish are helper T cells, and the effect is due to a loss of T cell membrane fluidity and reactivity to interleukins. Acclimatization to low temperatures can

also occur. For example, goldfish that are acclimatized at a low temperature may be able to produce a similar number of antibody-forming cells to those that have remained at a warmer temperature. The nature of the antigen is also critical in that certain T cell–dependent mitogens are ineffective at low temperatures, again implying that the target cell is a helper T cell. The temperature at which the animal is kept influences the rejection of allografts in all ectotherms.

Although it is well recognized that endotherms such as mammals develop a fever when infected, it is less apparent that ectotherms such as fish or reptiles also develop fever in response to infection. Ectotherms are unable to change their body temperature by physiological mechanisms. As a result, they cannot develop a fever if maintained in a constant temperature environment. If, however, they are maintained in an environment with cool and warm areas, they will cycle between these areas and maintain their body temperature within well-defined limits. For example, it has been observed that normal iguanas (*Dipsosaurus dorsalis*) maintain their temperature between 37° and 41° C. However, iguanas infected with the bacterium *Aeromonas hydrophila* modify their behavior so that they spend more time in the warm environment (Figure 38-13). As a result, their temperatures cycle

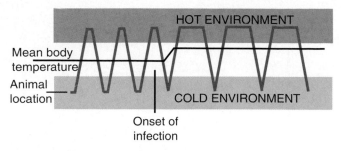

Figure 38-13. A fever can be induced in ectotherms by modifications in behavior. Simply spending more time in a warm environment will effectively raise average body temperature. This behavioral response occurs in response to microbial infection.

between 40° and 43° C. Once the bacterial infection is cured, the iguanas resume their normal behavior. Thus the iguanas effectively induce a fever by their behavior. A similar behavioral fever is seen in goldfish maintained in two interconnected tanks maintained at different temperatures. In response to microbial infection, the fish will choose to spend more time in the warmer water, thus effectively raising their body temperature. The benefits of this to ectotherms are obvious, because as pointed out above, their immune systems function much more efficiently at higher temperatures.

Some mammals hibernate, most notably bears, bats, and some rodents. At this time, their body temperature may fall. If bats are cooled to around 8° C, they cease antibody production, but rewarming permits rapid resumption of antibody synthesis. This cessation of the antibody response in hibernating bats may allow them to act as persistent carriers of viruses such as rabies.

SOURCES OF ADDITIONAL INFORMATION

Arason GJ: Lectins as defense molecules in vertebrates and invertebrates, *Fish Shellfish Immunol* 6:277-289, 1996.

Belov K, Hellman L, Cooper DW: Characterization of echidna IgM provides insights into the time of divergence of extant mammals, *Dev Comp Immunol* 26:831-839, 2002.

Cabanac M, Laberge F: Fever in goldfish is induced by pyrogens but not by handling, *Physiol Behav* 63:377-379, 1998.

Diaz M, Stanfield RL, Greenberg AS, Flajnik MF: Structural analysis, selection, and ontongeny of the shark new antigen receptor (IgNAR): identification of a new locus preferentially expressed in early development, *Immunogenetics* 54: 501-512, 2002.

Hanley PJ, Hook JW, Raftos DA, et al: Hagfish humoral defense protein exhibits structural and functional homology with mammalian structural components, *Proc Natl Acad Sci USA*, 89:7910-7914, 1992.

Hine PM: The granulocytes of fish, *Fish Shellfish Immunol* 2:79-98, 1992.

Holland MC, Lambris JD: The complement system in teleosts, *Fish Shellfish Immunol* 12:399-420, 2002.

Hordvik I: Identification of a novel immunoglobulin d transcript and comparative analysis of the genes encoding IgD in Atlantic salmon and Atlantic halibut, *Mol Immunol* 39: 85-91, 2002.

Johansson J, Aveskogh M, Munday B, Hellman L: Heavy chain V region diversity in the duck-billed platypus (*Ornithorhynchus anatinus*): long and highly variable complementarity-determining region 3 compensates for limited germline diversity, *J Immunol* 168:5155-5162, 2002.

Lee SY, Söderhäll K: Early events in crustacean innate immunity, *Fish Shellfish Immunol* 12:421-437, 2002.

Magor KE, Higgins DA, Middleton DL, Warr GW: One gene encodes the heavy chains for three different forms of IgY in the duck, *J Immunol* 153: 5549-5555, 1994.

Mansikka A: Chicken IgA H chains: implications concerning the evolution of H chain genes, *J Immunol* 149: 855-861, 1992.

Nonaka M, Smith SL: Complement system of bony and cartilaginous fish, *Fish Shellfish Immunol* 10:215-228, 2000.

Pilström L: The mysterious immunoglobulin light chain, *Dev Comp Immunol* 26:207-215, 2002.

Pilström L, Dengtén E: Immunoglobulin in fish—genes, expression and structure, *Fish Shellfish Immunol* 6:243-262, 1996.

Ratcliffe MJ, Jacobsen K: Rearrangement of immunoglobulin genes in chicken B cell development, *Sem Immunol* 6: 175-184, 1994.

Secombes CJ, Hardie LJ, Daniels G: Cytokines in fish: an update, *Fish Shellfish Immunol* 6:291-304, 1996.

Sunyer JO, Zarkadis IK, Lambris JD: Complement diversity: a mechanism for generating immune diversity? *Immunol Today* 19:519-523, 1998.

Vernersson M, Aveskogh M, Munday B, Hellman L: Evidence for an early appearance of modern postswitch immunoglobulin isotypes in mammalian evolution (II): cloning of IgE, IgG1, and IgG2 from a monotreme, the duck-billed platypus, *Ornithorhynchus anatinus*, *Eur J Immunol* 32: 2145-2155, 2002.

Warr GW: The immunoglobulin genes of fish, *Dev Comp Immunol* 19:1-12, 1995.

Warr GW, Magor KE, Higgins DA: IgY: clues to the origins of modern antibodies, *Immunol Today* 16:392-398, 1995.

Wilson R, Chen C, Ratcliffe NA: Innate immunity in insects: the role of multiple, endogenous serum lectins in the recognition of foreign invaders in the cockroach, *Blaberus discoidalis*, *J Immunol* 162:1590-1596, 1999.

APPENDIX

An Annotated List of Selected CD Molecules

NOTE: Of the 247 officially recognized CD molecules, many have no known function at this time, while many others do not play a significant role in the immune system. This list summarizes the key features of only the CD molecules described in the text.

CD1 A family of MHC class Id molecules that act as antigen-presenting molecules for lipids and glycolipids. Heterodimers of 49/12 kDa, they are found on thymocytes, macrophages, dendritic cells, and some B cells.

CD2 Also called LFA-2, this is a 67 kDa molecule found on T cells and some B cells. It is a cell adherence molecule whose ligands are CD58 (nonrodents) and CD48 (rodents only). CD2 was first recognized by its ability to bind sheep red blood cells to T cells to form characteristic rosettes.

CD3 The collective designation for the set of proteins that act as the major signal transduction molecules of the TCR. They are 16- to 28-kDa glycoproteins found only on T cells.

CD4 A specific receptor for MHC class II molecules, it plays a key role in the recognition of processed antigen by helper T cells. It is a 59-kDa glycoprotein found on helper T cells, thymocytes, and monocytes. CD4 is also a receptor for HIV.

CD5 A 67-kDa molecule whose ligand is CD72. It is found on a subset of B cells and on all T cells. If blocked, T cells no longer respond to antigen. Its expression on B cells varies among species. Thus it is found on all rabbit B cells and on a subpopulation of B cells (B-1a cells) in most species, including mice and humans, but it is not found on B cells in rats or dogs.

CD8 This 32-kDa dimeric glycoprotein serves as a specific receptor for MHC class I molecules. It is expressed on cytotoxic T cells and plays a key role in the recognition of endogenous antigen by these cells.

CD9 A glycoprotein of 22 to 27 kDa expressed on platelets, immature B cells, eosinophils, basophils, and activated T cells. It may be the receptor for FIV on cat T cells.

CD10 An endopeptidase of 100 kDa expressed on T and B cell precursors.

CD11 Also called LFA-1, this is a 180-kDa integrin α chain found on leukocytes. Three forms are known: 11a, 11b, and 11c. They play a key role in binding leukocytes to vascular endothelium.

CD14 A 55-kDa protein found on macrophages and granulocytes. It is the receptor for lipopolysaccharide-binding protein and therefore plays a key role in regulating the biological activities of this molecule.

CD15 A complex carbohydrate called Lewis-X. It is found on many cells, especially granulocytes. Its sialylated form, sialyl Lewis^x, is characteristic of NK cells. Its ligand is the selectin CD62.

CD16 Also called FcγRIII, this is a low-affinity receptor for IgG and for CD4. It is a 50- to 65-kDa dimer found on NK cells, granulocytes, and macrophages.

CD18 This is the integrin β_2 chain. A protein of 95 kDa, it is found on all leukocytes. It associates with the various forms of CD11. A defect in the CD18 gene is responsible for leukocyte adherence deficiency in calves.

CD19 A glycoprotein of 95 kDa expressed on B cells and their precursors but not on plasma cells. It is also expressed on dendritic cells. It is associated with CD21. CD19 plays a key role in regulating the B cell response to antigen.

CD21 A complement receptor also called CR2. It is a glycoprotein of 145 kDa found on B cells, some T cells, and dendritic cells. Its several ligands include CD23 and C3d. It regulates B cell responses in association with CD19.

CD22 Also called siglec-2, this is a B cell inhibitory receptor.

CD23 Also called FcϵRII, this receptor for IgE is a glycoprotein of 45 kDa found mainly on mature B cells. In its soluble form it regulates the production of IgE. It can also regulate B cell responses by binding to CD21.

CD25 The α chain of the IL-2 receptor. A glycoprotein of 55 kDa, CD25 associates with the IL-2Rβ chain (CD122). It is expressed on activated T cells, B cells, and monocytes. When it binds IL-2, it activates these cells.

CD28 The ligand for CD80 and CD86 expressed on activated B cells and other antigen-presenting cells. It is a homodimer of 45 kDa subunits found on most T cells. It plays a key role in regulating T cell responses.

CD29 The β_1 integrin chain, a protein of 130 kDa expressed on leukocytes and platelets. In conjunction with its α chain (one of the forms of CD49), it binds these cells to extracellular matrix proteins.

CD31 CD31 mediates adhesion between cells that express CD31 (for example, leukocytes to endothelial cells) in a homophilic manner (CD31 binds CD31 on the apposing cell). It regulates the phagocytosis of dead and dying cells.

CD32   A 40-kDa, medium-affinity IgG receptor that is also called FcγRII. Different forms of CD32 are expressed on macrophages, granulocytes, and B cells.

CD33   Siglec-3, a molecule expressed on immature hematopoietic stem cells. CD33 has carbohydrate-binding properties.

CD34   Also called sialomucin, CD34 is a 105- to 120-kDa glycoprotein expressed on endothelial cells, where it is a ligand for integrins.

CD35   A 160- to 250-kDa glycoprotein expressed on granulocytes, monocytes, B cells, NK cells, and primate erythrocytes. The receptor for the complement components C3b and C4b, it is also called CR1. This molecule is important in opsonization and the removal of immune-complexes from the body.

CD40   A 50-kDa member of the tumor necrosis factor receptor superfamily expressed on all antigen-presenting cells. Binding to its ligand CD40L (CD154) on activated helper T cells is essential for a successful antibody response and class switching.

CD41   An integrin α chain of 120 kDa expressed on platelets and macrophages. It associates with its β chain (CD61) and binds to fibrinogen.

CD43   Also called sialophorin or leukosialin, this 115-kDa glycoprotein is expressed on all T cells, as well as granulocytes, macrophages, NK cells platelets, and activated B cells. It serves as an antiadhesive molecule on leukocytes.

CD44   A 90-kDa glycoprotein expressed in large amounts on T and B cells, monocytes, and granulocytes, as well as a wide variety of other cells. It is the principal receptor for hyaluronic acid. As a result it mediates binding of these cells to high-endothelial venules.

CD45   A family of 190- to 220-kDa glycoproteins found on all cells of hematopoietic origin except red cells. Various isoforms of CD45 are generated by alternative splicing of three exons. They are all phosphotyrosine phosphatases, some of which are required for signaling through the TCR.

CD46   Also called membrane cofactor protein, this is a receptor for C3b and C4b. Once bound, these complement components are destroyed by factor I. CD46 is a 50-kDa glycoprotein expressed on T cells, B cells, monocytes, granulocytes NK cells, platelets, fibroblasts, endothelial cells, and epithelial cells but not on red cells.

CD48   A 47-kDa GPI-linked glycoprotein expressed on all blood lymphocytes. It is a ligand for CD2 and CD247 in rodents.

CD49   A family of 170-kDa integrin α chains that are associated with the CD29 β chain. They are expressed in various forms on leukocytes, platelets, and epithelial cells. Also called very late antigens (VLAs), their ligands are extracellular matrix proteins.

CD51   A 125-kDa integrin α chain found on platelets and endothelial cells. Its β chain is CD61, and its ligand is vitronectin.

CD54   Also called ICAM-1, this glycoprotein of 90 kDa is the ligand for the CD11a/CD18 and CD11b/CD18 integrins. It is expressed on a wide variety of cells, most notably vascular endothelial cells. It has also been reported to bind to CD43.

CD55   Also called decay-accelerating factor, this glycoprotein of 60 to 70 kDa blocks the assembly of C3 convertase and accelerates its disassembly, thus protecting normal cells against attack by complement. It is broadly distributed on many cell types.

CD56   In humans, CD56 is found on NK cells, where it appears to play an important role in NK cell–mediated cytotoxicity. In dogs, in contrast, CD56 is found exclusively on a subset (~10%-20%) of CD3$^+$ T cells. It is a glycoprotein of 180 kDa.

CD58   Also called LFA-3, this is a 65-kDa glycoprotein found on most cells, where it is a ligand for CD2. Sheep CD58 is expressed on red cells so that these will bind to T cells to form E-rosettes.

CD59   A small glycoprotein of 18 to 20 kDa expressed on leukocytes, vascular endothelium, and epithelial cells. Also called protectin, it acts as an inhibitor of the terminal complement pathway by binding to C8 and C9 and blocking the assembly of the membrane attack complex.

CD61   A β$_3$ integrin of 105 kDa that associates with CD41 to bind to extracellular matrix proteins. It is expressed on platelets and macrophages.

CD62   The selectins, a family of carbohydrate-binding glycoproteins expressed on platelet lymphocytes and endothelial cells. They bind to carbohydrate structures such as CD15s (sialyl Lewis^x) on neutrophils. CD62E is E-selectin (115 kDa), CD62L is L-selectin (75-80 kDa), and CD62P is P-selectin (150 kDa).

CD64   Also called FcγRI, this high-affinity IgG receptor is a glycoprotein of 72 kDa expressed on monocytes and interferon-stimulated granulocytes. It plays a key role in antibody-dependent cellular cytotoxicity.

CD66e   Also called carcinoembryonic antigen, this 180- to 200-kDa glycoprotein is expressed in large quantities by malignant intestinal cells. Its detection is therefore diagnostic for intestinal malignancy in humans.

CD71   A 95-kDa transferrin receptor expressed on activated leukocytes. It is required by dividing cells to import iron. It may also act as a selective IgA receptor.

CD72   Found on B cells (but not plasma cells), CD72 is a 42-kDa glycoprotein ligand for CD5. It may participate in an alternative pathway of B cell and T cell activation.

CD74   The γ or invariant chain of 32 kDa associated with intracellular MHC class II molecules. Found in all MHC class II–positive cells. It is believed to prevent the binding of endogenous peptides.

CD79   CD79a is an alternative name for the BCR signal-transducing peptide Ig-α, and CD79b is another name for Ig-β. Both are glycoproteins of 33 to 40 kDa.

CD80 Also called B7-1, this is a 60-kDa member of the immunoglobulin superfamily expressed on a subset of antigen-presenting B cells and macrophages. It is a high-affinity receptor for CD28 and CD152 (CTLA-4). The interaction of CD80 with its ligands is crucial to T cell communication with antigen-presenting cells.

CD81 Also called TAPA-1, CD81 is a widely expressed cell surface protein that regulates both B and T cell responses. On B cells it forms a complex with CD19, CD21, and Leu13 and is involved with costimulation of T cells.

CD85 A family of leukocyte Ig-like receptors (LIRs) or Ig-like transcripts (ILTs) expressed on macrophages, dendritic cells, and B cells. They act as receptors for MHC class I molecules.

CD86 Related to CD80 and also called B7-2, this is a 60-kDa glycoprotein expressed on antigen-presenting macrophages, activated B cells, and dendritic cells. Its ligands are CD28 and CD152 (CTLA-4). Like CD80, this receptor is critical for the interaction between T cells and antigen-presenting cells.

CD88 The C5a receptor found on granulocytes, macrophages, and mast cells. It is a 42-kDa glycoprotein.

CD89 This IgA receptor (FcαR) is a 50- to 70-kDa glycoprotein expressed on granulocytes, monocytes, and some subpopulations of T and B cells.

CD90 Otherwise known as Thy-1, this glycoprotein of 25 to 35 kDa is expressed on thymocytes and T cell in some species. It is also expressed on some brain cells.

CD91 The heat-shock protein receptor. This protein, expressed on macrophages, is important in the intracellular processing of these molecules.

CD94 One of the NK cell receptors. This 70 kDa glycoprotein is a C-type lectin that binds target cell MHC class I molecules.

CD95 Otherwise known as fas, this is a receptor for fas-ligand (CD95L or CD178) and a signaling component of an important cell death pathway. It is a 42-kDa glycoprotein found on myeloid and T cells. It plays a key role in the negative selection of self-reactive T cells.

CD102 Also called ICAM-2, a glycoprotein of 60 kDa expressed on vascular endothelial cells, resting lymphocytes, and monocytes but not neutrophils. It is the ligand for the integrin CD11a/CD18.

CD105 The TGF-β receptor, a glycoprotein of 95kDa expressed on endothelial cells.

CD106 Also called VCAM-1, a glycoprotein of 100 to 110 kDa expressed on endothelial cells. It is the ligand for CD49d/CD29 (VLA-4).

CD115 The M-CSF receptor is a 150-kDa glycoprotein expressed on macrophages and their precursors.

CD116 The α chain of the GM-CSF receptor is a 43-kDa glycoprotein found on granulocytes, monocytes, and eosinophils. It shares a common β chain with IL-3R and IL-5R.

CD117 Also called c-kit, this is the receptor for stem cell factor. It is an immunoglobulin superfamily tyrosine kinase of 145 kDa found on hematopoietic precursor cells.

CDw118 The receptor for IFN-α and IFN-β

CDw119 The IFN-γ receptor is a 90-kDa glycoprotein found on B cells, macrophages, monocytes, fibroblasts, and endothelial cells.

CD120 There are two TNF receptors (TNFR-I [CD120a] and TNFR-II [CD120b]). These are glycoproteins of 55 and 75 kDa, respectively, expressed on most cells. TNFR-I is found at higher levels on epithelial cells, whereas TNFR-II is more highly expressed on myeloid cells.

CD121 These are the two IL-1 receptors, IL-1RI (80 kDa) and IL-1RII (60 to 70 kDa), glycoproteins expressed on thymocytes, fibroblasts, keratinocytes, endothelial cells (type I), macrophages, and B cells (type II).

CD122 The IL-2R β chain. This 75-kDa glycoprotein is expressed on T cells, activated B cells, NK cells, and monocytes.

CD123 The IL-3 receptor α chain.

CD124 The IL-4 receptor, a glycoprotein of 87 kDa expressed on T and B cells, fibroblasts, endothelial cells, and stem cells.

CDw125 The IL-5 receptor α chain. A transmembrane glycoprotein of 60 kDa.

CD126 The α chain of the IL-6 receptor. An 80-kDa glycoprotein expressed on B cells, plasma cells, epithelial cells, and hepatocytes.

CD127 The IL-7 receptor is a glycoprotein of 75 kDa expressed on stem cells, T cells, and monocytes.

CDw128 The IL-8 receptors are 58- to 67 kDa-glycoproteins expressed on leukocytes and keratinocytes. Also called CXCR1 and 2.

CD130 The β chain of the IL-6 (with CD126) and IL-11 receptors is a 130-kDa glycoprotein found mainly on B cells but expressed at lower levels on most leukocytes, epithelial cells, hepatocytes, and fibroblasts.

CD131 A type I transmembrane protein of 120-140 kDa. It acts as the common β chain of the IL-3 (with CD123), IL-5 (with CD125), and GM-CSF (with CD123) receptors.

CD132 The common γ chain of IL-2 (with CD25 and CD122), IL-4 (with CD124), IL-7 (with CD127), IL-9 (with CD129), and IL-15 receptors. It is a transmembrane glycoprotein of 65-70 kDa.

CD134 A receptor that plays an important role in the survival and proliferation of CD4+ T cells. It is also found on CD8+ T cells, macrophages, and activated B cells. The feline homolog of CD134 is the primary receptor for feline immunodeficiency virus.

CD140 Platelet-derived growth factor (PDGF) receptor.

CD152 Found on activated T cells, this transmembrane glycoprotein of 46-50 kDa is also known as CTLA-4. It is the ligand for CD80 and CD86 and a negative regulator of T cell activation.

CD154 A 35-kDa member of the TNF family. Since it serves as the ligand for CD40, it is also called CD40L. Found on activated Th cells, it plays a key role in T cell activation by cross-linking with CD40 on antigen-presenting cells.

CD158 The KIR family of MHC class I receptors expressed on NK cells and T cell subsets. They play a key role in NK cell activation.

CD169 Siglec 1 or sialoadhesin, a 200 kDa macrophage lectin-like adhesion molecule that binds sialyated ligands.

CD172a A signal regulatory protein expressed on monocytes and a subset of dendritic cells.

CD178 The ligand for CD95 (Fas-ligand or CD95-L). A member of the tumor necrosis factor superfamily, this is a key molecule in the induction of cell death by apoptosis. It is a polymeric protein with 40 kDa subunits that is readily shed from cells.

CD206 A type I membrane protein of 160 kDa found on mature macrophages and immature dendritic cells. It is a C-type lectin that binds mannose-rich carbohydrates.

CD209 DC-SIGN, a C-type lectin found on dendritic cells. Its ligand is ICAM-3 (CD50) on T cells and other leukocytes (Chapter 6).

CDw210 IL-10R cytokine receptor.

CD212 IL-12R cytokine receptor.

CD213 A transmembrane protein of 65 kDa that acts as the IL-13R cytokine receptor α chain and a member of the IL-4 receptor complex.

CD217 IL-17R cytokine receptor.

CD220 Insulin receptor.

CD221 IGF1R cytokine receptor.

CD230 The prion protein (PrP). A large membrane protein found on neurons. The abnormal form of this protein (PrPsc) is a transmissible agent causing spongiform encephalopathies.

CD233 An erythrocyte membrane protein of 95-110 kDa that functions as an anion (chloride and bicarbonate) exchanger. Also called band 3 protein.

CD240 Rhesus blood group molecules in humans.

CD247 The T cell antigen receptor zeta (ζ) chain.

Activated macrophage A macrophage in a state of enhanced metabolic and functional activity.

Active immunity Immunity produced as a result of administration of an antigen, thus triggering an immune response.

Acute inflammation Rapidly developing inflammation of recent onset. It is characterized by tissue infiltration by neutrophils.

Acute phase proteins Proteins, synthesized by the liver, whose level in serum rises rapidly in response to acute inflammation and tissue damage.

Adjuvant Any substance that, when given with an antigen, enhances the immune response to that antigen.

Adoptive immunity Immunity that results from the transfer of cells from an immunized animal to an unimmunized recipient.

Affinity The strength of binding between two molecules such as an antigen and antibody. Usually expressed as an association constant (Ka).

Affinity maturation The progressive increase in antibody affinity for antigen that occurs during the course of an immune response as a result of somatic mutation in V genes.

Agammaglobulinemia The absence of gamma globulins in blood.

Agglutination The clumping of particulate antigens by antibody.

Agnatha A class of jawless fish. It includes the cyclostomes, an order containing the hagfish and lamprey.

Albumin The major serum protein of 60 kDa.

Alleles Different forms of a gene that occupy the same locus.

Allelic exclusion The expression of only one allelic protein by a cell from a heterozygous individual that has the genes to express both allelic proteins.

Allergens Antigens that provoke an IgE response and hence type I hypersensitivity (allergy).

Allergic contact dermatitis An inflammatory skin disease resulting from a type IV hypersensitivity reaction to skin cells modified by exposure to foreign chemicals.

Allergy Immediate (type I) hypersensitivity. An immune response characterized by the release of pharmacological agents as a result of mast cell and basophil degranulation following the binding of antigen to cell-bound IgE.

Allogeneic Genetically dissimilar animals of the same species.

Allograft An organ graft between two genetically dissimilar animals of the same species.

Allotype Antigenic (and structural) differences between the proteins of different individuals of the same species as a result of transcription of different alleles.

Alternative complement pathway The complement pathway triggered by the activation of C3 by the presence of an activating surface.

Amyloid An extracellular, amorphous, waxy protein deposited in the tissues of individuals with chronic inflammation or a myeloma.

Analog An organ or tissue that has the same function as another but is of different evolutionary origin.

Anamnestic response A secondary immune response.

Anaphylatoxins Complement fragments that stimulate mast cell degranulation and smooth muscle contraction.

Anaphylaxis A sudden, systemic, severe immediate hypersensitivity reaction resulting from rapid generalized mast cell and eosinophil degranulation.

Anergy The failure of a sensitized animal to respond to an antigen—a form of immunological tolerance.

Antibiotic A chemical compound, usually obtained from microorganisms, that can prevent growth or kill bacteria. Do not confuse this with antibody.

Antibody An immunoglobulin molecule synthesized on exposure to antigen, which can combine specifically with that antigen.

Antibody-dependent cellular cytotoxicity (ADCC) The killing of antibody-coated target cells by cytotoxic cells with surface Fc receptors.

Antigen Any foreign substance that can bind to specific lymphocyte receptors and so induce an immune response.

Antigen-presenting cells Cells that can ingest, process, and present antigen to antigen-sensitive cells in association with MHC class I and class II molecules.

Antigen processing The series of events that modify antigens so that they bind to MHC molecules and so can be recognized by antigen-sensitive cells.

Antigen-sensitive cells Cells that can bind and respond to specific antigen.

Antigenic determinant See Epitope.

Antigenic variation The progressive change in surface antigens exhibited by viruses, parasites, and some bacteria in order to evade destruction.

Antigenicity The ability of a molecule to be recognized by an antibody or lymphocyte.

Antiglobulin Antibody made against an immunoglobulin, usually by injecting immunoglobulin into an animal of another species.

Antiglobulin test A technique for detecting the presence of nonagglutinating antibody on the surface of a particle.

Antiserum   Serum that contains specific antibodies. Synonymous with immune globulin.

Antitoxin   Antiserum directed against a toxin and used for passive immunization.

Anurans   An order of advanced amphibians that includes the frogs and toads.

Apoptosis   The controlled self-destruction of a cell; one form of programmed cell death. (*Apoptosis* is a Greek word describing the falling away of petals from flowers or the leaves from trees).

Arthus reaction   Local inflammation due to a type III hypersensitivity reaction; it is induced by the injection of antigen into the skin of an immunized animal.

Asthma   A type I hypersensitivity disease characterized by a reduction in airway diameter, leading to difficulty in breathing (dyspnea).

Atopy   A genetically determined predisposition to develop clinical allergies.

Attenuation   The reduction of virulence of an infectious agent.

Autoantibodies   Antibodies directed against epitopes on normal body tissues.

Autoantigen   A normal body component that acts as an antigen.

Autoimmune disease   Disease caused by an immune attack against an individual's own tissues.

Autoimmunity   The process of mounting an immune response against a normal body component.

Autograft   A tissue or organ graft made between two sites within the same animal.

B lymphocytes (B cells)   Lymphocytes that have undergone a period of processing in the bursa or its mammalian equivalent. They are responsible for antibody production.

Bacille Calmette-Guérin (BCG) vaccine   An attenuated strain of *Mycobacterium bovis*. This may be used as a specific vaccine or as a nonspecific immune stimulator.

Bacterin   A preparation of killed bacteria used for immunization.

Basophil   A polymorphonuclear cell that contains granules with a high avidity for basic dyes such as hematoxylin. It participates in type I hypersensitivity reactions.

BCG   See Bacille Calmette-Guérin (BCG) vaccine.

Bence-Jones protein   Immunoglobulin light chains found in the urine of patients with myelomas. They precipitate out of solution when the urine is warmed and redissolve at higher temperatures.

Benign tumor   A tumor that does not spread from its site of origin.

Blastogenesis   The stimulation of cell division.

Blast cells   Cells before division when they have large amounts of cytoplasm.

Blocking antibody   A noncytotoxic, noncomplement activating antibody that, by coating cells, can protect them against immune destruction.

Blood groups   Antigens found on the surface of red blood cells. Their expression is inherited.

Bursectomy   Surgical removal of the bursa of Fabricius.

C3 convertases   Enzymes that can cleave native C3 into C3a and C3b fragments.

Capping   The clumping of surface structures such as antigens or receptors in a small area on the surface of a cell.

Capsid   The protein coat around a virus.

Carcinoma   A tumor originating from cells of epithelial origin.

Carrier   An immunogenic macromolecule to which a hapten may be bound, thus making the hapten immunogenic.

Cascade reactions   A linked series of enzyme reactions in which the products of one reaction catalyze a second reaction, and so forth.

CD molecule   A cell surface molecule classified according to the internationally accepted CD system. CD numbers are assigned to cell surface molecules based on their reactivity with a panel of monoclonal antibodies.

Cell-mediated cytotoxicity   The killing of target cells induced by contact with cytotoxic T cells, NK cells, or macrophages.

Cell-mediated immunity   A form of immune response mediated by T lymphocytes and macrophages; it can be conferred on an animal by adoptive transfer.

Cestodes   Parasitic tapeworms.

Chemokine   A family of proinflammatory and chemotactic cytokines with a characteristic sequence of four cysteine residues. They regulate the emigration of leukocytes from blood into tissues.

Chemotaxis   The directed movement of cells under the influence of a chemical concentration gradient.

Chimera   An animal that contains cells from two or more genetically different individuals.

Chondrichthyes   The class that contains the cartilaginous fishes, including sharks, skates, and rays.

Chromosome translocation   A form of mutation in which portions of two chromosomes switch position.

Chronic inflammation   Slowly developing or persistent inflammation characterized by tissue infiltration with macrophages and fibroblasts.

Class   The five major forms of immunoglobulin molecules common to all members of a species (see Isotype).

Class switch   The change in immunoglobulin class that occurs during the course of an immune response as a result of heavy chain gene rearrangement.

Classical complement pathway   The complement pathway triggered by activation of C1 by antigen-antibody complexes.

Clonal deletion   The elimination of self-reactive T cells in the thymus.

Clonal selection   A key concept in immunology. The proliferation of specific lymphocyte clones in response to a specific epitope. The response is triggered through specific antigen-binding receptors.

Clone   The progeny of a single cell.

Clonotype   A clone of B cells with the ability to bind a single epitope.

Cluster of differentiation (CD)   The set of monoclonal antibodies that recognize a single protein on a cell surface. A CD antigen is by extension, therefore, a defined protein on the surface of a cell.

Coelomocyte   A phagocytic cell found in the coelomic cavity of invertebrates.

Collectins   A family of carbohydrate-binding lectins that depend on calcium for their adhesion.

Colostrum   The secretion that accumulates in the mammary gland in the last weeks of pregnancy. It is very rich in immunoglobulins.

Combined immunodeficiency   A deficiency in both the T cell– and B cell–mediated components of the immune system.

Complement   A group of serum and cell-surface proteins activated by factors such as the combination of antigen and antibody and results in the generation of enzyme cascades that have a variety of biological consequences including cell lysis and opsonization.

Complementarity-determining region   Those areas within the variable regions of antibodies and T cell antigen receptors that bind to antigen and determine the molecule's antigen binding specificity. Synonymous with hypervariable region.

Concanavalin A (Con A)   A lectin extracted from the Jack bean that makes T cells divide.

Conglutinin   A bovine mannose-binding protein that also combines with C3b.

Constant domains   Structural domains with little sequence variability found in antibodies and TCRs.

Constant region   The portion of immunoglobulin and TCR peptide chains that consists of a relatively constant sequence of amino acids.

Contrasuppression   The suppression of suppressor cells by a population of contrasuppressor T cells. Contrasuppressor cells are distinct from helper cells.

Convertase   A protease that acts on a protein to cause its activation.

Cortex   The outer region of an organ such as the thymus or lymph node.

Corticosteroids   Steroid hormones released from the adrenal cortex that have profound effects on the immune system. Some corticosteroids may be synthetic in origin.

Costimulators   Molecules required to stimulate an antigen-sensitive cell simultaneously with antigen in order to initiate an effective immune response.

Cross-reaction   The reaction of an antibody or an antigen receptor directed against one antigen, with a second antigen. This occurs because the two antigens possess epitopes in common.

Cutaneous basophil hypersensitivity   A form of delayed hypersensitivity reaction in skin associated with an extensive basophil infiltration.

Cytokines   Proteins that mediate cellular interactions and regulate cell growth and secretion. As a result, they regulate many aspects of the immune system.

Cytolysis   Destruction of cells by immune processes.

Cytotoxic cell   A cell that can injure or kill other cells.

Delayed hypersensitivity   A cell-mediated inflammatory reaction in the skin, so called because it takes 24 to 48 hours to reach maximum intensity.

Dendritic cells   Cells that possess long cytoplasmic processes. Their primary role is to function as highly effective antigen-trapping and antigen-presenting cells.

Desensitization   The prevention of allergic reactions through the use of multiple injections of allergen.

Diapedesis   The emigration of cells from intact blood vessels during inflammation.

Disseminated intravascular coagulation   Activation of the clotting cascade within the circulation.

Disulfide bonds   Bonds that form between two cysteine residues in a protein. They may be either interchain (between two peptide chains) or intrachain (joining two parts of one chain).

Domain   Discrete structural units from which protein molecules are constructed. Their sizes and amino acid sequences are very diverse.

Dysgammaglobulinemia   The abnormal production of gamma globulins in blood.

Effector cell   A cell that is able to effect an immune response. These cells include cytotoxic T cells and natural killer cells.

Electrophoresis   The separation of the proteins in a complex mixture by subjecting them to an electrical potential.

ELISA   Enzyme-linked immunosorbent assay. An immunological test that uses enzyme-linked antiglobulins and substrate bound to an inert surface.

Endocytosis   The uptake of extracellular substances by cells.

Endogenous antigen   Foreign antigen synthesized within body cells. Examples include newly formed virus proteins.

Endosomes   Cytoplasmic vesicles formed by invagination of the outer cell membrane. They contain endocytosed substances.

Endothelium   The cells that line blood vessels and lymphatics.

Endotoxins   Lipopolysaccharide components of gram-negative bacterial cell walls.

Enhancement   Improved survival of grafts or tumor cells induced by some antibodies.

Eosinophil   A polymorphonuclear leukocyte containing characteristic granules that stain intensely with the dye eosin.

Eosinophilia   Increased numbers of eosinophils in the blood.

Epithelioid cells   Macrophages that accumulate around a tubercle and resemble epithelial cells in histological sections.

Epitope   A site on the surface of an antigen that is recognized by an antigen receptor. As a result, immune responses are directed against specific epitopes. Synonymous with antigenic determinant.

Erythema   Redness due to inflammation.

Eukaryotic organism   An organism characterized by cells possessing a distinct nucleus and containing both DNA and RNA.

Eutherians   The placental mammals; the order to which humans belong and a dominant life form on this planet.

Exocytosis   The export of material from a cell by the fusion of cytoplasmic vesicles with the outer cell membrane.

Exogenous antigen   A foreign antigen that originates at a source outside the body; for example, bacterial antigens.

Exon   A region within a gene that is expressed.

Exotoxins   Soluble protein toxins, usually produced by gram-positive bacteria, that have a specific toxic effect.

Fab fragment   The antigen-binding fragment of a partially digested antibody. It consists of light chains and the N-terminal halves of heavy chains.

Facultative intracellular organism   An organism that can, if necessary, grow within cells.

Fc receptor   A cell-surface receptor that specifically binds antibody molecules through their Fc region.

Fc region   That part of an immunoglobulin molecule consisting of the C-terminal halves of heavy chains. It is responsible for the biological activities of the molecule.

Fibronectin   A glycoprotein responsible for adhesion between cells. It also binds foreign material to cells and thus functions as an opsonin.

First-set reaction   The rejection of a first foreign tissue graft.

Fluorescent antibody   An antibody chemically attached to a fluorescent dye.

Framework regions   The parts of a variable region of immunoglobulins and TCRs that have a relatively constant amino-acid sequence and so form a structure on which the hypervariable, complementarity determining regions may be constructed.

G-proteins   Guanosine triphosphate (GTP)–binding proteins that act as signal transducers for many cell surface receptors.

Gamma (γ) globulins   Serum proteins that migrate toward the cathode on electrophoresis. They contain most of the immunoglobulins.

Gammopathies   Abnormal increases in gamma globulin levels.

Gel diffusion   An immunoprecipitation technique that involves letting antigen and antibody meet and precipitate in a clear gel such as agar.

Gene complex   A cluster of related genes occupying a restricted area of a chromosome.

Gene conversion   The exchange of blocks of DNA between different genes.

Gene segment   Another term for exon. It tends to be used exclusively to denote the exons that code for immunoglobulin and TCR V, D, and J regions.

Genes   Units of DNA that code for the amino acid sequence of a polypeptide chain.

Germinal center   A structure characteristic of many lymphoid organs, in which rapidly dividing B cells form a pale-staining spherical mass surrounded by a zone of dark-staining cells. This is the location where somatic mutation occurs and memory cells are generated.

Globulins   Serum proteins precipitated by the presence of a half-saturated solution of ammonium sulfate.

Glomerulonephritis   Pathological lesions in the glomeruli of the kidney.

Glycoform   Differing molecular forms of a protein resulting from differences in glycosylation.

Glycoprotein   A protein that contains carbohydrate.

Graft-versus-host disease   Disease caused by an attack of transplanted lymphocytes (usually in the form of a bone marrow allograft) on the cells of a histoincompatible and immunodeficient recipient.

Granulocyte   A myeloid cell containing prominent cytoplasmic granules. They include neutrophils, eosinophils, and basophils.

Granuloma   An inflammatory lesion characterized by chronic inflammation with mononuclear cell infiltration and extensive fibrosis.

Granzyme   A family of proteases found in the granules of cytotoxic T cells.

Growth factors   Molecules that promote cell growth.

Haplotype   The complete set of linked alleles within a gene complex. They are inherited as a group and determine a specific phenotype.

Hapten   A small molecule that cannot initiate an immune response unless first bound to an immunogenic carrier molecule.

Heat shock proteins   Proteins synthesized by cells in response to many different physiological stresses. Their function is to act as chaperones and carry proteins within different subcompartments of a cell.

Helminths   Worms, many of which are parasites and so stimulate immune responses.

Helper T cells   The subpopulation of T cells that promote immune responses by providing costimulation from cytokines and costimulatory receptors.

Hemagglutination   The agglutination of red blood cells.

Hematopoietic organ   An organ in which blood cells are produced.

Hemocytes   Phagocytic cells found in invertebrate hemolymph.

Hemolymph   The fluid that fills the body cavities of invertebrates. It has functions analogous to those of blood.

Hemolysin   An antibody that can lyse red blood cells in the presence of complement.

Hemolytic disease   Disease occurring as a result of the destruction of red blood cells by antibodies transferred to the young animal from its mother.

Herd immunity   Immunity conferred on a population as a result of the presence of immune individuals within that population.

Heterodimer A molecule consisting of two different subunits.

Heterophile antibodies Antibodies that react with epitopes found on a wide variety of unrelated molecules.

High endothelial venule A specialized blood vessel lined with high epithelium, found in the paracortex of lymph nodes and other lymphoid organs.

Hinge region The region between the first and second constant domains in some immunoglobulin molecules that permits them to bend freely.

Histiocytes Tissue macrophages.

Histocompatibility molecules Cell membrane proteins that are required to present antigen to antigen-sensitive cells.

Homodimer A molecule consisting of two identical subunits.

Homolog A part similar in structure, position, and origin to another organ.

Homology The degree of sequence similarity between two genes (nucleotide sequences) or two proteins (amino acid sequences).

Humoral immunity An immune response mediated by antibodies.

Hybridoma A cell line formed by the fusion of a myeloma cell with a normal antibody-producing cell.

Hypersensitivity An immunologically mediated damaging inflammatory response to a normally innocuous antigen.

Hypersensitivity pneumonitis Inflammation in the lung caused by a type III hypersensitivity reaction to inhaled antigen within the alveoli.

Hypervariable regions Areas within immunoglobulin or TCR variable regions where the greatest variations in amino acid sequence occur and which therefore bind antigens.

Hypogammaglobulinemia Low levels of gamma globulins in blood.

Idiotope An epitope located in the variable region of an immunoglobulin molecule.

Idiotype The collection of idiotopes on an immunoglobulin molecule.

Idiotype networks The series of reactions among idiotypes, antiidiotypes, and anti-antiidiotypes that play a role in controlling immune responses.

Immediate hypersensitivity The hypersensitivity reaction mediated by IgE and mast cells. Otherwise known as type I hypersensitivity.

Immune complex Another term for antigen-antibody complexes.

Immune elimination The removal of an antigen from the body by circulating antibodies and phagocytic cells.

Immune exclusion The prevention of absorption of antigens from body surfaces by immunoglobulin A.

Immune globulin An antibody preparation containing specific antibodies against a pathogen and used for passive immunization.

Immune paralysis Tolerance induced by very high doses of antigen.

Immune response genes MHC class II genes, so called because they regulate the ability of an animal to respond to specific antigens.

Immune stimulants Compounds, commonly bacterial in origin, that stimulate the immune system by promoting cytokine release from macrophages.

Immune surveillance The concept that lymphocytes survey the body for cancerous or abnormal cells and then eliminate them.

Immunity The state of resistance to an infection.

Immunization The administration of an antigen to an individual in order to confer immunity.

Immunoconglutinins Autoantibodies directed against activated complement components.

Immunodeficiency Diseases in which immune function is partially or totally deficient.

Immunodiffusion Another name for the gel diffusion technique.

Immunodominant The epitope on a molecule that provokes the most intense immune response.

Immunoelectrophoresis A procedure involving electrophoresis in gel followed by immunoprecipitation; it is used to identify the proteins in a complex solution such as serum.

Immunofluorescence Immunological tests that make use of antibodies conjugated to a fluorescent dye.

Immunogenetics That portion of immunology that deals with the direct effects of genes on the immune system.

Immunogenicity The ability of a molecule to elicit an immune response.

Immunoglobulin A glycoprotein with antibody activity.

Immunoglobulin superfamily A family of proteins that contain characteristic immunoglobulin domains.

Immunological paralysis A form of immunological tolerance in which an ongoing immune response is inhibited by the presence of large amounts of antigen.

Immunological synapse The area of contact between an antigen-presenting cell and a lymphocyte such as a T- or B-cell. Within the synapse, cell-surface molecules are arranged in a well-defined pattern designed to optimize signaling between the cells.

Immunoperoxidase Immunological test that makes use of antibodies chemically conjugated to the enzyme peroxidase.

Immunosuppression Inhibition of the immune system by drugs or other processes.

Inactivated vaccine A vaccine containing an agent that has been treated in such a way that it can no longer replicate in the host.

Incomplete antibody An antibody that can bind to a particulate antigen but cannot make it agglutinate.

Indurated Hardened.

Inflammation The responses of tissues to injury. These responses enhance tissue defenses and initiate repair.

Inflammatory macrophage A partially activated macrophage associated with microbial invasion, tissue damage, or inflammation.

Inoculation The administration of a vaccine by injection or scratching.

Integral membrane protein Cell surface proteins that are integral components of the cell membrane as opposed to proteins that are passively adsorbed to cell surfaces.

Integrins A family of adhesion proteins found on cell membranes that bind either to ligands on the surface of other cells or to connective tissue proteins such as fibronectin or collagen.

Interchain bond A bond between two different peptide chains. Usually formed by a disulfide linkage between two cysteine residues.

Interdigitating cell A form of dendritic cell found within lymphoid organs.

Interferons Cytokines that can interfere with viral replication. Some interferons play an important role in the regulation of immunity.

Interleukins Proteins that act as growth and differentiation factors for the cells of the immune system.

Intrachain bond A bond between two cysteine residues on a single peptide chain. Because disulfide bonds are short, its effect is to produce a fold in the peptide chain.

Intraepithelial lymphocytes Lymphocytes, mainly T cells, located among the epithelial cells in the intestinal wall.

Intron A region within a gene that separates exons and is not expressed.

Isoform Different molecular forms of a protein that are generated by differential processing of RNA transcripts of a single gene.

Isogeneic (syngeneic) Genetically identical.

Isograft A graft between two genetically identical animals.

Isotype These are closely related proteins that arise as a result of gene duplication. They are found in all animals of a species. Thus the classes and subclasses of immunoglobulins are actually isotypes.

Isotype switching The change in immunoglobulin class that occurs during the course of the immune response as a result of heavy chain gene switching.

J chain A short peptide that joins units in the polymeric immunoglobulins IgM and IgA.

Joining (J) gene segment A short gene segment that is located 3′ to the V gene segments in immunoglobulin and TCR V genes and codes for part of the variable region.

K antigens Capsular antigens of gram-negative bacteria.

Killer cell See Cytotoxic T cell and Natural killer cell.

Kinins Vasoactive peptides produced in injured or inflamed tissue.

Kupffer cells Macrophages lining the sinusoids of the liver.

Lactenins Bactericidal molecules in milk.

Lag period The interval between administration of antigen and the first detection of antibody.

Langerhans cells Dendritic cells found in the skin. They are effective antigen-presenting cells.

Lectin A protein that can bind specifically to a carbohydrate. Some lectins of plant origin can induce lymphocytes to divide.

Leukemia A cancer consisting of white cells that proliferate within the blood.

Leukocytes White blood cells. This general term covers all the nucleated cells of blood.

Leukopenia The absence of leukocytes.

Leukotrienes Vasoactive metabolites of arachidonic acid produced by the actions of lipoxygenase.

Ligand A generic term for the molecules that bind specifically to a receptor.

Linkage disequilibrium A situation in which a pair of genes is found in a population at an unexpectedly high frequency when compared with the frequency of the individual genes.

Linked recognition The necessity for lymphocytes to receive two simultaneous signals to be activated.

Locus The location of a gene in a chromosome.

Looping out A method of excising a segment of intervening DNA (intron) in order to join two gene segments (exons).

Lymph The clear tissue fluid that flows through lymphatic vessels.

Lymphadenopathy Literally, "disease of lymph nodes." In practice it is used to describe enlarged lymph nodes.

Lymphoblast A dividing lymphocyte.

Lymphocyte A small mononuclear cell with a round nucleus containing densely packed chromatin found in blood and lymphoid tissues. Most have only a thin rim of cytoplasm. They recognize foreign antigens through specialized receptors.

Lymphocyte trapping The trapping of lymphocytes within a lymph node during the node's response to antigen.

Lymphokine-activated killer (LAK) cells Lymphocytes activated by exposure to cytokines such as IL-2 in vitro.

Lymphokines Cytokines secreted by lymphocytes.

Lymphopenia Abnormally low numbers of lymphocytes in blood.

Lymphotoxins Cytotoxic cytokines secreted by lymphocytes.

Lysosomal enzymes The complex mixture of enzymes, many of which are proteases, found within lysosomes.

Lysosomes Cytoplasmic organelles found within phagocytic cells that contain a complex mixture of potent proteases.

Lysozyme An enzyme present in tears, saliva, and neutrophils. It attacks carbohydrates in the cell walls of gram-positive bacteria.

Macrophages Large phagocytic cells containing a single rounded nucleus.

Major histocompatibility complex   The gene region that contains the genes for the major histocompatibility molecules, as well as for some complement components and related proteins.

Malignant tumors   Tumors whose cells have a tendency to invade normal tissues and spread by lymphatics or blood to distant tissue sites.

Marsupials   The order containing the pouched mammals. These include not only the Australian forms, such as kangaroos and koalas, but also the opossums.

Maternal antibodies   Antibodies that originate in the mother but enter the bloodstream of her offspring either by transport across the placenta as in primates, or by adsorption of ingested colostrum in other mammals.

Medulla   The region in the center of lymphoid organs such as the thymus or lymph nodes.

Membrane attack complex   The complement protein structure that is embedded in target cell membranes, resulting in their lysis.

Memory cells   Lymphocytes formed as a result of exposure to antigen. They have the ability to mount an enhanced response to antigen as compared with lymphocytes that have not previously encountered antigen.

Memory response   The enhanced immune response that is triggered as a result of exposing a primed animal to antigen.

Mesangial cells   Modified muscle cells found within a glomerulus.

MHC molecules   Proteins coded for by genes located in the major histocompatibility complex (see Chapter 7).

MHC restriction   The necessity for a T cell to recognize an antigen in association with an MHC molecule. It is required for helper and cytotoxic T cells to recognize antigen and for helper T cells to cooperate with B cells.

Microglia   Macrophages resident within the brain.

Mitogen   Any substance that makes cells divide.

Mixed lymphocyte reaction   Lymphocyte proliferation induced by contact with foreign lymphocytes in vitro.

Modified live virus   A virus whose virulence has been reduced so that it can replicate in the host but cannot cause disease in normal animals.

Molecular mimicry   The development by parasites or other infectious agents of molecules whose structure closely resembles molecules found in their host. In this way the invaders may be able to evade destruction by the immune system or perhaps trigger autoimmunity.

Monoclonal   Originating from a single clone of cells.

Monoclonal antibody   Antibody derived from a single clone of cells and hence chemically homogeneous.

Monoclonal gammopathy   The appearance in serum of a high level of a monoclonal immunoglobulin. This is commonly, but not always, associated with the presence of a myeloma.

Monocytes   Immature macrophages found in the blood.

Monokines   Cytokines secreted by macrophages and monocytes.

Monomer   The basic unit of a molecule that can be assembled using repeating subunits.

Mononuclear cells   Those leukocytes with a single round nucleus; for example, lymphocytes and macrophages.

Mononuclear-phagocytic system   The cells that belong to the macrophage family and their precursors.

Monotremes   The order containing the least evolved egg-laying mammals. These include the platypus and the spiny anteaters (Echidna).

Myeloid system   All the granulocytes and their precursors. These precursor cells are found in the bone marrow.

Myeloma   A tumor of plasma cells.

Myeloma protein   The immunoglobulin product secreted by a myeloma cell.

Natural antibodies   Antibodies against foreign antigens found in serum in the absence of known antigenic stimulation from immunization or an infection. Most probably arise as a result of exposure to cross-reacting bacterial antigens.

Natural killer cells   Large granular lymphocytes that are found in normal, unsensitized individuals and that can recognize and kill abnormal cells such as tumor- and virus-infected cells.

Natural suppressor cells   A population of cells found in unimmunized individuals that have the ability to suppress some immune responses.

Necrosis   Cell death due to pathological causes.

Negative feedback   A control mechanism whereby the products of a reaction act to suppress their own production.

Negative selection   The killing of T cells that have the potential to react to self-antigens. A key mechanism in the prevention of autoimmunity.

Nematode   A roundworm.

Neutralization   Blockage of the activity of an organism or a toxin by antibody.

Neutropenia   Low numbers of neutrophils in blood.

Neutrophilia   High numbers of neutrophils in blood.

Neutrophils   Polymorphonuclear neutrophil granulocytes.

NK cells   Natural killer cells.

Noncovalent bonds   Chemical bonds, such as hydrogen or hydrophobic bonds, that can reversibly link peptide chains. They play a key role in the binding of antigen with antibodies or with T cell antigen receptors.

Normal flora   The microbial population consisting mainly of bacteria that colonize normal body surfaces. They play a key role in preventing invasion by pathogenic organisms.

Nucleocapsid   The key structural component of a virus consisting of the viral nucleic acid and its protective capsid coat.

Nude mice   A mutant strain of mice that have no thymus and are hairless.

O antigens   Somatic antigens of gram-negative bacteria.

Obligate intracellular parasite   An organism that is absolutely required to grow inside cells. Viruses are excellent examples.

Oncofetal antigens   Antigens found on fetal and tumor cells.

Oncogene   A gene whose protein product plays a key role in cell division. As a result, its uncontrolled production leads to excessive cell growth and tumor formation. Oncogenes may be found in normal cells, as well as in cancer-causing viruses.

Oncogenic virus   A virus that causes cancer.

Ontogeny   The embryonic development of an organ or animal.

Opportunistic pathogen   An organism that, although unable to cause disease in a healthy individual, may invade and cause disease in an individual whose immunological defenses are impaired.

Opsonin   A molecule that facilitates phagocytosis by coating foreign particles.

Optimal proportions   When antigen and antibody combine, this is the ratio of reactants that generates the largest immune complexes.

Osteichthyes   The class containing the bony fish. It includes several orders of fish, the most highly evolved of which are the teleosts. The teleosts include such typical fish as the goldfish, catfish, and trout.

Paracortex   The region located between the cortex and medulla of lymph nodes in which T cells predominate.

Paratopes   The antigen-combining sites on an immunoglobulin.

Passive agglutination   The agglutination of inert particles by antibody directed against antigen bound to their surface.

Passive immunization   Protection of one individual conferred by administration of antibody produced in another individual.

Pathogenesis   The mechanism of a disease.

Pathogenic organism   An organism that causes disease.

Perforin   A family of proteins made by T cells and NK cells (and the complement component C9) that, when polymerized, can insert themselves into target cell membranes and provoke cell lysis.

Phagocytes   Cells whose prime function is to eat foreign particles, especially bacteria. They include macrophages and related cells, neutrophils, and eosinophils.

Phagocytosis   The ability of some cells to ingest foreign particles. Literally, "eating by cells."

Phagolysosome   A structure produced by the fusion of a phagosome and a lysosome following phagocytosis.

Phagosome   The cytoplasmic vesicle that encloses an ingested organism.

Phenogroup   A set of blood group alleles that are consistently inherited as a group.

Phylogeny   The evolutionary history of a plant or animal species.

Phytohemagglutinin (PHA)   A lectin derived from the red kidney bean. It acts as a T-cell mitogen.

Pinocytosis   The endocytosis of small fluid droplets.

Plaque-forming cells   Antibody-secreting cells capable of forming plaques in a layer of red blood cells in the presence of complement.

Plasma   The clear fluid that forms the liquid phase of blood.

Plasma cell   A fully differentiated B cell capable of synthesizing and secreting large amounts of antibody.

Point mutation   A mutation resulting from an alteration in a single base in a gene.

Pokeweed mitogen (PWM)   A lectin derived from the pokeweed plant that stimulates T and B cells to divide.

Polyclonal gammopathies   The appearance in serum of a high level of immunoglobulins of many different specificities originating from many different clones.

Polymorphism   Inherited structural differences among proteins from allogeneic individuals as a result of multiple alternative alleles at a single locus.

Polymorphonuclear neutrophil granulocytes   Blood leukocytes possessing neutrophilic cytoplasmic granules and an irregular lobed nucleus.

Positive selection   The enhanced proliferation of cells within the thymus that can respond optimally to foreign antigen.

Precipitation   The clumping of soluble antigen molecules by antibody to reproduce a visible precipitate.

Premunition   A form of immunity seen in some parasitic conditions that depends on the continued presence of the parasite in the host.

Prevalence   The number of cases of a disease.

Primary binding tests   Serological assays that directly detect the binding of antigen and antibody.

Primary immune response   The immune response resulting from an individual's first encounter with an antigen.

Primary immunodeficiencies   Inherited immunodeficiency diseases.

Primary lymphoid organ   An organ that serves as a source of lymphocytes or in which lymphocytes mature.

Primary pathogen   An organism that can cause disease without first suppressing an individual's immune defenses.

Primary structure   The amino acid sequence of a protein.

Privileged sites   Locations within the body where foreign grafts are not rejected. A good example is the cornea of the eye.

Programmed cell death   Physiological killing of a cell. Morphologically, these cells show apoptosis.

Prokaryotic organism   An organism composed of cells whose genetic material is free in the cytoplasm and as a result do not contain a recognizable nucleus.

Prostaglandins   Biologically active lipid metabolites of arachidonic acid produced by the actions of the enzyme cyclooxygenase.

Protein kinase   An enzyme that phosphorylates proteins.

Proteasome A complex enzyme structure consisting of multiple different proteases. It can act on proteins to cleave them into small fragments.

Protooncogene A normal cellular gene that, when mutated, can result in a cell becoming malignant.

Prozone The inhibition of agglutination by the presence of high concentrations of antibody.

Pseudogenes DNA sequences that resemble functional genes but that cannot be transcribed.

Pyrogen A fever-causing substance.

Pyroninophilic Stained by the dye pyronin. This stain preferentially binds to RNA and thus a cell whose cytoplasm stains intensely with pyronin is rich in ribosomes and is therefore probably a protein-synthesizing cell.

Radioimmunoassay An immunological test that requires the use of an isotope-labeled reagent.

Reaginic antibody An antibody of the IgE class that mediates type I hypersensitivity.

Recombinant vaccine A vaccine containing antigen prepared by recombinant DNA techniques.

Respiratory burst The rapid increase in metabolic activity that occurs in phagocytic cells while particles are being ingested. It generates potent oxidants that can kill invading microorganisms.

Reticuloendothelial system All the cells in the body that take up circulating colloidal dyes. Many are macrophages. This term is best avoided because it is not a true body system.

Retrovirus An RNA virus that employs the enzyme reverse transcriptase to convert its RNA into DNA.

Reverse transcriptase An enzyme that reversely transcribes RNA to DNA. It is found in retroviruses such as FIV.

Rheumatoid factor An autoantibody directed against epitopes on the immunoglobulin Fc region. Classically found in the blood of patients with rheumatoid arthritis.

Rosettes The structure formed when several red blood cells bind to the surface of another cell in suspension.

Sarcoma A tumor arising from cells of mesodermal origin.

Second-set reaction The rapid rejection of an organ or tissue graft by a previously sensitized host.

Secondary binding tests Serological tests that detect the consequences of antigen-antibody binding such as agglutination and precipitation.

Secondary immune response An enhanced immune response that results from second or subsequent exposure to an antigen.

Secondary immunodeficiencies Immunodeficiency diseases resulting from a known, nongenetic cause.

Secondary infections Infections by organisms that can invade only a host whose defenses are first weakened or destroyed by other infectious organisms.

Secondary lymphoid organ A lymphoid organ whose function is to trap and respond to foreign antigens.

Secondary response The response of a sensitized animal to foreign antigen.

Secondary structure The way in which a peptide chain is made up of structural components such as α-helices and β-pleated sheets.

Secretory component A protein produced by mucosal epithelial cells; it functions as an IgA receptor and, on binding to IgA, protects IgA against proteases in the intestine.

Selectin A family of cell surface adhesion proteins that bind cells to glycoproteins on vascular endothelium.

Self-cure The elimination of intestinal worms by a localized type I hypersensitivity reaction in the intestinal tract.

Sensitization The triggering of an immune response by exposure to an antigen.

Septic shock A severe disease condition that results from the massive release of cytokines such as TNF as a result of infection with large numbers of gram-negative bacteria.

Seroconversion The appearance of antibodies in blood, indicating the onset of an infection.

Serology The science of antibody detection.

Serum The clear, yellow fluid that is expressed when blood has clotted and the clot contracts.

Serum sickness A type III hypersensitivity response to the administration of foreign serum as a result of the development of immune complexes in the bloodstream.

Signal transduction The transmission of a signal through a receptor to a cell by means of a series of linked reactions.

Skin test A diagnostic procedure that induces a local inflammatory response following intradermal inoculation of an antigen or allergen.

Somatic antigens Antigens associated with bacterial bodies.

Somatic mutation Mutations that occur in somatic rather than germ line cells. In immunology, this refers to the extensive mutations that occur in the V genes of B cells during the course of an immune response.

Specificity A term that describes the ability of a test to give true positive reactions.

Splice The joining of two DNA or RNA segments (exons) together.

Stem cell A cell that can give rise to many different differentiated cell lines.

Stimulation index A measure of the extent to which a cell population is stimulated to divide. It is the ratio of thymidine uptake in a stimulated cell population to the thymidine uptake in an unstimulated population.

Subclass Different immunoglobulin isotypes closely related within a specific class.

Subisotype See Subclass.

Substrate modulation A method of controlling enzyme activity seen in the complement system, by which a protein cannot be cleaved by a protease until it first binds to another protein.

Superantigen   A molecule that, as a result of its ability to bind to certain TCR variable regions, can cause certain T cells to divide.

Superfamily   A grouping of protein molecules that share common structures. For example, the members of the immunoglobulin superfamily all contain characteristic immunoglobulin domains.

Suppressor cells   Lymphocytes (usually T cells) that are claimed to suppress the response of other cells to antigen.

Syncytium   The fusion of many cells into one large cytoplasmic mass containing multiple nuclei. Usually the result of viral action.

Syndrome   A group of symptoms that together are characteristic of a specific disease.

Syngeneic (isogeneic)   Genetically identical.

T lymphocyte   A lymphocyte that has undergone a period of processing in the thymus and is responsible for mediating cell-mediated immune responses.

Tertiary binding tests   Serological tests that measure the protective ability of an antibody in living animals.

Tertiary structure   The way in which the peptide chains of a protein are folded together.

Thoracic duct   The major lymphatic vessel that collects the lymph, draining the lower portion of the body.

Thymectomy   Surgical removal of the thymus.

Thymocytes   Developing lymphocytes in the thymus.

Thymus-dependent antigen   An antigen that requires the assistance of T helper cells to provoke an immune response.

Thymus-independent antigen   An antigen that can activate B cells and trigger an antibody response without help from T cells.

Titer   The reciprocal of the highest dilution of a serum that gives a reaction in an immunological test.

Titration   The measurement of the level of specific antibodies in a serum, achieved by testing increasing dilutions of the serum for antibody activity.

Tolerance   The inability of an animal to mount an immune response against a specific antigen.

Tolerogen   A substance that induces tolerance.

Toxic shock   A disease resulting from exposure to large amounts of staphylococcal superantigen.

Toxoid   Nontoxic derivatives of toxins used as antigens.

Transcription   The conversion of a DNA nucleotide sequence into an RNA nucleotide sequence by complementary base pairing.

Transduction   The conversion of a signal from one form to another.

Translation   The conversion of the RNA nucleotide sequence into an amino acid sequence in a ribosome.

Transporter protein   Proteins that bind fragments of endogenous antigen and carry them to newly assembled MHC class I molecules in the endoplasmic reticulum.

Trematode   A helminth known as a fluke. Trematodes are important human and animal parasites.

Tubercle   A persistent inflammatory response to the presence of mycobacteria in the tissues.

Tuberculin   An extract of tubercle bacilli used in a diagnostic skin test for tuberculosis.

Tumor necrosis factors   Macrophage and lymphocyte-derived cytokines that can exert a direct toxic effect on neoplastic cells.

Tunicates   Complex marine invertebrates possessing characteristic outer cuticular coverings, whose embryonic stages possess features that resemble those found in some vertebrates.

Tyrosine kinase   An enzyme that phosphorylates tyrosine residues in proteins. It plays a key role in signal transduction.

Urodeles   The most primitive order of amphibians; it includes the newts and salamanders.

Urticaria   An erythematous and edematous skin reaction due to type I hypersensitivity and associated with intense itching.

Vaccination   The administration of an antigen (vaccine) to stimulate a protective immune response against an infectious agent. The term originally referred specifically to protection against smallpox. It is synonymous with immunization.

Vaccine   A suspension of living or inactivated organisms used as an antigen to confer immunity.

Variable region   That part of the immunoglobulin or TCR peptide chains in which the amino acid sequence shows significant variation among molecules.

Variolation   An early method of protecting an individual against smallpox by inoculation with live smallpox virus.

Vasculitis   Inflammation of blood vessel walls.

Viral interference   The inhibition of virus invasion of a cell by the presence of a competing virus or gene.

Virgin lymphocyte   A lymphocyte that has not previously encountered antigen.

Virion   A virus particle.

Virulence   The ability of an organism to cause disease.

Xenograft   A graft between two animals of different species.

Xenohybridoma   A hybridoma formed by fusing plasma cells and myeloma cells from two different species (for example, mouse and bovine).

INDEX

Page numbers followed by b indicate boxed material;
those followed by f indicate figure; those followed by t
indicate table.

477